Dictionary of Biomedical Sciences

Dictionary of Biomedical Sciences

Peter J. Gosling

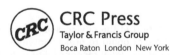

CRC Press
Taylor & Francis Group
Boca Raton London New York

CRC Press is an imprint of the
Taylor & Francis Group, an **informa** business
A TAYLOR & FRANCIS BOOK

Publisher's note
This book has been prepared from camera-ready copy supplied by the author

First published 2002 by Taylor & Francis

Published 2021 by CRC Press
Taylor & Francis Group
6000 Broken Sound Parkway NW, Suite 300
Boca Raton, FL 33487-2742

© 2002 by Peter J. Gosling
CRC Press is an imprint of Taylor & Francis Group, an Informa business

No claim to original U.S. Government works

ISBN 13: 978-0-415-23723-9 (pbk)
ISBN 13: 978-0-415-24138-0 (hbk)

Visit the Taylor & Francis Web site at
http://www.taylorandfrancis.com

and the CRC Press Web site at
http://www.crcpress.com

British Library Cataloguing in Publication Data
A catalogue record for this book is available from the British Library

Library of Congress Cataloging in Publication Data
A catalog record for this book has been requested

Preface

Why write a dictionary of biomedical science? After all, several medical and science dictionaries have been published in the last few years. To answer that question it is first necessary to consider what is meant by 'biomedical science'. Biomedical science involves and relates biological, medical and physical science. Biomedical scientists must be familiar with a great number of technical terms, many of which are from disciplines other than their own speciality, including anatomy, audiology, biochemistry, biology, chemistry, computing science, cytology, genetics, haematology, histology, mathematics, medicine, microbiology, molecular biology, microscopy, mycology, parasitology, pharmacology, physics, physiology, radiology, statistics, virology, and so on. So the answer to the initial question is that the dictionaries published to date do not provide the mix of terminology within a single volume that is required of biomedical scientists and none have had the aims of the present dictionary.

The aim of the present dictionary is to define not just terms from one field of biomedical science but as many as possible of those terms from related disciplines that pop out of the page whenever one reads anything on biomedical science. In fact, were it not that the title is awkward this volume would have been called "A Dictionary for Biomedical Scientists".

Although the dictionary contains no extended essays, and it is not intended to be a dictionary of medical laboratory scientific techniques, formulae and methods, I have, however, tried to give enough material on each term to allow the reader to grasp both its meaning and its significance. By its very nature therefore it was not my intention nor could the dictionary hope to comprehensively cover all the terms used in all disciplines of biomedical science. The expert in any of the disciplines touched upon in compiling this dictionary will undoubtedly find omissions. Those seeking such comprehensive coverage of terms of any particular discipline would do better to consult a volume more specifically targeted to their needs. However it was my intention that the *Dictionary of Biomedical Sciences* should provide the breadth of knowledge to make it both an informative and useful volume for students and experts alike.

Acknowledgements

I must acknowledge the constant encouragement and support that my family, Betty and Jim Martin, and Paul and Kathy Gosling, have freely provided, without which this work would not have been accomplished.

Notes on use

The order of headings is based on the alphabetical sequence of letters in the term, ignoring spaces, hyphens, accents, and numerals. (Thus A-band is to be found between ABA and aberration).

No headings are inverted, for example, there is an entry under gamma radiation, and not under radiation, gamma.

Headings defined appear in bold type and cross-references appear in SMALL CAPITALS.

Plurals formed by the addition of 's' have not usually been regarded, but abnormal formations may be given.

The term 'abbreviations' includes contracted and shortened forms of words and phrases, and acronyms and initials. I have followed the common practice of omitting the full point after each initial in abbreviations but have used them when a word has been truncated. (Thus AAM has no full points but chemo. does).

Throughout the dictionary I have supplied American spellings to words where they differ from those in current use in the United Kingdom.

A

A (1,2 physics) An abbreviation for 1 'A'mplitude. 2 An abbreviation for 'A'mpere.

Aa (chemistry) An abbreviation of 'A'bsolute 'a'lcohol.

AA (society) An abbreviation for 'A'lcoholics 'A'nonymous.

AAA (1 chemistry; 2 society) 1 Amino-acid lysine. 2 An abbreviation of 'A'merican 'A'ssociation of 'A'natomists.

AAAN (education) An abbreviation of 'A'merican 'A'cademy of 'A'pplied 'N'utrition.

AAAS (society) An abbreviation of 'A'merican 'A'ssociation for the 'A'dvancement of 'S'cience.

AAB (society) An abbreviation of 'A'ssociation of 'A'pplied 'B'iologists.

AABB (society) An abbreviation of 'A'merican 'A'ssociation of 'B'lood 'B'anks.

AACC (society) An abbreviation of 'A'merican 'A'ssociation of 'C'linical 'C'hemists.

AACT (education) An abbreviation of 'A'merican 'A'cademy of 'C'linical 'T'oxicology.

AAFS (education) An abbreviation of 'A'merican 'A'cademy of 'F'orensic 'S'ciences.

A-alpha fibre (histology) An alternative term for ALPHA MOTOR NEURON. (*USA*: A-alpha fiber).

AAM (society) An abbreviation of 'A'merican 'A'ssociation for 'M'icrobiology.

AAPCC (society) An abbreviation of 'American 'A'ssociation of 'P'oison 'C'ontrol 'C'enters.

AAPS (society) An abbreviation of 'A'merican 'A'ssociation for the 'P'romotion of 'S'cience.

AAS (1,2, education; 3 physics) An abbreviation of 1 'A'ustralian 'A'cademy of 'S'cience. 2 An abbreviation of 'A'ssociate in 'A'pplied 'S'cience. 3 An abbreviation of 'A'tomic 'A'bsorption 'S'pectrometry.

AASH (physiology/ biochemistry) An abbreviation of 'A'drenal 'A'ndrogen-'S'timulating 'H'ormone.

AAVS (society) An abbreviation of 'A'merican 'A'nti-'V'ivisection 'S'ociety.

a/b (pathogenicity and epidemiology) An abbreviation of 'a'ir'b'orne. Also termed abn.

AB (1 medical; 2 haematology) 1 An abbreviation of 'A'sthmatic 'B'ronchitis. 2 A human BLOOD type of the ABO GROUP.

ABA (biochemistry) An abbreviation of 'A'drenergic 'B'locking 'A'gent.

1

A-band (histology) One of the alternating bands of extrafusal MUSCLE FIBRE (*USA*: muscle fiber), seen through a MICROSCOPE as a dark band, which corresponds to the thick MYOSIN filaments.

ABC (physiology/biochemistry) An abbreviation of 'A'TP-'B'inding 'C'assette.

ABD (governing body) An abbreviation of 'A'merican 'B'oard of 'D'ermatology.

abd (radiology) An abbreviation of 'a'verage 'b'ody 'd'ose.

abdom. (anatomy) An abbreviation of 'abdom'en or 'abdom'inal.

abdomen (abdom.) (anatomy) The part of the trunk between the THORAX and the PELVIS. It is separated above from the THORAX by a muscular partition called the DIAPHRAGM, and below by the PELVIC floor. The structures which make up the abdominal wall are SKIN, fat of varying thickness, MUSCLE, another layer of fat, and the thin, slippery MEMBRANE called the PERITONEUM which lines the abdominal cavity. The PERITONEUM, which is rather like wet cellophane, covers ill the internal organs in the abdominal cavity. The abdomen contains the STOMACH, and most of the organs of the digestive system *i.e.* the small and LARGE INTESTINE with the APPENDIX and CAECUM, and the LIVER and PANCREAS. Other abdominal organs include the kidneys, the ADRENAL GLANDS, the SPLEEN, and some large and important BLOOD VESSELS including the AORTA and the INFERIOR VENA CAVA. The PROSTATE GLAND in the male and the UTERUS, ovaries and FALLOPIAN TUBES in the female are in the PELVIS below the abdominal cavity.

Abell-Kendall Method (biochemistry) A chemical method of CHOLESTEROL ANALYSIS. PRECIPITATION of CHOLESTEROL esters after an initial extraction separates esterified from free CHOLESTEROL, permitting measurement of only the free FRACTION.

aberration (1 physics; 2 genetics) 1 The production of an IMAGE with coloured (*USA*: colored) fringes that occurs because the FOCAL LENGTH of a LENS is different for different colours of LIGHT (CHROMATIC ABERRATION), so that the LENS focuses different colours in different planes; or the production of an IMAGE that is not sharp when a beam of LIGHT falls on the edges as well as on the centre (*USA*: center) of a LENS (SPERICAL ABERRATION). 2 Change in the number or the structure of chromosomes in a CELL.

See also MUTATION.

ABFT (governing body) An abbreviation of 'A'merican 'B'oard of 'F'orensic 'T'oxicology.

abiogenesis (biology) Theory of the ORIGIN of life which states that living organisms gradually formed from non-living material.

See also SPONTANEOUS GENERATION.

abiotic (biology) Nonliving; in biomedical science used primarily for the nonliving parts of ecosystems, or of the ENVIRONMENT in general.

ablation (medical) Surgical removal of an ORGAN or part of an ORGAN.

ABMT (governing body) An abbreviation of 'A'merican 'B'oard of 'M'edical 'T'oxicology.

abn (pathogenicity) An abbreviation of 'a'ir'b'or'n'e. Also termed a/b.

abnormal (general terminology) Departing from normality. The term is usually used for departures from normality in an undesirable direction rather than in a desirable one.

ABO (1 governing body; 2 haematology) 1 An abbreviation of 'A'merican 'B'oard of 'O'phthalmology/ 'O'pticianry/ 'O'rthodontics/ 'O'tolaryngology; 2 A CLASSIFICATION of human BLOOD. *See* ABO BLOOD GROUPS.

ABO blood groups (haematology) A system of classifying BLOOD GROUPS. BLOOD is classified in various ways. The most common classifications are by the agglutinogens in red BLOOD corpuscles (factors A and B) and by the RHESUS FACTOR. BLOOD can therefore have either FACTOR (Group A and Group B) or both factors (Group AB) or neither (Group O) and each of these groups can be Rhesus negative or POSITIVE. It is medically important, because in a BLOOD transfusion the DONOR's ABO BLOOD GROUP must be compatible with the RECIPIENT's or rejection will occur.

abortion (medical) The expulsion of the FOETUS (*USA*: fetus) from the UTERUS before the end of PREGNANCY, especially during the first twenty-eight weeks of PREGNANCY when it is not likely to survive birth. A natural abortion is often termed a MISCARRIAGE.

abortus fever (medical/ bacteriology) BRUCELLOSIS.

ABP (1 governing body; 2 haematology, 3 biochemistry) 1 An abbreviation of 'A'merican 'B'oard of 'P'athology/ 'P'ediatrics/ 'P'edodontics/ 'P'eridontology/ 'P'rosthodontics. 2 An abbreviation of 'A'rterial 'B'lood 'P'ressure. 3 An

abbreviation of 'A'ndrogen-'B'inding 'P'rotein.

ABR (governing body) An abbreviation of 'A'merican 'B'oard of 'R'adiology.

abrasion (medical) The AREA from which the surface layer of the SKIN has been rubbed.

abs. (general terminology) An abbreviation of 'abs'olute/ 'abs'orbent/ 'abs'tract.

abs. visc. (physics) An abbreviation of 'abs'olute 'visc'osity.

abscess (medical/ microbiology) Painful swollen localised AREA where pus forms. An abscess forms in the tissues as the result of irritation, usually because of BACTERIAL INFECTION. Increased BLOOD flow leads to EFFUSION of FLUID into the TISSUE spaces and the collection of a great number of WHITE BLOOD CELLS. The AREA of INFECTION becomes cut off from the healthy TISSUE and in time the dead WHITE BLOOD CELLS, BACTERIA and exuded FLUID form pus. The earliest outward sign of abscess formation on the surface of the body is a painful and tender AREA of redness. As the abscess becomes localised and pus forms, so the AREA of redness becomes more sharply defined, and its centre (*USA*: center) begins to soften. Usually the pus tracks to the AREA of least resistance, which in the case of a surface abscess or boil is the surface of the body. If left, the abscess will eventually burst and DISCHARGE, but often much pain and illness can be avoided if it is lanced or incised as soon as it has localised and pus has formed. While abscesses on the surface of the body are caused by INFECTION entering through a small cut or through the tiny lubricating GLANDS of the SKIN or HAIR follicles, internal abscesses can be caused by the entry of a foreign body as in the case of knife or bullet WOUNDS, or, in the lungs, by the accidental inhalation of food or a TOOTH. Other internal abscesses are caused by the spread of local infections, as in a burst APPENDIX which causes a PELVIC abscess, or the spread of INFECTION from the MIDDLE EAR to the BRAIN. The GROWTH of ANAEROBIC BACTERIA is often favoured by the ENVIRONMENT inside an abscess and they are frequently the underlying cause of the INFECTION.

abscissa (mathematics) The horizontal CO-ORDINATE of a GRAPH, conventionally called the X-AXIS. *See* CARTESIAN CO-ORDINATES.

absgiute value (mathematics) A number or value expressed regardless of its sign.

absol. (gerneral terminology) An abbreviation of 'absol'ute.

absolute alcohol (chemistry) ETHANOL (ETHYL ALCOHOL) that contains no more than 1 per cent WATER.

absolute configuration (chemistry) Arrangement of groups about an asymmetric ATOM. *See* CONFIGURATION.

absolute humidity (physics) Amount of WATER VAPOUR in a given VOLUME of AIR, also called VAPOUR CONCENTRATION.

See also RELATIVE HUMIDITY.

absolute temperature (physics) Funda-mental TEMPERATURE SCALE used in theoretical physics and chemistry. It is expressed in either KELVIN or degrees Rankine (corresponding respectively to the Celsius and Fahrenheit scales). On both these scales, zero is taken as ABSOLUTE ZERO. Also termed thermody-namic TEMPERATURE.

absolute threshold (physiology) The lowest INTENSITY of a STIMULUS at which it can be detected. It is usually measured by determining the INTENSITY at which the STIMULUS is detected on 50 per cent of presentations.

absolute unit (physics) UNIT defined in terms of units of fundamental quantities such as length, time, MASS and ELECTRIC CHARGE or CURRENT.

absolute value (mathematics) Numerical value of a REAL NUMBER irrespective of whether it is POSITIVE or negative. Also termed: modulus (or mod) x, where x is the number.

absolute zero (physics) Lowest TEMPERATURE theoretically possible, at which a substance has no HEAT ENERGY whatever. It corresponds to -273.15 C, or zero on the KELVIN scale.

absorbance (chemistry) A measure of the amount of LIGHT absorbed by a SOLUTION. The difference between the amount of incident LIGHT and transmitted LIGHT expressed mathematically is referred to as the ABSORBANCE of the SOLUTION.

absorbance rate (chemistry) Rate at which a LIQUID is absorbed by a SOLID.

See also ABSORPTION.

absorbed dose (biochemistry) The amount of a chemical that enters the body of an exposed organism.

absorptance (α) (physics) Ability of a medium to absorb RADIATION. It is the ratio of the total RADIATION absorbed by a medium to the total RADIATION arriving at its surface. Also termed: ABSORPTIVITY.

absorption (1 physics; 2 biochemistry; 3 medical) 1 ACTION of taking a LIQUID into a SOLID. 2 The uptake of WATER or dissolved chemicals by CELLS or organisms. 3 Taking substances into the body, such as proteins or fats which have been digested from food and are taken into the bloodstream from the STOMACH and intestines.

absorption factor (biochemistry) That FRACTION of a chemical coming into contact with an organism that is absorbed via the SKIN, respiratory system or GASTROINTESTINAL tract and enters the body of the organism.

absorption spectrum (physics) The proportion of incident LIGHT of each WAVELENGTH absorbed when passed through a selectively absorbing medium.

absorptivity (physics) *See* ABSORPTANCE.

abstr. (general terminology) An abbreviation of 'abstr'act.

abt (general terminology) An abbreviation of 'ab'ou't'.

ABT (governing body) An abbreviation of 'A'merican 'B'oard of 'T'oxicology.

AC (1 physics; 2 computing; 3 employment) 1 An abbreviation of 'A'lternating 'C'urrent. 2 An abbreviation of 'A'nalogue 'C'omputer. 3 An abbreviation of 'A'nalytical 'C'hemist.

ac (1 advisory body; 2 physics) 1 An abbreviation of 'a'dvisory 'c'ommittee. 2 An abbreviation of 'a'lternating 'c'urrent.

Ac (chemistry) CHEMICAL SYMBOL for ACTINIUM.

ac. (general terminology) An abbreviation of 'ac'tivity.

Acad. sci. (education) An abbreviation of 'Acad'emy of 'sci'ence.

acanthosis (medical/ histology) Thickening of the inner layer of CELLS of the EPIDERMIS by ABNORMAL increase in the number of CELLS.

acaricide (parasitololgy) PESTICIDE which kills mites.

acarus (parasitololgy) A GENUS of mites which often live as PARASITES on the external surface of larger animals. They cause various SKIN diseases such as itch and mange.

acceleration (1 genetics; 2 physics) 1 The appearance of a structure in EMBRYOGENESIS earlier than in ancestral forms. The opposite is retardation. 2 A rate of change of velocity; its SI UNITS are ms^{-2} (metres per second per second).

accelerator (1 chemistry; 2 biology; 3 physics) 1 An alternative term for CATALYST. 2 A substance that increases the effectiveness of an ENZYME. 3 Machine that increases the KINETIC ENERGY of an OBJECT or PARTICLE, *e.g.* a PARTICLE accelerator.

acceptable daily intake (ADI) (toxicology/ pharmacology) The ESTIMATED amount of a substance that can be ingested daily during life without causing appreciable adverse effects. It is expressed in mg/ kg body-WEIGHT/ day.

access time (computing) PERIOD of time required for reading out of, or writing into, a COMPUTER's MEMORY.

accidental host (parasitology) An ANIMAL HOST to a PARASITE which is not the usual HOST SPECIES for that PARASITE.

acclimatization (biology) Way in which an organism adapts to a different or changing ENVIRONMENT (*e.g.* the thin AIR at higher altitudes).

accolé (microbiology) Early ring form of *Plasmodium falciparum* found at margin of red CELL.

accommodation (physiology) The process by which the LENS of the EYE brings images to a sharp FOCUS on the RETINA. The LENS of the EYE is made of elastic TISSUE so that its shape can be altered by contraction of the CILIARY MUSCLE which surrounds it. When the MUSCLE contracts the LENS becomes more CONVEX, and as it relaxes the LENS becomes less CONVEX.

accreditation (quality standards) Certification of the expertise of individuals and establishments WORKING in biomedical sciences. Accreditation is performed by several organisations who establish standards and accredit on the basis of education, experience, and accomplishments.

accumulator (1 computing; 2 physics) 1 The part of the CENTRAL PROCESSOR that executes logical or arithmetic operations. 2 An alternative term for a SECONDARY CELL, or STORAGE BATTERY.

accuracy (quality standards) *See* QUALITY CONTROL.

ACDP (advisory committee) An abbreviation of 'A'dvisory 'C'ommittee on 'D'angerous 'P'athogens.

ACE (1 biochemistry; 2 education; 3 chemistry) An abbreviation of 1

'A'ngiotensin 'C'onverting 'E'nzyme. 2 An abbreviation of 'A'dvisory 'C'entre for 'E'ducation. 3 An abbreviation of 'A'lcohol-'C'hloroform-'E'ther.

acellular (biology) Not made up of CELLS; in particular, describing an organism that is not divided into separate CELLS.

acentric chromosome (genetics) A CHROMOSOME with no CENTROMERE. This may be merely a large part of a CHROMOSOME that has broken off from another one. Acentrics tend to get lost because they cannot be manoeuvred during the NORMAL CELL-DIVISION process.

acet. (chemistry) An abbreviation of 'acet'one.

acetal (chemistry) $CH_3CH(OC_2H_5)_2$ Colourless (*USA*: colorless) VOLATILE LIQUID ORGANIC COMPOUND. Also termed: 1,1- diethoxyethane.

acetaldehyde (biochemistry) CH_3CHO Colourless (*USA*: colorless) LIQUID ORGANIC COMPOUND with a pungent odour (*USA*: odor); a simple ALDEHYDE made by the OXIDATION of ETHANOL (ETHYL ALCOHOL). Produced physiologically in significant quantities in individuals taking isulfiram who have also ingested ETHANOL. Also termed: acetic ALDEHYDE; ETHANAL.

acetaldol (chemistry) An alternative term for ALDOL.

acetamide (chemistry) CH_3CONH_2 Colourless (*USA*: colorless) DELIQUESCENT CRYSTALLINE ORGANIC COMPOUND, with a 'mousy' odour (*USA*: odor). Also termed: ethanamide.

acetaminophen (pharmacology) The standard name in the *USA* for paracetamol.

acetate (1,2 chemistry) 1 SALT of ACETIC ACID (ETHANOIC ACID) in which the terminal HYDROGEN ATOM is substituted by a METAL ATOM; *e.g.* COPPER acetate $Cu(CH_3COO)_2$. 2 ESTER of ACETIC ACID in which the terminal HYDROGEN ATOM is substituted by a RADICAL, *e.g.* ETHYL ACETATE $CH_3COOC_2H_5$. Also termed: ETHANOATE.

acetazolamide (physiology/ pharmacology) A carbonic anhydrase inhibitor that has wide-ranging actions in the body. It reduces the formation of aqueous humour in the eye, acts as a DIURETIC, and has use in treatment of glaucoma and OEDEMA (*USA*: edema) respectively. It has also been used as an ANTI-EPILEPTIC DRUG, in treatment of premenstrual syndrome, and in the prevention of motion sickness.

acetic acid (chemistry) CH_3COOH Colourless (*USA*: colorless) LIQUID CARBOXYLIC ACID, with a pungent odour (*USA*: odor) and acidic properties. It is the acid in vinegar. Also termed: ETHANOIC ACID.

acetone (biochemistry) CH_3COCH_3 Colourless (*USA*: colorless), VOLATILE LIQUID ORGANIC COMPOUND, formed during the DEGRADATION of fats as well as a widely manufactured SOLVENT. It is a simple KETONE. May be found in the URINE, primarily in severe cases of DIABETES, sometimes in CHRONIC wasting diseases such as CANCER, and after prolonged vomiting. It has a CHARACTERISTIC SMELL which can often he detected in the breath of patients in diabetic coma. Also termed: 2-propanone.

acetonitrile (chemistry) CH_3CN Colourless LIQUID ORGANIC COMPOUND, with a pleasant odour (*USA*: odor). Also termed: METHYL CYANIDE.

acetonuria (biochemistry) The presence of ACETONE in the URINE, which gives it a sweet CHARACTERISTIC SMELL.

acetophenone (chemistry) $C_6H_5COCH_3$ Colourless LIQUID ORGANIC COMPOUND, with a sweet pungent odour (*USA*: odor). Also termed: phenyl methyl KETONE.

acetyl chloride (chemistry) CH_3COCl Colourless (*USA*: colorless), highly refractive LIQUID ORGANIC COMPOUND, with a strong odour (*USA*: odor). Also termed: ETHANOYL CHLORIDE.

acetylcholinesterase stain (histology) Histochemical enzymatic staining technique.

acetylcholine (ACH) (biochemistry) White HYGROSCOPIC CRYSTALLINE ORGANIC COMPOUND. The CHOLINE ESTER of ACETIC ACID which is synthesised from CHOLINE and acetyl CoA by the mitochondrial ENZYME CHOLINE acetyltransferase. ACh is released in vertebrates as the NEUROTRANSMITTER for cholinergic neurons in the CENTRAL NERVOUS SYSTEM, in addition to several other PERIPHERAL locations, including NEUROMUSCULAR JUNCTIONS; preganglionic neurons in both divisions of the AUTONOMIC NERVOUS SYSTEM; parasympathetic postganglionic neurons; and a few sympathetic postganglionic neurons. CHOLINE, but not ACh, is absorbed into NERVE terminals by a specific, high-AFFINITY, SODIUM- and ENERGY-dependent process. This high-AFFINITY uptake process is specific to cholinergic NERVE terminals, is tightly coupled to ACh SYNTHESIS, is the rate-LIMITING STEP for ACh levels. Cholinergic receptors (cholinoceptors), that mediate the effects of ACh, are generally classified as nicotinic or muscarinic, based on their binding preferences for

NICOTINE and muscarine, respectively. Receptors can be blocked by such agents as d-tubocurarine, decamethonium, ATROPINE and scopolamine. ACh is hydrolysed to CHOLINE and ACETATE by acetylcholinesterase.

acetylcholine acetyl-hydrolase (biochemistry) See ACETYLCHOLINESTERASE.

acetylcholinesterase (ACHE) (biochemistry) An ENZYME that hydrolyses the NEUROTRANSMITTER ACETYLCHOLINE (ACh) to CHOLINE and ACETATE, thereby terminating the ACTION of ACh. It is found extensively throughout the NERVOUS SYSTEM, as well as in many non-nervous tissues.

acetyl Co-A (pharmacology) An abbreviation of ACETYL 'CO'ENZYME A.

acetyl coenzyme A (acetyl Co-A) (physiology/ biochemistry) A derivative of pantothenic acid acetyl coenzyme A is an intermediate in many key metabolic processes, particularly in the transfer of the products of glycolysis to the KREB'S CYCLE and in FATTY ACID METABOLISM.

acetylene (chemistry) C_2H_2 Colourless (USA: colorless) organic GAS with an ETHER-like odour (USA: odor) (when pure), used as a fuel and in organic SYNTHESIS. It is the simplest alkyne (OLEFIN). Also termed: ETHYNE.

acetylide (chemistry) Type of carbide resulting from the INTERACTION of ACETYLENE and a SOLUTION of a heavy METAL SALT. Most acetylides are unstable and explosive. Also termed: ethynide.

acetylsalicyllic acid (biochemistry) See ASPIRIN.

ACFAS (education) An abbreviation of 'A'ssociation 'C'anadienne 'F'rannçaise *pour l'A'vancement des 'S'ciences*. [French-Canadian, meaning 'Assossication for the Advancement of Science'.]

ACH (biochemistry) An abbreviation of 'A'CETYL'CH'OLINE.

ACHE (biochemistry) An abbreviation of 'A'CETYL'CH'OLIN'E'STERASE.

Achilles tendon (anatomy) The TENDON, which runs from the great muscles of the calf to the calcancum, the BONE which forms the heel, and draws the foot downwards about the hinge of the ankle.

achlorhydria (biochemistry) A condition where the GASTRIC JUICES do not contain HYDROCHLORIC ACID. It is found in 4 to 5 per cent of NORMAL people in whom it produces no ill effects, but it is a common symptom of those with STOMACH CANCER or PERNICIOUS ANAEMIA (USA: pernicious anemia).

achondroplasia (medical/ genetics) A genetic disease caused by a DOMINANT ALLELE. Easily recognisable at birth, the features of the disease are very short limbs and a large HEAD but usually a small nose. Adults grow to a height of 4 feet (1.2 m) or less. Achondroplastics are perfectly healthy and have NORMAL intelligence, fertility and so on. About one baby in 50,000 is born with achondroplasia. Some 80 per cent of them have NORMAL parents, which means that the achondroplasia GENE must arise by a new MUTATION in these cases, which appears to occur more often when the father is over the age of 30.

achromatic lens (optics) COMBINATION of two or more lenses that has a FOCAL LENGTH that is the same for two or more different wavelengths of LIGHT. This arrangement largely overcomes CHRO-MATIC ABERRATION.

A chromosomes (genetics) The NORMAL chromosomes in a EUKARYOTE. Occasionally extra chromosomes occur, which are known as B chromosomes.

acid (chemistry) Member of a CLASS of chemical compounds whose AQUEOUS SOLUTIONS contain HYDROGEN IONS. SOLUTIONS of acids have a PH of less than 7. STRONG ACIDS dissociate completely (into ions) in SOLUTION; WEAK ACIDS only partly dissociate. An acid neutralizes a BASE to form a SALT, and reacts with most metals to liberate HYDROGEN GAS.

acidaemia (biochemistry/ haematology) Abnormally high BLOOD acidity (low PH). (*USA*: acidemia).

See also ACIDOSIS.

acid anhydride (chemistry) Member of a GROUP of ORGANIC COMPOUNDS, GENERAL FORMULA RCOOCOR" (where R and R" are alkyl radicals), that can be regarded as a CARBOXYLIC ACID from which a MOLECULE of WATER has been removed.

acid/base balance (bichemistry/ haematology) The ratio of acidic to BASIC ions in a SOLUTION. *In vivo* the acid/BASE BALANCE is controlled physiologically, and disturbances can have profound effects. CARBON DIOXIDE is transported in the BLOOD primarily as BICARBONATE ions (HCO_3-), the BICARBONATE ION being formed in the RED BLOOD CELL by carbonic anhydrase. BICARBONATE is important in maintaining BLOOD PH at 7.4. Disturbances in acid/BASE BALANCE affect BLOOD PH, giving rise to ACIDOSIS or ALKALOSIS.

acid chloride (chemistry) Member of a GROUP of VOLATILE pungent-smelling ORGANIC COMPOUNDS, GENERAL FORMULA RCOCl (where R is an alkyl RADICAL), much used in organic SYNTHESIS.

acid-fast (microbiology/ histology) CHARACTERISTIC of certain BACTERIA, such as mycobacteria, which involves resistance to decolourisation (*USA*: decolorization) by acids when stained by an ANILINE dye, such as carbol fuchsin.

acidic oxide (chemistry) OXIDE of a NON-METAL, usually an ANHYDRIDE, that reacts with WATER to form an ACID; *e.g.* SULPHUR DIOXIDE (*USA*: SULFUR DIOXIDE), SO_2, reacts to form SULPHUROUS ACID (*USA*: SULFUROUS ACID), H_2SO_3.

See also BASIC OXIDE.

acidosis (biochemistry/ haematology) A condition in which the PH of the BLOOD is acidic beyond the NORMAL range (7.35 to 7.45). Acidosis may result from the generation of excess ACID and the resultant disturbance of the ACID/BASE BALANCE, as occurs in DIABETES and renal disease; or from failure to expire CARBON DIOXIDE, which may occur in pneumonia, emphysema and congestive HEART failure.

acid phosphatase (biochemistry) A lysosomal ACID hydrolase that hydrolyses phosphoric ACID esters. It is important in the ABSORPTION and METABOLISM of carbohydrates, nucleotides and phospholipids. SERUM levels of acid phosphatase become elevated in patients with METASTATIC prostatic CARCINOMA, BENIGN prostatic HYPERTROPHY, prostatitis, Paget's disease and metastases to BONE and LIVER from breast CARCINOMA.

acid phosphatase stain (histology) Histochemical enzymatic staining technique.

acid picro mallory stain (histology) A histological staining technique that may be used to make CONNECTIVE TISSUE visible under the MICROSCOPE.

acid salt (chemistry) SALT formed when not all the replaceable HYDROGEN atoms of an ACID are substituted by a METAL or its equivalent; *e.g.* SODIUM HYDROGENCARBONATE (BICARBONATE), $NaHCO_3$, diammonium hydrogenphosphate, $(NH_4)-2HPO_4$.

acid value (AV) (chemistry) Measure of the amount of free FATTY ACID present in fat or oil, indicated by the number of milligrams of POTASSIUM HYDROXIDE required to neutralize the FATTY ACIDS in 1g of the substance being tested.

acini (histology) GROUP of small sacs or cavities lined with secreting CELLS in a GLAND. [Greek, meaning 'bunch of grapes'.] Sing; 'acinus'.

acipimox (pharmacology) A drug administered orally in cases of hyperlipidaemia (*USA*: hyperlipidemia), to reduce or change the proportions of various LIPIDS in the bloodstream. It acts, similar to nicotinic acid, by inhibiting synthesis of LIPIDS in the LIVER.

ack. (literature terminology) An abbreviation of 'ack'nowledge. Also termed ackt.

ackt (literature terminology) *See* ack.

ACM (advisory committee) An abbreviation of 'A'dvisory 'C'ommittee on 'M'utagenesis.

ACME (computing) An abbreviation of 'A'dvanced 'C'omputer for 'ME'dical research.

ACMT (education) An abbreviation of 'A'merican 'C'ollege of 'M'edical 'T'echnologists.

acne vulgaris (medical) A CHRONIC SKIN disease affecting the SEBACEOUS GLANDS of the face, shoulders, back or chest. It occurs most often in people between the ages of 14 and 20. The medical name for a blackhead is comedo; comedones are found not only in the acne of puberty but also as a result of exposure of the SKIN to oil and grease.

aconitase (biochemistry) The ENZYME that reversibly interconverts CITRIC ACID, *cis*-aconitic ACID and isoCITRIC ACID in the CITRIC ACID (KREBS) CYCLE by DEHYDRATION and HYDRATION reactions.

ACOP (quality standards) An abbreviation of 'A'pproved 'C'ode 'O'f 'P'ractice.

ACOS (advisory committee) An abbreviation of 'A'dvisory 'C'ommittee 'O'n 'S'afety.

acoustic (physics) Pertaining to sound waves.

acoustic nerve tumour (medical/histology) A FIBROUS TISSUE TUMOUR which forms on the ACOUSTIC NERVE, one of the CRANIAL NERVES which connects the BRAIN with the EAR. As it grows it presses upon the BRAIN STEM and on the other CRANIAL NERVES which originate there causing giddiness, double vision, deafness, weakness of one side of the face, and various other signs that points to its presence. (*USA*: acoustic nerve tumor).

acoustic pressure (audiology) The VARIATION in the PRESSURE of a medium as a sound is conducted through it. The human EAR is sensitive to sound PRESSURE variations of as little as 0.0001 dyne per square centimetre (*USA*: dyne per square centimeter) and to about a million-fold range of pressures.

acoustic radiations (audiology) The pathways running from the MEDIAL geniculate bodies to the AUDITORY CORTEX, which transmit information about sounds.

acoustics (physics) The scientific study of the physical properties of sound.

ACP (society) An abbreviation of 'A'ssociation of 'C'linical 'P'athologists.

acquired characteristics (microbiology/ biology) Physical or behavioural (*USA*: behavioral) characteristics that are acquired during INTERACTION of an organism and its ENVIRONMENT during its lifetime (*e.g.* scars following WOUNDS), and which cannot be genetically transferred to any offspring.

See also LAMARCKISM.

acquired immune deficiency syndrome (AIDS) (medical/ virology) VIRUS disease more commonly known by its abbreviation AIDS. A disease caused by the HIV (human immunodeficiency) VIRUS, transmitted through the exchange of body fluids such as BLOOD or SEMEN.

acridine (chemistry) A mutagenic COMPOUND occurring in coal tar that has been used in the manufacture of dyes and intermediates. Derivatives are used as antiseptics *e.g.* acriflavin, and antimalarial drugs. ACRIDINE is a strong irritant to MUCOUS MEMBRANES and SKIN, and it causes sneezing on inhalation.

acridine orange (chemistry) A dye used to stain NUCLEIC ACIDS. It fluoresces at 530 nm when intercalated into double-stranded DNA, or at 640 nm when ionically bound to single-stranded DNA. It produces MUTATIONS, some involving reading frame shifts, although its carcinogenicity is uncertain.

acriflavine (chemistry/ pharmacology) Orange CRYSTALLINE ORGANIC COMPOUND used as an ANTISEPTIC. Also termed: 2,8-diaminoACRIDINE methochloride.

acroanaesthesia (medical) Loss of sensation in one or more of the bodily extremities. (*USA*: acroanesthesia).

acrocentric chromosome (genetics) A CHROMOSOME whose CENTROMERE is towards one end.

acrolein (chemistry) $CH_2 = CHCHO$ Colourless (*USA*: colorless) LIQUID ORGANIC COMPOUND, with a pungent odour (*USA*: odor). Also termed: 2-propenal.

acromegaly (medical/ biochemistry) A condition produced by over-SECRETION of the PITUITARY GROWTH HORMONE, commonly as the result of a TUMOUR (*USA*: tumor) of the PITUITARY GLAND. GIGANTISM occurs in cases were ACROMEGALY occurs early in life, before the bones have stopped growing. TREATMENT is directed toward restoring the LEVEL of GROWTH HORMONE to NORMAL and preventing further GROWTH of the PITUITARY TUMOUR (*USA*: pituitary tumor), and may be achieved by RADIOTHERAPY, surgery or the use of the drug bromocriptine.

acrosome (biology) Cap-like structure at the tip of ANIMAL SPERM CELLS. It contains ENZYMES that dissolve the MEMBRANE of the OVUM during FERTILIZATION.

acrylamide (chemistry) A substance used in the preparation of clear GEL for use in

ACRYLAMIDE GEL ELECTROPHORESIS. Humans exposed to ACRYLAMIDE MONOMER, but not its polymers, are vulnerable to neurotoxic injury. Although ACUTE high doses can result in an encephalopathy that is apparently reversible, repeated smaller doses are cumulative and result in a distal sensorimotor axonopathy.

acrylamide gel electrophoresis (chemistry) A technique using an ACRYLAMIDE GEL for the electrophorectic separation of proteins and RNA according to their MOLECULAR WEIGHT. The MONOMER can be cast in the form of sheets or cylinders by polymerisation *in situ* to give a clear GEL.

acrylic resin (chemistry/ OPTICS) TRANSPARENT thermoplastic formed by the POLYMERIZATION of ESTER or AMIDE derivatives of acrylic ACID. The resins are used to make artificial fibres (*USA*: fibers) and for optical purposes, such as making lenses (*e.g.* Acrilan, PERSPEX).

acrylonitrile (chemistry) $CH_2 = CHCN$ Colourless (*USA*: colorless) LIQUID NITRILE used in manufacture of ACRYLIC RESINS. Also termed: vinyl cyanide, propenonitrile.

ACS (society) An abbreviation of 'A'merican 'C'hemical 'S'ociety.

ACT (1 advisory committee; 2, 3 education) 1 Abbreviation of 'A'dvisory 'C'ouncil on 'T'echnology. 2 Abbreviation of 'A'ssociate of the 'C'ollege of 'T'echnology. 3 An abbreviation of 'A'merican 'C'ollege of 'T'oxicology.

ACTH (biochemistry) An abbreviation of 'A'dreno'C'ortico'T'rophic 'H'ormone. (*USA*: Adrenocorticotropic HORMONE).

actin (histology) A PROTEIN whose INTERACTION with MYOSIN forms ACTO-MYOSIN in skeletal MUSCLE. It exists in two forms: G-ACTIN, which is globular, and its POLYMER, F-ACTIN, which is fibrous.

actinic radiation (physics/ chemistry) ELECTROMAGNETIC RADIATION (particularly ULTRAVIOLET RADIATION) that can cause a CHEMICAL REACTION.

actinide (chemistry) Member of a SERIES of elements in GROUP IIIB of the PERIODIC TABLE, of ATOMIC NUMBERS 90 to 103 (ACTINIUM, at. no. 89, is sometimes also included). All ACTINIDES are RADIOACTIVE. Also termed: actinoid.

actinium (chemistry) Ac RADIOACTIVE ELEMENT in GROUP IIIB of the PERIODIC TABLE (usually regarded as one of the ACTINIDES); it has several isotopes, with half-lives of up to 21.7 years. It results from the DECAY of URANIUM-235. At. no. 89; r.a.m. 227 (most STABLE ISOTOPE).

actinomycetes (microbiology) GROUP of mostly saprophytic BACTERIA that are characterized by branching MULTICELLULAR filaments (hyphae).

actinomycin D (microbiology) A CYTOTOXIC ANTIBIOTIC produced by *Streptomyces parvullus*. ACTINOMYCIN D inhibits DNA-dependent RNA SYNTHESIS and DNA SYNTHESIS. In humans, it produces BONE MARROW suppression, GASTROINTESTINAL toxicity and the possibility of anaphalaxis.

action (physics) An alternative term for FORCE.

action current (physiology) *See* ACTION POTENTIAL.

action potential (physiology) The change in POTENTIAL across the MEMBRANE of a MUSCLE or NERVE CELL that generates an

IMPULSE along its length. Also termed ACTION CURRENT.

See also ALL-OR-NONE RESPONSE.

activated charcoal (chemistry) CHARCOAL that, after PYROLYSIS during manufacture, has been subjected to steam or AIR at high TEMPERATURE, which makes it an effective absorber of substances.

activation energy (chemistry) Amount of ENERGY required to initiate the breaking and re-formation of CHEMICAL BONDS, and thus to start a CHEMICAL REACTION.

active immunity (immunology) An IMMUNITY to a disease that has been acquired through previous exposure to it. *Contrast* passive IMMUNITY.

See also IMMUNE SYSTEM.

active mass (chemistry) CONCENTRATION of a substance that is involved in a CHEMICAL REACTION.

active site (biochemistry) Part of an ENZYME that firstly specifically binds the SUBSTRATE(s) and secondly catalyses PRODUCT formation. The ACTIVE SITE consists of two or more often overlapping regions that recognize and bind the SUBSTRATE(s) and then catalyse the ensuing reactions. The initial binding of the SUBSTRATE involves the formation of non-COVALENT BONDS (*e.g.* HYDROGEN BONDS, IONIC BONDS, HYDROPHOBIC INTERACTIONS) with chemical groups at the ACTIVE SITE. During CATALYSIS, COVALENT BONDS may be formed, and then broken, as part of the REACTION mechanism. The chemical groups involved in CATALYSIS include the chemically reactive sidechains of the AMINO ACIDS HISTIDINE, LYSINE, ARGININE, SERINE, THREONINE, TYROSINE, CYSTEINE,

GLUTAMIC ACID and aspartic ACID, and for some ENZYMES a COENZYME or cofactor.

active site (biochemistry) Part of an ENZYME MOLECULE to which its SUBSTRATE is bound during CATALYSIS.

active transport (biochemistry/ physiology) The various ENERGY-requiring processes that permit the movement of chemicals/ ions across biological membranes. All ACTIVE TRANSPORT systems require metabolic ENERGY; can be inhibited by chemicals that affect ENERGY METABOLISM; are selective in terms of the molecules transported; are saturable; and can transport chemicals against a CONCENTRATION GRADIENT. *Contrast* DIFFUSION.

actomyosin (physiology) Substance formed from the association of ACTIN and MYOSIN in skeletal MUSCLE, upon which the contraction mechanism is based.

acupuncture (medical) A method of TREATMENT used in Chinese medicine for the TREATMENT of pain, to produce anaesthesia (*USA*: anesthesia), or to treat various general illnesses. It consists of puncturing the surface of the body with needles at traditionally established sites. The needles may be rotated, vibrated or electrically stimulated. There is evidence to suggest that pain can be relieved by ACUPUNCTURE, and an explanation sought in Western terms is that needling has been shown to increase BLOOD levels of naturally occurring substances called endorphins, which are known to be concerned in the relief of pain.

acute (1 medical; 2 mathematics) 1 Any process which has a sudden onset and has a relatively brief duration. *Contrast*

CHRONIC. 2 Describing an angle of less than 90 degrees.

acute abdomen (medical) The condition in which the patient is suffering from ACUTE severe pain in the ABDOMEN. This is typical in such cases as appendicitis, perforated ulcers, and ACUTE INFLAMMATION of the GALL-BLADDER.

acute brain disorder (medical) Any organic BRAIN disorder that is temporary, and from which the patient makes a full recovery.

acute tolerance (pharmacology) Development of TOLERANCE to a drug after only one or a few doses. *Contrast* CHRONIC TOLERANCE.

acyclic (chemistry) Not CYCLIC; describing a chemical COMPOUND that does not contain a ring of atoms in its molecular structure.

acyclovir (pharmacology/ microbiology) A SYNTHETIC antiviral drug. It acts as an inhibitor of DNA SYNTHESIS, and is active against the VIRUS of HERPES simplex (HSV), but less so against the VIRUS of HERPES ZOSTER (HVZ). ACYCLOVIR is phosphorylated by HERPES-specific thymidine kinases, resulting in the formation of acyclo-GTP, that inhibits viral DNA polymerase 10 to 30 times more efficiently than it does cellular DNA polymerase. Acyclo-GTP is incorporated into viral DNA causing TERMINATION of strand SYNTHESIS. *See* HERPES.

acyl group (chemistry) Part of an ORGANIC COMPOUND that has the FORMULA RCO; where R is a HYDROCARBON GROUP. (*e.g.* acetyl GROUP CH_3CO-).

ad hoc. (General terminology) Unprincipled, particularly of explanations constructed *post hoc.* to explain DATA.

ADA (1 chemistry; 2 society) 1 An abbreviation of 'A'cetone-'D'icarboxylic 'A'cid. 2 An abbreviation of 'A'merican/ 'A'ustralian 'D'ental 'A'ssociation.

adaptation (1, 2 biology; 3 physiology) 1 CHARACTERISTIC of an organism which improves that organism's chance of survival in its ENVIRONMENT. 2 Change in the BEHAVIOUR (*USA*: behavior) of an organism in RESPONSE to environmental conditions. 3 Change in the sensitivity of a sensory mechanism after it has been exposed to a particular continuous STIMULUS. This allows the mechanism to adjust the sensitivity scale according to the LEVEL of the STIMULUS; *e.g.* the process by which the EYE is able to adjust to varying intensities of LIGHT.

adaptive radiation (biology) Mechanism of EVOLUTION in which a single ancestor gives rise to a number of SPECIES that coexist but occupy different ECOLOGICAL NICHEs. Also termed: divergent EVOLUTION.

adaptive value (genetics) The amount of increase or decrease in reproductive fitness that a given GENOTYPE or MUTATION confers, relative to other GENOTYPES and in a particular ENVIRONMENT.

ADCC (histology/ immunology) An abbreviation of 'A'ntibody-'D'ependent 'C'ellular 'C'ytotoxicity.

adder (computing) Part of a COMPUTER that adds digital signals (addend, augend and a carry DIGIT) to produce the sum and a carry DIGIT.

addiction (medical/ biochemistry) DEPENDENCE on the use of a drug such as

ALCOHOL, HEROIN, or cocaine. The habits of drug takers may be such as to LEAD to grave deterioration in their general physical as well as mental health.

Addison's disease (medical/ biochemistry) A degenerative illness caused by deficiency of adrenocortical HORMONE. It is characterised by weakness, vomiting, anorexia, HYPERTENSION, IRRITABILITY, and other symptoms. The HORMONE deficiency is caused by destruction of the suprarenal GLANDS due to AUTO-IMMUNE DISEASE, TUBERCULOSIS or TUMOURS (*USA*: tumors) leading to loss of the HORMONES which are essential to life. The disease is rare in childhood or old age.

addition reaction (chemistry) CHEMICAL REACTION in which one substance combines with another to form a third. without any other substance being produced. The term is most commonly used in ORGANIC CHEMISTRY; *e.g.* for the REACTION between HYDROGEN BROMIDE (HBr) and ETHYLENE (ETHENE, $CH_2 = CH_2$) to form ETHYL BROMIDE (bromoethane, C_2H_5Br).

See also SUBSTITUTION REACTION.

additive effect (biochemistry) The combined effect of two or more chemicals, this being equal to the sum of the individual effects.

additive variance (genetics) The COMPONENT of GENETIC VARIANCE that is due to the ADDITIVE EFFECT of two or more genes on the trait in question, *i.e.* excluding any dominance or INTERACTION.

address (1, 2 computing) 1 identity of a location's position in a MEMORY or store. 2 specification of an OPERAND's location.

adduct (biochemistry) A chemical moiety that has become covalently bound to a large MOLECULE such as DNA or PROTEIN. The term may cover both the chemical and the portion of the MACROMOLECULE with which it is combined.

adenine (molecular biology) One of the four nitrogenous bases which form the CORE of both DNA and RNA. It pairs with THYMINE (T) in DNA, and URACIL (U) in RNA. Also termed: 6-aminopurine.

See also REPLICATION.

adenitis (medical) INFLAMMATION of a GLAND. Usually applied to INFLAMMATION of the lymphatic GLANDS.

adenocarcinoma (histology) A MALIGNANT tumor arising from EPITHELIUM and comprising MALIGNANT CELLS CHARACTERISTIC of the TISSUE from which it arises. Due to profound degeneration of MORPHOLOGY accompanying MALIGNANT TRANSFORMATION in the CANCER CELLS, the TISSUE of ORIGIN of a disseminated ADENOCARCINOMA often cannot be determined.

adenofibroma (histology) A TUMOUR (*USA*: tumor) composed of CONNECTIVE TISSUE with glandular elements.

adenohypophysis (biochemistry) The ANTERIOR portion of the HYPOPHYSIS (PITUITARY), which secretes a VARIETY of tropic HORMONES in RESPONSE to the releasing factors (releasing HORMONES) secreted by the HYPOTHALAMUS. HORMONES of the ADENOHYPOPHYSIS are adrenocorticotrophic HORMONE (ACTH), FOLLICLE-STIMULATING HORMONE (FSH), LUTEINIZING HORMONE (LH), PROLACTIN, somatotrophin (GROWTH HORMONE), and THYROID-STIMULATING HORMONE (TSH).

adenoids (anatomy) Pair of LYMPH GLANDS, more prominent in children than in adults, present at the back of the nose, which may become enlarged as the result of CHRONIC INFECTION and obstruct the free passage of AIR. INFECTION and enlargement of the ADENOIDS is associated with CHRONIC tonsillitis and recurrent colds.

adenoma (histology) A TUMOUR (*USA*: tumor), usually BENIGN, arising from EPITHELIUM and containing CELLS CHARACTERISTIC of the TISSUE from which it arises. The term is most often applied to TUMOURS (*USA*: tumors) of GLANDS or of mucosal EPITHELIUM (*e.g.* the lining of the mouth, bronchial tree, intestines, etc.).

adenomyoma (histology) A BENIGN TUMOUR (*USA*: tumor) made up of GLANDS and MUSCLE.

adenomyosis (histology) Ectopic endometrium in the MUSCLE.

adenopathy (medical) Disease of a GLAND.

adenosine (biochemistry) COMPOUND consisting of the BASE ADENINE linked to the SUGAR RIBOSE. Its phosphates are important ENERGY carriers in biochemical processes.

adenosine deaminase (ADA) (biochemistry/ immunology) An ENZYME involved in the IMMUNE SYSTEM. Lack of it is one of the causes of severe combined immune deficiency.

adenosine diphosphate (ADP) (biochemistry) The PRECURSOR of ADENOSINE TRIPHOSPHATE, formed by the addition of an extra PHOSPHATE GROUP. ENERGY is released when it is formed from ADENOSINE TRIPHOSPHATE (ATP). It is converted back to ATP during RESPIRATION.

adenosine monophosphate (AMP) (biochemistry) A NUCLEOTIDE that is part of the ATP ENERGY CYCLE that supplies ENERGY to drive reactions that require input of FREE ENERGY, such as MUSCLE contraction. FREE ENERGY is liberated when ATP is hydrolysed to AMP and pyrophosphate. The AMP can be recycled to ADP via adenylate KINASE and oxidative PHOSPHORYLATION.

adenosine triphosphatase (atpase) stain (histology) ENZYME histochemical staining technique.

adenosine triphosphate (ATP) (biochemistry) A chemical COMPOUND found in all living CELLS, essential in the production of PROTEIN and a source of cellular ENERGY. It carries the chemical ENERGY obtained from the oxygenation of food. When it is converted to ADENOSINE DIPHOSPHATE and then ADENOSINE MONOPHOSPHATE, the REACTION releases ENERGY that is used in the CELL'S METABOLISM, to energise GROWTH, muscular contraction, or the SODIUM PUMP, etc.

adenosis (medical) Any disease or disorder of the GLANDS.

adenovirus (virology) One of a GROUP of VIRUSES first isolated from human adenoid TISSUE, that contain DNA and are found in a number of animals, including human beings. They cause infections of the respiratory tract, (*e.g.* LARYNGITIS and some kinds of pneumonia), conjunctival infections and may induce cancerous TUMOURS (*USA*: tumors).

ADH (biochemistry) An abbreviation of 'A'nti'D'iuretic 'H'ormone.

See also VASOPRESSIN.

adhesion (physics) Attraction between different substances (at the atomic or molecular LEVEL); *e.g.* between WATER particles and GLASS, creating a MENISCUS.

See also COHESION.

ADI (pharmacology) An abbreviation of 'A'cceptable 'D'aily 'I'ntake.

adiabatic process (physics) Process that occurs without interchange of HEAT with the surroundings.

adipose tissue (histology) TISSUE that contains CELLS specialized for the STORAGE of fat. It gives INSULATION and acts as an ENERGY reserve.

adiposis (histology) An ABNORMAL accumulation of fatty TISSUE in the body.

ADMA (pharmacology) An abbreviation of 'A'merican 'D'rug 'M'anufacturers' 'A'ssociation.

admittance (Y) (physics) Property that allows the flow of ELECTRIC CURRENT across a POTENTIAL DIFFERENCE; the RECIPROCAL of IMPEDANCE.

ADP (biochemistry) An abbreviation of 'A'denosine 'D'i'P'hosphate.

ADR (biochemistry/ toxicology) An abbreviation of 'A'dverse 'D'rug 'R'eaction.

adrenal cortex (anatomy) Outer part of the ADRENAL GLAND.

adrenal gland (anatomy/ biochemistry) ENDOCRINE GLAND that occurs in vertebrates (in mammals there are two GLANDS, located on the kidneys). Each GLAND has two sections: the central MEDULLA, which secretes the HORMONES ADRENALINE (*USA*: epinephrine) and NORADRENALINE (*USA*: norepinephrine); and the outer CORTEX, which secretes certain STEROID HORMONES. Also termed: suprarenal GLAND.

adrenaline (biochemistry) HORMONE secreted by the MEDULLA of the ADRENAL GLAND and at some NERVE endings of the SYMPATHETIC NERVOUS SYSTEM. It is produced when the body prepares for violent physical ACTION. Its effects include increased HEARTBEAT, raised levels of SUGAR (GLUCOSE) in the BLOOD and improved MUSCLE ACTION. Also termed: adrenalin. (*USA*: epinephrine).

adrenergic drugs (biochemistry) Substances, such as AMPHETAMINE, that increase activity at ADRENERGIC synapses.

adrenergic (biochemistry) Releasing or stimulated by ADRENALINE (*USA*: epinephrine) or NORADRENALINE (*USA*: norepinephrine). The term is applied to the SYMPATHETIC NERVOUS SYSTEM.

adrenocorticotrophic hormone (ACTH) (biochemistry) PROTEIN released by the ANTERIOR PITUITARY. It controls SECRETION from the CORTEX of the ADRENAL GLAND. Also termed: CORTICOTROPHIN.

adsorbent (physics) Substance on which ADSORPTION takes place.

adsorption (physics) Accumulation of molecules or atoms of a substance (usually a GAS) on the surface of another substance (a SOLID or a LIQUID).

Advisory Committee on Dangerous Pathogens (ACDP) (advisory committee) A UK Government committee which advises the Health and Safety Commission, the Health and Safety Executive and Health and Agriculture Ministers, as required, on all aspects of hazards and risks to workers and others from exposure to pathogens. The ACDP was SET up in 1981 following a second outbreak of LABORATORY-acquired small-pox and was the successor to the Dangerous Pathogens Advisory GROUP.

Advisory Committee on Mutagenesis (ACM) (advisory committee) Canadian expert committee to advise the Canadian government on the evaluation and regulation of chemical mutagens.

-aemia (haematology) Suffix pertaining to the BLOOD. (*USA*: -emia).

aerobic (microbiology) Pertaining to an organism that requires free OXYGEN, or to the uptake of OXYGEN by an organism. AEROBIC CELLS or organisms require OXYGEN and depend upon the pathways of AEROBIC RESPIRATION *i.e.* GLYCOLYSIS to PYRUVATE, TRICARBOXYLIC ACID CYCLE and ELECTRON TRANSPORT system, for their ENERGY generation. *See* AEROBIC RESPIRATION.

aerobic respiration (biochemistry) Process by which CELLS obtain ENERGY from the OXIDATION of fuel molecules by MOLECULAR OXYGEN with the formation of CARBON DIOXIDE and WATER. This process yields more ENERGY than ANAEROBIC RESPIRATION.

See also GLYCOLYSIS; KREBS CYCLE.

aerogenic (microbiology) GAS producing. *Contrast* ANAEROGENIC.

aerosol (1, 2 physics) 1 SUSPENSION of particles of a LIQUID or SOLID in a GAS; a type of COLLOID. Haze and cloud are the commonest atmospheric AEROSOLs, with fall speeds much less than 10 mm/sec. 2 Device used to produce such a SUSPENSION.

aerosol transmission (microbiology) Person-to-person transmission of disease agents via AEROSOLised droplets. Many respiratory diseases are transmitted in this way.

aerotolerant (microbiology) Ability of an ANAEROBIC MICRO-ORGANISM to grow in AIR, albeit usually poorly, especially after ANAEROBIC ISOLATION.

aesthesiometer (physiology/ physics) A device for measuring SKIN sensitivity, usually by determining the two-point THRESHOLD.

aetiology (1, 2 epidemiology) 1 The cause or causes of a disease. 2 Study of the causes of a disease. (*USA*: etiology).

See also EPIDEMIOLOGY.

AFAS (society) An abbreviation of '*A*'ssociation '*F*'rançaise pour l''*A*'vancement des '*S*'ciences. [French, meaning 'Association for the Advancement of the Sciences'.]

AFD (physics) An abbreviation of '*A*'ccelerated '*F*'reeze '*D*'ried.

afferent (anatomy) Leading towards (*e.g.* towards an ORGAN of the body); the term is particularly used of various NERVEs and BLOOD VESSELs.

See also EFFERENT.

affinity (1 chemistry; 2 biology) 1 The tendency of some substances to combine chemically with others *e.g.* the likelihood of a SUBSTRATE binding to an ENZYME, a LIGAND binding to a RECEPTOR, or an ANTIBODY combining site with a single antigenic DETERMINANT. 2 A similarity of structure or form between different SPECIES of plants or animals.

affinity labelling (chemistry) A procedure for identifying or quantifying receptors by covalently binding a high AFFINITY LIGAND to the RECEPTOR. Binding can be achieved by either using a LIGAND possessing a chemical GROUPING capable of covalently binding to the RECEPTOR directly, or by allowing a cross-linking REAGENT to covalently bind to both the LIGAND and the RECEPTOR.

aflatoxin (mycology) One of a FAMILY of mycotoxins, including CARCINOGENS and HEPATOTOXICANTS, produced by the mould (*USA*: mold) *Aspergillus flavus* and related FUNGI. AFLATOXINS are found as contaminants in both human foodstuffs and ANIMAL feed, particularly in corn and peanuts. The extent of AFLATOXIN contamination is a FUNCTION of environmental conditions at the time of harvest and STORAGE conditions. Although generally a LIVER CARCINOGEN, there are SPECIES differences. CARCINOGENESIS is believed to be initiated when this potent ELECTROPHILE reacts with DNA, and HEPATOTOXICITY when it reacts with proteins to cause either fatty LIVER or LIVER necrosis.

AFNOR (quality standards) An abbreviation of *'A'ssociation 'F'rançaisede 'Nor'malisation,* French Standards Association.

AFP (biochemistry) An abbreviation of 'a'lpha'f'eto'p'rotein.

african swine fever (virology) A DNA VIRUS with icosahedral SYMMETRY, enveloped, within the VIRUS FAMILY Iridoviridae.

after birth (medical) PLACENTA and membranes expelled in the third stage of LABOUR (*USA*: LABOR).

afterdischarge (physics) Electrical activity in a neuron continuing for a brief time after the STIMULUS has stopped.

AFTM (society) An abbreviation of 'A'merican 'F'oundation of 'T'ropical 'M'edicine.

ag. feb. (medical) An abbreviation of *'ag'grediente feb're.* [Latin, meaning 'when the FEVER increases'.]

AGA (society) An abbreviation of 'A'merican 'G'enetic 'A'ssociation.

agar (microbiology) Complex POLYSACCHARIDE obtained from seaweed, especially that of the GENUS *Gelidium*. It resists the digestive ACTION of BACTERIA, and is therefore used by BACTERIOLOGISTS to make a medium on which cultures can be grown. It is commonly combined with broth or BLOOD for this purpose. Also termed: AGAR-AGAR.

ageing (physiology) The phenomenon of progressive failure of self-repair of an organism.

agglutination (physiology) Clumping or sticking together, *e.g.* of RED BLOOD CELLS from incompatible BLOOD GROUPS, or of BACTERIA. AGGLUTINATION is commonly used as an END POINT in immunological tests.

agglutinin (immunology) ANTIBODY that causes AGGLUTINATION. The term commonly refers to such an ANTIBODY in a person's BLOOD PLASMA that reacts with the RED BLOOD CELLS of another person's BLOOD.

aggr. (general terminology) An abbreviation of 'aggr'egate.

agit. (general terminology) Abbreviation of 'agit'atum. [Latin, meaning 'shaken'.]

aglm (general terminology) An abbreviation of 'ag'g'l'o'm'erate.

agonist (physiology/ pharmacology) Substances or drugs which possess intrinsic activity. The responses to AGONISTs may be prevented or reduced by ANTAGONISTS. See ANTAGONIST.

agranulocytosis (haematology) BLOOD disorder in which there is a deficiency of granulocytes. It may be accompanied by mouth ulcers and a sore THROAT, and a much reduced resistance to INFECTION. It has been found to be associated with the toxic side effects on the BONE MARROW of various drugs, but the commonest are those used in the chemotherapeutic TREATMENT of CANCER. Monitoring patients at risk by conducting regular BLOOD counts enables the offending drug to be withdrawn immediately if there is any suspicion that the white CELL count has dropped. The condition is sometimes fatal due to the impaired IMMUNE SYSTEM.

agv (chemistry) An abbreviation of 'a'niline 'g'entian 'v'iolet.

agw (measurement) An abbreviation of 'a'ctual 'g'ross 'w'eight.

AHF (1 chemistry; 2 haematology; 3 microbiology) 1 An abbreviation of 'A'nhydrous 'H'ydro'F'luoric acid. 2 'A'nti-'H'aemophilic (USA: antihemophilic) 'F'actor. 3 An abbreviation of 'A'rgentine 'H'aemorrhagic 'F'ever (USA: Argentine hemorrhagic fever).

AHG (physiology/ biochemistry) An abbreviation of 'A'nti'H'aemophilic 'G'lobulin (USA: antihemophilic globulin).

ahr (EPIDEMIOLOGY/ risk ANALYSIS) An abbreviation of 'a'cceptable 'h'azard 'r'ate.

AIBS (society) An abbreviation of 'A'merican 'I'nstitute of 'B'iological 'S'ciences.

AID (1 medical/ microbiology; 2 medical) 1 An abbreviation of 'A'cute 'I'nfectious 'D'isease. 2 An abbreviation of 'A'rtificial 'I'nsemination by 'D'onor.

AIDS (medical/ virology) An abbreviation of 'A'cquired 'I'mmune 'D'eficiency 'S'yndrome.

Aids-related complex (ARC) (medical/ virology) The medical condition of a debilitated HIV-POSITIVE person not diagnosed with AIDS.

See also AIDS.

AIP (society) An abbreviation of 'A'merican 'I'nstitute of 'P'hysics.

air (chemistry) MIXTURE of gases that forms the EARTH's ATMOSPHERE. Its composition varies slightly from place to place - particularly with regard to the amounts of CARBON DIOXIDE and WATER VAPOUR it contains - but the AVERAGE composition of dry AIR is (percentages by VOLUME): NITROGEN 78. 1 per cent; OXYGEN 20.9 per cent; agon 0.9 per cent; other gases 0.1 per cent.

AIS (education) An abbreviation of 'A'ssociate of the 'I'nstitute of 'S'tatisticians.

AIST (education) An abbreviation of 'A'ssociate of the 'I'nstitute of 'S'cience and 'T'echnology.

AIT (society) An abbreviation of 'A'merican 'I'nstitute of 'T'echnology.

AIWM (society) An abbreviation of 'A'merican 'I'nstitute of 'W'eights and 'M'easures.

AIWMA (education) An abbreviation of 'A'ssociate Member of the 'I'nstitute of 'W'eights and 'M'easures 'A'dministration.

ak (medical) An abbreviation of 'a'bove 'k'nee.

akinesia (medical) Loss of muscular responsiveness, arrest of motion.

Al (chemistry) The CHEMICAL SYMBOL for ELEMENT 13, aluminum.

-al (chemistry) Suffix usually denoting that an ORGANIC COMPOUND is an ALDEHYDE.

al. (chemistry) An abbreviation of 'al'cohol.

Ala (physiology/ biochemistry) An abbreviation of 'Ala'nine.

ALAC (society/ quality standards) An abbreviation of 'A'merican association for ACCREDITATION of 'L'aboratory 'A'nimal 'C'are.

ALAD (biochemistry/ haematology) An abbreviation of 'A'mino'L'evulinic 'A'cid 'D'ehydratase. *See* FREE ERYTHROCYTE PROTOPORPHYRIN.

alanine (Ala) (biochemistry) $CH_3C(NH_2)$-COOH AMINO ACID commonly found in proteins. Also termed: 2-aminoPROPANOIC ACID.

albinism (genetics) A genetically determined condition in which there is no pigmentation in the SKIN, HAIR, eyes, etc. It is commonly caused by a RECESSIVE ALLELE; the corresponding NORMAL ALLELE codes for the ENZYME tyrosinase which is one step in the production of MELANIN, the PIGMENT that usually gives these tissues their COLOUR (*USA*: color). Albino humans are healthy but they must avoid bright sunlight which damages their SKIN and eyes.

albumen (biochemistry) White of an EGG.

albumin (biochemistry/ haematology) A GROUP of proteins characterised by their HEAT COAGULATION characteristics and SOLUBILITY in DILUTE SALT solutions. Although found in most tissues and SPECIES, they are best known from mammalian BLOOD. SERUM ALBUMINS together form the most abundant CLASS of BLOOD proteins, and are mainly responsible for keeping the OSMOTIC PRESSURE CONSTANT in the circulation, and facilitates the transport of fats, HORMONES, haptens and drugs. ALBUMINS vary in their composition, but all contain CARBON, HYDROGEN, NITROGEN, OXYGEN and SULPHUR (*USA*: sulfur). ALBUMINS are colloidal and do not pass through parchment membranes or the membranes of NORMAL living CELLS; they are coagulated by HEAT, following which they become INSOLUBLE in WATER until treated with CAUSTIC ALKALIS (*USA*: caustic alkalies) or MINERAL ACIDS; they are precipitated by various chemicals such as ALCOHOL, tannin, NITRIC ACID and mercury perchloride.

albuminuria (biochemistry) A condition where ALBUMIN is found in the URINE, which it is not normally present in as it does not pass through the KIDNEY CELLS unless they are damaged *e.g.* by NEPHRITIS or INFLAMMATION of the KIDNEYS.

It is usually a sign of KIDNEY disease, but also sometimes of HEART failure.

albumose (biochemistry) An INTERMEDIATE PRODUCT in the DIGESTION of PROTEIN.

alcian blue stain (histology) Histological staining technique for ACID mucins.

alcian blue/ PAS stain (histology) Histological staining technique for ACID and NEUTRAL mucins.

alcian blue/safranine stain (histology) Histological staining technique for different types of mast cell.

alcohol (1, 2 chemistry) 1 Member of a large CLASS of ORGANIC COMPOUNDS that contain one or more hydroxyl (-OH) groups. A PRIMARY ALCOHOL has the GENERAL FORMULA R - CH_2OH, where R is an ALKYL GROUP (or H in the case of METHANOL). A secondary ALCOHOL has the FORMULA RR'CHOH, and a tertiary ALCOHOL has the FORMULA RR'R" OH. ALCOHOLs with two -OH groups are diols. ALCOHOLs react with acids to form esters. 2 The term ALCOHOL is often used to refer specifically to ETHANOL.

alcohol dehydrogenase (biochemistry) An ENZYME that catalyses the conversion of ALCOHOLS to ALDEHYDES or KETONES. The ENZYME is found in the SOLUBLE FRACTION of LIVER, KIDNEY and LUNG, and is the most important ENZYME involved in the METABOLISM of foreign ALCOHOLS. It is a DIMER, the subunits of which can occur in several forms, thus giving rise to a large number of variants of the ENZYME.

alcohol withdrawal (medical) An ACUTE mental disorder caused by withdrawal from ALCOHOL, and marked by tremor, nausea, sweating, anxiety, IRRITABILITY, and depressed mood.

alcoholics anonymous (AA) (society) An international organisation, started in the US in 1935, for helping people to stop drinking and for rehabilitating them.

alcoholism (medical) ADDICTION to ALCOHOL. A condition in which there is CHRONIC or periodic drinking of a compulsive nature.

aldehyde (chemistry) Member of a large CLASS of ORGANIC COMPOUNDS that have the GENERAL FORMULA RCHO, where R is an ALKYL GROUP or ARYL GROUP. ALDEHYDES may be made by the controlled OXIDATION of ALCOHOLS. Their systematic names end with the suffix -al (e.g. the systematic name of ACETALDEHYDE, CH_3CHO, is ETHANAL). All are REDUCING AGENTS, and undergo addition, CONDENSATION and polymerisation reactions. When oxidised, they form CARBOXYLIC ACIDS.

aldehyde dehydrogenase (biochemistry) An ENZYME that catalyses the formation of acids from ALIPHATIC and aromatic ALDEHYDES.

aldehyde fuchsin stain (histology) Histological staining technique for pancreatic islet CELLS.

aldehyde oxidase (biochemistry) A FLAVOPROTEIN, also containing molybdenum, that is found in the SOLUBLE FRACTION of LIVER CELLS. Its primary role appears to be the OXIDATION of ENDOGENOUS ALDEHYDES.

aldimine (biochemistry) See SCHIFF'S BASE.

aldol (chemistry) $CH_3CHOHCH_2CHO$ Viscous LIQUID ORGANIC COMPOUND. It is an ALDEHYDE, a CONDENSATION PRODUCT of acetaldehyde (ETHANAL). Also termed: ACETALDOL; beta-hydroxy-butyraldehyde.

aldol reaction (chemistry) CONDENSATION REACTION between two ALDEHYDE or two KETONE molecules that produces a MOLECULE containing an ALDEHYDE (-CHO) GROUP and an ALCOHOL (-OH) GROUP, hence *ald-ol* REACTION.

aldose (chemistry) Type of SUGAR whose molecules contain an ALDEHYDE (-CHO) GROUP and one or more ALCOHOL (-OH) groups.

aldosterone (biochemistry) A HORMONE secreted by the CORTEX of the ADRENAL GLAND. Its FUNCTION is to control the SALT BALANCE of the body, promoting by its ACTION on the KIDNEY the retention of SODIUM ions and WATER and the EXCRETION of POTASSIUM ions.

aldosterone antagonists (pharmacology) DIURETICS such as POTASSIUM canrenoate that act by blocking the action of the normal minerlocorticoid HORMONE aldosterone. They are useful in treating OEDEMA (*USA*: EDEMA) associated with aldosteronism, LIVER failure and certain HEART conditions.

aleppo boil (medical/ microbiology) A common name for cutaneous LEISH-MANIASIS.

algae (biology) Simple plants, which may be UNICELLULAR or MULTICELLULAR (*e.g.* some seaweeds). ALGAe contain a VARIETY of photosynthetic pigments, and are present in many habitats; most are aquatic.

algebra (mathematics) Branch of mathematics that deals with the general properties of numbers by means of abstract symbols.

algesimeter (physiology/ physics) An instrument, containing a calibrated needle, used to determine people's sensitivity to pain.

alginic acid (chemistry) $(C_6H_8O_6)_n$ Yellowish-white organic SOLID, a POLYMER of mannuronic ACID in the PYRANOSE ring form, that occurs in brown seaweeds. Even very DILUTE solutions of the ACID are extremely viscous, and because of this property it has many industrial applications.

ALGOL (computing) Acronym for the early high-level COMPUTER programming language 'ALGO'rithmic 'L'anguage, used for manipulating mathematical and scientific DATA.

algorithm (computing) Operation or SET of operations that are required to effect a particular calculation or to manipulate DATA in a certain way, usually to solve a specific problem. The term is commonly used in the context of COMPUTER programming.

alicyclic compound (chemistry) Member of a CLASS of organic chemicals that possess properties of both ALIPHATIC COMPOUNDs and CYCLIC compounds.

alimentary canal (anatomy) Tube in the body of animals along which food passes, and in which the food is subjected to physical and chemical DIGESTION and is absorbed. Also termed: digestive tract; enteric canal; GUT.

aliphatic compound (chemistry) An ORGANIC COMPOUND (HYDROCARBON) whose molecules contain a main chain of CARBON atoms, as opposed to ring structures. The chain of CARBON atoms may be straight or branched, and the componds saturated or UNSATURATED. The CLASS includes ALKANES, ALKENES and alkynes and their derivatives.

alizarin (chemistry) $C_6H_4(CO)_2C_6H_2(OH)_2$ Orange-red CRYSTALLINE ORGANIC COMPOUND important in the manufacture of dyes. Also termed: 1,2-dihydroxy-anthraquinone.

alizarin red stain (histology) Histological staining technique for CALCIUM deposits.

alk. (chemistry) An abbreviation of 'alk'aline.

alkali (chemistry) A chemical COMPOUND, usually oxides, hydroxides, or carbonates and bicarbonates of metals. Alkalis (*USA*: alkalies) that combine with ACID in WATER to form SALTS, hence neutralising the ACID. [pl. ALKALIS (*USA*: alkalies)] *See* PH.

alkali metal (chemistry) One of the elements in GROUP IA of the PERIODIC TABLE. They are LITHIUM, SODIUM, POTASSIUM, RUBIDIUM, CAESIUM (*USA*: cesium) and FRANCIUM, which are all soft silvery metals that react vigorously with WATER and occur naturally only as their compounds.

alkaline (chemistry) Having a PH between 7 and 14.

alkaline congo red stain (histology) Histological TISSUE staining technique for amyloid.

alkaline earth (chemistry) One of the metallic elements in GROUP IIA of the PERIODIC TABLE. They are BERYLLIUM, MAGNESIUM, CALCIUM, STRONTIUM, BARIUM and RADIUM.

alkaline phosphatase (biochemistry) An ENZYME that hydrolyses PHOSPHATE monoesters. It has an ALKALINE PH optimum. An elevation of its activity in the SERUM usually indicates obstructive JAUNDICE, Paget's disease or BONE CARCINOMA.

alkaline phosphatase stain (histology) Immunohistochemical staining technique.

alkaloid (pharmacology) One of a GROUP of NITROGEN-containing ORGANIC COMPOUNDS found in plants, many of which have pharmacological effects on the NERVOUS SYSTEM and form the basis of many drugs. Common ALKALOIDS are ATROPINE from the belladonna plant, cocaine from coca leaves, CAFFEINE from tea and coffee, MORPHINE, CODEINE and other drugs from the OPIUM in the poppy, NICOTINE from tobacco, QUININE and QUINIDINE from Peruvian bark, STRYCHNINE from nux vomica seeds. Most ALKALOIDS are CRYSTALLINE solids with a very bitter TASTE; they are sparingly SOLUBLE in WATER, but usually SOLUBLE in organic solvents such as ETHANOL, ETHER and TRICHLOROMETHANE. The majority are very toxic both by inhalation and ingestion.

alkalosis (biochemistry/ haematology) A condition in which the PH of the BLOOD is ALKALINE beyond the NORMAL range, usually above 7.8, due to a disturbance in the ACID/BASE BALANCE. *Contrast* ACIDOSIS.

alkane (chemistry) Member of a GROUP of saturated ALIPHATIC COMPOUNDS that have the GENERAL FORMULA C_nH_{2n+2}; *e.g.* methane (CH_4), ETHANE (C_2H_6), etc. Also termed: paraffin.

alkaptonuria (medical) A genetic disease in which a defective enzyme leads to the accumulation of a coloured (*USA*: colored) polymer molecule. This binds to the collagen of cartilage, making it brittle and easily worn away. The result is a form of osteoarthritis.

alkene (chemistry) Member of a GROUP of UNSATURATED ALIPHATIC COMPOUNDS that have CARBON-to-CARBON DOUBLE BONDS and the GENERAL FORMULA C_nH_{2n}; *e.g.* ETHENE (ETHYLENE, C_2H_4), PROPENE (propylene, C_3H_6), etc. Also termed: OLEFIN.

alkoxyalkane (chemistry) An alternative term for an ETHER.

alkyl group (chemistry) GROUP formed by removing a HYDROGEN ATOM from an ALIPHATIC COMPOUND. *e.g.* methane (CH_4) and ETHANE (C_2H_6) form methyl (CH_3 -) and ETHYL (C_2H_5 -) groups, respectively. It is a HYDROCARBON RADICAL.

alkyl halide (chemistry) An ORGANIC COMPOUND of GENERAL FORMULA RX, where R is an ALKYL GROUP and X is a HALOGEN. Also termed: HALOGENOALKANE.

alkylating agents (biochemistry) Chemicals that can add ALKYL GROUPs to DNA, a REACTION that can result either in mispairing of bases or in CHROMOSOME breaks. Thus ALKYLATING AGENTS such as N-dimethyinitrosamine are frequently CARCINOGENS and/or mutagens.

alkylation (chemistry) CHEMICAL REACTION that introduces an ALKYL GROUP into an ORGANIC COMPOUND (by either addition or substitution).

alkyllaryl sulphide *See* THIOETHER.

ALL (medical/ haematology) An abbreviation of 'A'cute 'L'ymphocytic 'L'eukaemia (*USA*: Acute Lymphocytic Leukemia).

allantois (biology) Membranous sac that develops in the embryos of reptiles, birds and mammals. It is involved in the STORAGE of waste and the provision of food and OXYGEN. In reptiles and birds, it grows to surround the EMBRYO in the shell; in mammals it becomes incorporated into the PLACENTA.

allele (genetics) One of a pair of genes situated at the same location on HOMOLOGOUS CHROMOSOMES that controls a specific inherited trait. If the two ALLELEs are identical, the individual is a HOMOZYGOTE, in respect of that LOCUS, and if they are different, the individual is a HETEROZYGOTE. Each GENE may have a very large number of alternative ALLELEs, since an ALLELE need only differ from the original form by one BASE-pair out of thousands. Also termed 'ALLELOMORPH'. *See* MUTATION.

allele-specific oligonucleotides (ASO) (chemistry) SYNTHETIC DNA probes used to detect single BASE MUTATIONS. These probes, usually about 18 BASE-PAIRS long but sometimes as long as 80 BASE-PAIRS, can be used to detect the presence or absence of the sequence in question (perhaps a disease-producing MUTANT) in a SAMPLE of natural DNA: when a quantity of the NUCLEOTIDE is added to the natural SAMPLE, it will bind if it can find its exact complementary sequence, but not otherwise, being accurate to a single BASE. In a case such as sickle-CELL ANAEMIA (*USA*: sickle-cell anemia), where the exact sequence of the MUTATION site is known, an ALLELE-specific oligonucleotide is an efficient way of detecting the presence of the MUTATION, and is used in prenatal diagnosis.

allelic exclusion (immunology) An assembly of functional IMMUNOGLOBULIN heavy or LIGHT chain genes on only one of the two HOMOLOGOUS CHROMOSOMES for each chain. This arrangement ensures that a given B CELL makes only one unique functional

ANTIBODY after DNA rearrangement. The ALLELEs encoding the IMMUNOGLOBULIN genes on the 'unused' CHROMOSOME are excluded from the rearrangement process by an unknown mechanism.

allelic series (genetics) The SET of ALLELEs available for a given LOCUS.

allelomorph (genetics) *See* ALLELE.

allergen (immunology) Any substance that is capable of eliciting an ALLERGIC RESPONSE. Allergens are usually proteins, and include foods, ANIMAL DANDER, POLLEN from flowers, trees and weeds, and so on.

See also ALLERGY, ALLERGIC RESPONSE.

allergenicity (immunology) The POTENTIAL of a COMPOUND to provoke an ALLERGIC RESPONSE.

allergic response (immunology) A physiological response occurring when an ANTIGEN makes contact with mast cells of the IMMUNE SYSTEM. This contact triggers the release of histamine, which induces local inflammation and produces symptoms of asthma, hay fever or the swelling of insect bites. *See* ALLERGY.

allergic shellfish poisoning (immunology) Allergic REACTION that can result in certain individuals after the ingestion of shellfish that contain powerful sensitising agents. Such poisoning is rarely fatal.

allergy (immunology) ABNORMAL sensitivity of the body to a substance (known as an ALLERGEN). Contact with the ALLERGEN causes symptoms such as SKIN rashes, watery eyes, and sneezing. Hay FEVER is a widespread ALLERGY to the POLLEN of certain plants.

allometry (genetics) Differential GROWTH of one part of the body compared to another or to the body as a whole.

allophene (genetics) An organism that has received a transplant of foreign CELLS, such as in a patient who receives a BONE-MARROW transplant to replace their own defective MARROW TISSUE. The transplanted CELLS have their own GENOTYPE different from the HOST's, and they make their own GENE PRODUCTs.

allopurinol (pharmacology/ biochemistry) A drug used to reduce the formation of URIC ACID in the TREATMENT of GOUT.

all-or-none response (physiology) The RESPONSE of excitable TISSUE (*e.g.* some NERVE CELLS) that occurs in full only at or above a certain LEVEL of STIMULUS, the THRESHOLD, but not at all below that LEVEL.

See also ACTION POTENTIAL.

allosterism (biochemistry) The modulation or regulation of the activity of a PROTEIN through reversible changes in the physical CONFORMATION of the PROTEIN.

allotrope (chemistry) One of the forms of an ELEMENT that exhibits ALLOTROPY.

allotropy (chemistry) Existence of different structural forms of an ELEMENT. *e.g.* graphite and diamond are ALLOTROPES of CARBON.

alloy (chemistry) Metallic substance that is made up of two or more elements (usually metals); *e.g.* brass (COPPER and ZINC), bronze (COPPER and TIN), solder (LEAD and TIN) and steel (IRON and CARBON).

allozyme (biochemistry/ genetics) One of the variant forms of an ENZYME coded for by ALLELES at a given LOCUS.

allyl group (chemistry) $CH_2 = CHCH_2$- UNSATURATED HYDROCARBON RADICAL found in compounds such as allylbromide.

alpha decay (radiology) RADIOACTIVE DISINTEGRATION of a substance with the emission of ALPHA PARTICLES.

alpha level (statistics) The probability that the outcome of a statistical test will reject a HYPOTHESIS when it is in fact true. *Compare* significance LEVEL.

alpha motor neuron (histology) A large motor neuron that innervates EXTRAFUSAL FIBRES (*USA*: fibers) thus causing skeletal muscles to contract.

alpha particles (radiology) Heavy particles composed of two protons and two neutrons of IONIZING RADIATION produced by some modes of RADIOACTIVE DECAY *e.g.* DECAY of PLUTONIUM, with little penetrative POWER, but damaging when in contact with living TISSUE such as occurs following inhalation or ingestion. They have little penetrative POWER.

alpha radiation (radiology) IONIZING RADIATION consisting of a stream of ALPHA PARTICLES.

alpha ray (radiology) An alternative term for ALPHA RADIATION.

alpha rhythm (physiology) Pattern of electrical activity in the BRAIN (as recorded by an ELECTROENCEPHALOGRAPH) that is CHARACTERISTIC of a person who is awake, but relaxed and inactive.

alpha-amylase (biochemistry) An ENZYME that hydrolyses 1,4-GLUCOSIDE linkages of STARCH to form a MIXTURE of dextrins, tri- and di-saccharides, and GLUCOSE. Levels of this ENZYME can rise during renal failure and fall following hepatobilary toxicity.

alpha-fetoprotein (AFP) (biochemistry) PROTEIN found in high concentrations in foetal (*USA*: fetal) SERUM. Transfers to AMNIOTIC FLUID and maternal BLOOD in increased amounts when there is a DEFECT in the developing NERVOUS SYSTEM of the growing FOETUS (*USA*: fetus) such as spina bifida or anencephaly. Samples of the AMNIOTIC FLUID can be taken by the process of AMNIOCENTESIS early in the second three months of PREGNANCY in cases where it is thought to be advisable, and ANALYSIS carried out. High levels may indicate a foetal (*USA*: fetal) abnormality such as spina bifida. Alpha-fetoprotein is also found in increased quantities in the BLOOD of adult patients suffering from certain MALIGNANT tumours (*USA*: tumors).

alphanumeric (computing) Describing characters or their codes that represent letters of the alphabet or NUMERALS, particularly in COMPUTER applications.

alprazolam (pharmacology) A benzodiazepine drug, which is used as an ANXIOLYTIC drug, administered orally, in the short-term treatment of anxiety.

ALS (medical) An abbreviation of 'A'myotrophic 'L'ateral 'S'clerosis.

ALT (biochemistry) An abbreviation of 'AL'anine amino'T'ransferase.

alteplase (pharmacology) A tissue-type plasminogen activator which is used therapeuticlly as a fibrinolytic drug, as when administered by injection or infusion, it has the property of breaking up blood clots.

alternate angle (mathematics) In geometry, one of a pair of angles on opposite sides of a line (TRANSVERSAL) that cuts two other lines; the angles are between the other lines and the TRANSVERSAL. If the two other lines are parallel, the ALTERNATE ANGLES are equal.

See also CORRESPONDING ANGLE.

alternating current (a.c.) (physics) ELECTRIC CURRENT that reverses its direction of flow in periodic cycles (measured in hertz). Mains ELECTRICITY in Britain alternates at a rate of 50 cycles per second; its FREQUENCY is 50 Hz.

alternative medicine (medical) The term applied to systems of TREATMENT which cannot be accepted by orthodox medical practitioners because they cannot be ratified by accepted scientific methods.

alternative splicing (genetics) The production of multiple MESSENGER RNAs from a single TRANSCRIPTION UNIT.

alternator (physics) Generator that produces ALTERNATING CURRENT (a.c.) by rotating coils in a MAGNETIC FIELD.

altruism (biology) Category of ANIMAL BEHAVIOUR (*USA*: behavior), especially common among social insects, in which older individuals tend to sacrifice themselves, losing their lives if necessary, in ORDER that offspring and younger individuals may survive or otherwise benefit.

Alu family (genetics) A SET of highly repetitive DNA elements dispersed throughout the human GENOME; each member is about 300 BASE-pairs in length, and is repeated 300,000 times, the copies being scattered around the chromosomes. The Alu sequence copies make up some 3 per cent of the total human DNA. The copies exist in slightly varying forms, and it is the COMBINATION of these variants that gives the individuality analysed in GENETIC FINGERPRINTING. The Alu sequence got its name from that of the restriction endonuelease, *Alu I,* by which it was isolated.

alum (1, 2 chemistry) 1 $Al_2(SO_4)_3.K_2SO_4.24H_2O$ ALUMINIUM POTASSIUM SULPHATE (*USA*: aluminium potassium sulfate), a white CRYSTALLINE substance (that occurs naturally as kalinite) used in leather-making and as a mordant in dyeing. 2 Any of a GROUP of salts with an ANALOGOUS composition to ALUM (*i.e.* a double SULPHATE of a TRIVALENT and MONOVALENT METAL with 24 molecules of WATER OF CRYSTALLIZATION).

alum. (chemistry) An abbreviation of 'ALUM'inium.

alumina (chemistry) An alternative term for ALUMINIUM OXIDE.

aluminate (chemistry) Type of SALT formed when ALUMINIUM OXIDE or HYDROXIDE dissolves in a strong ALKALI.

aluminium Al (chemistry) Silvery-white metallic ELEMENT in GROUP IIIA of the PERIODIC TABLE. It occurs (as ALUMINO-SILICATES) in many rocks and clays and in bauxite, its principal ore, from which it is extracted by ELECTROLYSIS. It is a LIGHT METAL, protected against corrosion by a surface FILM of OXIDE. Its ALLOYS are used in the aerospace industry and in lightweight structures. At. no. 13; r.a.m. 26.9815.

aluminium chloride (chemistry) $AlCl_3$ White or yellowish DELIQUESCENT SOLID, covalently bonded when ANHYDROUS, which fumes in moist AIR. It is used as a CATALYST in the cracking of petroleum HYDROCARBONS.

aluminium hydroxide (pharmacology) An antacid which is relatively insoluble in water and has a long duration of action when retained in the STOMACH. It can also be used to treat hyperphoshataemia (*USA*: hyperphoshatemia).

aluminium oxide (chemistry) Al_2O_3 White CRYSTALLINE AMPHOTERIC COMPOUND, the principal source of ALUMINIUM, which occurs as the mineral corundum and in bauxite. A thin surface FILM of ALUMINIUM OXIDE gives ALUMINIUM and its ALLOYS their corrosion-resistant properties. Such films can be created by ANODIZING. Also termed: ALUMINA.

aluminium sulphate (chemistry) $Al_2(SO_4)_3$ White CRYSTALLINE COMPOUND, used as a flocculating agent in WATER TREATMENT and sewage works, as a mordant in dyeing, as a size in paper-making and as a foaming agent in fire extinguishers. (*USA*: ALUMINIUM SULFATE).

aluminosilicate (chemistry) Common chemical COMPOUND in minerals and rocks (*e.g.* clays, mica) consisting of ALUMINA and silica with WATER and various bases; such compounds are also formed in GLASS and various ceramics.

alveolar clearance (physiology) Particles that reach the alveoli are cleared by two principal routes: 1 by PHAGO-CYTOSIS and removal either via the mucociliary process or via the LYMPHATIC SYSTEM; 2 by dissolution of the particles, with the dissolved material passing either to the BLOOD stream or the LYMPHATIC SYSTEM.

alveolar macrophage (haematology/ immunology) A CELL-type in the LUNG that kills and engulfs MICRO-ORGANISMS as well as secreting antimicrobial substances. The ALVEOLAR MACROPHAGE may also secrete ENZYMES involved in the LYSIS of LUNG TISSUE.

See also PHAGOCYTOSIS.

alveolus (1, 2 anatomy) 1 MINUTE sac in the VERTEBRATE LUNG. There are vast numbers of alveoli, and most of the exchange of gases between AIR and BLOOD takes place within them. *See also* RESPIRATION. 2 In zoology the term is also used for any small indent or sac in the surface of an ORGAN.

Alzheimer's disease (medical) Progressive neurodegenerative disease, usually of people in their fifties and beyond, producing severe intellectual, sensory, and motor deterioration, and ultimately death. CHARACTERISTIC neuropathological features in the BRAIN include amyloid plaques (PROTEIN deposits) and neurofibrillary tangles. The disease is named after the Bavarian physician, Alois Alzheimer (1864-1915).

AM (physics) An abbreviation of 'a'mplitude 'm'odulation.

Am (1 chemistry; 2 physics) 1 CHEMICAL SYMBOL for AMERICIUM. 2 An abbreviation of 'am'meter.

AMA (1 general terminology; 2, 3 governing body) 1 An abbreviation of 'A'gainst 'M'edical 'A'dvice. 2 An abbreviation of 'A'ustralian 'M'edical 'A'ssociation. 3 An abbreviation of 'A'merican 'M'edical 'A'ssociation.

amalgam (chemistry) MIXTURE of MERCURY with one or more other metals, used for dental fillings.

amantadine hydrochloride (pharmacology) A drug administered orally to treat PARKINSON'S disease. It also has antiviral activity and has been used to prevent infection with specific influenzae viruses and in the treatment of HERPES VARICELLA ZOSTER VIRUS (HVZ).

AMBAC (education) An abbreviation of 'A'ssociate 'M'ember of the 'B'ritish 'A'ssociation of 'C'hemists.

amber codon (genetics) One of the three NONSENSE CODONs in DNA that code for 'stop' and therefore signal the TERMINATION of the PROTEIN being synthesised. Amber is UAG. *See* PROTEIN SYNTHESIS.

ambient (physics) Environmental or surrounding conditions *e.g.* AMBIENT TEMPERATURE.

amenorrhoea (medical) Absence or stoppage of the menstrual flow. May be primary, *i.e.* never menstruated, or secondary *i.e.* after previous MENSTRUATION. The commonest cause of amenorrhoea is PREGNANCY. *See* MENSTRUATION. (*USA*: amenorrhea).

American Academy of Clinical Toxicology (AACT) (education) An organisation of professionals active in clinical toxicology or teaching and/or research related to clinical toxicology.

American Academy of Forensic Sciences (AAFS) (society) A society to encourage the study of all aspects of forensic science.

American Association for the Advancement of Science (society) A US professional society whose members are from all branches of science, medicine and engineering.

American Standard Code for Information Interchange (ASCII) (computing) A standard format for representing characters in differing COMPUTER programs.

americium Am (chemistry) RADIOACTIVE ELEMENT in GROUP IIIB of the PERIODIC TABLE (one of the ACTINIDEs). It has several isotopes, with half-lives of up to 7,650 years. It is used as a source of alpha-particles. At. no. 95; r.a.m. 243 (most STABLE ISOTOPE).

amethocaine hydrochloride (pharmacology) A local anaesthetic drug administered by topical application, to treat localised pain and irritation and in ophthalmic treatments.

amide (chemistry) Member of a GROUP of organic chemical compounds in which one or more of the HYDROGEN atoms of AMMONIA (NH_3) have been replaced by an ACYL GROUP (-RCO). In primary amides one, in secondary amides two and in tertiary amides three of the hydrogens have been so replaced. Also termed: alkanamides.

amiloride hydrochloride (pharmacology) A weak DIURETIC drug that is administered orally and has the property of retaining the body's POTASSIUM. It is therefore frequently used in combination with other DIURETICs, such as the THIAZIDES that are prone to cause a loss of POTASSIUM from the body. It has use in treatment of OEDEMA (*USA*: EDEMA), ascites in LIVER cirrhosis, as an ANTI-HYPERTENSIVE and in treatment of congestive HEART FAILURE.

aminase (biochemistry) One of a GROUP of ENZYMES that can catalyse the HYDROLYSIS of amines.

amination (chemistry) Transfer of an AMINO GROUP (- NH$_2$) to a COMPOUND.

amine (chemistry) Member of a GROUP of organic chemical substances in which one or more of the HYDROGEN atoms of AMMONIA (NH$_3$) have been replaced by a HYDROCARBON GROUP. In primary amines one, in secondary amines two and in tertiary amines three hydrogens have been so replaced.

amino acid (biochemistry) The building blocks of proteins, AMINO ACIDS are ORGANIC COMPOUNDS that contain an acidic CARBOXYL GROUP (-COOH) and a BASIC AMINO GROUP (-NH$_2$). Twenty AMINO ACIDS are commonly found in proteins in animals, and about 100 more that are rare and found only in plants. Those that can be synthesized by a particular organism are known as 'non-essential'; 'essential' AMINO ACIDS must be obtained from the ENVIRONMENT, usually from food. The ESSENTIAL AMINO ACIDS for humans are: ISOLEUCINE, LEUCINE, LYSINE, methionme, PHENYLALANINE, THREONINE, TRYPTOPHAN and VALINE.

amino group (biochemistry) Chemical GROUP with the GENERAL FORMULA -NRR', where R and R' may be HYDROGEN atoms or organic radicals; the commonest form is -NH$_2$. Compounds containing AMINO GROUPS include amines and AMINO ACIDS.

aminobenzene (chemistry) An alternative term for ANILINE.

aminobutyric acid transaminase (biochemistry) An ENZYME found in mitochondria that is responsible for the DEGRADATION of GABA by transferring its AMINO GROUP to alpha-ketoglutaric ACID, which is an INTERMEDIATE in the KREBS CYCLE, yielding succinic semialdehyde and GLUTAMIC ACID.

aminoisovaleric acid (chemistry) An alternative term for VALINE.

aminophylline (pharmacology) A bronchodilator drug that can be administered orally or by injection and used as an acute ANTI-ASTHMATIC or a bronchitis treatment for severe attacks.

aminoplastic resin (chemistry) SYNTHETIC RESIN derived from the REACTION of UREA, THIOUREA or melamine with an ALDEHYDE, particularly FORMALDEHYDE (METHANAL).

aminotoluene (chemistry) An alternative term for TOLUIDINE.

amiodarone hydrochloride (pharmacology) An anti-arrhymic drug which may be administered orally or by injection to treat certain severe irregularities of the HEARTBEAT, although it has many side-effects and is potentially toxic.

amitriptyline hydrochloride (pharmacology) An ANTIDEPRESSANT drug of the tricyclic group. It may be administered orally or by injection and has marked sedative properties, which may be of benefit to agitated or violent patients, but has pronounced ANTICHOLINERGIC side-effects.

AML (medical/ haematology) An abbreviation of 'A'cute 'M'yelocytic 'L'eukaemia (*USA*: ACUTE Myelocytic Leukemia).

AMM (1, 2 society) 1 An abbreviation of 'A'ssociation of 'M'edical 'M'icrobiologists. 2 An abbreviation of *'A'ssociation 'M'édicale 'M'ondiale* [French, meaning 'World Medical Association'.]

ammeter (physics) An instrument for measuring ELECTRIC CURRENT, usually calibrated in AMPERES. The common moving-coil AMMETER is a type of galvanometer.

AMML (medical/ haematology) An abbreviation of 'A'cute 'M'yelo'M'onocytic 'L'eukaemia (USA: ACUTE Myelomonocytic Leukemia).

ammonia (chemistry) (NH_3) A colourless (*USA*: colorless) GAS with a pungent odour (*USA*: odor), detectable by humans down to concentrations of 53 ppm. Inhalation of the VAPOUR arising from a SOLUTION of AMMONIA, while uncomfortable, is not dangerous, but inhalation of the GAS can cause oedema (*USA*: edema) of the lungs and bronchitis but this is rarely serious. It is formed naturally by the BACTERIAL DECOMPOSITION of proteins, purines and UREA; made in the LABORATORY by the ACTION of ALKALIS (*USA*: alkalies) on ammonium salts; or synthesized commercially by FIXATION OF NITROGEN. LIQUID AMMONIA is used as a REFRIGERANT. The GAS is the starting material for making NITRIC ACID and NITRATES.

ammonia solution (chemistry) An alternative term for AMMONIUM HYDROXIDE.

ammonium carbonate (chemistry) $(NH_4)_2CO_3$ Unstable white CRYSTALLINE COMPOUND which decomposes spontaneously to produce AMMONIA, used in smelling salts. The substance known in industry as AMMONIUM CARBONATE is usually a double SALT consisting of ammonium HYDROGENCARBONATE (BICARBONATE) and ammonium aminomethanoate (carbamate). Also termed: sal volatile.

ammonium chloride (chemistry) NH_4Cl Colourless (*USA*: colorless) or white CRYSTALLINE COMPOUND, used in dry batteries, as a flux in soldering and as a mordant in dyeing.

ammonium hydroxide (chemistry) NH_4OH ALKALI made by dissolving AMMONIA in WATER, giving a SOLUTION that probably contains hydrates of AMMONIA. It is used for making soaps and fertilizers. 880 AMMONIA is a saturated AQUEOUS SOLUTION of AMMONIA (DENSITY 0.88 g cm^{-3}). Also termed: AMMONIA SOLUTION.

ammonium ion (chemistry) The ION NH_4^+, which behaves like a METAL ION.

ammonium nitrate (chemistry) NH_4NO_3 Colourless (*USA*: colorless) CRYSTALLINE COMPOUND, used as a fertilizer and in explosives.

ammonium phosphate (chemistry) $(NH_4)_3PO_4$ Colourless (*USA*: colorless) CRYSTALLINE COMPOUND, used as a fertilizer (when it adds both NITROGEN and PHOSPHORUS to the soil).

ammonium sulphate (chemistry) $(NH_4)_2SO_4$ White CRYSTALLINE COMPOUND, much used as a fertilizer. (*USA*: AMMONIUM sulfate).

amnesia (medical) Loss of MEMORY, a symptom occurring in a number of BRAIN disorders such as early ALZHEIMER'S DISEASE or increased PRESSURE from a TUMOUR (*USA*: tumor).

amniocentesis (histology) Test in which a SAMPLE of AMNIOTIC FLUID is taken from the AMNION surrounding a FOETUS (*USA*: fetus). The CELLS that this contains are examined for FOETAL (*USA*: fetal) ABNORMALITIES.

amnion (histology) Innermost MEMBRANE that envelops an EMBRYO or FOETUS (*USA*:

fetus) (in mammals, reptiles and birds) and encloses the FLUID-filled amniotic cavity.

amniotic fluid (anatomy) LIQUID that occurs in the AMNION surrounding a FOETUS (*USA*: fetus).

amoeba (biology) Single-celled organism, a protozoan, that moves and feeds by the projection of pseudopodia. (*USA*: ameba).

amoebiasis (medical/ microbiology) An INFECTION caused by AMOEBA (*USA*: ameba), which can result in amoebic dysentery (USA: amebic dysentery). (*USA*: amebiasis).

amoebocyte (cytology) CELL that demonstrates amoeboid movement. Such CELLS may be present in body fluids, such as the BLOOD of invertebrates.

See also AMOEBA.

AMOL (medical/ haematology) An abbreviation of 'A'cute 'MO'nocytic 'L'eukaemia (*USA*: ACUTE Monocytic Leukemia).

amorphous (biology) Without clear shape or structure.

amp (measurement) An abbreviation of 'amp'ere/ 'amp'erage.

AMP (biochemistry) An abbreviation of 'a'denosine 'm'ono'p'hosphate.

ampere (A) (measurement) SI UNIT of ELECTRIC CURRENT. It was named after the French physicist André Marie Ampère (1775-1836).

Ampère's law (physics) Relationship that gives the MAGNETIC INDUCTION at a point due to a given CURRENT in terms of the CURRENT elements and their positions relative to the point. Also termed: Laplace LAW.

amphetamine (pharmacology) Drug that stimulates the CENTRAL NERVOUS SYSTEM. It was once much used for the TREATMENT of depression and to lessen appetite, but is now seldom prescribed because of its addictive properties.

amphoteric (chemistry) Describing a chemical COMPOUND with both BASIC and acidic properties e.*g*. ALUMINIUM OXIDE, Al_2O_3, dissolves in acids (behaving like a BASE) to form ALUMINIUM salts and dissolves in ALKALIS (*USA*: alkalies) (acting like an acid) to form acuminates.

amplifier (1 physics; 2 microbiology) 1 A device that can magnify a physical quantity, such as electrical CURRENT or mechanical FORCE. An electronic AMPLIFIER increases the AMPLITUDE of the input signal, to produce a GAIN. 2 A HOST that epidemiologically serves the FUNCTION of increasing the size of the PATHOGEN population.

amplitude (physics) A term used in defining a LIGHT WAVE. The distance between the peak and trough. The higher the AMPLITUDE, the more intense the LIGHT and the more ENERGY produced at that WAVELENGTH.

amputation (medical) The removal of part of the body, usually a limb.

AMT (1, 2 education) 1 An abbreviation of 'A'cademy of 'M'edicine, 'T'oronto; 2 An abbreviation of 'A'ssociate in 'M'edical 'T'echnology.

AMU (physics) An abbreviation of 'a'tomic 'm'ass 'u'nit.

33

AMV (society) An abbreviation of *'A'sso-ciation 'M'ondiale 'V'itirinaire.* [French, meaning 'World Veterinary Association'.]

amyl group (chemistry) C_5H_{11}- MONO-VALENT ALKYL GROUP. Also termed: PENTYL GROUP.

amyl nitrite (chemistry) $C_5H_{11}ONO$ Pale brown VOLATILE LIQUID ORGANIC COMPOUND, often used in medicine to DILATE the BLOOD VESSELs of patients with some forms of HEART disease (*e.g.* ANGINA).

amylase (biochemistry) Member of a GROUP of ENZYMES that digest STARCH or GLYCOGEN to DEXTRIN, MALTOSE and GLUCOSE. AMYLASES are found in the salivary GLANDS and the PANCREAS, and MICRO-ORGANISMS. Also termed: DIASTASE.

amylose (chemistry) POLYSACCHARIDE, a POLYMER of GLUCOSE, that occurs in STARCH.

amylum (chemistry) An alternative term for STARCH.

anabolic steroid (biochemistry/ pharma-cology) COMPOUND that is concerned with ANABOLISM. Commonly used ANABOLIC STEROIDs are SYNTHETIC male SEX HORMONES (ANDROGENs) which promote PROTEIN SYNTHESIS (hence their use by some athletes wishing to build up MUSCLE).

See also STEROID.

anabolism (physiology) PHASE of METABO-LISM that is concerned with the building up (or BIOSYNTHESIS) of molecules.

See also CATABOLISM.

anaemia (medical/ haematology) General term for any disorder in which the BLOOD HAEMOGLOBIN (*USA*: hemoglobin) CON-CENTRATION is below NORMAL. Causes may include BLOOD loss, increased intra-vascular destruction of BLOOD CELLS or decreased production of BLOOD CELLS. (*USA*: anemia)

anaerobe (microbiology) Organism that respires anaerobically. *See* ANAEROBIC RESPIRATION.

anaerobic (microbiology) Living in the absence of free OXYGEN.

anaerobic respiration (biology) Process by which organisms obtain ENERGY from the breakdown of food molecules in the absence of OXYGEN (*e.g.* FERMENTATION). This process yields less ENERGY than AEROBIC RESPIRATION.

anaerogenic (microbiology) Non-GAS-producing. *Contrast* AEROGENIC.

anaesthetic (pharmacology) Drug that induces overall insensibility (general ANAESTHETIC [*USA*: general anesthetic]) or loss of sensitivity in one AREA (local ANAESTHETIC [*USA*: local anesthetic]). (*USA*: anesthetic).

analeptic (pharmacology) Any stimulant drug such as CAFFEINE and AMPHETAMINE, excluding the specific antidepressant drugs.

analgesia (medical) The relief of pain in the conscious patient.

analgesic (pharmacology) Drug that relieves pain without causing loss of consciousness.

analog computer (computing) COMPUTER that represents numerical values by continuously VARIABLE physical quantities (*e.g.* VOLTAGE, CURRENT). *Contrast* DIGITAL COMPUTER.

analogidigital converter (computing) A device that converts the output of an ANALOG COMPUTER into digital signals for a DIGITAL COMPUTER.

analogous (biology) Describing features that have similar functions which have developed completely independently.

See HOMOLOGOUS.

analysis *See* CHROMATOGRAPHY; QUALITATIVE ANALYSIS; QUANTITATIVE ANALYSIS; VOLUMETRIC ANALYSIS.

analysis of variance (ANOVA) (statistics) A statistical procedure for testing hypotheses about population means in which the overall VARIABILITY in samples of DATA is split into additive components associated with the INDEPENDENT VARIABLES.

analytic reagent (AR) (chemistry) Grade of chemical.

analytical geometry (mathematics) An alternative term for CO-ORDINATE geometry.

anaphase (cytology/ genetics) Stage in MITOSIS and moiosis (CELL DIVISION) in which chromosomes migrate to opposite poles of the CELL by means of the spindle.

anaphylaxis (medical/ immunology) A sudden severe REACTION (an ALLERGY) to a drug or venom, requiring urgent medical TREATMENT. Also termed: anaphylactic shock.

anaplasia (histology) A CHARACTERISTIC of tumor TISSUE in which there is loss of differentiation of CELLS and of their orientation to one another within the TISSUE and with respect to adjacent TISSUE.

anastomosis (1 histology; 2 medical) 1 Natural VESSEL that connects two BLOOD VESSELS. 2 Artificially made connection between two body tubes (*e.g.* in the GUT).

anat. (anatomy) An abbreviation of 'Anat'omy/ 'Anat'omical.

anatomy (anatomy) The study of the structural forms of the body and its parts.

And gate (computing) COMPUTER LOGIC ELEMENT that combines two binary input signals to produce one output signal according to particular rules. Also termed: AND ELEMENT.

androblastoma (histology/ biochemistry) ANDROGEN secreting TUMOUR (*USA*: tumor) of the OVARY.

androgen (physiology/ pharmacology) Term used to describe the predominantly male (steroid) sex HORMONES, which stimulate the development of male sex characteristics. In men, they are produced primarily by the testes and the main form is called TESTOSTERONE. However, ANDROGENS are produced in both men and women by the adrenal glands and in women small quantities are also secreted by the ovaries. An excessive amount in women causes masculinization. Forms of the natural HORMONES and a number of synthetic ANDROGENS including TESTOSTERONE and mesterolone, are used therapeutically to correct hormonal deficiency, and can also be used as ANTICANCER treatments for cancers linked to sex HORMONES, *e.g.* breast cancer in women.

androgen insensitivity syndrome (genetics) A condition occurring in some chromosomal males in which the TESTES develop, but because the organs are insensitive to TESTOSTERONE, most of the bodily characteristics are female, including the external genitalia. Such people are usually brought up as females and tend to behave as females.

androgenisation (medical) The TRANSFORMATION of any bodily structure or part of the BRAIN into those typical of a male rather than of a female.

androsterone (biochemistry) A breakdown PRODUCT OF TESTOSTERONE, which acts as an ANDROGEN.

-ane (chemistry) Suffix usually denoting that an ORGANIC COMPOUND is an ALKANE or CYCLOALKANE; *e.g.* methane, cyclohexane.

anergy (immunology) Absence of REACTION to antigens or ALLERGENS.

anes. (biochemistry) An abbreviation of 'anes'thetic.

aneuploidy (genetics) The condition in which the number of CHROMOSOMES in a CELL is not an exact multiple of the HAPLOID number. The loss of one or more chromosomes, or the presence of extra chromosomes can bring about the condition. One form of ANEUPLOIDY is TRISOMY, in which there are three copies of a CHROMOSOME: a well-known example is DOWN'S SYNDROME, also called TRISOMY 21, in which there are three copies of CHROMOSOME 21.

aneurin (biochemistry) An alternative term for THIAMINE (VITAMIN B$_1$).

angina (medical) Spasmodic, choking or suffocating pain. The word is now applied to the disease causing the pain, *e.g.* VINCENT'S ANGINA and ANGINA pectoris. The former named after the physician and BACTERIOLOGIST, J. H. Vincent (1862-1950).

angiogenesis (medical/ haematology) The formation of new BLOOD VESSELs.

angiogram (radiography) X-RAY picture produced following the injection of an X-RAY OPAQUE dye into an ARTERY.

angioma (histology/ haematology) A BENIGN (non-MALIGNANT) TUMOUR (*USA*: tumor) consisting of BLOOD VESSELs (HAEMANGIOMA; *USA*: hemANGIOMA) or LYMPH vessels (lymphANGIOMA). These tumours may occur in any part of the body where these types of vessels are found.

angiotensin converting enzyme (ACE) (physiology/ biochemistry) An enzyme that converts angiotensin I to the potent VASOPRESSOR form, angiotensin II.

angle of incidence (physics) Angle that a RAY or any other straight line makes with the NORMAL to a surface at which it arrives.

angle of reflection (physics) Angle made by a RAY with the NORMAL to a surface from which it is reflected at the point of REFLECTION.

angle of refraction (physics) Angle made by a RAY refracted at a surface separating two media with the NORMAL to the surface at the point of REFRACTION.

See also LAWS OF REFRACTION OF LIGHT.

angstrom (Å) (measurement) UNIT of WAVELENGTH for ELECTROMAGNETIC RADIATION, including VISIBLE LIGHT and X-RAYS, equal to 10^{-10} m, or 0.1 nm. It was named after the Swedish physicist Anders Ångstrom (1814-74).

anhyd. (chemistry) An abbreviation of 'anhyd'rous. Also termed anhydr.

anhydride (chemistry) Chemical COMPOUND formed by removing WATER from another COMPOUND (usually an acid); *e.g.* an ACID ANHYDRIDE or ACIDIC OXIDE.

anhydrite (chemistry) Naturally occurring CALCIUM SULPHATE (*USA*: CALCIUM sulfate), used to make fertilizers.

See also GYPSUM.

anhydrous (chemistry) Describing a substance that is devoid of moisture, or lacking WATER OF CRYSTALLIZATION.

aniline (chemistry) $C_6H_5NH_2$ Colourless (*USA*: colorless) oily LIQUID ORGANIC COMPOUND, one of the BASIC chemicals (feedstock) used in the manufacture of dyes, pharmaceuticals and plastics. Also termed: AMINOBENZENE; PHENYLamine.

animal (biology) Member of a large KINGDOM of organisms that feed heterotrophically on other organisms or organic MATTER. Animals are usually capable of movement and react quickly to stimuli (because they have SENSE ORGANS and a NERVOUS SYSTEM). ANIMAL CELLS have limited GROWTH, no chlorophyll, and are surrounded by a CELL MEMBRANE.

animal starch (chemistry) An alternative term for GLYCOGEN.

anion (physics) A negatively charged PARTICLE, which in an ELECTRIC FIELD will migrate toward the POSITIVE POLE. *See* ANODE.

anisocytosis (haematology) The condition in which there is excessive VARIATION in size between individual ERYTHROCYTES.

anisogamy (genetics) The production of two unequal-sized types of gametes in a SPECIES. It is the system used by all higher eukaryotes, including humans, in which the OVUM is much larger than the SPERM. *Contrast* ISOGAMY.

anisotropic (physics) Describing a substance that has different properties with respect to velocity of LIGHT transmission, CONDUCTIVITY of HEAT and ELECTRICITY, and compressibility in different directions of its MATRIX.

ankylosing spondylitis (medical) A human disease probably caused by a VIRUS but with an ELEMENT of genetic susceptibility. The symptoms are the fusing together of the vertebrae of the SPINE, starting from the lowest, but even though there may be almost no movement in the back, the patient is usually well enough to LEAD a NORMAL life. Men are affected four times more often than women, and there is often more than one case in a FAMILY. The FACTOR that makes someone liable to develop ANKYLOSING SPONDYLITIS seems to be linked with a GENE in the hla complex, part of the IMMUNE SYSTEM: almost all cases of the condition are in people with HLA type B27, though this type occurs in only 3 or 4 per cent in the population. The HLA genes may be directly involved in the disease, in causing an attack on the body's own tissues, or they may only be genetic markers linked very closely to the real genetic factor. *See* GENETIC CODE.

ankylosis (medical) Fixation or near-fixation of a JOINT normally freely movable, brought about by disease, injury or surgical operation. Common causes of ANKYLOSIS are TUBERCULOSIS, rheumatoid ARTHRITIS or septic ARTHRITIS, in which conditions the bones become bound together by scar TISSUE. JOINT deformities caused by fractures can also result in ANKYLOSIS, and fixation of a JOINT may follow if it is kept immobilised for a long time.

annealing (biochemistry/ molecular biology) The reassociation of complementary strands of DNA after they have been denatured, usually by melting at a high TEMPERATURE. The annealed strands can either be original complementary strands or they can be any two strands that have enough BASE-pairs matching for reassociation to occur. This HYBRIDIZATION of DNA is one technique used in GENETIC ENGINEERING. ANNEALING can also occur between a strand of DNA and a strand of RNA. *See* denaturation.

anode (physics) An ELECTRODE that is positively charged relative to another with a CURRENT flowing between the two; it attracts anions. *Contrast* CATHODE.

See also ELECTROLYSIS.

anodizing (chemistry) Process of coating a METAL (*e.g.* ALUMINIUM) with a thin layer of OXIDE by ELECTROLYSIS.

anon. (literary terminology) An abbreviation of 'anon'ymous, used with capital as attribution of unknown authorship

anorexia nervosa (medical) Pathological and CHRONIC FASTING, occurring most frequently in adolescent girls; it is usually accompanied by AMENORRHOEA (*USA*: amenorrhea), sickness, weakness, severe WEIGHT loss, and psychological disturbance.

anosmia (medical) Complete loss of the sense of SMELL.

ANOVA (statistics) An abbreviation of 'AN'alysis 'O'f 'VA'riance.

anoxaemia (haematology) Less than the NORMAL amount of OXYGEN in the BLOOD. (*USA*: anoxemia). *See* ANOXIA.

anoxia (medical) Condition where body tissues receive inadequate amounts of OXYGEN. ANOXIA may result from low atmospheric OXYGEN PRESSURE, ANAEMIA (*USA*: anemia), INTERFERENCE with BLOOD flow or the inability of tissues to utilize OXYGEN normally.

ANP (physiology/ biochemistry) An abbreviation of 'A'trial 'N'atriuretic 'P'eptide.

ANS (anatomy) An abbreviation for 'A'utonomic 'N'ervous 'S'ystem.

ANSL (quality standards) An abbreviation of 'A'ustralian 'N'ational 'S'tandards 'L'aboratory.

antacid (pharmacology) Substance used medicinally to combat excess STOMACH ACID (*e.g.* various compounds of MAGNESIUM).

antagonist (pharmacology) Substances that have no pharmacological actions in their own right, but that have profound actions because they actually physically occupy receptors, thus blocking, those that normally allow natural mediators, or sometimes synthetic drugs, to have an effect. Many widely used drugs in medicine are ATAGONISTS, used to prevent the actions of mediators within the body, thereby 'switching off' systems that are not functioning correctly, such as in the disease states caused by excessive amounts of NEUROTRANSMITTERS and HORMONES. Examples of ANTAGONISTS include BETA-BLOCKERS, that prevent the action of adrenaline and NORADRENALINE by blocking the receptors called BETA-ADRENOCEPTORS, and ANTIHISTAMINES that inhibit the effects in the body of the local HORMONE histamine by blocking receptors called H_1 receptors.

See also AGONIST.

anterior (biology) Near the HEAD of an ANIMAL.

See also POSTERIOR.

anthracene (chemistry) $C_{14}H_{10}$ White SOLID AROMATIC COMPOUND whose molecules consist of three BENZENE RINGS fused in line.

anthraquinone (chemistry) $C_6H_4(CO)_2C_6H_4$ Yellow CRYSTALLINE ORGANIC COMPOUND important in the manufacture of dyes.

anthrax (medical/ microbiology) BACTERIAL disease that affects many animals, including human beings, and which is frequently fatal. The disease-causing BACTERIUM can form spores, and remain dormant in the soil or on stored ANIMAL hides for many years.

anthropoid (biology) Man-like. Members of the suborder Anthropoidea, which consists of monkeys, apes and man.

anthropology (biology) Study of the human RACE. Physical anthropology is concerned with human EVOLUTION, social anthropology with BEHAVIOUR (USA: behavior).

anti-androgens (pharmacology) Drugs that inhibit the actions of ANDROGENS.

anti-angina drugs (pharmacology) Drugs that relieve the intense pain of angina pectoris originating from the heart due to insufficient blood supply to the heart muscle.

anti-arrhythmic drugs (pharmacology) Drugs that strengthen and regularise a HEARTBEAT that is unsteady or not showing its usual pattern of activity.

anti-asthmatic drugs (pharmacology) Drugs used to relieve the symptoms of bronchial asthma or prevent recurrent attacks.

antibiotic (pharmacology) Member of a GROUP of chemical substances that are byproducts of METABOLISM in certain MICRO-ORGANISMS. Antibiotics cause the destruction of other MICRO-ORGANISMS, and are used as drugs to kill BACTERIA.

antibody (immunology) Highly specific MOLECULE produced by the IMMUNE SYSTEM in RESPONSE to the presence of an ANTIGEN, which it neutralizes.

See also acquired IMMUNITY.

anticancer agents (pharmacology) Drugs used to treat cancer, most of which are cytotoxic i.e. they act by interfering with CELL replication or production, so preventing the growth of new cancerous TISSUE. They are usually administered in combination in a series of treatments known collectively as CHEMOTHERAPY.

anticholinergic drugs (pharmacology) Drugs used to inhibit the action, release or production of the NEUROTRANSMITTER ACETYLCHOLINE.

anticoagulant (pharmacology/ haematology) An agent that prevents BLOOD from clotting. Anticoagulants are used to prevent the formation of clots in the veins after operation and, in cases where it is known that clotting has occurred, to prevent further extension of the clot. WARFARIN which can be given orally and HEPARIN which requires INTRAVENOUS infusion are examples of therapeutic anticoagulants.

anticodon (genetics) The three adjacent nucleotides in a transfer-RNA MOLECULE that are complementary to, and BASE PAIR with, the three complementary nucleotides of a codon in a messenger-RNA MOLECULE. *See* PROTEIN SYNTHESIS; GENETIC CODE.

anticonvulsant drugs (pharmacology) Drugs used to prevent the onset of epileptic seizures or to reduce their severity should they occur.

antidepressants (pharmacology) Drugs used to control the psychiatric illness of depression. The three classes of drugs that are most commonly used are the selective SEROTONIN re-uptake inhibitors (SSRIs), tricyclic antidepressants, and the monoamine OXIDASE inhibitors (MAOIs).

antidiuretic hormone (ADH) (biochemistry) HORMONE secreted from the POSTERIOR PITUITARY and synthesized in the HYPOTHALAMUS. In mammals it stimulates the reABSORPTION of WATER in the KIDNEY, and thus diminishes the VOLUME of URINE produced.

See also VASOPRESSIN.

antidote (pharmacology) A COMPOUND that is administered in ORDER to counteract the effect of a POISON. ANTIDOTES may be specific, exerting their effect through a mechanism related to the mechanism of ACTION of the TOXICANT, or non-specific, counteracting the symptoms of toxicity in a manner not clearly related to the mechanism of ACTION.

antiemetics (pharmacology) Drugs that suppress vomiting. The chief ANTIEMETICS are the phenothiazines, such as chlorpromazine, perphenazine, prochlorperazine or promethazine.

anti-epileptic drugs (pharmacology) Drugs used to prevent the occurrence of epileptic seizures.

antigen (immunology) A substance that elicits an IMMUNE RESPONSE. Usually a PROTEIN MOLECULE that the body's IMMUNE SYSTEM recognizes as 'foreign', but they may be other macromolecules (*e.g.* BACTERIA, transplanted TISSUE).

See also ANTIBODY.

antihistamine (pharmacology) Chemical substance that inhibits the ACTION of HISTAMINE by blocking its site of ACTION. It may be used to treat an ALLERGY.

antihypertensive (pharmacology) A drug used to treat raised BLOOD PRESSURE (HYPERTENSION).

anti-inflammatory drugs (pharmacology) Drugs used to reduce the body's INFLAMMATORY RESPONSE to for instance injury, infection or presence of foreign proteins.

antilogarithm (mathematics) Number that is represented by a LOGARITHM.

antimony Sb (chemistry) Blue-white semimetallic ELEMENT in GROUP VA of the PERIODIC TABLE. It is used to impart hardness to LEAD-TIN ALLOYS and as a DONOR impurity in semiconductors. Its compounds, used as pigments, are poisonous. At. no. 51; r.a.m. 121.75.

antinauseant drugs (pharmacology) Drugs used to prevent or minimise the sensation of nausea and to reduce any subsequent vomiting.

antineopastics (pharmacology) *See* ANTI-CANCER agents.

antioxidant (biochemistry) Chemicals that hinder OXIDATION, frequently serving as FREE RADICAL scavengers *e.g.* VITAMINS C and E. Most antioxidants are ORGANIC COMPOUNDS. Natural ones are found in vegetable oils and in some fruits.

antiparallel (genetics) The orientation of DNA strands in a duplex. One strand runs 5' to 3' in one direction whereas the complementary strand runs 5' to 3' in the opposite direction. By virtue of the POLARITY of DNA, the two strands are therefore ANTIPARALLEL.

antiparticle (physics) SUBATOMIC PARTICLE that corresponds to another PARTICLE of equal MASS but opposite ELECTRIC CHARGE (*e.g.* a POSITRON is the ANTIPARTICLE of the ELECTRON).

antirheumatic drugs (pharmacology) Drugs used to relieve the pain and inflammation of rheumatism and arthritis, and sometimes other musculoskeletal disorders.

antisense RNA (genetics) An RNA transcript having the POLARITY complementary to that of normally transcribed RNA.

antiseptic (pharmacology) Substance that prevents sepsis by killing BACTERIA or preventing their GROWTH. Also termed: germicide.

antiserum (immunology) BLOOD SERUM containing antibodies, used in vaccines to treat or prevent a disease or to combat ANIMAL venom (*e.g.* snakebite).

antispasmodic drugs (pharmacology) Drugs used to relieve spasm in smooth muscle such as those in the respiratory tract or intestinal wall.

antisympathetic drugs (pharmacology) Drugs that act at some site within the SYMPATHETIC NERVOUS SYSTEM to reduce its overall effect.

antithyroid drugs (pharmacology) Drugs used in the treatment of over-activity of the THYROID gland.

antitoxin (immunology) Type of ANTIBODY against a TOXOID produced in the body by a disease organism or by VACCINATION.

antrum (1, 2 anatomy) 1 Cavity in a BONE (*e.g.* a SINUS). 2 Part of the STOMACH next to the pyloris.

anus (anatomy) POSTERIOR opening of the ALIMENTARY CANAL, through which the undigested residue of DIGESTION is passed.

anx (literary term) An abbreviation of 'an'ne'x'.

anxiolytic drugs (pharmacology) Agents which alleviate anxiety without inducing sedation. The most widely used anxiolytic drugs are the benzodiazepines, such as DIAZEPAM and chlordiazepoxide.

ANZAAS (education) An abbreviation of 'A'ustralian and 'N'ew 'Z'ealand 'A'ssociation for the 'A'dvancement of 'S'cience.

ANZIC (education) An abbreviation of 'A'ssociate of the 'N'ew 'Z'ealand 'I'nstitute of 'C'hemists.

aorta (anatomy) Principal ARTERY that takes oxygenated BLOOD from the HEART to all parts of the body other than the lungs.

a.-part. (radiology) An abbreviation of 'a'lpha -'part'icle.

apatite (chemistry) Mineral that consists mainly of CALCIUM PHOSPHATE, used as a source of PHOSPHORUS and for making fertilizers.

APC (physiology/ biochemistry) An abbreviation of 'A'ctivated 'P'rotein 'C'.

aperture (optics) Effective DIAMETER of a LENS or LENS system. Its RECIPROCAL is the f-number.

apex (physics) Point on a SOLID or plane figure that is farthest from its BASE. *e.g.* the pointed top of a pyramid.

Apgar score (medical) A method of assessing the condition of a newborn infant by assigning 0 to 2 points to the quality of HEART rate, RESPIRATION, COLOUR (*USA*: color), tone and REFLEX activity at one and five minutes of life. The method is named after the physician Virginia Apgar (1909-74).

APH (1 medical; 2 biochemistry) 1 An abbreviation of 'A'nte'P'artum 'H'aemorrhage (*USA*: antepartum hemorrhage), bleeding during PREGNANCY or LABOUR (*USA*: labor). 2 An abbreviation of 'A'nterior 'P'ituitary 'H'ormone.

APHA (society) An abbreviation of 'A'merican 'P'ublic 'H'ealth 'A'ssociation.

apical growth (biology) An alternative term for primary GROWTH.

APML (medical/ haematology) An abbreviation of 'A'cute 'P'ro'M'yelocytic 'L'eukaemia (*USA*: ACUTE Promyelocytic Leukemia).

apnoea (medical) Cessation of BREATHING for short periods of time. (*USA*: apnea).

apoenzyme (biochemistry) PROTEIN part of an ENZYME that consists of a PROTEIN and a non-PROTEIN portion.

apomorphine hydrochloride (pharmacology) An anti-PARKINSON'S drug that has similar actions to bromocriptine. It is chemically related to morphine, though it is not an ANALGESIC and has been used as an emetic.

apoprotein (biochemistry) PROTEIN part of any complex or CONJUGATED PROTEIN.

apoptosis (physiology) The process of programmed CELL death.

apothecary ounce (measurement) UNIT of WEIGHT, 1/12 of a pound (apothecary). 1 oz ap. = 1.0971 oz (AVOIRDUPOIS) = 31.103481 grams. Also termed: ounce, troy.

APP (biochemistry) An abbreviation of 'A'myloid 'P'recusor 'P'rotein.

app. (1, 2, 3, 4, general terminology) 1 An abbreviation of 'app'aratus (also termed appar.; apparat.). 2 An abbreviation of 'app'arent. 3 'app'lied (also termed appl.). 4 'app'roximate (also termed approx.).

apparat. (general terminology) *See* app.

apparent depth (physics) Perceived depth of a LIQUID, which is different from its actual depth because of the REFRACTION OF LIGHT.

appd. (general terminology) An abbreviation of 'app'rove'd'.

appendix (anatomy) Vestigial outgrowth of the caccum in some mammals. In human beings its full name is VERMIFORM APPENDIX.

appl. (1, 2 general terminology) 1 An abbreviation of 'appl'icable. 2 An abbreviation of 'appl'ied.

applications program (computing) COMPUTER PROGRAM written by the user for a specific purpose, *e.g.* RECORD-keeping or stock control.

approx. (general terminology) *See* app.

apps (literary terminology) An abbreviation of 'app'endice's'.

appx (literary terminology) An abbreviation of 'app'endi'x'.

aprotinin (pharmacology) An inhibitor of proteolytic ENZYMES and has antifibrinolytic activity, because it prevents thrombosis by an action on the blood clot formation system.

APST (society) An abbreviation of 'A'ssociation of 'P'rofessional 'S'cientists and 'T'echnologists.

APTT (haematology) An abbreviation of 'A'ctivated 'P'artial 'T'hromboplastin 'T'ime.

APUD cells (physiology/ biochemistry) An abbreviation of 'A'mine 'P'recursor 'U'ptake and 'D'ecarboxylation CELLS.

aq. (chemistry) An abbreviation of 'aq'ueous/ *'aq'ua.* [Latin, meaning 'WATER'.]

AQL (quality standards) An abbreviation of 'A'cceptable 'Q'uality 'L'evel.

aqua fortis (chemistry) Obsolete term for concentrated NITRIC ACID.

aqua regia (chemistry) MIXTURE of one part concentrated NITRIC ACID to three parts concentrated HYDROCHLORIC ACID, so called because it dissolves the 'noble' metals GOLD and PLATINUM.

aqueous (chemistry) Dissolved in WATER, or chiefly consisting of WATER.

aqueous humour (anatomy) The LIQUID between the LENS and CORNEA of the EYE.

aqueous solution (chemistry) SOLUTION in which the SOLVENT is WATER.

Ar (chemistry) The CHEMICAL SYMBOL for ARGON.

arabinose (chemistry) $C_5H_{10}O_5$ CRYSTALLINE PENTOSE SUGAR derived from plant POLYSACCHARIDES (such as gums).

arachnoid layer (anatomy) The middle of the three layers of TISSUE that enclose the CENTRAL NERVOUS SYSTEM. Named after its resemblance to a spider's web. *See* MENINGES.

arachnoid membrane (histology) One of the three thin membranes that cover the BRAIN, the other two being the pia mater and the dura mater.

aragonite (chemistry) Fairly unstable mineral form of CALCIUM CARBONATE ($CaCO_3$).

ARBD (medical) An abbreviation of 'A'lcohol-'R'elated 'B'irth 'D'efects.

arborization (anatomy) The branching of NERVE CELLS.

Arboviruses (microbiology) A GROUP of VIRUSES transmitted by arthropods. Examples include the causative agents of dengue, sandfly FEVER, St Louis encephalitis, western equine encephalitis and YELLOW FEVER. The GENOME is single-stranded RNA.

ARC (medical/ virology) An abbreviation of 'A'IDS-'R'elated 'C'omplex.

Archimedes' principle (physics) When a body is immersed in a FLUID it has an apparent loss in WEIGHT equal to the WEIGHT of the FLUID it displaces. It was named after the ancient Greek mathematician Archimedes (c.287-212BC).

arc (mathematics) Part of a curve. The length of an ARC of a circle, RADIUS r, that subtends an angle of θ degrees at the centre (*USA*: center) is given by $2\pi r\theta/360$ (equal to $r\theta$ if the angle is in radians).

ARDS (physiology/ biochemistry) An abbreviation of 'A'dult 'R'espiratory 'D'istress 'S'yndrome.

area (mathematics) Measure of the size of a surface.

areola (1, 2 anatomy) 1 Part of the IRIS of the EYE, bordering the pupil. 2 Dark SKIN on the breast surrounding a nipple.

areolar tissue (histology) CONNECTIVE TISSUE made up of CELLS separated by bundles of FIBRES (*USA*: fibers) embedded in MUCIN.

ARF (medical) An abbreviation of 'A'cute 'R'enal 'F'ailure.

Arg. (biochemistry) An abbreviation of 'Arg'inine.

arginine (chemistry) $C_6H_{14}N_4O_2$ Colourless (*USA*: colorless) CRYSTALLINE ESSENTIAL AMINO ACID of the alpha-ketoglutaric ACID FAMILY.

argon Ar (chemistry) An INERT GAS ELEMENT in GROUP 0 of the PERIODIC TABLE (the RARE GASes). It makes up 0.93 per cent of AIR (by VOLUME), from which it is extracted. It is used to provide an INERT ATMOSPHERE in electric lamps and DISCHARGE tubes, and for welding reactive metals (such as ALUMINIUM). At. no. 18; r.a.m. 39.948.

ARIC (education) An abbreviation of 'A'ssociate of the 'R'oyal 'I'nstitute of 'C'hemistry.

arithmetic mean (statistics) A measure of central tendency, obtained by dividing the sum of a SET of numbers by the number in the SET. *Contrast* GEOMETRIC MEAN; MEDIAN; MODE.

arithmetic mean average (statistics) of a collection of numbers obtained by dividing the sum of the numbers by the quantity of numbers.

arithmetic progression (mathematics) Sequence of numbers for which there is a CONSTANT COMMON DIFFERENCE, d, such that the difference between any two successive terms is equal to d. *e.g.* for the ARITHMETIC PROGRESSION 2, 9, 16, 23, 30, the COMMON DIFFERENCE is 7. If the nth term of the SERIES is given by $[a + (n - 1)d]$, the sum of n terms is $n[2a + (n - 1)d]/2$.

See also GEOMETRIC PROGRESSION.

arithmetic series (mathematics) SERIES whose terms form an ARITHMETIC PROGRESSION.

arithmetic unit (computing) Part of a COMPUTER'S CENTRAL PROCESSOR that performs arithmetical operations (addition, subtraction, multiplication, DIVISION).

aromatase (biochemistry) The name given to an ENZYME catalysing the aromatization of the A-ring of the STEROID NUCLEUS during the conversion of ANDROGENS to oestrogens (*USA,* estrogens).

aromatic compound (chemistry) Member of a large CLASS of organic chemicals that exhibit AROMATICITY, the simplest of which is BENZENE.

aromaticity (chemistry) Presence in an organic chemical of five or more CARBON atoms joined in a ring that exhibits DELOCALIZATION of electrons, as in BENZENE and its compounds. All the CARBON-CARBON bonds are equivalent.

array (computing) An ordered pattern of symbol strings having one or more dimensions.

arrhythmia (medical) Irregular HEART beat.

arsenate (chemistry) SALT or ESTER of ARSENIC ACID (H_3AsO_4). Also termed: arsenates).

arsenic acid (chemistry) H_3AsO_4 Tribasic ACID from which ARSENATEs are derived. an AQUEOUS SOLUTION of ARSENIC(V) OXIDE, As_2O_5. Also termed: ORTHOARSENIC ACID; ARSENIC(V) ACID.

arsenic As (chemistry) SILVER-grey semimetallic ELEMENT in GROUP VA of the PERIODIC TABLE which exists as several ALLOTROPES. It is extracted from SULPHIDE (*USA:* sulfide) ores (*e.g.* arsenopyrite) and is used in ALLOYS, as a DONOR impurity in semiconductors and in insecticides and drugs; its compounds are very poisonous. The substance known as WHITE ARSENIC is ARSENIC(III) OXIDE (arsenious OXIDE), As_4O_6. At. no. 33; r.a.m. 74.9216.

arsenide (chemistry) COMPOUND formed from ARSENIC and another METAL; *e.g.* IRON(III) [FERRIC] ARSENIDE, $FeAs_2$.

arsenious acid (chemistry) H_3AsO_3 Tribasic ACID from which arsenates are derived; an AQUEOUS SOLUTION of ARSENIC(III) OXIDE (arsenious OXIDE, WHITE ARSENIC), As_4O_6. Also termed: ARSENIC(III) ACID; arsenous ACID.

arsenite (chemistry) SALT or ESTER of ARSENIOUS ACID (H_3AsO_3). Also termed: ARSENATE(III).

arsine (chemistry) H_3As Colourless (*USA:* colorless) highly poisonous GAS with an unpleasant odour (*USA:* odor). Organic derivatives, in which ALKYL GROUPS replace one or more HYDROGEN atoms, are also called ARSINES. Also termed: ARSENIC(III) HYDRIDE.

arteriole (anatomy) Small ARTERY.

artery (anatomy) BLOOD VESSEL that carries oxygenated BLOOD from the HEART to other tissues. An exception is the PULMONARY ARTERY, which carries deoxygenated BLOOD to the lungs.

arthritis (medical) INFLAMMATION of the joints and the surrounding tissues.

artificial insemination (1, 2 medical) 1 Artificial IMPLANTATION of SPERM-containing SEMEN into the female CERVIX. 2 Transfer of a fertilized OVUM from the reproductive tract of one female to that of a HOST mother.

artificial intelligence (AI) (computing) The study of how to make computers perform intelligently.

artificial radioactivity (radiology) RADIO-ACTIVITY in a substance that is not normally RADIOACTIVE. It is created by bombarding the substance with IONIZING RADIATION. Also termed: INDUCED RADIO-ACTIVITY.

ARV (virology) An abbreviation of 'A'IDS-'R'elated 'V'irus.

aryl group (chemistry) RADICAL that is derived from a COMPOUND exhibiting AROMATICITY by the removal of one HYDROGEN ATOM. *e.g.* phenyl, C_6H_5 derived from BENZENE.

arylation (chemistry) The chemical addition of an ARYL GROUP to another MOLECULE.

As (chemistry) The CHEMICAL SYMBOL for ELEMENT 33, ARSENIC.

asap (general terminology) An abbreviation of 'a's 's'oon 'a's 'p'ossible.

asb (chemistry) An abbreviation of 'asb'estos.

ASB (society) An abbreviation of 'A'merican 'S'ociety of 'B'acteriologists.

asbestos (chemistry) Fibrous VARIETY of a number of rock-forming silicate minerals that are HEAT-resistant and chemically INERT.

ASc. (education) An abbreviation of 'A'ssociate in 'Sc'ience.

ASc.W (society) An abbreviation of 'A'ssociation of 'Sc'ientific 'W'orkers.

ASCII (computing) An abbreviation of 'A'merican 'S'tandard 'C'ode for 'I'nformation 'I'nterchange.

ascites (medical) ABNORMAL accumulation of FLUID from the BLOOD in the peritoneal cavity, occurring in HEART, LIVER and KIDNEY FAILURE.

ascitic fluid (medical) Serous FLUID in peritoneal cavity.

Ascomycetes (mycology) Important CLASS of FUNGI in which the SPORE-producing body is an ASCUS. It includes morels, truffles, the fungal part of most lichens, and many yeasts. Also termed: ASCOMYCOTINA.

Ascomycotina (mycology) An alternative term for ASCOMYCETES.

ascorbic acid (VITAMIN C) (biochemistry) $C_6H_8O_6$ A white CRYSTALLINE, WATER-SOLUBLE VITAMIN that has seven known biochemical roles including acting as cofactor in TYROSINE METABOLISM. ASCORBIC ACID is necessary for, amongst other things, formation of BONE, and CARTILAGE. Lack of the VITAMIN leads to scurvy in humans. The principal sources of ASCORBIC ACID in the diet are fruits and vegetables.

ascus (mycology) CELL in FUNGI in which HAPLOID spores are formed. *See* ASCOMYCETES.

aseptic (microbiology) Referring to being free from PATHOGENIC MICRO-ORGANISMS (particularly BACTERIA).

asexual reproduction (biology) REPRO-DUCTION that does not involve gametes or

FERTILIZATION. There is a single parent, and all offspring are genetically identical. This commonly occurs in prokaryotes, and also FUNGI, PROTOZOA and some plants. BACTERIA normally reproduce asexually, but are also capable of a form of SEXUAL REPRODUCTION known as CONJUGATION. *See* CLONE.

See also VEGETATIVE PROPAGATION.

ASGBI (society) An abbreviation of 'A'natomical 'S'ociety of 'G'reat 'B'ritain and 'I'reland.

Asherman's syndrome (medical) AMENOR-RHOEA (*USA*: amenorrhea) due to ADHESIONS in the uterine cavity.

Asn (biochemistry) An abbreviation of 'As'paragi'n'e.

ASN (statistics) An abbreviation of 'A'verage 'S'ample 'N'umber.

Asp. (biochemistry) An abbreviation of 'Asp'artic acid.

aspartame (chemistry) Artificial sweetener (a dipeptide) that is 200 times as sweet as ordinary SUGAR (SUCROSE), but does not have the bitter aftertaste CHARACTERISTIC of SACCHARIN.

ASPCA (society) An abbreviation of 'A'merican 'S'ociety for 'P'revention of 'C'ruelty to 'A'nimals.

Aspergillosis (medical/ mycology) INFECTION of the lungs with *Aspergillus* SPECIES, a type of FUNGUS.

ASPET (society) An abbreviation of 'A'merican 'S'ociety for 'P'harmacology and 'E'xperimental 'T'herapeutics.

asphyxia (medical) Suffocation. It can be brought about by obstruction to the AIR-passages, by lack of OXYGEN in the AIR, or by gases which interfere with the use of OXYGEN by the body, such as CARBON MONOXIDE.

aspiration (medical) The removal of fluids by suction.

aspirator (physics) Apparatus that produces suction in ORDER to draw a GAS or LIQUID from a VESSEL or cavity.

aspirin (pharmacology) $CH_3COO.C_6H_4-COOH$ Drug that is commonly used as an ANALGESIC, antipyretic (to reduce FEVER) and anti-inflammatory. Also termed: acetylsalicyllic acid.

assimilation (biochemistry) Process of turning food into body substances after it has been digested (*e.g.* in animals excess GLUCOSE is turned into GLYCOGEN or fat, AMINO ACIDS are made into proteins).

Assoc.Sc. (education) An abbreviation of 'Assoc'iate in 'Sc'ience. Also termed Assoc.Sci.

association (general term) A connection.

Association of the British Pharmaceutical Industry (ABPI) (association) A UK trade association that aims to ensure that medicinal and related products are of the highest quality and are readily available for the TREATMENT of human and ANIMAL disease.

associative (mathematics) Describing a two-stage mathematical operation of the type $a * (b * c)$ whose result does not depend on the ORDER in which the operation is carried out; *e.g.* the multiplication 5 x (6 x 7) gives the same result as (5 x 6) x 7, and thus multiplication is associative. DIVISION, however, is not; *e.g.* 40 ÷ (20 ÷ 4) does not equal (40 ÷ 20) ÷ 4.

See also COMMUTATIVE.

AST (biochemistry) An abbreviation of 'AS'partate amino'T'ransferase.

astatine At (chemistry) RADIOACTIVE ELEMENT in GROUP VIIA of the PERIODIC TABLE (the halogens). It has several isotopes, of half-lives of 2×10^{-6} sec to 8 hr. Because of their short half-lives, they are available in only MINUTE quantities. At. no. 85; r.a.m. 210 (most STABLE ISOTOPE).

aster phase (genetics) An alternative term for METAPHASE.

astigmatism (1 medical; 2 optics) 1 The refractive error PRODUCT by a CORNEA that is more CONVEX in some directions than others, so that lines or edges in different orientations cannot simultaneously be brought into FOCUS on the RETINA. 2 Failure of an optical system, such as a LENS or a mirror, to FOCUS the IMAGE of a point as a single point.

ASTM (society) An abbreviation of 'A'merican 'S'ociety for 'T'esting and 'M'aterials.

astrocyte (histology) One of the many types of non-NEURONE CELL found within the NERVOUS SYSTEM, the name being derived from the star-like appearance. Astrocytes support the FUNCTION of neurones. Also termed astroglia.

astrocytosis (medical/ histology) An increase in numbers and size of ASTROCYTES as a result of traumatic BRAIN damage or in neurodegenerative disease.

astroglia (histology) *See* ASTROCYTE.

asymptomatic (medical) Not showing any signs or symptoms of disease whether disease is present or not.

asymptote (mathematics) In geometry and CO-ORDINATE geometry, a line that a curve approaches closer and closer but never reaches.

asystole (medical) Absence of HEARTBEAT.

at. no. (physics) An abbreviation of 'at'omic number.

at. wt. (physics) An abbreviation of 'at'omic 'w'eigh't'.

ataxia (medical) Inability to control motor coordination caused by damage to the CENTRAL NERVOUS SYSTEM, *e.g.* by drugs, disease, or lesions.

ATG (haematology) An abbreviation of 'A'nti'T'hymocyte 'G'lobulin.

atheroma (medical/ haematology) The thickening of the wall or the FATTY DEGENERATION occurring in the walls of the larger arteries in atherosclerosis. Scar TISSUE which limits BLOOD circulation and predisposes to THROMBOSIS.

atheroselerosis (medical/ haematology) An accumulation of LIPID deposits within or beneath the surfaces of BLOOD VESSELs that partially occludes the LUMEN of the VESSEL and roughens its interior surface. This reduces BLOOD flow to tissues, increases the chance of PLATELET aggregation and BLOOD COAGULATION by increasing the turbulence within the BLOOD, and increases the chances of OCCLUSION by trapping a circulating BLOOD clot. If CALCIUM becomes deposited in the atherosclerotic plaques, then arteriosclerosis ('hardening of the arteries') results. Certain diets may contribute to atherosclerosis, as may CHROMIUM deficiency or excess COPPER.

atlas (anatomy) The first (CERVICAL) VERTEBRA, which joins the SKULL to the SPINE and articulates with the AXIS, allowing nodding movements of the HEAD.

Atm. (physiology/ physics) An abbreviation of 'Atm'osphere.

atmosphere (1 physics; 2 measurement) 1 AIR or gases surrounding the EARTH or other heavenly body. The EARTH's ATMOSPHERE extends outwards several thousand kilometres, becoming increasingly rarefied until it merges gradually into space. *See* AIR. 2 (atm.) UNIT of PRESSURE, equal to 101,325 pascals (equivalent to 760 mm Hg).

atmospheric pressure (physics) FORCE exerted on the surface of the EARTH (and any other planetary body), and on the organisms that live there, by the WEIGHT of the ATMOSPHERE. Its standard value at sea-LEVEL is 1.01325×10^5 Nm^{-2}, and it decreases with altitude, but is subject to local and temporary VARIATION. It is measured with a BAROMETER.

ATN (medical) An abbreviation of 'A'cute 'T'ubular 'N'ecrosis.

atom (chemistry) Fundamental PARTICLE that is the BASIC UNIT of MATTER. An ATOM consists of a positively charged NUCLEUS surrounded by negatively charged electrons restricted to orbitals of a given ENERGY LEVEL. Most of the MASS of an ATOM is in the NUCLEUS, which is composed principally of protons (positively charged) and neutrons (electrically

NEUTRAL); HYDROGEN is exceptional in having merely one PROTON in its NUCLEUS. The number of electrons is equal to the number of protons, and this is the ATOMIC NUMBER. The chemical BEHAVIOUR (*USA*: behavior) of an ATOM is determined by how many electrons it has, and how they are transferred to, or shared with, other atoms to form CHEMICAL BONDs.

See also RELATIVE ATOMIC MASS; ISOTOPE; MOLECULE; SUBATOMIC PARTICLE; VALENCE.

atomic mass (chemistry) An alternative term for ATOMIC WEIGHT.

See also RELATIVE ATOMIC MASS.

atomic mass unit (AMU) (chemistry) Arbitrary UNIT that is used to express the MASS of individual atoms. The standard is a MASS equal to 1/12 of the MASS of a CARBON ATOM (the CARBON-12 ISOTOPE). A MASS expressed on this standard is called a RELATIVE ATOMIC MASS (r.a.m.), symbol A_r. ATOMIC MASS UNIT is also termed dalton.

atomic number (at. no.) (chemistry) Number equal to the number of protons in the NUCLEUS of an ATOM of a particular ELEMENT, symbol Z. Also termed: PROTON NUMBER.

atomic orbital (chemistry) WAVE FUNCTION that characterizes the BEHAVIOUR (*USA*: behavior) of an ELECTRON when orbiting the NUCLEUS of an ATOM. It can be visualized as the region in space occupied by the ELECTRON.

atomic weight (at. wt.) (chemistry) Relative MASS of an ATOM given in terms of ATOMIC MASS UNITs. *See* RELATIVE ATOMIC MASS.

atomicity (chemistry) Number of atoms in one MOLECULE of an ELEMENT; *e.g.* ARGON has an ATOMICITY of 1, NITROGEN 2, OZONE 3.

ATP (biochemistry) An abbreviation of 'A'denosine 'T'ri'P'hosphate.

ATPD (physics) An abbreviation of 'A'mbient 'T'emperature and 'P'ressure, 'D'ry.

ATPS (physics) An abbreviation of 'A'mbient 'T'emperature and 'P'ressure, 'S'aturated with water vapour (*USA*: vapor).

atrium (anatomy) One of the thin-walled upper chambers of the HEART. Also termed: AURICLE.

atrophy (medical) A wasting away, or decrease in the size and FUNCTION of a CELL, TISSUE, or ORGAN.

atropine (1 toxicology; 2 pharmacology) 1 White CRYSTALLINE poisonous ALKALOID that occurs in deadly nightshade. Also termed: belladonna. 2 A muscarinic ANTAGONIST. This powerful ANTICHO-LINERGIC drug is able to depress certain functions of the autonomic nervous system and is therefore a useful ANTISPASMODIC drug. It can also be used to cause a long-lasting dilation of the pupil of the eye for ophthalmic procedures.

attenuated (microbiology) Weakened, reduced in VIRULENCE (*e.g.* live poliovirus VACCINE).

attenuation (physics) Loss of strength of a physical quantity (*e.g.* a radio signal or an ELECTRIC CURRENT) caused by ABSORPTION or scattering.

Au (chemistry) The symbol for the ELEMENT GOLD. [From the Latin, 'aurum'.]

AUC (statistics) An abbreviation of 'A'rea 'U'nder 'C'urve.

audiology (audiology) The scientific study of hearing.

auditory canal (anatomy) Tube that leads from the OUTER EAR to the EAR DRUM (tympanum).

auditory nerve (histology) NERVE that carries impulses concerned with hearing from the INNER EAR to the BRAIN.

auditory (medical) Relating to the EAR or hearing.

Auger effect (chemistry) Radiationless ejection of an ELECTRON from an ION. It is named after the French physicist Pierre Auger (1899-1993). Also termed: AUTOIONIZATION.

AUL (haematology) An abbreviation of 'A'cute 'U'ndifferentiated 'L'eukaemia (*USA*: ACUTE Undifferentiated Leukemia).

auranofin (pharmacology) A disease modifying ANTIRHEUMATIC and ANTI-INFLAMMATORY drug containing gold. It is administered orally to treat severe progressive rheumatoid arthritis.

auric (chemistry) TRIVALENT GOLD. Also termed: GOLD(III); GOLD(3+).

auricle (anatomy) An alternative term for ATRIUM.

aurous (chemistry) MONOVALENT GOLD. Also termed: GOLD(I); GOLD(1+).

autism (medical) BRAIN disorder that develops in infancy and which is characterized by extreme learning difficulties and a lack of responsiveness to other people.

autocatalysis (chemistry) Catalytic REACTION that is started by the products of a REACTION that was itself catalytic. *See* CATALYST.

autoclave (laboratory equipment) Airtight container that heats and sometimes agitates its contents under high-PRESSURE steam. Autoclaves are usually used for STERILIZATION or industrial processing.

autogamy (biology) Uniting of gametes produced by the same CELL. Also termed: self-FERTILIZATION.

auto-immune diseases (medical/ immunology) A wide range of conditions *e.g.* rheumatoid arthritis, ulcerative colitis, and so on, in which destructive inflammation of various body tissues is caused by antibodies produced because the body has ceased to regard the affected part as 'self'.

autoionization (chemistry) Spontaneous IONIZATION of excited atoms, molecules or fragments of an ION. Also termed: pre-IONIZATION.

See also AUGER EFFECT.

autolysis (biochemistry) Breakdown of the contents of an ANIMAL or plant CELL by the ACTION of ENZYMES produced within that CELL.

autonomic nervous system (ANS) (physiology) In vertebrates, the part of the NERVOUS SYSTEM that is not under voluntary control and carries NERVE IMPULSES to the SMOOTH MUSCLES, GLANDS, HEART and other organs. It is subdivided

into the parasympathetic and SYMPATHETIC NERVOUS SYSTEMS.

auto-oxidation (chemistry) OXIDATION caused by the unaided ATMOSPHERE.

autopsy (medical) The examination of a body after death, so that physicians can arrive at a true diagnosis of the cause of death.

autoradiography (radiology) Technique for photographing a specimen by injecting it with RADIOACTIVE material so that it produces its own IMAGE on a photographic FILM or plate.

autosome (genetics) Any CHROMOSOME other than one of the SEX CHROMOSOMES.

autotroph (biology) Organism that lives using AUTOTROPHISM.

autotrophism (biology) In BACTERIA and green plants, the ability to build up food materials from simple substances, *e.g.* by PHOTOSYNTHESIS.

See also HETEROTROPHISM.

AV (chemistry) An abbreviation of 'A'cid 'V'alue.

avalanche diode (physics) An alternative term for ZENER DIODE.

A-V difference (physiology/ biochemistry) An abbreviation of 'A'rterio'V'enous concentration 'difference' of any given substance.

average (statistics) Number that is representative of a collection of numbers; *e.g.* an ARITHMETIC MEAN, GEOMETRIC MEAN, MODE or MEDIAN.

Avg (statistics) An abbreviation of 'av'era'g'e.

AV node (physiology/ biochemistry) An abbreviation of 'A'trioV'entricular 'node'.

Avogadro constant (L or N_A) (chemistry) Number of particles (atoms or molecules) in a mole of a substance. It has a value of 6.02253×10^{23}. It was named after the Italian scientist Amedeo Avogadro (1776-1856). Also termed: AVOGADRO'S NUMBER.

Avogadro's law (chemistry) Under the same conditions of PRESSURE and TEMPERATURE, equal volumes of all gases contain equal numbers of molecules. Also termed: Avogadro's HYPOTHESIS.

Avogadro's number (chemistry) An alternative term for AVOGADRO CONSTANT.

avoirdupois (measurements) System of weights based on a pound (symbol lb), equivalent to 2.205kg, and subdivided into 16 ounces, or 7,000 grains. In science and medicine it has been almost entirely replaced by SI UNITS. *See* AVOIRDUPOIS OUNCE.

avoirdupois ounce (measurement) UNIT of WEIGHT, 1/16 of a pound. 1 oz = 28.349527 grams. *See* AVOIRDUPOIS.

AVP (physiology/ biochemistry) An abbreviation of 'A'rginine 'V'aso'P'ressin.

AVS (society) An abbreviation of 'A'nti-'V'ivisection 'S'ociety.

AV valves (physiology) An abbreviation of 'A'trioV'entricular 'valves' of HEART.

aw (chemistry) An abbreviation of 'a'tomic 'w'eight.

A/W (measurement) An abbreviation of 'A'ctual 'W'eight.

axiom (philosophy) Principle that is taken as true, without needing PROOF.

See also HYPOTHESIS; LAW; THEOREM.

axis (1 mathematics; 2 biology; 3 anatomy) 1A line of significant reference for a GRAPH or figure; *e.g.* x- and y-axes in CARTESIAN CO-ORDINATES. 2 Central line of SYMMETRY of an organism. 3 The second (CERVICAL) VERTEBRA, which articulates with the ATLAS and allows the HEAD to turn from side to side.

axon (histology) Long, thread-like outgrowth of a NERVE CELL (NEURONE), the main FUNCTION of which is to carry impulses away from the CELL.

azathioprine (pharmacology) A powerful cytotoxic and immunosuppressant drug that may be administered orally or by injection. It is used to reduce tissue rejection in transplant recipients as well as to treat patients with several autoimmune diseases, myasthenia gravis, rheumatoid arthritis and ulcerative colitis.

azeotrope (chemistry) MIXTURE of two liquids that boil at the same TEMPERATURE.

azide (chemistry) One of the ACYL GROUP of compounds, or salts, derived from hydrazoic ACID (N_3H). Most azides are unstable, and heavy METAL azides are explosive.

azo compound (chemistry) ORGANIC COMPOUND of GENERAL FORMULA R-N = N-R', in which R and R' are usually aromatic groups.

azo dye (chemistry) Member of a CLASS of dyes that are derived from compounds containing an AMINO GROUP and have an -N = N- LINKAGE in their molecules. They are intensely coloured (*USA*: colored) (usually red, brown or yellow) and account for a large proportion of the SYNTHETIC dyes produced. AZO DYES can be made as ACID, BASIC, direct or mordant dyes. Their use as food colourants (*USA*: colorants) has been questioned because of their possible effects on sensitive people, particularly children.

azomethine (biochemistry) *See* SCHIFF'S BASE.

AZT (pharmacology) An abbreviation of 'AZ'ido'T'hymidine.

B

B (1 chemistry; 2 haematology) 1 The CHEMICAL SYMBOL for ELEMENT 5, BORON. 2 A BLOOD type. *See* ABO BLOOD GROUPs.

B App. Sc. (education) An abbreviation of 'B'achelor of 'App'lied 'Sc'ience.

B cell (immunology/ haematology) An abbreviation of 'b'eta CELL.

B Hy. (education) An abbreviation of 'B'achelor of 'Hy'giene/ Public Health.

B Med Biol. (education) An abbreviation of 'B'achelor of 'Med'ical 'Biol'ogy.

B Med Sc. (education) An abbreviation of 'B'achelor of 'Med'ical 'Sc'ience.

B Sc. App. (education) An abbreviation of 'B'achelor of 'App'lied 'Sc'ience.

b. pt (physics) An abbreviation of 'b'oiling 'p'oin't'.

B. Sc. (education) Bachelor of Science; - (LA) Bachelor of Science (LABORATORY Assistant); - (Med.) Bachelor of Science in Medicine; - (Med. Lab. Tech.) Bachelor of Science in Medical LABORATORY Technology; - (Med. Sci.) Bachelor of Science in Medical Sciences; - (M.L.S.) Bachelor of Science in Medical LABORATORY Science; - (Nutr.) Bachelor of Science in Nutrition; - (Pharm.) Bachelor of Science in Pharmacy; - (R.T.) Bachelor of Science in Radiologic Technology; - (Vet.) Bachelor of Science in Veterinary Science, - (Vet.Sc. & A.1A.) Bachelor of Science in Veterinary Science and ANIMAL Husbandry.

Ba (chemistry) The CHEMICAL SYMBOL for ELEMENT 56, BARIUM.

BA Sc. (education) An abbreviation of 'B'achelor of 'A'pplied 'Sc'ience.

BAAS (education) An abbreviation of 'B'ritish 'A'ssociation for the 'A'dvancement of 'S'cience.

BAC (1 biochemistry; 2 society) 1 An abbreviation of 'B'lood 'A'lcohol 'C'oncentration. 2 An abbreviation of 'B'ritish 'A'ssociation of 'C'hemists.

Bacillus (bacteriology) The name originally used in bacteriology to MEAN any ROD-shaped as opposed to a round MICRO-ORGANISM. It is now properly used to denote only one GENUS of SPORE-producing BACTERIA, one member of which is *BACILLUS anthracis* the causative organism of ANTHRAX.

Bacille Calmette-Guérin (BCG) (immunology) A VACCINE used against TUBERCULOSIS. It was named after two French BACTERIOLOGISTs, Albert Calmette (1863-1933) and Camille Guérin (1872-1961).

bacillus cereus (bacteriology) a gram-POSITIVE, an AEROBIC BACILLUS that produces toxins that cause foodpoisoning. They include a THERMOLABILE TOXIN causing DIARRHOEA (*USA*: diarrhea) and a thermostable TOXIN causing EMESIS.

back emf (physics) ELECTROMOTIVE FORCE produced in a CIRCUIT that opposes the main flow of CURRENT; *e.g.* in an ELECTROLYTIC CELL because of POLARIZATION or in an ELECTRIC MOTOR because of ELECTROMAGNETIC INDUCTION.

backbone (anatomy) An alternative term for VERTEBRAL COLUMN.

background radiation (radiology) RADIATION from natural sources, including outer space (cosmic RADIATION) and RADIOACTIVE substances on the EARTH (*e.g.* in igneous rocks such as granite).

backing store (computing) COMPUTER store that is larger than the main (immediate access) MEMORY, but with a longer ACCESS TIME.

baclofen (pharmacology) A skeletal muscle relaxant drug that is administered orally to relax muscles that are in spasm, particularly when caused by injury or by a disease of the CENTRAL NERVOUS SYSTEM.

bact. (bacteriology) An abbreviation of 'bact'eria/ 'bact'erial/ 'bact'eriology.

bacteraemia (bacteriology) The condition of having BACTERIA in the bloodstream. (*USA*: bacteremia).

bacteria (bacteriology) A large GROUP of single-celled microscopic organisms. They can occur either free-living in AIR, WATER, soil, etc; or they may be parasitic upon a HOST plant or ANIMAL. Only a minority cause any disease, and more are actually useful to their hosts, *e.g.* in breaking down food as part of the digestive process. The three BASIC shapes are *BACILLUS* (ROD), *spirillum* (spiral) and *COCCUS* (spherical), but some BACTERIA may link up to form chains or clumps. Multiplication is fast, usually by FISSION. Between them, the various SPECIES can utilize almost any type of organic MOLECULE as food and inhabit almost any ENVIRONMENT. Some can even use

inorganic elements such as SULPHUR (*USA*: sulfur).The activities of some BACTERIA are of great significance to man, *e.g.* FIXATION OF NITROGEN in certain plants, as agents of DECAY, and their medical importance as disease-causing agents (pathogens). Much genetical research is done on BACTERIA because, being prokaryotes, they have simple genetic machinery. Sing. 'BACTERIUM'. *See* ESCHERICHIA COLI.

bacterial (bacteriology) Refering to BACTERIA or caused by BACTERIA.

bacterial endocarditis (medical/ bacteriology) BACTERIAL INFECTION of the endocardium.

bacterial strain (bacteriology) A distinct VARIETY of BACTERIA.

bactericidal (bacteriology) The ACTION of a substance which destroys BACTERIA.

bactericide (bacteriology) A substance which kills BACTERIA.

See also BACTERIOSTATIC.

bacteriocins (bacteriology) PROTEIN ANTIBIOTIC-like substances produced by some BACTERIA, which are lethal to other strains of BACTERIA, generally those closely related to the producer organism.

bacteriological (bacteriology) Pertaining to bacteriology.

bacteriological warfare (bacteriology) War where one side tries to kill or affect the people of the enemy side by infecting them with BACTERIA.

bacteriologist (bacteriology) A scientist who specialises in the study of BACTERIA.

bacteriology (microbiology) The scientific study of BACTERIA, their effects on organisms, including humans, and their uses in agriculture and industry (*e.g.* in biotechnology).

bacteriolysin (bacteriology) A PROTEIN, usually an IMMUNOGLOBULIN, which destroys BACTERIAL CELLS.

bacteriolysis (bacteriology) The destruction of BACTERIAL CELLS.

bacteriolytic (bacteriology) A substance which can destroy BACTERIA.

bacteriophage (bacteriology) VIRUS that infects BACTERIA. When inside a CELL it replicates using its HOST'S ENZYMES; the release of new VIRUSES may disintegrate the CELL. Bacteriophages have been used extensively in research on genes. Also termed: PHAGE.

bacteriostatic (bacteriology) Substance that inhibits the GROWTH of BACTERIA without killing them.

See also BACTERICIDE.

bacterium (bacteriology) The singular form of BACTERIA. *See* BACTERIA.

bacteriuria (bacteriology) Presence of BACTERIA in URINE.

BAFM (society) An abbreviation of 'B'ritish 'A'ssociation of 'F'orensic 'M'edicine.

Baker's cyst (medical/ histology) Swelling filled with SYNOVIAL FLUID, at the back of the knee, caused by weakness of the JOINT MEMBRANE. Named after the physician, W. M. Baker (1838-96).

baker's dermatitis (medical/ immunology) Irratation of the SKIN caused by handling YEAST. Also termed baker's itch.

baker's itch (medical/ immunology) *See* BAKER'S DERMATITIS.

baking soda (chemistry) An alternative term for SODIUM HYDROGENCARBONATE (SODIUM BICARBONATE).

balance (1 physics; 2 physiology) 1 Apparatus for weighing things accurately; types include a beam BALANCE, spring BALANCE, torsion BALANCE and substitution BALANCE. 2 Sense supplied by organs within the SEMICIRCULAR CANALS of the INNER EAR.

balanitis (medical) INFLAMMATION of the glans of the PENIS.

balanoposthitis (medical) INFLAMMATION of the foreskin and the end of the PENIS.

Balmer series (physics) Visible atomic SPECTRUM of HYDROGEN, consisting of a unique SERIES of ENERGY emission levels which appears as lines of red, blue and blue-violet LIGHT. It is the key to the discrete ENERGY LEVELs of electrons.

bals. (microscopy) An abbreviation of 'bals'am.

balsam (microscopy) Vegetable RESIN combined with oil, *e.g.* Canada balsam, used in preparing slides for microscopy, which comes from the balsam fir of North America.

bar (measurement) UNIT of PRESSURE defined as 10^5 newtons per square METRE; equal to approximately one ATMOSPHERE.

bar chart (statistics) GRAPH that has vertical or horizontal bars whose lengths are proportional to the quantities they represent.

See also PIE CHART.

bar code (general terminology) Information about a PRODUCT coded as a SERIES of thick and thin parallel lines printed on it (or on a LABEL attached to it), which can be scanned and 'read' by a machine.

See also CHARACTER recognition.

barbiturate (pharmacology) SEDATIVE and hypnotic drug derived from BARBITURIC ACID.

barbituric acid (pharmacology) $C_4H_4N_2O_3$ DIBASIC ORGANIC ACID that gives rise to BARBITURATE drugs.

barium Ba (chemistry) SILVER-white metallic ELEMENT in GROUP IIA of the PERIODIC TABLE (the ALKALINE EARTHS), obtained mainly from the mineral barytes (BARIUM SULPHATE [*USA*: barium sulfate]). Its SOLUBLE compounds are poisonous, and used in fireworks; its INSOLUBLE compounds are used in pigments and medicine. At. no. 56; r.a.m. 137.34.

barium sulphate (chemistry) $BaSO_4$ White CRYSTALLINE INSOLUBLE powder, used as a PIGMENT and as the basis of 'BARIUM meal' to show up structures in X-RAY diagnosis (because it is OPAQUE to X-RAYS). It occurs as the mineral barytes (also called barite). (*USA*: barium sulfate).

barograph (physics) Type of BAROMETER that produces a chart recording changes in ATMOSPHERIC PRESIURE over a PERIOD of time.

barometer (physics) Instrument for measuring ATMOSPHERIC PRESSURE, much used in meteorology.

Barr body (genetics) Condensed X-CHROMOSOME, seen in female CELLS of mammals, due to one or other of the two X-CHROMOSOMES in each CELL being inactivated.

BAS (education) An abbreviation of 'B'achelor of 'A'pplied 'S'cience.

basal ganglion (anatomy) Region of GREY MATTER within the WHITE MATTER that forms the inner part of the CEREBRAL HEMISPHERES of the BRAIN.

basal metabolic rate (BMR) (physiology) Minimum amount of ENERGY on which the body can survive, measured by OXYGEN consumption and expressed in kilojoules per UNIT body surface.

basal nucleus (anatomy) Also known as basal ganglia, a body of GREY MATTER (NERVE TISSUE) located deep within the CEREBRAL HEMISPHERES of the BRAIN, and concerned with movement.

base (1 chemistry; 2, 3, 4 mathematics; molecular biology) 1 A member of a CLASS of chemical compounds whose AQUEOUS SOLUTIONS contain OH⁻ ions. A BASE neutralizes an ACID to form a SALT. *See also* ALKALI. 2 The horizontal line upon which a geometric figure stands. 3 The starting number for a numerical or logarithmic system; *e.g.* binary NUMERALS have the BASE 2, COMMON LOGARITHMS are to the BASE 10. 4 Number on which an EXPONENT operates; *e.g.* in 5^2, 5 is the BASE (and 2 the EXPONENT). 5 One of the nucleotides of DNA or RNA (*i.e.* ADENINE, CYTOSINE, GUANINE, THYMINE or URACIL).

base metals (chemistry) Metals that corrode, oxidize or tarnish on exposure to AIR, moisture or HEAT; *e.g.* COPPER, IRON, LEAD.

base pair (Bp) (molecular biology) Used as a UNIT of length to describe a sequence of DNA.

base pairing (molecular biology) Specific pairing between complementary nucleotides in double-stranded DNA or RNA by hydrogen bonding; *e.g.* in DNA GUANINE pairs with CYTOSINE, and ADENINE pairs with THYMINE.

See also PURINE; PYRIMIDINE.

basic (chemistry) Having a tendency to release HYDROXIDE (OH⁻) ions. *See* BASE.

basic oxide (chemistry) Metallic OXIDE that reacts with an ACID to form a SALT and WATER.

See also ACIDIC OXIDE.

basic salt (chemistry) SALT that contains HYDROXIDE (OH⁻) ions; *e.g.* BASIC LEAD CARBONATE, $2PbCO_3.Pb(OH)_2$.

battery (physics) Device for producing ELECTRICITY (DIRECT CURRENT) by chemical ACTION; Also termed: CELL. *See* DANIELL CELL; DRY CELL; PRIMARY CELL; SECONDARY CELL.

See also SOLAR CELL.

BBA (medical) An abbreviation of 'B'orn 'B'efore 'A'rrival.

BBC (chemistry) An abbreviation of 'B'romo-'B'enzyl 'C'yanide.

BBT (physiology) An abbreviation of 'B'asal 'B'ody 'T'emperature.

BC (education) An abbreviation of 'B'achelor of 'C'hemistry.

BCG (immunology) An abbreviation of 'B'ACILLUS 'C'ALMETTE-'G'UERIN (VACCINE).

BCMA (governing body) An abbreviation of 'B'ritish 'C'olumbia 'M'edical 'A'ssociation.

BDA (society) An abbreviation of 'B'ritish 'D'ental / 'D'iabetic 'A'ssociation (now Diabetes UK).

BDH (chemistry) An abbreviation of 'B'ritish 'D'rug 'H'ouses.

BDNF (physiology/ biochemistry) An abbreviation of 'B'rain-'D'erived 'N'eurotrophic 'F'actor.

Be (chemistry) CHEMICAL SYMBOL for BERYLLIUM.

Beckmann thermometer (physics) MERCURY THERMOMETER used for accurately measuring very small changes or differences in TEMPERATURE. The scale usually covers only 6 or 7 degrees. It was named after the German chemist Ernst Beckmann (1853-1923).

becquerel (Bq) (measurement) SI UNIT of RADIOACTIVITY, equal to the number of atoms of a RADIOACTIVE substance that disintegrate in one second. It was named after the French physicist Antoine Henri BECQUEREL (1852-1908). 1 Bq = 2.7 x 10⁻¹¹ curies (the former UNIT of RADIOACTIVITY).

Beer's law (physics) Concerned with the ABSORPTION of LIGHT by substances, it states that the FRACTION of incident LIGHT absorbed by a SOLUTION at a given WAVELENGTH is related to the thickness of the absorbing layer and the CON-

CENTRATION of the absorbing substance. Also termed: Beer Lambert LAW.

beet sugar (chemistry) An alternative term for SUCROSE.

behaviour (medical) Way of acting. (*USA*: behavior).

behavioural scientist (medical) A person who specialises in the study of BEHAVIOUR. (*USA*: behavioral scientist).

bel (B) (measurement) UNIT representing the ratio of two amounts of POWER, *e.g.* of sound or an electronic signal, equal to 10 decibels. It was named after the American inventor Alexander Graham Bell (1847-1922).

Benedict's test (biochemistry) Food test used to detect the presence of a REDUCING SUGAR by the addition of a SOLUTION containing SODIUM CARBONATE, SODIUM citrate, POTASSIUM THIOCYANATE, COPPER SULPHATE (*USA*: copper sulfate) and POTASSIUM FERROCYANIDE. A change in COLOUR (*USA*: color) from blue to red or yellow on boiling indicates a POSITIVE result. It was named after the American chemist S. Benedict (1884-1936).

See also FEHLING'S TEST.

benign (medical/ histology) Describing a TUMOUR (*USA*: tumor) that does not spread or destroy the TISSUE where it is located; not MALIGNANT; not recurrent; favourable for recovery.

See also MALIGNANT.

benzaldehyde (chemistry) C_6H_5CHO Colourless (*USA*: colorless) aromatic ALDEHYDE, with a SMELL of almonds, used as a flavouring, in perfumes and as an INTERMEDIATE in making dyes.

benzene (chemistry) C_6H_6 Colourless (*USA*: colorless) inflammable LIQUID HYDROCARBON, simplest of the AROMATIC COMPOUNDS. It is used as a SOLVENT and in the manufacture of plastics.

benzene-1,3-diol (chemistry) $C_6H_4(OH)_2$ An alternative term for RESORCINOL.

benzene ring (chemistry) CYCLIC (closed-chain) arrangement of six CARBON atoms, as in a MOLECULE of BENZENE. Molecules containing one or more BENZENE RINGS DISPLAY aromatic CHARACTER. *See* AROATICITY.

benzocaine (pharmacology) A local anaesthetic drug administered by topical application for the relief of pain in the skin surface or MUCOUS MEMBRANES.

benzodiazepine (pharmacology) Member of a GROUP of drugs used as ANTIDEPRESSANTS and anticonvulsants.

benzoic acid (chemistry) C_6H_5COOH White CRYSTALLINE ORGANIC COMPOUND, used as a food preservative because it inhibits the GROWTH of yeasts and moulds (*USA*: molds).

benzole (chemistry) An alternative term for BENZENE.

benzpyrene (chemistry) CYCLIC ORGANIC COMPOUND, found in coal-tar and tobacco smoke, which has strong CARCINOGENIC properties.

benzpyrrole (chemistry) An alternative term for INDOLE.

BER (physiology) An abbreviation of 'B'asic 'E'lectric 'R'hythm.

berkelium Bk (chemistry) RADIOACTIVE ELEMENT in GROUP IIIB of the PERIODIC TABLE (one of the ACTINIDES). It has several isotopes, with half-lives of up to 1,400 years, made by alpha-particle bombardment of AMERICIUM-241. At. no. 97; r.a.m. 247 (most STABLE ISOTOPE).

Bernoulli's theorem (physics) At any point in a tube through which a LIQUID is flowing the sum of the POTENTIAL, kinetic and PRESSURE energies is CONSTANT. Also termed: Bernoulli's principle. It was named after the Swiss mathematician and physicist Daniel Bernoulli (1700-82).

beryllium Be (chemistry) SILVER-grey metallic ELEMENT in GROUP IIA of the PERIODIC TABLE (the ALKALINE EARTHS). It is used for windows in X-RAY TUBES and as a moderator in nuclear reactors. At. no. 4; r.a.m. 9.0122.

beta-adrenoceptors (physiology/ pharmacology) Receptor sites at which NORADRENALINE and other HORMONES act to cause muscle to contract or relax.

beta-blocker (pharmacology) Drugs that block beta-adrenergic receptors, used to treat HYPERTENSION (HIGH BLOOD PRESSURE).

beta decay (radiology) DISINTEGRATION of an unstable RADIOACTIVE NUCLEUS that involves the emission of a BETA PARTICLE. It occurs when a NEUTRON emits an ELECTRON and is itself converted to a PROTON, resulting in an increase of one PROTON in the NUCLEUS concerned and a corresponding decrease of one NEUTRON. This leads to the formation of a different ELEMENT (*e.g.* BETA DECAY of CARBON-14 produces NITROGEN).

betamethasone (pharmacology) A corticosteroid that has ANTI-INFLAMMATORY properties. It is used in the treatment of many kinds of inflammation, particularly inflammation associated with SKIN conditions such as eczema and psoriasisis.

beta particle (radiology) High-velocity ELECTRON emitted by a RADIOACTIVE NUCLEUS undergoing BETA DECAY.

beta radiation (radiology) RADIATION, consisting of BETA PARTICLES (electrons), due to BETA DECAY.

beta ray (radiology) Stream of BETA PARTICLES.

bethanechol chloride (pharmacology) A parasympathomimetic drug administered orally to stimulate motility in the INTESTINES and to treat urinary retention.

bezafibrate (pharmacology) A LIPID-lowering drug administered orally to reduce levels, or change the proportions of various LIPIDs in the bloodstream of patients with hyperLIPIDaemia (*USA*: hyperLIPIDemia).

betz cells (cytology) The large pyramidal cells of the motor cortex of the brain. Named after the Ukrainian anatomist Vladimir Betz (1834-94).

BFO (physics) An abbreviation of 'B'eat-'F'requency 'O'scillator.

BGP (physiology/ biochemistry) An abbreviation of 'B'one 'G'la 'P'rotein.

bibl. (literary terminology) An abbreviation of 'bibl'iographer/ bibl'iographical/ bibl'iography. Also termed bibliog.

bicarb. (chemistry) An abbreviation of 'bicarb'onate of SODA.

bicarbonate (chemistry) An alternative term for HYDROGENCARBONATE.

biceps (anatomy) Two-headed MUSCLE in the arm or thigh.

bichromate (chemistry) An alternative term for DICHROMATE.

biconcave (optics) Describing a LENS that is CONCAVE on both surfaces.

biconvex (optics) Describing a LENS that is CONVEX on both surfaces.

bilateral symmetry (physiology) Type of SYMMETRY in which a shape is symmetrical about a single AXIS or plane (each half being a mirror IMAGE of the other). *E.g.* most vertebrates are bilaterally symmetrical.

See also RADIAL SYMMETRY.

bile (biochemistry) ALKALINE MIXTURE of substances produced by the LIVER and stored in the GALL BLADDER, which passes it to the DUODENUM, where it emulsifies fats (preparing them for DIGESTION) and neutralizes ACID. Its (yellowish) COLOUR (*USA*: color) is due to BILE pigments (*e.g.* BILIRUBIN).

bile duct (anatomy) A tube that carries BILE from the GALL BLADDER to the DUODENUM.

bilharzia (parasitology) Disease that affects human beings and domestic ANIMALS in some subtropical regions, which results from an INFESTATION by one of the parasitic BLOOD FLUKES belonging to the GENUS *Schistosoma*. The larvae of the FLUKES develop inside freshwater snails and become free-swimming organisms which can attach themselves to a wading mammal, penetrating the SKIN and entering the bloodstream. Also termed: SCHISTOSOMIASIS.

biliary (anatomy) To do with BILE or the GALL BLADDER.

bilirubin (biochemistry) Major PIGMENT in BILE, formed in the LIVER by the breakdown of HAEMOGLOBIN (*USA*: hemoglobin). Its accumulation causes the symptom JAUNDICE.

billion (measurement) Number now generally accepted as being equivalent to 1,000 million (10^9). Formerly in Britain a BILLION was regarded as a million million (10^{12}).

binary code (mathematics) An alternative term for BINARY NOTATION.

binary compound (chemistry) Chemical that consists of two elements.

binary fission (physiology) Method of REPRODUCTION employed by many single-celled organisms, in which the so-called mother CELL divides in half (by MITOSIS), forming two identical, but independent, DAUGHTER CELLS. It is a type of ASEXUAL REPRODUCTION.

binary notation (mathematics) Number system to the BASE 2, involving only two digits, 0 and 1. Instead of the units, tens, hundreds, etc; of the DECIMAL SYSTEM, units, twos, fours, eights, etc; are used. Thus, *eg;* 8 is given as 1000 and 9 as 1001. BINARY NOTATION is important in ELECTRONICS and computers because the 0 and 1 can be represented by a CIRCUIT being 'on' or 'off'. Also termed: BINARY CODE; BINARY SYSTEM.

binary system (mathematics) An alternative term for BINARY NOTATION.

binding energy (physics) ENERGY required to cause a NUCLEUS to decompose into its constituent NEUTRONS and PROTONS.

binomial (mathematics) POLYNOMIAL that has two variables, *e.g.* $(x + 2y)^2$.

binomial nomenclature (biology) System by which organisms are identified by two Latin names. The first is the name of the GENUS (GENERIC name), the second is the name of the SPECIES (specific name), *e.g. HOMO SAPIENS.* Also termed: LINNAEAN SYSTEM (after the Swedish biologist Carolus Linnaeus, 1707-78).

See also CLASSIFICATION.

binomial theorem (mathematics) FORMULA for calculating the POWER of a BINOMIAL without complicated multiplication.

bioassay (biochemistry) Method for quantitatively determining the CONCENTRATION of a substance by its effect on living organisms, *e.g.* its effect on the GROWTH of BACTERIA.

biochemistry (biochemistry) Study of the chemistry of living organisms.

biodegradation (biology) Breakdown or DECAY of substances by the ACTION of living organisms, especially saprophytic BACTERIA and FUNGI. Through BIODEGRADATION, organic MATTER is recycled.

bioenergetics (physiology) Study of the transfer and utilization of ENERGY in living systems.

See also ATP.

bioengineering (biology) Application of engineering science and technology to living systems.

biofeedback (physiology) Method of controlling a bodily process (*e.g.* HEARTBEAT) that is not normally subject to voluntary control by making the person

concerned aware of measurements from instruments monitoring that process.

biogenesis (biology) Theory that living organisms may originate only from other living organisms, as opposed to the theory of SPONTANEOUS GENERATION.

See also ABIOGENESIS.

biological clock (biology) Hypothetical mechanism in plants and animals that controls periodic changes in internal functions and BEHAVIOUR (*USA*: behavior) independently of ENVIRONMENT, *e.g.* diurnal rhythms and hibernation patterns.

biology (biology) Study of living organisms.

bioluminescence (physiology) Emission of VISIBLE LIGHT by living organisms, *e.g.* certain BACTERIA, FUNGI, fish and insects. The LIGHT is produced by ENZYME reactions in which chemical ENERGY is converted to LIGHT.

biomass (biology) Total MASS of living MATTER in a given ENVIRONMENT or food chain LEVEL.

biometry (biology) Application of mathematical and statistical methods to the study of living organisms.

bionic (bioengineering) Describing an artificial device or system that has the properties of a living one.

biophysics (biology) Use of ideas and methods of physics in the study of living organisms and processes.

biopsy (histology) Small SAMPLE of CELLS or TISSUE removed from a living subject for LABORATORY examination (usually as an aid to diagnosis).

biorhythm (physiology) One of the CYCLIC pattern of 'highs' and 'lows' which some people believe govern each person's emotional, physical and intellectual BEHAVIOUR (*USA*: behavior). Most scientists are sceptical because the idea is based on the individual's subjective perceptions of these qualities.

biosynthesis (biology) Formation of the major molecular components of CELLS, *e.g.* proteins, from simple components.

biotechnology (biotechnology) Utilization of living organisms for the production of useful substances or processes, *e.g.* in FERMENTATION and milk production.

biotin (biochemistry) COENZYME that is involved in the transfer of CARBONYL GROUPS in biochemical REACTIONS, such as the METABOLISM of fats; one of the B VITAMINS.

bisacodyl (pharmacology) A stimulant laxative administered orally or topically as suppositories to promote defecation and relieve constipation. It can be used to evacuate the colon prior to rectal examination or surgery.

bismuth Bi (chemistry) Silvery-white metallic ELEMENT in GROUP VA of the PERIODIC TABLE. It is used as a LIQUID METAL COOLANT in nuclear reactors and as a COMPONENT of low-MELTING POINT LEAD ALLOYS. Its SOLUBLE compounds are poisonous; its INSOLUBLE ones are used in medicine. At. no. 83. r.a.m. 208.9806.

bisulphate (chemistry) An alternative term for HYDROGENSULPHATE (*USA*: hydrogensulfate). (*USA*: bisulfate).

bisulphite (chemistry) An alternative term for HYDROGENSULPHITE (*USA*: hydrogensulfite). (*USA*: bisulfite).

bit (computing) An abbreviation of 'bi'nary digi't'; either 1 or 0, the only two digits in BINARY NOTATION. Amount of information that is required to express choice between two possibilities. The term is commonly applied to a single DIGIT of BINARY NOTATION in a COMPUTER.

See also BYTE.

biuret test (biochemistry) Test used to detect peptides and proteins in SOLUTION by TREATMENT of biuret ($NH_2CONHCONH_2$) with COPPER SULPHATE (*USA*: copper sulfate) and ALKALI to give a purple COLOUR (*USA*: color).

bivalent (chemistry) Having a VALENCE of two. Also termed: DIVALENT.

bkgd (general terminology) An abbreviation of 'b'ac'kg'roun'd'.

bladder (anatomy) A membranous sac containing GAS or FLUID, *e.g.* the GALL BLADDER and urinary BLADDER.

See also VESICLE.

blastocyst (biology) A stage in the EMBRYOGENESIS of mammals, prior to IMPLANTATION. It is the first stage at which there is any differentiation among the ball of CELLS. The BLASTOCYST consists of an outer layer of protective CELLS (the trophectoderm) surrounding a FLUID filled cavity containing the inner CELL MASS that goes on to develop as the EMBRYO. The human BLASTOCYST is about 0.15 mm in DIAMETER.

blastula (histology) Hollow sphere composed of a single layer of CELLS produced by CLEAVAGE of a fertilized OVUM in animals.

bleach (chemistry) Substance used for removing COLOUR (*USA*: color) from, *e.g.* cloth, paper and straw. A common BLEACH is a SOLUTION of SODIUM CHLORATE(I) (SODIUM HYPOCHLORITE), NaClO, although HYDROGEN PEROXIDE, SULPHUR DIOXIDE (*USA*: sulfur dioxide), CHLORINE, OXYGEN and even sunlight are also used as bleaches. All are OXIDIZING AGENTs.

bleaching powder (chemistry) White powder containing CALCIUM CHLORATE(I) (CALCIUM HYPOCHLORITE), Ca(OCl)$_2$, made by the ACTION of CHLORINE on CALCIUM HYDROXIDE (slaked LIME). When treated with DILUTE ACID it generates CHLORINE, which acts as a BLEACH.

blind spot (biology) AREA on the RETINA of the VERTEBRATE EYE which, because it is at the point of entry of the OPTIC NERVE, is without LIGHT sensitive CELLS and is thus blind.

blood (haematology) FLUID in the bodies of animals that circulates and transports OXYGEN and nutrients to CELLS, and carries waste products from them to the organs of EXCRETION. It also transports HORMONES and the products of DIGESTION. Essential for maintaining uniform TEMPERATURE in warmblooded animals, BLOOD is made up mainly of ERYTHROCYTES, LEUCOCYTES, platelets, WATER and proteins.

See also HAEMOCYANIN; HAEMOGLOBIN.

blood cells (haematology) *See* ERYTHROCYTES; leueocytes.

blood clotting (pharmacology) *See* HAEMOSTASIS.

blood count (haematology) A count of the number of red and WHITE BLOOD CELLS and platelets.

blood group (haematology) *See* ABO BLOOD GROUPS.

blood plasma (haematology) FLUID part of BLOOD in which BLOOD CELLS are suspended. It contains PLASMA PROTEINS, UREA, sugars and salts.

blood poisoning (medical/ microbiology) An alternative term for SEPTICAEMIA (*USA*: septicemia).

blood pressure (physiology) PRESSURE of BLOOD flowing in the arteries. It varies between the higher value of the systolic PRESSURE (when the HEART's ventricles are contracting and forcing BLOOD out of the HEART) and the lower value of the diastolic PRESSURE (when the HEART is filling with BLOOD). It is affected by exercise, emotion and various drugs.

blood serum (haematology) FLUID part of BLOOD from which all BLOOD CELLS and FIBRIN have been removed. It may contain antibodies, and such serums are used as vaccines.

blood sugar (biochemistry) The ENERGY-generating SUGAR GLUCOSE, whose LEVEL in the BLOOD is controlled by the HORMONE INSULIN.

blood vascular system (anatomy) System consisting of the HEART, arteries, veins and capillaries. The HEART acts as a central muscular PUMP which propels oxygenated BLOOD from the lungs along arteries to the tissues; deoxygenated BLOOD is carried along veins back to the HEART and lungs.

blood vessel (anatomy) An ARTERY, VEIN, or CAPILLARY. Many BLOOD VESSELs have muscular walls, whose contraction and relaxation aids BLOOD flow.

blue vitriol (chemistry) An alternative term for the HYDRATED form of COPPER(II) SULPHATE (*USA*: copper (II) sulfate).

blue-green alga (microbiology) An alternative term for a member of the CYANOPHYTA.

BLWA (society) An abbreviation of 'B'ritish 'L'aboratory 'W'are 'A'ssociation.

BM (medical) An abbreviation of 'B'owel 'M'ovement.

BMA (governing body) An abbreviation of 'B'ritish 'M'edical 'A'ssociation.

BMJ (literary terminology) An abbreviation of 'B'ritish 'M'edical 'J'ournal.

BMR (physiology) An abbreviation of 'B'asal 'M'etabolic 'R'ate.

BMS (society) An abbreviation of 'B'ritish 'M'ycological 'S'ociety.

BNP (physiology/ biochemistry) An abbreviation of 'B'rain 'N'atriuretic 'P'eptide.

body-centred cube (crystallography) Crystal structure that is CUBIC, with an ATOM at the centre of each cube. Each ATOM is surrounded by eight others. (*USA*: body-centered cube).

boiling point (b.p.) (physics) TEMPERATURE at which a LIQUID boils freely turning into a VAPOUR; its VAPOUR PRESSURE then equals the external PRESSURE.

boils (medical/ microbiology) Staphylococcal infections of the HAIR follicles of the SKIN. A painful red nodule appears which grows bigger and then breaks down in the middle for pus to appear. In a few days it usually discharges and

heals. An interconnecting collection of BOILS is called a carbuncle. Recurrent BOILS may be associated with DIABETES MELLITUS.

bond (chemistry) Link between two atoms in a MOLECULE. *See* CO-ORDINATE BOND; COVALENT BOND; IONIC BOND.

bond energy (chemistry) ENERGY involved in BOND formation.

bond length (chemistry) Distance between the nuclei of two atoms that are chemically bonded.

bone (anatomy) The skeletal substance of vertebrates. It consists of CELLS called osteocytes distributed in a MATRIX of COLLAGEN fibres (*USA*: collagen fibers) impregnated with a complex SALT (BONE SALT), mainly CALCIUM PHOSPHATE, for hardness. CELLS are connected by fine channels that permeate the MATRIX. Larger channels contain BLOOD VESSELS and NERVES. Some bones are hollow and contain BONE MARROW. There are about 206 bones in an adult human SKELETON.

bone marrow (haematology) The soft haematopoietic (*USA*: hematopoietic) TISSUE that has STEM CELLS capable of differentiating into ERYTHROCYTES, LEUCOCYTES (*USA*: leukocytes) or platelets (THROMBOCYTES).

boracic acid (chemistry) An alternative term for BORIC ACID.

borax (chemistry) $Na_2B_4O_7.\ 10H_2O$ A white AMORPHOUS COMPOUND, SOLUBLE in WATER, which occurs naturally as TINCAL. It is used in the manufacture of enamels and HEAT-resistant GLASS. Also termed: DISODIUM TETRABORATE; SODIUM BORATE.

boric acid (chemistry) H_3BO_3 White CRYSTALLINE COMPOUND, SOLUBLE in WATER, which occurs naturally in volcanic regions of Italy. It has ANTISEPTIC properties. Also termed: BORACIC ACID.

Bornholm disease (medical/ virology) An INFECTION caused by the Coxsakie VIRUS B, which usually lasts about a week. There may be FEVER with a headache and sometimes a sore THROAT, and it may occur in EPIDEMIC form. It gets its name from being first described as occurring on the Danish island Bornholm.

boron B (chemistry) AMORPHOUS, NON-metallic ELEMENT in GROUP IIIA of the PERIODIC TABLE. Because of its high NEUTRON ABSORPTION it is used for control rods in nuclear reactors. Important compounds include BORAX and BORIC ACID. At. no. 5; r.a.m. 10.81.

borosilicate glass (chemistry) HEAT-resistant GLASS of low thermal expansion, made by adding BORON OXIDE (B_2O_3) to GLASS during manufacture.

botulism (toxicology/ bacteriology) A severe form of FOOD POISONING. An often fatal disorder caused by eating food contaminated with a TOXIN produced by the BACTERIUM *Clostridium botulinum* (which is destroyed by adequate cooking). Botulinus TOXIN is one of the most potent poisons known.

bowel (anatomy) An alternative term for INTESTINE.

Bowman's capsule (anatomy) Dense ball of CAPILLARY BLOOD VESSELS that cover the closed end of every NEPHRON in the KIDNEY. From it leads the uriniferous tubule. It was named after the British physician William Bowman (1816-92).

Boyle's law (physics) At CONSTANT TEMPERATURE the VOLUME of a GAS V is inversely proportional to its PRESSURE p; *i.e.* pV = a CONSTANT. It was named after the Irish chemist Robert Boyle (1627-91).

bp (genetics) An abbreviation of 'b'ase-'p'air.

brain (anatomy) Principal collection of NERVE CELLS that form the ANTERIOR part of the CENTRAL NERVOUS SYSTEM, consisting (in mammals) of a moist pinkish-grey MASS protected by the bones of the CRANIUM (SKULL). It receives, mostly via SPINAL NERVES from the SPINAL CORD but also via CRANIAL NERVES from organs in the HEAD, sensory information through AFFERENTS carrying the output of SENSE ORGANS and it sends out instructions along efferents (*e.g.* motor NERVES) to the EFFECTOR organs (*e.g.* muscles). It is also the centre (*USA*: center) of intellect and MEMORY (so that BEHAVIOUR (*USA*: behavior) can be based on past experience), and is responsible for the coordination of the whole body.

See also CEREBELLUM; CEREBRUM; CORTEX.

brain stem (anatomy) Part of the BRAIN at the end of the SPINAL CORD, consisting of the midbrain, MEDULLA OBLONGATA and pons.

brainwave (physiology) Pattern of electrical activity in the BRAIN as revealed by an ELECTROENCEPHALOGRAPH. Alpha waves correspond to wakefulness with eyes closed, beta waves to wakefulness with eyes open and delta waves to deep sleep.

branched chain (chemistry) Side GROUP(s) attached to the main chain in the MOLECULE of an ORGANIC COMPOUND.

breastbone (anatomy) An alternative term for STERNUM.

breathing (physiology) An alternative term for RESPIRATION, but often restricted to the physical actions of inhalation and exhalation.

bretylium tosylate (pharmacology) An ANTISYMPATHETIC class of drug that administered by injection, is an ADRENERGIC neurone blocker, preventing the release of NORADRENALINE from sympathetic nerves. It can be used in ANTI-ARRHYTHMIC treatment of abnormal HEART rhythms in resuscitation.

BRI (education) An abbreviation of 'B'iological/ 'B'rain 'R'esearch 'I'nstitute.

Bright's disease (medical) ACUTE NEPHRITIS. Named after the physician, Richard Bright (1789-1858).

brine (chemistry) Concentrated SOLUTION of COMMON SALT (SODIUM CHLORIDE).

British thermal unit (BTU) (measurement) Amount of HEAT required to raise the TEMPERATURE of 1 pound of WATER through 1°F. 1 BTU = 1,055 joules.

Broca's area (anatomy) Speech centre (*USA*: center) of the BRAIN. It was named after the French surgeon Paul Broca (1824-80).

brom. (chemistry) An abbreviation of 'brom'ide.

bromide (chemistry) BINARY COMPOUND containing BROMINE; a SALT of HYDRO-BROMIC ACID.

bromide paper (photography) LIGHT-sensitive paper coated with an EMULSION containing SILVER BROMIDE, used for making black-and-white photographic prints and enlargements.

bromine Br (chemistry) Dark red LIQUID non-metallic ELEMENT in GROUP VIIA of the PERIODIC TABLE (the halogens), extracted from sea-WATER. It has a pungent SMELL. Its compounds are used in PHOTOGRAPHY and as anti-knock additives to petrol. At. no. 35; r.a.m. 79.904.

bromocriptine (pharmacology) An ergot alkaloid drug that is administered orally in patients primarily to treat Parkinsonism, but not the parkinsonian symptoms caused by certain drug therapies. It acts by stimulating the DOPAMINE receptors in the BRAIN. It additionally inhibits prolactin secretion by the pituitary gland and may be used for a variety of conditions including delayed puberty caused by hormonal insufficiency; to relieve certain menstrual disorders and to reduce or halt lactation in galactorrhoea.

bronchiole (anatomy) Terminal AIR-conducting tube (1mm in DIAMETER) of mammalian lungs, arising from secondary subdivision of a BRONCHUS and terminating in alveoli.

bronchus (anatomy) One of the two AIR-carrying divisions of the TRACHEA (windpipe) into the lungs. The bronchi become inflamed in the disorder bronchitis.

brown ring test (chemistry) LABORATORY test for NITRATES in SOLUTION. An acidic SOLUTION of IRON(II) SULPHATE (*USA*: iron(II) sulfate) (FERROUS SULPHATE [*USA*: ferrous sulfate]) is added to the suspected NITRATE SOLUTION in a test-tube, and concentrated SULPHURIC ACID (*USA*: sulfuric acid) carefully poured down the inside of the tube. A brown ring at the junction of the liquids indicates the presence of a NITRATE.

Brownian movement (physics) Random motion of particles of a SOLID suspended in a LIQUID or GAS, caused by collisions with molecules of the suspending medium. It was named after the British botanist Robert Brown (1773-1858). Also termed: Brownian motion.

brucellosis (medical/ bacteriology) An infectious disease, caused by bacteria of the genus *Brucella*, and contracted by eating infected meat and dairy products or by contact with the secretions of sheep, goats or cows. Named after the British pathologist Sir David Bruce (1855-1931).

BS (1 education; 2 society; 3 quality standards) 1 An abbreviation of 'B'achelor of 'S'cience/ 'S'urgery. 2 An abbreviation of 'B'iochemical/ 'B'iometric/ 'B'iological 'S'ociety. 3 An abbreviation of 'B'ritish 'S'tandard.

BSAVA (society) An abbreviation of 'B'ritish 'S'mall 'A'nimals 'V'eterinary 'A'ssociation.

BSc (education) An abbreviation of 'B'achelor of 'Sc'ience.

bsc (general terminology) An abbreviation of 'b'a's'i'c'.

BSCC (society) An abbreviation of 'B'ritish 'S'ociety for 'C'linical 'C'ytology.

BSCP (quality standards) Abbreviation of 'B'ritish 'S'tandard 'C'ode of 'P'ractice.

BSI (quality standards) An abbreviation of 'B'ritish 'S'tandards 'I'nstitution.

BSIRA (society) An abbreviation of 'B'ritish 'S'cientific 'I'nstrument 'R'esearch 'A'ssociation.

BSP (society) Abbreviation of 'B'achelor of 'S'cience in 'P'harmacy.

BSRA (society) Abbreviation of 'B'ritish 'S'ociety for 'R'esearch on 'A'geing.

BTPS (physics) An abbreviation of 'B'ody 'T'emperature and 'P'ressure, 'S'aturated with water vapour (*USA*: vapor).

BTX (1 chemistry; 2 toxicology) 1 An abbreviation of 'b'enzene, 't'oluene and 'x'ylene. 2 An abbreviation of 'B'atracho'T'o'X'in.

bty (physics) An abbreviation of 'b'at't'er'y'.

bubo (medical) The swelling of a lymphatic GLAND or GROUP of GLANDS, particularly in the groin or the armpit.

buccal (anatomy) Pertaining to the cheek and mouth.

buccal cavity (anatomy) Mouth cavity in front of the opening of the PHARYNX, where in mammals food is usually chewed and subjected to the initial stages of DIGESTION.

budding (biology) Method of ASEXUAL REPRODUCTION employed by yeasts and simple ANIMAL organisms.

budesonide (pharmacology) A corticosteroid drug with ant-inflammatory, ant-allergic and ANTI-ASTHMATIC properties. It may be administered by inhalation to prevent attacks of asthma and rhinitis and topically to treat severe inflammatory skin disorders such as psoriasis and eczema.

buffer (1 chemistry; 2 computing) 1 A SOLUTION that resists changes in pH on DILUTION or on the addition of ACID or

ALKALI. 2 A temporary store for DATA in transit between the CENTRAL PROCESSOR and an OUTPUT DEVICE.

buffy coat (haematology) Layer of WHITE BLOOD CELLS and platelets above RED BLOOD CELL MASS when BLOOD is sedimented.

bug (1 parasitology; 2 computing) 1 BLOOD-sucking insect of the ORDER Hemiptera. 2 Error in a COMPUTER PROGRAM or a fault in HARDWARE.

bumetanide (pharmacology) A powerful DIURETIC drug which can be administered orally or by injection and is used to treat OEDEMA (*USA*: edema), particularly pulmonary OEDEMA. It is one of the class of LOOP DIURETICS.

BUN (biochemistry/ haematology) An abbreviation of 'B'lood 'U'rea 'N'itrogen.

Bunsen burner (laboratory equipment) GAS burner that efficiently mixes AIR with the fuel GAS, commonly used for heating in laboratories. It was named after the German chemist Robert Bunsen (1811-99).

bupivacaine hydrochloride (pharmacology) A local anaesthetic drug administered by injection that has a long duration of action. It is an amide and chemically related to lignocaine hydrochloride.

burette (laboratory equipment) A long vertical graduated GLASS tube with a tap, used for the addition of controlled and measurable volumes of liquids (*e.g.* in making titrations in VOLUMETRIC ANALYSIS).

Burkitts lymphoma (medical/ histology) A TUMOUR (*USA*: tumor) of the LYMPH GLANDS, common in some parts of West Africa. It appears to be triggered by a VIRUS INFECTION and is one of the commonest cancers found in people with AIDS. Named after the surgeon, Denis Parsons Burkitt (1911-93).

Bursa (anatomy) A closed sac lined with SYNOVIAL MEMBRANE containing FLUID placed where there may be friction between structures such as tendons and bones so that they can move easily over each other. Sometimes they become inflamed, as the result of either injury or INFECTION, a condition called bursitis.

Bursa of fabricius (immunology) Lymphoid ORGAN which processes B-LYMPHOCYTES.

bus (computing) A pathway connecting the components of a COMPUTER, usually shared by several components.

bushel (measurement) UNIT for measuring dry goods by VOLUME, equal to 4 pecks and equivalent to 8 gallons or 36.369 LITRES (in Britain) or 35.238 LITRES (United States).

buspirone hydrochloride (pharmacology) An antiolytic drug which is used for short-term treatment of anxiety. It is administered orally and acts by stimulating SEROTONIN receptors in the BRAIN.

butane (chemistry) C_4H_{10} Gaseous ALKANE, used as a portable supply of fuel.

butanedioic acid (chemistry) An alternative term for SUCCINIC ACID.

butanol (chemistry) C_4H_9OH Colourless (*USA*: colorless) LIQUID ALCOHOL that exists in four isomeric forms. Also termed: BUTYL ALCOHOL.

butyl alcohol (chemistry) An alternative term for BUTANOL.

BV (haematolgy) An abbreviation of 'B'lood 'V'olume.

BVA (society) An abbreviation of 'B'ritish 'V'eterinary 'A'ssociation.

bw (1 microbiology; 2 medical) An abbreviation of 'b'iological 'w'arfare. 2 An abbreviation of 'b'irth'w'eight.

bwd (general terminology) An abbreviation of 'b'ack'w'ar'd'.

by-product (biotechnology) Incidental or secondary PRODUCT of manufacture.

byte (computing) A number of binary digits that FUNCTION as a UNIT, *e.g.* in the store of a COMPUTER. The term is sometimes limited to a UNIT consisting of eight binary digits.

C

C (1 chemistry; 2 measurement) 1 CHEMICAL SYMBOL for CARBON. 2 An abbreviation of 'C'elsius.

C$_{H2O}$ (physiology) A symbol for Free water 'C'learance.

CA (1 medical; 2, 3 biochemistry) An abbreviation for 1 'C'hronological 'A'ge. 2 An abbreviation for 'ca'techolamine. 3 An abbreviation of 'C'ellulose 'A'cetate.

Ca (chemistry) The CHEMICAL SYMBOL for CALCIUM.

ca. (1 physics; 2 Literature terminology) 1 An abbreviation of 'ca'thode. 2 An abbreviation of 'c'irc'a'. [Latin, meaning about].

cabergoline (pharmacology) An antiparkinsonism drug that is administered orally with similar properties to BROMOCRIPTINE.

CAD (medical) An abbreviation of 'C'oronary 'A'rtery 'D'isease.

cad (medical) An abbreviation of 'cad'aver. Also termed cadav.

CADE (computing) An abbreviation of 'C'omputer 'A'ssisted 'D'ata 'E'valuation.

cadmium Cd (chemistry) Silvery-white metallic ELEMENT in GROUP IIB of the PERIODIC TABLE. It is used in control rods for nuclear reactors and as a corrosion-resistant electroplating on steel articles. Its compounds are used as yellow or red pigments. At. no. 48; r.a.m. 112.40.

cADPR (physiology/ biochemistry) An abbreviation of 'c'yclic 'A'denosine 'D'is'P'hosphate 'R'ibose.

caecum (anatomy) Pouch or pocket, such as one at the junction of the small and LARGE INTESTINES from which hangs the APPENDIX.

caesium Cs (chemistry) Soft reactive metallic ELEMENT in GROUP IA of the PERIODIC TABLE (the ALKALI METALS), a major FISSION PRODUCT of URANIUM. It is used in PHOTOELECTRIC CELLS. The ISOTOPE CAESIUM-137 is used in RADIOTHERAPY. At. no. 55; r.a.m. 132.9055. (*USA*: cesium)

caesium clock (physics) Atomic clock used in the SI UNIT definition of the second. (*USA*: cesium clock).

CAF (medical) An abbreviation of 'C'ardiac 'A'ssessment 'F'actor.

caffeine (pharmacology) White ALKALOID with a bitter TASTE, obtained from coffee beans, tea leaves, kola nuts, or by chemical SYNTHESIS. It is a diuretic and a stimulant to the CENTRAL NERVOUS SYSTEM.

cal (measurement) An abbreviation of 'cal'orie (small).

Cal (measurement) An abbreviation of 'Cal'orie.

calamine (chemistry) ZINC ore whose main constituent is ZINC OXIDE.

calciferol (biochemistry) Fat-SOLUBLE VITAMIN formed in the SKIN by the ACTION of sunlight, which controls levels of CALCIUM in the BLOOD. Also termed: VITAMIN D.

calcification (histology) Depositing of CALCIUM salts in body TISSUE, a NORMAL process in the formation of bones and TEETH but ABNORMAL in the formation of calculi ('stones').

See also CARTILAGE.

calcitonin (biochemistry) HORMONE secreted in vertebrates that controls the release of CALCIUM from BONE. In mammals it is secreted by the THYROID GLAND. Also termed: thyrocalcitonin.

calcium **Ca** (chemistry) SILVER-white metallic ELEMENT in GROUP IIA of the PERIODIC TABLE (the ALKALINE EARTH). The fifth most abundant ELEMENT on the EARTH, it occurs mainly in CALCIUM CARBONATE minerals; it also occurs in bones and TEETH. At. no. 20; r.a.m. 40.08.

calcium carbonate (chemistry) $CaCO_3$ White powder or colourless (*USA*: colorless) crystals, the main constituent of CHALK, limestone and marble.

calcium chloride (chemistry) $CaCl_2$ White CRYSTALLINE COMPOUND, which forms several hydrates, used to control dust, as a de-icing agent and as a REFRIGERANT. The ANHYDROUS SALT is DELIQUESCENT and is employed as a DESICCANT.

calcium hydrogencarbonate (chemistry) $CaHCO_3$ White CRYSTALLINE COMPOUND, STABLE only in SOLUTION and the cause of temporary HARDNESS OF WATER. Also termed: CALCIUM BICARBONATE.

calcium hydroxide (chemistry) $Ca(OH)_2$ White CRYSTALLINE powder which gives an ALKALINE AQUEOUS SOLUTION known as limewater, used as a test for CARBON DIOXIDE (which turns it cloudy). Also termed: CALCIUM HYDRATE; HYDRATED LIME; CAUSTIC LIME; slaked LIME.

calcium oxide (chemistry) CaO White CRYSTALLINE powder made commercially by roasting limestone (CALCIUM CARBONATE). It is used to make CALCIUM HYDROXIDE. Also termed: LIME, QUICKLIME.

calcium phosphate (chemistry) $Ca_3(PO_4)_2$ White CRYSTALLINE SOLID which makes up the mineral COMPONENT of bones and TEETH, and occurs as the mineral APATITE. It is produced commercially as BONE ash and BASIC slag. Treated with SULPHURIC ACID (*USA*: sulfuric acid) it forms the fertilizer known as superphosphate.

calcium sulphate (chemistry) $CaSO_4$ White CRYSTALLINE COMPOUND which occurs as the minerals ANHYDRITE and (as the DIHYDRATE) GYPSUM, used to make PLASTER OF PARIS. It is the cause of permanent HARDNESS OF WATER. It is used in making ceramics, paint, paper and SULPHURIC ACID (*USA*: sulfuric acid), and is the substance in blackboard CHALK. (*USA*: calcium sulfate).

calculus (1 mathematics; 2 medical/ biochemistry) AREA of mathematics that deals with INTEGRATION and differentiation. 2 Hard accretion (a 'stone') of CALCIUM salts and other compounds that forms in the kidneys and urinary tract, GALL BLADDER, BILE DUCTS or salivary GLANDS.

caleancus (anatomy) Heel-bone; the major BONE of the foot. Also termed: calcaneum.

calibration (1, 2 measurements) 1 Measuring scale on a scientific instrument or apparatus. 2 Method of putting a scale on a scientific instrument, usually by checking it against fixed quantities or standards.

californium Cf (chemistry) RADIOACTIVE ELEMENT in GROUP IIIB of the PERIODIC TABLE (one of the ACTINIDES), produced by alpha-PARTICLE bombardment of CURIUM-242; it has several isotopes, with half-lives of up to 800 years. At. no. 98; r.a.m. 251 (most STABLE ISOTOPE).

calliper (1 equipment; 2 medical) 1 Measuring instrument that resembles a large pair of geometrical dividers; there are internal and external versions. 2 METAL brace that supports an injured or paralysed leg, keeping the leg rigid and helping to support the WEIGHT of the body.

calomel (chemistry) An alternative term for MERCURY(I) CHLORIDE.

calomel half-cell (physics) An ELECTRODE consisting of MERCURY, MERCURY(I) CHLORIDE and POTASSIUM CHLORIDE SOLUTION, employed as a reference ELECTRODE because it has a known CONSTANT POTENTIAL. Also termed: CALOMEL ELECTRODE; CALOMEL reference ELECTRODE.

calorie (measurement) Amount of HEAT required to raise the TEMPERATURE of 1 g of WATER by 1°C at one ATMOSPHERE PRESSURE; equal to 4.184 joules.

See also CALORIE.

Calorie (measurement) Amount of HEAT required to raise the TEMPERATURE of 1 kg of WATER by 1°C at one ATMOSPHERE PRESSURE; equal to 4.184 kilojoules. It is used as an UNIT of ENERGY of food (when it is sometimes spelled with a small *c*). Also termed: KILOCALORIE; large CALORIE.

See also CALORIE.

calorific value (physics) Quantity of HEAT liberated on the complete COMBUSTION of a UNIT WEIGHT or UNIT VOLUME of fuel.

calorimeter (physics/ chemistry) Apparatus for measuring HEAT quantities generated in or evolved by materials in processes such as CHEMICAL REACTIONS, changes of state and SALVATION. The technique is known as calorimetry.

CAM (physiology/ biochemistry) An abbreviation of 'C'ell 'A'dhesion 'M'olecule.

CaMKII (physiology/ biochemistry) Abbreviation of 'Ca'$^{2+}$/cal'M'odulin-dependent 'K'inase II.

cAMP (biochemistry) An abbreviation of 'c'yclic 'A'denosine 'M'ono'P'hosphate.

camphor (chemistry) Naturally-occurring ORGANIC COMPOUND with a penetrating aromatic odour (*USA*: odor). Also termed: gum CAMPHOR; 2-camphanone.

cancer (medical/ histology) Disorder that results when body CELLS undergo unrestrained DIVISION, because of a breakdown in the NORMAL control of cellular processes, to form a MALIGNANT TUMOUR (*USA*: malignant tumor). CANCER may spread by METASTASIS, when TUMOUR CELLS (*USA*: tumor cells) leave their original position and invade other tissues.

candela (cd) (measurement) SI UNIT of LUMINOUS INTENSITY.

C and G (education) An abbreviation of 'C'ity and 'G'uilds.

candle power (cp) (measurement) LUMINOUS INTENSITY expressed in candelas (formerly in INTERNATIONAL CANDLES).

cane-sugar (chemistry) An alternative term for SUCROSE.

canine tooth (anatomy) Pointed TOOTH in most mammals, adapted for stabbing and tearing food. There are two canines in each JAW. Also termed: EYE-TOOTH.

Cannizzaro reaction (chemistry) The formation of an ALCOHOL and an ACID SALT by the REACTION between certain ALDEHYDES and strong ALKALIS (*USA*: alkalies). The REACTION was named after the Italian chemist Stanislao Cannizzaro (1826-1910).

canonical form (chemistry) *See* MESOMERISM.

cap. (general terminology) An abbreviation of 'cap'acity.

capacitance (physics) Ratio of the CHARGE on one of the conductors of a CAPACITOR (there being an equal and an opposite CHARGE on the other CONDUCTOR) to the POTENTIAL DIFFERENCE between them. The SI UNIT of CAPACITANCE is the farad.

capacitor (physics) Device that can store CHARGE and introduces CAPACITANCE into an electrical CIRCUIT. Also termed: CONDENSER; ELECTRICAL CONDENSER.

capacity (general terminology) The amount necessary to fill a container or VESSEL.

capillarity (physics) A phenomenon resulting from SURFACE TENSION that causes low-DENSITY liquids to flow along narrow (CAPILLARY) tubes or soak into porous materials. Also termed: CAPILLARY ACTION.

capillary (1 physics; 2 anatomy) 1 Any narrow tube, in which CAPILLARITY can occur. 2 Finest VESSEL of the BLOOD VASCULAR SYSTEM in vertebrates. Large numbers of capillaries are present in tissues. Their walls are composed of a single layer of CELLS through which exchange of substances, *e.g.* OXYGEN, occurs between the tissues and BLOOD.

caprylic acid (chemistry) An alternative term for OCTANOIC ACID.

capsule (1 bacteriology; 2 anatomy) 1 In certain BACTERIA, a gelatinous EXTRACELLULAR ENVELOPE, which in some cases confers protective properties on the CELL. 2 Sheath of MEMBRANE that surrounds an ORGAN or AREA of TISSUE; *e.g.* the synovial CAPSULE that surrounds the moving parts of joints.

captopril (pharmacology) A powerful ACE inhibitor which is administered orally and used as an ANTIHYPERTENSIVE and in HEART FAILURE treatment.

carbachol (pharmacology) A parasympathomimetic drug which is administered orally, by injection, or through eye drops in the treatment of glaucoma to lower pressure in the eyeball, and which is also used to treat urinary retention.

carbamazepine (pharmacology) An ANTICONVULSANT and ANTI-EPILEPTIC drug with is administered orally or by suppositories. It is used to prevent most forms of epilepsy, to relieve the pain of trieminal neuralgia, in the management of manic-depressive illnesses and in the treatment of diabetes insipidus.

carbamide (chemistry) An alternative term for UREA.

carbanion (chemistry) Transient negatively charged organic ION that has one more ELECTRON than the corresponding FREE RADICAL.

carbene (chemistry) Organic RADICAL that contains DIVALENT CARBON.

carbimazole (pharmacology) A drug that acts as an indirect HORMONE ANTAGONIST, by inhibiting the production of the THYROID HORMONEs by the THYROID gland. It is thus administered orally in cases of thyrotoxicosis to reduce the excess of THYROID HORMONEs in the blood.

carbocyclic (chemistry) Describing a CYCLIC ORGANIC COMPOUND consisting of aromatic rings containing only CARBON and HYDROGEN atoms. Also termed: HOMOCYCLIC.

carbohydrate (chemistry) COMPOUND of CARBON; HYDROGEN and OXYGEN that contains a SACCHAROSE GROUP or its first REACTION PRODUCT, and in which the ratio of HYDROGEN to OXYGEN is 2:1 (the same as in WATER). CELLULOSE, STARCH and all sugars are common carbohydrates. Digestible carbohydrates in the diet are a good source of ENERGY.

carbolic acid (chemistry) An alternative term for PHENOL.

carbon black (chemistry) Finely divided form of CARBON obtained by the incomplete COMBUSTION or thermal DECOMPOSITION of natural GAS or petroleum oil.

carbon C (chemistry) Non-metallic ELEMENT in GROUP IVA of the PERIODIC TABLE which exists as several ALLOTROPES (including diamond and graphite). It occurs in all living things and its compounds are the basis of ORGANIC CHEMISTRY. It is the principal ELEMENT in coal and petroleum. Its nonORGANIC COMPOUNDs include the oxides CARBON MONOXIDE (CO) and CARBON DIOXIDE (CO_2), carbides and carbonates. CARBON is used for making electrodes, brushes for ELECTRIC MOTORS, CARBON fibres (*USA*: carbon fibers) and in steel. Diamonds are used as gemstones and industrially as abrasives. Its ISOTOPE CARBON-14 is the basis of radiocarbon dating. *See* BETA DECAY. At. no. 6; r.a.m. 12.001.

carbon dioxide CO_2 (chemistry) Colourless (*USA*: colorless) GAS formed by the COMBUSTION of CARBON and its ORGANIC COMPOUNDs, by the ACTION of acids on carbonates, and as a PRODUCT of FERMENTATION and RESPIRATION. It is a raw material of PHOTOSYNTHESIS. It is used in fire extinguishers, in fizzy (carbonated) drinks, as a COOLANT in nuclear reactors and, as SOLID CARBON DIOXIDE (DRY ICE), as a REFRIGERANT. The accumulation of CARBON DIOXIDE in the ATMOSPHERE creates the greenhouse effect.

carbon disulphide (chemistry) CS_2 LIQUID chemical, used as a SOLVENT for oils, fats and rubber and in paint-removers. (*USA*: carbon disulfide).

carbon monoxide (chemistry) CO Colourless (*USA*: colorless) odourless (*USA*: odorless) poisonous GAS produced by the incomplete COMBUSTION of CARBON or its compounds. It is used in the chemical industry as a REDUCING AGENT.

carbon tetrachloride (chemistry) An alternative term for TETRACHLOROMETHANE.

carbonate (chemistry) SALT of CARBONIC ACID (H_2CO_3), containing the ION CO_3^{2-}.

Carbonates commonly occur as minerals (*e.g.* CALCIUM CARBONATE) and are readily decomposed by acids to produce CARBON DIOXIDE.

See also HYDROGENCARBONATE.

carbonation (chemistry) Addition of CARBON DIOXIDE under PRESSURE to a LIQUID.

carbonic acid (chemistry) H_2CO_3 ACID formed by the COMBINATION of CARBON DIOXIDE and WATER. Its salts are carbonates.

carbonic anhydrase inhibitors (pharmacology) Drugs that have enzyme-inhibitor actions against the enzyme carbonic anhydrase, which is distributed widely throughout the body and that has a fundamental role in controlling the acid-base balance (pH). Some are used as weak DIURETICS such as acetazolamide, which is useful in reducing fluid in the anterior of the eye in treatment of glaucoma.

carbonium ion (chemistry) Positively charged fragment that arises from the HETEROLYTIC FISSION of a COVALENT BOND involving CARBON.

carbonyl chloride (chemistry) An alternative term for PHOSGENE.

carbonyl compound (chemistry) Chemical containing the RADICAL CO (CARBONYL GROUP), formed when CARBON MONOXIDE combines with a METAL (*e.g.* NICKEL carbonyl, $Ni(CO)_4$).

carbonyl group (chemistry) The GROUP =CO. *See* CARBONYL COMPOUND.

carboprost (pharmacology) A drug which may be administered by injection to treat haemorrhage (*USA*: hemorrhage)

following childbirth, which is caused by tonal loss in the muscles of the uterus. It is an analogue of prostaglandin which is a local HORMONE naturally involved in controlling the muscles of the uterus.

carboxyl group (chemistry) The organic GROUP -COOH, CHARACTERISTIC of CARBOXYLIC ACIDs. Also termed: carboxy GROUP, OXATYL GROUP.

carboxylic acid (chemistry) ORGANIC ACID that contains the CARBOXYL GROUP, -COOH (*e.g.* acetic (ethanoic) ACID, CH_3COOH).

carbylamine (chemistry) An alternative term for ISOCYANIDE.

carcinogen (toxicology) A substance capable of inducing a CANCER. Most CARCINOGENS are also mutagens, and this is thought to be their principal mode of action.

carcinogenesis (medical) The causation of cancer.

carcinogenic (toxicology) Causing cancer or capable of causing cancer.

carcinoma (medical/ histology) CANCER in epithelial TISSUE.

card punch (computing) Machine for punching coded sets of holes in punched cards, to be fed through a CARD READER for inputting DATA into a COMPUTER.

card reader (computing) COMPUTER INPUT DEVICE that reads DATA off punched cards.

cardiac (anatomy) Relating to the HEART.

cardiac glycosides (pharmacology) A class of drugs derived from the leaf of the *Digitalis* foxgloves, which includes DIGOXIN and DIGITOXIN. These drugs increase the force of contraction of the HEART and so have been used for their cardiac stimulant actions to increase the force in treatment of congestive HEART FAILURE.

cardiac muscle (anatomy) Specialized STRIATED MUSCLE, found only in the HEART, that continually contracts rhythmically and automatically (*i.e.* it is myogenic).

See also CARDIAC MUSCLE.

cardinal number (mathematics) Number of elements in a SET (*e.g.* all sets with 5 elements have the CARDINAL NUMBER 5); in everyday terms, an ordinary counting number.

See also ORDINAL NUMBER.

cardiogram (physiology) An alternative term for an ELECTROCARDIOGRAM.

cardiovascular system (anatomy) HEART and the NETWORK of BLOOD VESSELs that circulate BLOOD around the body.

Caro's acid (chemistry) An alternative term for peroxomonosulphuric(VI) ACID (*USA*: peroxomonosulfuric acid), H_2SO_5 (perSULPHURIC ACID [*USA*: persulfuric acid]).

carotene (biochemistry) PIGMENT that belongs to the carotenoids, a PRECURSOR of RETINOL (VITAMIN A).

carotenoid (biology/ chemistry) Member of a GROUP of pigments found in *e.g.* carrots, which can absorb LIGHT during PHOTOSYNTHESIS. They also aid in the protection of prokaryotes from damage by LIGHT.

See also CAROTENE.

carotid artery (anatomy) Either of two main arteries that carry BLOOD from the HEART to the HEAD.

carotid body (physiology) RECEPTOR located between the internal and external carotid arteries. It is sensitive to changes in the CARBON DIOXIDE and OXYGEN content of the BLOOD, and sends impulses to the respiratory and BLOOD-vascular centres (*USA*: centers) in the BRAIN to adjust these levels if necessary.

carpal (anatomy) BONE in the foot and wrist of tetrapods. There are 10-12 carpals in most animals; in human beings there are eight.

carpus (anatomy) The wrist, consisting of eight bones in human beings.

carrier (1 EPIDEMIOLOGY; 2 medical) 1 Somebody who carries pathogens (*e.g.* BACTERIA, VIRUSES) and can pass them on to others, although not necessarily themselves having symptoms of the disease. 2 VECTOR (in medicine).

See also COENZYME.

Cartesian co-ordinates (mathematics) System for locating a point, P, by specifying its distance from axes at right-angles, which intersect at a point, O, called the ORIGIN. For a point on a plane, the distance from the horizontal or X-AXIS is called the ORDINATE of P; the distance from the Y-AXIS is called the ABSCISSA. The point's CARTESIAN CO-ORDINATES are (*x, y*). They were named after the French mathematician Rene Descartes (1596-1650).

cartilage (anatomy) In animals that have a bony SKELETON, pre-BONE TISSUE occurring in young animals that becomes hard through CALCIFICATION. It also occurs in some parts of the SKELETON of adults, where it is structural (*e.g.* forming EAR flaps and the LARYNX) or provides a cushioning or lubricating effect during movement (*e.g.* intervertebral discs, CARTILAGE at the ends of bones in joints). In some animals, *e.g.* sharks, rays and related fish (Chondrichthyes), the whole SKELETON is composed of CARTILAGE even in the adult. Also termed: gristle.

carvedilol (pharmacology) A BETA-BLOCKER drug which can be administered orally as an ANTIHYPERTENSIVE.

casein (biochemistry) PROTEIN that occurs in milk which serves to store AMINO ACIDS as nutrients for the young of mammals.

CAT (radiology) An abbreviation of 'C'omputerised 'A'xial 'T'omography.

catabolism (biochemistry) The part of METABOLISM concerned with the breakdown of complex ORGANIC COMPOUNDS into simple molecules for the release of ENERGY in living organisms.

See also ANABOLISM.

catalysis (chemistry) The ACTION of a CATALYST.

catalyst (chemistry) Substance that increases the rate of a CHEMICAL REACTION without itself undergoing any permanent chemical change. Some reactions take place so slowly without a CATALYST that they are rendered virtually impossible.

See also ENZYME.

catecholamine (biochemistry) Member of a GROUP of amines that include NEUROTRANSMITTERS (*e.g.* DOPAMINE) and HORMONES (*e.g.* ADRENALINE [*USA*: epinephrine]).

cathode (physics) Negatively-charged ELECTRODE in an ELECTROLYTIC CELL or BATTERY.

cathode rays (physics) Stream of electrons produced by the CATHODE (negative ELECTRODE) of an evacuated DISCHARGE tube (such as a CATHODE-RAY TUBE).

cathode-ray oscilloscope (CRO) (physics) Apparatus based on a CATHODE-RAY TUBE which provides a visible IMAGE of one or more rapidly varying electrical signals.

cathode-ray tube (physics) VACUUM tube that allows the direct observation of the BEHAVIOUR (*USA*: behavior) of CATHODE RAYS. It is used as the picture tube in television receivers, radar displays, visual DISPLAY units (VDUs) of computers and in CATHODE-RAY OSCILLOSCOPES.

cation (chemistry) Positively charged ION, which travels towards the CATHODE during ELECTROLYSIS.

cauda equina (anatomy) Sheaf of NERVE roots that arise from the lower end of the SPINAL CORD and serve the lower parts of the body.

caudal vertebra (anatomy) One of the SET of vertebrae nearest to the BASE of the SPINAL COLUMN.

caustic (chemistry) Describing ALKALINE substances that are corrosive towards organic MATTER.

caustic lime (chemistry) An alternative term for CALCIUM HYDROXIDE.

caustic potash (chemistry) An alternative term for POTASSIUM HYDROXIDE.

caustic soda (chemistry) An alternative term for SODIUM HYDROXIDE.

CBC (haematology) An abbreviation of 'C'omplete 'B'lood and differential 'C'ount.

CBF (physiology) An abbreviation of 'C'erebral 'B'lood 'F'low.

CBG (physiology/ biochemistry) An abbreviation of 'C'orticosteroid-'B'inding 'G'lobulin.

C Biol. (education) An abbreviation of 'C'hartered 'Biol'ogist.

CBR (statistics) An abbreviation of 'C'rude 'B'irth 'R'ate.

CBS (society) An abbreviation of 'C'anadian 'B'iochemical 'S'ociety.

CBW (general terminology) chemical and biological warfare.

cc (measurement) *See* c cm.

CCD (physics) An abbreviation of 'c'harge-'c'oupled 'd'evice.

CCE (chemistry) An abbreviation of 'C'arbon-'C'hloroform 'E'xtract.

CCF (medical) An abbreviation of 'C'hronic 'C'ardiac 'F'ailure.

cc hr (measurement) An abbreviation of 'c'ubic 'c'entimetres per 'h'ou'r'(*USA*: CUBIC centimeters per hour).

CCK-PZ (physiology/ biochemistry) An abbreviation of 'C'hole'C'ysto'K'inin-'P'ancreo'Z'ymin.

cckw (general terminology) An abbreviation of 'c'ounter'c'loc'k''w'ise. Also termed ccw.

c cm (measurement) An abbreviation of 'c'ubic 'c'enti'm'etre (*USA*: CUBIC centimeter). Also termed cc or millilitre (*USA*: milliliter).

CCRU (education) An abbreviation of 'C'ommon 'C'old 'R'esearch 'U'nit.

cc sec (measurement) An abbreviation of 'c'ubic 'c'entimetres per 'sec'ond (*USA*: CUBIC centimeters per second).

CCU (medical) An abbreviation of 'C'oronary 'C'are 'U'nit.

CD (1 haematology; 2 medical) 1 An abbreviation of 'C'luster 'D'ifferentiating type antigens. 2 An abbreviation of 'C'aesarean 'D'elivery.

Cd (chemistry) CHEMICAL SYMBOL for CADMIUM.

cd (measurement) An abbreviation of 'c'an'd'ela.

CD4 (immunology) A CELL surface PROTEIN, usually on helper T-LYMPHOCYTES, that recognizes foreign antigens on ANTIGEN-presenting CELLS.

CDC (governing body) An abbreviation of 'C'enters for 'D'isease 'C'ontrol and Prevention.

CDNA (genetics) An abbreviation of 'C'omplementary 'D'eoxyribo'N'ucleic 'A'cid.

CDR (statistics) An abbreviation of 'C'rude 'D'eath 'R'ate.

CE (1chemistry; 2 statistics) An abbreviation of 'C'arbon 'E'quivalent. 2 An abbreviation of 'C'onstant 'E'rror.

Ce (chemistry) CHEMICAL SYMBOL for CERIUM.

cell (biology) Fundamental UNIT of living organisms. It consists of a MEMBRANE bound compartment, often microscopic in size, containing PROTOPLASM. Although a CELL is not independent of its ENVIRONMENT, all bioCHEMICAL REACTIONs of METABOLISM necessary for life (within a favourable ECOLOGICAL NICHE) are located either within the PROTOPLASM, within or associated with the CELL MEMBRANE, or within the local ENVIRONMENT surrounding the CELL (which may be modified by secretory substances). In all CELLS the NUCLEUS contains NUCLEIC ACIDs (*e.g.* DNA) essential for the SYNTHESIS of new proteins. CELLS may be highly specialized for their particular FUNCTION and grouped into tissues, *e.g.* MUSCLE CELLS.

cell body (cytology) Part of a NERVE CELL that contains the CELL NUCLEUS and other CELL components from which an AXON extends.

cell differentiation (cytology) Way in which previously undifferentiated CELLS change structurally and take on specialized roles during GROWTH and development (*e.g.* becoming LIVER CELLS or BONE CELLS).

cell division (cytology) Splitting of CELLS in two by DIVISION of the NUCLEUS (MITOSIS) and DIVISION of the CYTOPLASM after duplication of the CELL contents.

See also MEIOSIS.

cell membrane (cytology) *See* PLASMA MEMBRANE.

cellulose (biology) Major POLYSACCHARIDE of plants found in CELL walls and in some ALGAe and FUNGI. It is composed of GLUCOSE units aligned in long parallel chains, and gives CELL walls their strength and rigidity.

Celsius scale (measurement) TEMPERATURE SCALE on which the FREEZING POINT of WATER is 0°C and the BOILING POINT is 100°C. It is the same as the formerly used CENTIGRADE SCALE, and a DEGREE Celsius is equal to a UNIT on the KELVIN scale. To convert a Celsius TEMPERATURE to KELVIN add 273.15 (and omit the DEGREE sign). To convert a Celsius TEMPERATURE to a Fahrenheit one, multiply by 9/5 and add 32. It was named after the Swedish astronomer Anders Celsius (1701-44).

cent. (measurement) An abbreviation of 'cent'igrade.

centigrade scale (measurement) Former name for the CELSIUS SCALE.

central nervous system (CNS) (anatomy) The CONCENTRATION of nervous TISSUE responsible for co-ordination of the body. In vertebrates it is highly developed to form the BRAIN and SPINAL CORD. The CNS processes information from the SENSE ORGANS and effects a RESPONSE, *e.g.* MUSCLE movement.

central processor (computing) HEART of a DIGITAL COMPUTER which controls and coordinates all the other activities of the machine, and performs logical processes on DATA loaded into it according to PROGRAM instructions it holds.

centre of curvature (optics) Geometric centre of a spherical mirror. (*USA*: center of curvature).

centre of mass (physics) Point at which the whole MASS of an OBJECT may be considered to be concentrated. Also termed: centre of gravity (*USA*: center of gravity). (*USA*: center of mass).

centrifugal force (physics) Outward FORCE on any OBJECT moving in a circular path.

See also CENTRIPETAL FORCE.

centrifuge (laboratory equipment) Instrument used for the separation of substances by SEDIMENTATION through rotation at high speeds, *e.g.* the separation of components of CELLS. SEDIMENTATION varies according to the size of the COMPONENT.

centriole (cytology) Cylindrical body present in the MICROTUBULE organizing centre (*USA*: center) of most ANIMAL CELLS. During MITOSIS it forms the poles of the spindle.

centripetal force (physics) FORCE, directed towards the centre (*USA*: center), that causes a body to move in a circular path. For an OBJECT of MASS m moving with a speed v in a curve of RADIUS OF CURVATURE r, it is equal to mv^2/r.

centromere (genetics) Region on a CHROMOSOME that attaches to the spindle during CELL DIVISION.

cerebellum (anatomy) Front part of hindbrain. It is important in BALANCE and muscular co-ordination.

cerebral cortex (anatomy) Outer region of the CEREBRAL HEMISPHEREs of the BRAIN that contains densely packed NERVE CELLS which are interconnected in a complex manner.

cerebral hemisphere (anatomy) Paired expansions of the ANTERIOR end of the FOREBRAIN. The FOREBRAIN is enormously enlarged by these expansions.

cerebrospinal fluid (CSF) (anatomy) LIQUID that fills the cavities of the BRAIN, which are continuous with each other and the central canal of the SPINAL CORD. The FLUID nourishes and removes secretions from the tissues of the CENTRAL NERVOUS SYSTEM (CNS).

cerebrum (anatomy) Part of FOREBRAIN which expands to form the CEREBRAL HEMISPHERES.

Cerenkov counter (radiology) Method of measuring RADIOACTIVITY by utilizing the effect of CERENKOV RADIATION.

Cerenkov radiation (radiology) LIGHT emitted when charged particles pass through a TRANSPARENT medium at a velocity which is greater than that of LIGHT in the medium. It was named after the Soviet physicist Pavel Cerenkov (1904-90).

cerium Ce (chemistry) Steel-grey metallic ELEMENT in GROUP IIIB of the PERIODIC TABLE (one of the LANTHANIDES). It is used in lighter flints, catalytic converters for car exhausts and GAS mantles. At. no. 58; r.a.m.140.12.

cerumen (biochemistry) WAX that forms in the EAR.

cervical (anatomy) Relating to the neck or to the CERVIX of the womb.

cervical vertebra (anatomy) VERTEBRA in the neck region of the SPINAL COLUMN, concerned with movements of the HEAD.

cervix (anatomy) Neck, usually referring to the neck of the UTERUS (womb) at the inner end of the VAGINA.

Cf (measurement) An abbreviation of 'c'ubic 'f'eet.

CF (medical) An abbreviation of 'C'ystic 'F'ibrosis.

CFBS (society) An abbreviation of 'C'anadian 'F'ederation of 'B'iological 'S'ciences.

CFC (chemistry) An abbreviation of 'c'hloro'f'luoro'c'arbon.

CFF (physiology) An abbreviation of 'C'ritical 'F'usion 'F'requency.

CFU (microbiology) An abbreviation of 'C'olony 'F'orming 'U'nit.

c ft (measurement) An abbreviation of 'c'ubic 'f'ee't'/ 'f'oo't'.

CFTR (physiology/ biochemistry) An abbreviation of 'C'ystic 'F'ibrosis 'T'ransmembrane conductance 'R'egulator.

cg (measurement) An abbreviation of 'c'enti'g'ram. Also termed cgm.

CGI (education) An abbreviation of 'C'ity and 'G'uilds 'I'nstitute.

cgm (measurement) *See* cg.

cGMP (physiology/ biochemistry) An abbreviation of 'c'yclic 3',5'-'G'uanosine 'M'ono'P'hosphate.

CGP (physiology/ biochemistry) An abbreviation of 'C'horionic 'G'rowth HORMONE-'P'rolactin.

CGRP (physiology/ biochemistry) An abbreviation of 'C'alcitonin 'G'ene-'R'elated 'P'eptide.

cgs (measurement) An abbreviation of 'c'entimetre 'g'ram 's'econd. (*USA*: centimeter gram second).

Ch D (education) An abbreviation of 'D'octor of 'Ch'emistry.

Chagas disease (medical/ microbiology) South American trypanosomiasis, a disease spread by the cone-nosed or assassin reduviid bug. The organism is *Trypanosma cruzi* and the disease is a major cause of heart damage and heart failure in endemic areas. Named after the Brazilian physician Carlos Chagas (1879-1934).

chain of infection (epidemiology) A SERIES of infections that are directly or immediately connected to a particular source.

chain reaction (physics/ chemistry) Nuclear or CHEMICAL REACTION in which the products ensure that the REACTION continues (*e.g.* COMBUSTION).

chalk (chemistry) Mineral form of CALCIUM CARBONATE ($CaCO_3$), a soft white limestone derived from the skeletons of microscopic marine animals.

character (genetics) VARIATION caused by a GENE; an inherited trait.

characteristic (mathematics) INTEGER part of a LOGARITHM; *e.g.* the LOGARITHM (to the BASE 10) of 200 is 2.3010, in which 2 is the CHARACTERISTIC.

charcoal (chemistry) Form of CARBON made from incomplete burning of ANIMAL or vegetable MATTER.

charge (physics) *See* ELECTRIC CHARGE; ELECTRON CHARGE.

charge-coupled device (CCD) (physics) Semiconductor device used in television cameras, video cameras and astronomical telescopes to produce an electronic signal from an optical IMAGE.

charge/mass ratio (physics) Fundamental physical CONSTANT, the ratio of an ELECTRON'S CHARGE to its MASS e/m_e, equal to 1.758796×10^{11} C kg^{-1} (coulombs per KILOGRAM).

Charles's law (physics) At a given PRESSURE, the VOLUME of an ideal GAS is directly proportional to its ABSOLUTE TEMPERATURE. It was named after the French physicist Jacques Charles (1746-1823).

See also KINETIC THEORY.

chelate (chemistry) Chemical COMPOUND in which a central METAL ION forms part of one or more organic rings of atoms. The formation of these compounds is useful in many contexts, *e.g.* medicine, in which chelating agents are administered to counteract poisoning by certain heavy metals. They can also act to BUFFER the CONCENTRATION of METAL ions (*e.g.* IRON and CALCIUM) in natural biological systems.

chemical bond (chemistry) LINKAGE between atoms or ions within a MOLECULE. A CHEMICAL REACTION and the input or output of ENERGY are involved in the formation or destruction of a CHEMICAL BOND.

See also COVALENT BOND. IONIC BOND.

chemical combination (chemistry) Union of two or more chemical substances to form a different substance or substances.

chemical equation (chemistry) Way of expressing a CHEMICAL REACTION by placing the formulas of the reactants to the left and those of the products to the right, with an equality sign or directional arrow in between. The number of atoms of any particular ELEMENT are the same on each side of the equation (when the REACTION is in EQUILIBRIUM). *E.g.* the CHEMICAL EQUATION for the COMBINATION of HYDROGEN and OXYGEN to form WATER is written as: $2H_2 + O_2 \rightarrow 2H_2O$

chemical equilibrium (chemistry) The balanced state of a CHEMICAL REACTION, when the CONCENTRATION of reactants and products remain CONSTANT.

See also EQUILIBRIUM CONSTANT.

chemical formula (chemistry) Method of representing the chemical composition of a single substance that uses the CHEMICAL SYMBOLS of the atoms, and indicates the numbers of those atoms, in a MOLECULE of the substance *e.g.* the CHEMICAL FORMULAe of WATER, CALCIUM CARBONATE and ETHANE are H_2O, $CaCO_3$ and C_2H_6.

chemical potential (chemistry) Measure of the tendency of a CHEMICAL REACTION to take place.

chemical reaction (chemistry) Process in which one or more substances react to form a different substance or substances.

chemical symbol (chemistry) Letter or letters that represent the name of a chemical ELEMENT, or one ATOM of it in a CHEMICAL FORMULA, *e.g.* the symbols of CARBON, and CHLORINE are C, and Cl. The symbol may be based on the ELEMENT'S

Latin, not English, name; *e.g.* Au for GOLD (*aurum*), Fe for IRON (*ferrum*).

chemiluminescence (chemistry/ biochemistry) LUMINESCENCE that results from a CHEMICAL REACTION (*e.g.* the OXIDATION of PHOSPHORUS in AIR). In living organisms it is termed BIOLUMINESCENCE.

chemistry (chemistry) The study of elements and their compounds, particularly how they behave in CHEMICAL REACTIONS.

chemo. (medical) An abbreviation of 'CHEMO'THERAPY.

chemoreceptor (physiology) CELL that fires a NERVE IMPULSE in RESPONSE to stimulation by a specific type of chemical substance; *e.g.* the TASTE BUDS on the TONGUE and OLFACTORY bulbs in the nose contain chemoreceptors that provide the SENSES of TASTE and SMELL.

chemotaxis (biology) RESPONSE of organisms to chemical stimuli; *e.g.* the movement of BACTERIA towards nutrients.

chemotherapy (pharmacology) TREATMENT of a disorder with drugs that are designed to destroy pathogens or cancerous TISSUE.

chiasma (1 genetics; 2 anatomy) 1 Point along the CHROMATID of a HOMOLOGOUS CHROMOSOME at which connections occur during crossing-over or exchange of genetic material in MEIOSIS. 2 Crossing-over point of the OPTIC NERVES in the BRAIN.

chile saltpetre (chemistry) Old name for impure SODIUM NITRATE.

chimaera (genetics) Genetic MOSAIC or organism composed of genetically different tissues arising *e.g.* from MUTATION or mixing of CELL types of different organisms. It can be achieved by incorporating DONOR CELLS at an early stage of embryonic development of the RECIPIENT.

Chinese restaurant syndrome (medical) Headache, nausea, a tight or burning sensation in the face, head and chest and sometimes dizziness and diarrhoea (*USA*: diarrhea) coming on one or two hours after a meal containing a large amount of MONOSODIUM GLUTAMATE.

chirality (chemistry) Property of a MOLECULE that has a CARBON ATOM attached to four different atoms or groups, and which can therefore exist as a pair of OPTICALLY ACTIVE stercoisomers (whose molecules are mirror images of each other). Commonly called 'handedness', CHIRALITY is significant in the biological activity of molecules, in some of which the righthanded version is active and the left-handed version is not, or vice versa (*e.g.* many pheromones).

chitin (biochemistry) POLYSACCHARIDE found in the exoskeleton of arthropods, giving it hard waxy properties.

chloral (chemistry) An alternative term for TRICHLOROETHANAL.

chloral hydrate (chemistry) An alternative term for TRICHLOROETHANEDIOL.

chlorate (chemistry) SALT of chloric ACID ($HClO_3$).

chloride (chemistry) BINARY COMPOUND containing CHLORINE; a SALT of HYDROCHLORIC ACID (HCl).

chlorination (1 chemistry; 2 microbiology) 1 REACTION between CHLORINE and an

ORGANIC COMPOUND to form the corresponding chlorinated COMPOUND; *e.g.* the CHLORINATION of BENZENE produces chlorobenzene, C_6H_5Cl. 2 TREATMENT of a substance with CHLORINE; *e.g.* to disinfect it.

chlorine Cl (chemistry) Gaseous non-metallic ELEMENT in GROUP VIIA of the PERIODIC TABLE (the HALOGENS), obtained by the ELECTROLYSIS of SODIUM CHLORIDE (COMMON SALT). It is a green-yellow poisonous GAS with an irritating SMELL, used as a disinfectant and BLEACH and to make CHLORINE containing organic chemicals. At. no. 17; r.a.m. 35.453.

chlorofluorocarbon (chemistry) FLUORO-CARBON that has CHLORINE atoms in place of some of the FLUORINE atoms. Chlorofluorocarbons and fluorocarbons have similar properties, and are used as AEROSOL propellants and refrigerants.

chloroform (chemistry) An alternative term for TRICHLOROMETHANE.

chloroquine (pharmacology) An antimalarial drug which can be administered orally, by injection or infusion to prevent and treat contraction of malaria.

chlorothiazide (pharmacology) A DIURETIC drug of the THIAZIDE class, which can be administered orally as an ANTIHYPER-TENSIVE and in the treatment of OEDEMA (*USA*: edema) and congestive HEART FAILURE.

chlorpromazine hydrochloride (pharmacology) An antipsychotic drug which can be administered orally, by injection or topically as suppositories in the treatment of schizophrenia and other psychoses. It can also be used as an anxolytic, ANTINAUSEANT and ANTIEMETIC.

chlorpropamide (pharmacology) A drug of the sulphonylurea type which can be administered orally in diabetic treatment of non-insulin-dependent diabetes.

chlortalidone (pharmacology) A DIURETIC related to the THIAZIDES which can be administered orally to treat hypertension, OEDEMA (*USA*: edema) and diabetes insipidus.

cholesterol (biochemistry) STEROL found in ANIMAL tissues, a LIPID-like substance that occurs in BLOOD PLASMA, CELL MEMBRANES and NERVES, and may form gallstones. High levels of CHOLESTEROL in the BLOOD are connected to the onset of ATHEROSELEROSIS, in which fatty materials are deposited in patches on ARTERY walls and can restrict BLOOD flow. Many steroids are derived from CHOLESTEROL.

choline (biochemistry) $HOC_2H_4N(CH_3)_3OH$ ORGANIC COMPOUND that is a constituent of the NEUROTRANSMITTER ACETYLCHOLINE and some fats. It is one of the B VITAMINS.

chondriosome (cytology) An alternative term for MITOCHONDRION.

chlordiazepoxide (pharmacology) A benzodiazepine drug which can be administered orally as an ANXIOLYTIC.

chorion (biology) The MEMBRANE that surrounds an implanted BLASTOCYST and the EMBRYO and FOETUS (*USA*: fetus) that develop from it.

chorionic gonadotrophin (biochemistry) HORMONE produced by the PLACENTA during PREGNANCY. Its presence in the URINE is the basis of many kinds of PREGNANCY testing.

chorionic villus sampling (biochemistry) Testing during early PREGNANCY of small samples of TISSUE taken from the CHORION for the presence of FOETAL (*USA*: fetal) ABNORMALITIES.

See also AMNIOCENTESIS.

choroid (histology) Layer of pigmented CELLS, rich in BLOOD VESSELs, between the RETINA and SCLEROTIC of the EYE.

chromatic aberration (physics/ genetics) *See* ABERRATION.

chromatid (genetics) One of two thread-like parts of a CHROMOSOME, visible during PROPHASE of MEIOSIS or MITOSIS, when the CHROMOSOME has duplicated. Chromatids are separated during ANAPHASE.

chromatin (biochemistry) BASIC PROTEIN that is associated with EUKARYOTIC chromosomes, visible during certain stages of CELL duplication.

chromatography (chemistry) Method of separating a MIXTURE by carrying it in SOLUTION or in a GAS stream through an absorbent. The separated substances may be extracted by ELUTION.

chromium Cr (chemistry) SILVER-grey metallic ELEMENT in GROUP VIB of the PERIODIC TABLE (a TRANSITION ELEMENT), obtained mainly from its ore chromite. It is electroplated onto other metals (particularly steel) to provide a corrosion-resistant decorative finish, and ALLOYed with NICKEL and IRON to make stainless steels; its compounds are used in pigments and dyes. At. no. 24; r.a.m. 51.996.

chromophore (chemistry) A chemical GROUPING that causes compounds to have

COLOUR (*USA*: color) (*e.g.* the -N=N-GROUP in an AZO DYE).

chromosome map (genetics) Diagram showing the positions of various genes on appropriate chromosomes.

chromosome (genetics) Structure within the NUCLEUS of a CELL that contains PROTEIN and the genetic DNA. Chromosomes occur in pairs in DIPLOID CELLS (ordinary body CELLS); HAPLOID CELLS (gametes or SEX CELLS) have only one CHROMOSOME in their nuclei. The number of chromosomes varies in different SPECIES. During CELL DIVISION, each CHROMOSOME doubles and the two duplicates separate into the two new DAUGHTER CELLS.

chronic (medical) Describing a condition or disorder that is long-standing, and often difficult to treat. *Compare* ACUTE.

chronic obstructive pulmonary disease (COPD) (medical) A progressive irreversible condition characterised by airway obstruction, the most common cause of which is smoking.

chyle (biochemistry) Milky FLUID resulting from the ABSORPTION of fats in the LACTEALS of the SMALL INTESTINE; it is removed by the LYMPHATIC SYSTEM.

chyme (physiology) Partly digested food that passes from the STOMACH into the DUODENUM and SMALL INTESTINE.

Ci (measurement) An abbreviation of 'C'ur'i'e.

ciliary body (histology) Ring of TISSUE that surrounds the LENS of the EYE. It generates the AQUEOUS HUMOUR and contains CILIARY MUSCLES, which are used in ACCOMMODATION.

ciliary muscle (histology) MUSCLE that controls the LENS of the EYE and thus achieves ACCOMMODATION.

cilium (cytology) Small HAIR-like structure that moves rhythmically on the surface of a CELL or the whole EPITHELIUM. Cilia usually cover the surface of a CELL and cause movement in the FLUID surrounding it. They are used for locomotion by some single-celled aquatic organisms.

See also FLAGELLUM.

cimetidine (pharmacology) A histamine$_2$-ANTAGONIST which can be administered orally, by injection or infusion as an ulcer-healing drug.

cinnarizine (pharmacology) An ANTI-HISTAMINE drug which can be administered orally as an ANTINAUSEANT and ANTIEMETIC, that also has vasodilator properties.

ciprofibrate (pharmacology) A LIPID-lowering drug which can be administered orally in hyperlipidaemia (*USA*: hyperlipidemia) to reduce the levels, or change the proportions, of various LIPIDs in the bloodstream.

circ. (physics) An abbreviation of 'circ'uit.

circadian rhythm (physiology) Cyclical VARIATION in the physiological, metabolic or behavioural (*USA*: behavioral) aspects of an organism over a PERIOD of about 24 hours; *e.g.* sleep patterns. It may arise from inside an organism or be a RESPONSE to a regular CYCLE of some external VARIATION in the ENVIRONMENT. Also termed: diurnal rhythm.

See also BIOLOGICAL CLOCK.

circuit (physics) An electrical term for the path that an ELECTRIC CURRENT flows along.

circuit breaker (physics) Safety device in an electric CIRCUIT that interrupts the CURRENT flow in the event of a fault.

See also FUSE.

circulatory system (physiology) In animals, transport system that maintains a CONSTANT flow of TISSUE FLUID in sealed vessels to all parts of body *e.g.* in the BLOOD VASCULAR SYSTEM, OXYGEN and food materials dissolved in BLOOD diffuse into each CELL; waste products, including CARBON DIOXIDE, diffuse out of the CELLS and into the BLOOD.

See also LYMPHATIC SYSTEM.

circum. (measurement) An abbreviation of 'circum'ference.

circumference (measurement) Boundary of a circle, equal in length to π times the DIAMETER (or 2π times the RADIUS).

cisapride (pharmacology) A motility stimulant which can be administered orally to release the NEUROTRANSMITTER acetylcholine from the nerves of the STOMACH and INTESTINE to treat conditions such as oesophageal reflux.

cistron (molecular biology) Functional UNIT of a DNA chain that controls PROTEIN manufacture.

cit. (literary terminology) An abbreviation of 'cit'ed.

citric acid (chemistry) $C_6H_8O_7$ Hydroxy-triCARBOXYLIC ACID, present in the juices of fruits and made by fermenting residues from SUGAR refining. It is important in the

KREBS CYCLE, and is much used as a flavouring and in medicines.

citric acid cycle (biochemistry) An alternative term for KREBS CYCLE.

C-J disease (medical) An abbreviation of 'C'reutzfeldt-'J'acob disease. Also termed CJD.

CK (biochemistry) An abbreviation of 'C'reatine 'K'inase.

Cl (chemistry) CHEMICAL SYMBOL for CHLORINE.

Claisen condensation (chemistry) A CHEMICAL REACTION in which two molecules combine to give a COMPOUND containing a KETONE GROUP and an ESTER GROUP. It was named after the German chemist Ludwig Claisen (1851-1930).

class (biology) In biological CLASSIFI- CATION, one of the groups into which a PHYLUM is divided, and which is itself divided into orders; *e.g.* Mammalia (mammals), Aves (birds).

classical physics (physics) Physics prior to the introduction of QUANTUM THEORY and a knowledge of RELATIVITY.

classification (biology) The placing of living organisms into a SERIES of groups according to similarities in structure, physiology, biochemistry, and other characteristics. The smallest GROUP is the SPECIES. Similar SPECIES are placed in a GENUS, similar GENERA are grouped into families, families into orders, orders into classes, classes into phyla (or divisions in plants), and phyla into kingdoms. Modern CLASSIFICATION is usually intended to reflect degrees of evolutionary relation- ship, although not all experts agree on single CLASSIFICATION schemes for animals or for plants.

See also BINOMIAL NOMENCLATURE.

clathrate (chemistry) Chemical structure in which one ATOM or MOLECULE is 'encaged' by a structure of other molecules, and not held by CHEMICAL BONDS.

See also CHELATE.

clavicle (anatomy) In vertebrates, the ANTERIOR BONE of the VENTRAL side of the shoulder girdle. Also termed: COLLARBONE.

cleavage (1 biology; 2 chemistry; 3 biochemistry) 1 A SERIES of mitotic divisions of a fertilized OVUM. 2 The splitting of a crystal structure along a certain plane parallel to a POTENTIAL crystal face. 3 The splitting of CHEMICAL BONDS (*e.g.* PROTEASE ENZYMES cleave PEPTIDE BONDS from proteins to release AMINO ACID residues).

clinical thermometer (medical) Type of (MERCURY) THERMOMETER used for taking body TEMPERATURE. It measures only a small range of temperatures.

CLIP (physiology/ biochemistry) An abbreviation of 'C'orticotropin-'L'ike 'I'ntermediate-lobe 'P'olypeptide.

clitoris (anatomy) MASS of erectile TISSUE in female mammals, the equivalent of the PENIS in males, situated in front of the opening of the VAGINA.

CLL (haematology) An abbreviation of 'C'hronic 'L'ymphocytic 'L'eukaemia. (*USA*: CHRONIC Lymphocytic Leukemia).

clobazam (pharmacology) A benzodiaze- pine drug which can be administered orally as an ANXIOLYTIC in the treatment of anxiety.

clofibrate (pharmacology) A LIPID-lowering drug which can be administered orally in hyperlipidaemia (*USA*: hyperlipidemia) to reduce the levels, or change the proportions, of various LIPIDS in the bloodstream.

clomiphene citrate (pharmacology) A sex HORMONE anAGONIST which prevents the action of OESTROGENS thus increasing secretion of gonadotrophins and causing ovulation. It can be administered orally as a fertility treatment in women whose condition is linked to the persistent presence of OESTROGENS and a consequent failure to ovulate.

clonazepam (pharmacology) A benzodiazepine drug which can be administered orally, by injection or infusion, as an ANTICONVULSANT and ANTI-EPILEPTIC in the treatment of epilepsy.

clone (genetics) One of many descendants produced by ASEXUAL REPRODUCTION. Members of a CLONE have identical genetic constitution.

clonidine hydrochloride (pharmacology) An ANTISYMPATHETIC class of drug that decreases the release of NORADRENALINE from sympathetic nerves. It can be administered orally or by injection in ANTIHYPERTENSIVE treatment and anti-migraine treatment.

clotting factor (haematology) PROTEIN-like structure, *e.g.* THROMBIN and FIBRINOGEN, that induces BLOOD COAGULATION when a BLOOD VESSEL is broken.

clozapine (pharmacology) An antipsychotic drug which can be administered orally in the treatment of schizophrenia.

Clozapine can cause potentially serious side-effects including agranulocytosis and neutropenia.

Cm (chemistry) CHEMICAL SYMBOL for CURIUM.

cm (measurement) An abbreviation of 'c'enti'm'etre (*USA*: centimeter).

CMA (1 education; 2 society) 1 An abbreviation of 'C'ertified 'M'edical 'A'ssistant. 2 An abbreviation of 'C'hemical 'M'anufacturers 'A'ssociation.

CML (medical/ haematology) An abbreviation of 'C'hronic 'M'yelocytic 'L'eukaemia. (*USA*: CHRONIC Myelocytic Leukemia).

cmpd (chemistry) An abbreviation of 'c'o'mp'oun'd'.

CMRO$_2$ (physiology/ biochemistry) An abbreviation of 'C'erebral 'M'etabolic 'R'ate for 'O'xygen.

CMV (virology) An abbreviation of 'C'yto'M'egalo'V'irus.

CNS (medical) An abbreviation of 'C'entral 'N'ervous 'S'ystem.

CNTF (physiology) An abbreviation of 'C'iliary 'N'euro'T'rophic 'F'actor.

co. (anatomy) An abbreviation of 'co'lon.

Co (chemistry) CHEMICAL SYMBOL for COBALT.

CoA (physiology/ biochemistry) An abbreviation of 'Co'enzyme 'A'.

coagulation (1 haematology; 2 biochemistry; 3 chemistry) 1 The process by which bleeding is arrested. THROMBIN is produced in the absence of antithrombin from the COMBINATION of prothrombin and CALCIUM ions. This interacts with SOLUBLE FIBRINOGEN to PRECIPITATE it as the INSOLUBLE BLOOD PROTEIN FIBRIN, which forms a mesh of fine threads over the WOUND. BLOOD CELLS become trapped in the mesh and form a clot. 2 Irreversible setting of PROTOPLASM on exposure to HEAT or POISON. 3 PRECIPITATION of colloids, *e.g.* proteins, from solutions.

cobalt Co (chemistry) SILVER-white magnetic metallic ELEMENT in GROUP VIII of the PERIODIC TABLE, used in ALLOYS to make cutting tools and magnets. The RADIOACTIVE ISOTOPE Co-60 is used in RADIOTHERAPY. At. no. 27; r.a.m. 58.9332.

COBOL (computing) An acronym of 'CO'mmon 'B'usiness 'O'riented 'L'anguage, a COMPUTER programming language designed for commercial use.

cocaine (pharmacology) A central nervous system stimulant that rapidly causes dependence. It may be used therapeutically as a topically applied local anaesthetic.

coccus (bacteriology) Spherical-shaped BACTERIUM. Cocci may join together to form clumps (staphylococci) or chains (streptococci).

coccyx (anatomy) Bony structure in primates and amphibians, formed by FUSION of tail vertebrae; *e.g.* in human beings it consists of three to five vestigial vertebrae at the BASE of the SPINE.

cochlea (anatomy) Spirally coiled part of the INNER EAR in mammals. It translates sound-induced vibrations into NERVE IMPULSEs that travel along the AUDITORY NERVE to the BRAIN, where they are interpreted as sounds.

Cockeroft-Walton generator (physics) High-VOLTAGE DIRECT CURRENT generator used for accelerating nuclear particles to high speeds. It was named after the British scientist John Cockcroft (1897-1967) and the Irish physicist Ernest Walton (1903-95).

codeine (pharmacology) Pain-killing drug (a NARCOTIC ANALGESIC), the methyl DERIVATIVE of MORPHINE.

coefficient (1 mathematics; 2 physics) 1 In an ALGEBRAic expression, the numerical FACTOR by which the VARIABLE is multiplied; *e.g.* in 5xy, the COEFFICIENT of xy is 5. 2 Number or parameter that measures some specified property of a given substance; *e.g.* COEFFICIENT of friction, COEFFICIENT of VISCOSITY.

coefficient of variation (statistics) A measurement of the amount of VARIATION within a population. It equals the STANDARD DEVIATION expressed as a PERCENTAGE of the value of the MEAN.

coenzyme (biochemistry) ORGANIC COMPOUND essential to catalytic activities of ENZYMES without being utilized in the REACTION. Coenzymes usually act as carriers of INTERMEDIATE products, *e.g.* ATP.

COHb (physiology/ biochemistry) An abbreviation of 'C'arbonmon'O'xy'-H'aemoglo'b'in (*USA*: carbon oxyhemoglobin).

coherent units (measurement) System of units in which the desired units are obtained by multiplying or dividing BASE units, with no numerical CONSTANT involved.

See also SI UNITS.

cohesion (physics) Attraction between similar particles (atoms or molecules of the same substance); *e.g.* between WATER molecules to create SURFACE TENSION.

See also ADHESION.

colestipol hydrochloride (pharmacology) A resin that binds bile acids and lowers LDL-cholesterol that is used as a LIPID-lowering drug which can be administered orally in hyperlipidaemia (*USA*: hyperlipidemia) to reduce the levels, or change the proportions, of various LIPIDS in the bloodstream.

colestyramine (pharmacology) A resin that binds bile acids in the gut that, similarly to COLESTIPOL HYDROCHLORIDE, is used as a LIPID-lowering drug which can be administered orally in hyperlipidaemia (*USA*: hyperlipidemia) to reduce the levels, or change the proportions, of various LIPIDS in the bloodstream.

collagen (biochemistry) Fibrous PROTEIN CONNECTIVE TISSUE that binds together bones, ligaments, CARTILAGE, muscles and SKIN.

collarbone (anatomy) An alternative term for the CLAVICLE.

colloid (physics) Form of MATTER that consists of small particles, about 10^{-4} to 10^{-6} mm across, dispersed in a medium such as AIR or WATER. Common colloids include AEROSOLS (*e.g.* fog, mist) and gels (*e.g.* GELATIN, rubber). A non-colloidal substance is termed a CRYSTALLOID.

colon (anatomy) LARGE INTESTINE, in which the main FUNCTION is the ABSORPTION of WATER from FAECES (*USA*: FECES).

colony (bacteriology) BACTERIAL GROWTH on a SOLID medium that forms a visible MASS.

colorimeter (physics/ chemistry) Instrument for measuring the COLOUR (*USA*: color) INTENSITY of a medium such as a coloured SOLUTION (which can be related to CONCENTRATION and therefore provide a method of QUANTITATIVE ANALYSIS). The technique is termed colorimetry.

colostrum (biology) Yellowish milky FLUID secreted from the mammalian breast immediately before and after childbirth. It contains more antibodies and leucocytes (and less fat and carbohydrates) than true milk, which follows within a few days.

colour blindness (medical) Inability to distinguish between certain colours. It is a CONGENITAL abnormality that affects 6 per cent of human males and 1 per cent of females. The most common DEFECT is red-green COLOUR BLINDNESS, which results in observation of both colours in grey, blue or yellow, depending on the amount of yellow and blue present in the LIGHT. (*USA*: color blindness)

colour (physics) Visual sensation or perception that results from the ADSORPTION of LIGHT ENERGY of a particular WAVELENGTH by the cones of the RETINA of the EYE. There are two or more types of CONE, each of which are sensitive to different wavelengths of LIGHT. The BRAIN combines NERVE IMPULSES from these cones to produce the perception of COLOUR. The COLOUR of an OBJECT thus depends on the WAVELENGTH of LIGHT it reflects (other wavelengths being absorbed) or transmits. (*USA*: color)

columbium (chemistry) Former name of NIOBIUM.

combination (mathematics) Any selection of a given number of objects from a SET, irrespective of their ORDER. The number of combinations of r objects that can be obtained from a SET of n objects (usually written ${}_nC_r$) is $n!/[r!(n - r)!]$. (The symbol ! stands for FACTORIAL.)

combustion (chemistry) Burning; the rapid OXIDATION of a substance accompanied by HEAT, LIGHT and flame. Usually the OXIDIZING AGENT is OXYGEN (often from AIR).

commensalism (biology) Close relationship between two organisms from which one benefits and the other neither benefits nor suffers.

See also, PARASITISM; SYMBIOSIS.

common denominator (mathematics) Same DENOMINATOR assigned to fractions (formerly with different ones) so that they can be added or subtracted; *e.g.* to subtract 1/3 from 1/2 the fractions are first assigned the COMMON DENOMINATOR of 6, becoming 2/6 and 3/6, and subtracted to give 1/6; using the same method they can be added (to give 5/6).

common difference (mathematics) Difference between any two consecutive terms of an ARITHMETIC PROGRESSION.

common logarithm (mathematics) LOGARITHM to the BASE 10.

common salt (chemistry) An alternative term for SODIUM CHLORIDE.

commutative (mathematics) A term describing a mathematical operation of the type $a * b$ whose result does not depend on the order in which the operation is carried out. *E.g.* the addition $7 + 2$ has the same result as $2 + 7$, so addition is COMMUTATIVE. Subtraction is not; *e.g.* $7 - 2$ is not the same as $2 - 7$.

See also ASSOCIATIVE.

competition (biology) The struggle within a community between organisms of the same or different SPECIES for survival.

See also NATURAL SELECTION.

compiler (computing) COMPUTER PROGRAM that converts a source language into MACHINE CODE (readable by the COMPUTER).

complementary deoxyribonucleic acid (CDNA) (genetics) Single-stranded DNA complementary to an RNA; it is synthesized *in vitro* by using the RNA as a template for the ACTION of reverse transcriptase.

complex compound (chemistry) An alternative term for a CO-ORDINATION COMPOUND.

complex ion (chemistry) CATION bonded by means of a CO-ORDINATE BOND.

complex number (mathematics) Number written in the form $x + iy$, where x and y are REAL NUMBERS and i is the SQUARE ROOT of -1 (*i.e.* $i^2 = -1$).

component (1 mathematics; 2 chemistry) 1 The resolved part of a VECTOR quantity in a particular direction, usually one of a pair at right-angles. 2 One of the substances in a system.

composite (physics) Material composed of two or more other materials that give a COMBINATION with better properties than any of the components individually; *e.g.* glass fibre (*USA*: glass fiber) or carbon fibre (*USA*: carbon fiber) reinforced plastic RESIN.

compound (chemistry) Substance that consists of two or more elements chemically united in definite proportions by WEIGHT. Also termed: chemical COMPOUND.

Compton effect (physics) REDUCTION in the ENERGY of a PHOTON as a result of its INTERACTION with a FREE ELECTRON. Some of the PHOTON's ENERGY is transferred to the ELECTRON. It was named after the American physicist Arthur Compton (1892-1962).

Compton wavelength (physics) WAVELENGTH associated with a SUBATOMIC PARTICLE, dependent on its MASS. For an ELECTRON it is 2.42621×10^{-12} m; for a PROTON 1.321398×10^{-15} m.

computer (computing) Electronic device that can accept DATA, apply a SERIES of logical operations to it (obeying a PROGRAM), and supply the results of these operations. *See* ANALOG COMPUTER; DIGITAL COMPUTER.

computerized axial tomography (CAT) scan (radiology) A technique for producing X-RAY pictures of cross-sectional 'slices' through the BRAIN and other parts of the body.

COMT (physiology/ biochemistry) An abbreviation of 'C'atechol-'O'-'M'ethyl'-T'ransferase.

concave (optics) Describing a surface that curves inwards (as opposed to one that is CONVEX).

concentration (chemistry) Strength of MIXTURE or SOLUTION. Concentrations can be expressed in very many ways; *e.g.* parts per million (for traces of a substance), PERCENTAGE (*i.e.* parts per hundred by WEIGHT or VOLUME), gm or kg per LITRE of SOLVENT or per LITRE of SOLUTION, moles per LITRE of SOLUTION (MOLARITY), moles per kg of SOLVENT (molality), or in terms of normality. *See* NORMAL.

See also SOLUBILITY.

condensation (1 physics; 2 chemistry) 1 Change of a GAS or VAPOUR into a LIQUID or SOLID by cooling. 2 CONDENSATION REACTION.

condensation pump (laboratory equipment) An alternative term for DIFFUSION PUMP.

condensation reaction (chemistry) A CHEMICAL REACTION in which two or more small molecules combine to form a larger one, often with the elimination of a simpler substance, usually WATER.

condenser (1 chemistry; 2 physics; 3 optics) 1 An apparatus for changing a VAPOUR into a LIQUID (by cooling it and causing CONDENSATION). 2 An alternative term for a CAPACITOR. 3 A LENS or mirror that concentrates a LIGHT source.

conditioned reflex (physiology) ANIMAL's RESPONSE to a NEUTRAL STIMULUS that learning has associated with a particular effect; *e.g.* a rat may learn (be conditioned) to press a lever when hungry because it associates this ACTION with receiving food.

conductance (physics) Ability to convey ENERGY as HEAT or ELECTRICITY. Electrical CONDUCTANCE, measured in siemens, is the RECIPROCAL of resistance. Also termed: CONDUCTIVITY.

conduction band (physics) ENERGY range in a semiconductor within which electrons can be made to flow by an applied ELECTRIC FIELD.

conductor (1, 2 physics) 1 Material that allows HEAT to flow through it by conduction. 2 Material that allows ELECTRICITY to flow through it; a CONDUCTOR has a low resistance.

cone (cytology) LIGHT-sensitive NERVE CELL present in the RETINA of the EYE of most vertebrates; it can detect COLOUR (*USA*: color).

See also ROD.

configuration (1 physics; 2 chemistry) 1 The arrangement of electrons about the NUCLEUS of an ATOM. Also termed: ELECTRON CONFIGURATION. 2 The arrangement in space of the atoms in a MOLECULE.

conformation (chemistry) Particular shape of a MOLECULE that arises through the NORMAL rotation of its atoms or groups about SINGLE BONDS.

congenital (medical) Dating from birth or before birth. CONGENITAL conditions may be caused by environmental factors or be inherited.

conjugated (chemistry) Describing an ORGANIC COMPOUND that has alternate single and double or TRIPLE BONDs.) *e.g.* buta-1, 3-diene, $H_2C = CH\text{-}CH = CH_2$.

conjugation (biology) Form of REPRO-DUCTION that involves the permanent or temporary union of two isogametes, *e.g.* in certain green ALGAe. In PROTOZOA, two individuals partly FUSE, exchanging nuclear materials. When separated, each CELL divides further to give uninucleate spores which eventually develop into full adults.

conjunctiva (histology) Layer of protective MUCUS-secreting EPIDERMIS that covers the CORNEA on the eyeball and is continuous with the inner lining of the eyelids of vertebrates.

connective tissue (histology) Strong TISSUE that binds organs and tissues together. It consists of a GLYCOPROTEIN MATRIX containing COLLAGEN in which CELLS, fibres (*USA*: fibers) and vessels are embedded. The most widespread CONNECTIVE TISSUE is arcolar TISSUE.

conservation of energy (physics) LAW that states that in all processes occurring in an isolated system the ENERGY of the system remains CONSTANT.

See also THERMODYNAMICS, LAWS OF.

conservation of mass (physics) Principle which states that the products of a purely CHEMICAL REACTION have the same total MASS as the reactants.

constant (measurement) Quantity that remains the same in all circumstances; *e.g.* in the expression $2y = 5x^2$, the numbers 2 and 5 are constants (and x and y are variables).

continuous wave (physics) ELECTRO-MAGNETIC WAVE of CONSTANT AMPLITUDE.

contractile vacuole (biology) Membranous sac within a single-celled organism (*e.g.* AMOEBA (*USA*: ameba) and other protozoans) which fills with WATER and suddenly contracts, expelling its contents from the CELL. It carries out OSMO-REGULATION and EXCRETION.

convection (physics) Transport of HEAT by the movement of the heated substance (usually a FLUID such as AIR or WATER).

converging lens (optics) LENS capable of bringing LIGHT to a FOCUS; a CONVEX LENS.

convex (optics) Describing a surface that is rounded outwards (as opposed to one that is CONCAVE).

coolant (physics) LIQUID or GAS that removes HEAT by CONVECTION.

co-ordinate bond (chemistry) Type of COVALENT BOND that is formed by the donation of a lone pair of electrons from one ATOM to another. Also termed: DATIVE BOND.

co-ordination compound (chemistry) Chemical COMPOUND that has CO-ORDINATE BONDS. Also termed: complex; COMPLEX COMPOUND.

co-ordination number (chemistry) Number of nearest neighbours of an ATOM or an ION in a chemical COMPOUND.

COPD (medical) Abbreviation of 'C'hronic 'O'bstructive 'P'ulmonary 'D'isease.

copper Cu (chemistry) Reddish metallic ELEMENT in GROUP IB of the PERIODIC TABLE (a TRANSITION ELEMENT) which occurs as the free METAL (native) and in various ores, chief of which is chalcopyrite. The METAL is a good CONDUCTOR of ELECTRICITY and is used for making wire, pipes and coins. Its chief ALLOYS are brass and bronze. Its compounds are used as pesticides and pigments. COPPER is an important TRACE ELEMENT in many plants and animals. At. no. 29; r.a.m. 63.546.

copper(I) (chemistry) An alternative term for CUPROUS.

copper(II) chloride (chemistry) $CuCl_2$ Brown covalently bonded COMPOUND, which forms a green CRYSTALLINE DIHYDRATE. It is used in fireworks to give a green flame and to remove SULPHUR (*USA*: sulfur) in the refining of petroleum. Also termed: CUPRIC CHLORIDE.

copper(II) (chemistry) An alternative term for CUPRIC.

copper(II) carbonate (chemistry) $CuCO_3$ Green CRYSTALLINE COMPOUND which occurs (as the BASIC SALT) in the minerals azurite and malachite. It is also a COMPONENT of verdigris, which forms on COPPER and its ALLOYS exposed to the ATMOSPHERE.

copper(II) oxide (chemistry) CuO INSOLUBLE black SOLID, used as a PIGMENT. Also termed: CUPRIC OXIDE; COPPER OXIDE.

copper(II) sulphate (chemistry) $CuSO_4$ White HYGROSCOPIC COMPOUND, which forms a blue CRYSTALLINE PENTAHYDRATE, $CuSO_4.5H_2O$, used as a wood preservative, FUNGICIDE, dyestuff and in electroplating. Also termed: CUPRIC SULPHATE (*USA*: cupric sulfate); BLUE VITRIOL. (*USA*: copper(II) sulfate).

copper(I) oxide (chemistry) Cu_2O INSOLUBLE red powder, used in rectifiers and as a PIGMENT. Also termed: CUPROUS OXIDE; COPPER OXIDE; CUPRITE; red COPPER OXIDE.

core (1 physics; 2 computing) 1 Magnetic material at the centre (*USA*: center) of a SOLENOID or within the windings of a transformer. 2 ELEMENT in a COMPUTER MEMORY consisting of a piece of magnetic material that can retain a permanent POSITIVE or negative ELECTRIC CHARGE until a CURRENT passes through it (when the CHARGE changes POLARITY).

cornea (histology) TRANSPARENT CONNECTIVE TISSUE at the front surface of the EYE of vertebrates, overlying the IRIS. Togther with the LENS, it focuses incoming LIGHT onto the RETINA.

cornification (histology) An alternative term for KERATINIZATION.

coronary vessels (anatomy) Arteries and veins that carry the BLOOD supplying the HEART MUSCLE in vertebrates.

coronene (chemistry) Aromatic ORGANIC COMPOUND which consists of six (or seven) BENZENE RINGS fused to form a circle.

corpus callosum (histology) Thick bundle of NERVE FIBRES (*USA*: nerve fibers) in the middle of the BRAIN that connects the two CEREBRAL HEMISPHERES.

corpus luteum (histology/ biochemistry) Yellow body formed in the OVARY of female mammals which produces the HORMONE PROGESTERONE. It develops from the Graaflan FOLLICLE after OVULATION. If FERTILIZATION does not occur, the CORPUS LUTEUM degenerates.

corresponding angle (mathematics) In geometry, one of a pair of angles on the same side of a line (TRANSVERSAL) that cuts two other lines; the angles are between the TRANSVERSAL and the other lines. If the two other lines are parallel, the corresponding angles are equal.

See also ALTERNATE ANGLE.

corrosive sublimate (chemistry) An alternative term for MERCURY(II) CHLORIDE.

cortex (anatomy) Outer layer of a structure, *e.g.* the outer layer of CELLS of the ADRENAL GLAND or BRAIN.

See also MEDULLA.

corticosteroid (biochemistry) HORMONE secreted by the ADRENAL CORTEX, which controls SODIUM and WATER METABOLISM as well as GLYCOGEN formation.

corticotrophin (biochemistry) An alternative term for ADRENOCORTICOTROPHIC HORMONE (ACTH).

cortisol (pharmacology) *See* HYDRO-CORTISONE.

cortisone (biochemistry/ pharmacology) HORMONE isolated from the ADRENAL CORTEX, used in the TREATMENT of rheumatoid ARTHRITIS and other inflammatory conditions. Also termed: 17-hydroxy- 11-dehydrocorticosterone.

costal (anatomy) Concerning the ribs.

coulomb (C) (measurement) SI UNIT of ELECTRIC CHARGE, defined as the quantity of ELECTRICITY transported by a CURRENT of 1 AMPERE in 1 second. It was named after the French physicist Charles Coulomb (1736-1806).

counter (1 physics; 2 computing) 1 An electronic apparatus for detecting and counting particles, usually by making them generate pulses of ELECTRIC CURRENT; the actual counting CIRCUIT is a scaler. 2 Any device that accumulates totals (*e.g.* of repeated PROGRAM loops or cards passing through a punched CARD READER).

couple (physics) A pair of equal and parallel forces acting in opposite directions upon an OBJECT. This produces a turning effect (torque) equal to one of the forces times the distance between them.

coupling (physics) Connection between two oscillating systems.

covalent bond (chemistry) CHEMICAL BOND that results from the sharing of a pair of electrons between two atoms.

See also CO-ORDINATE BOND; IONIC BOND.

covalent compound (chemistry) Chemical COMPOUND in which the atoms are covalently bonded.

covalent radius (chemistry) Effective RADIUS of an ATOM involved in a COVALENT BOND.

Cowper's gland (anatomy) One of a pair of small GLANDS located below the PROSTATE GLAND and connected to the URETHRA which produces FLUID for SEMEN. It was named after the British anatomist William Cowper (1666-1709).

Coxsackie virus (virology) Member of a GROUP of VIRUSES that cause inflammatory diseases in human beings. It was named after the city in New York state where it was first found.

CP (medical) An abbreviation of 'C'erebral 'P'alsy.

CPD (1 education; 2 haematology) An abbreviation of 'C'ontinuing 'P'rofessional 'D'evelopment. 2 An abbreviation of 'C'itrate-'P'hosphate-'D'extrose anticoagulant.

cpd (chemistry) An abbreviation of 'c'om'p'oun'd'.

C peptide (physiology/ biochemistry) An abbreviation of 'C'onnecting 'peptide'.

CPR (physiology/ medical) An abbreviation of 'C'ardio'P'ulmonary 'R'esuscitation.

cps (measurement) An abbreviation of 'c'ycles 'p'er 's'econd.

CR (physiology) An abbreviation of 'C'onditioned 'R'eflex.

Cr. (physiology/ biochemistry) An abbreviation of 'Cr'eatinine.

cranial (anatomy) Relating to the CRANIUM and BRAIN.

cranial nerve (histology) One of the 10 to 12 pairs of NERVES connected directly with a VERTEBRATE'S BRAIN and supplying the SENSE ORGANS, muscles of the HEAD and neck and abdominal organs. Together with the SPINAL NERVES they make up the PERIPHERAL NERVOUS SYSTEM.

cranium (anatomy) Part of the SKULL that encloses and protects the BRAIN, consisting of eight fused bones in human beings.

cream of tartar (chemistry) An alternative term for POTASSIUM hydrogentartrate.

creatine (biochemistry) $NH_2C(NH)N(CH_3)$-CH_2COOH White CRYSTALLINE AMINO ACID present in MUSCLE, where it plays an important role in MUSCLE contraction. It is broken down to CREATININE.

creatinine (biochemistry) $C_4H_7N_3O$ HETEROCYCLIC CRYSTALLINE SOLID formed by the breakdown of CREATINE and excreted in URINE.

Creutzfeldt-Jacob disease (medical) A rapidly progressive transmissible disease of the nervous system associated with an abnormal protein called a prion, which causes death within a few months of onset. Named after the German psychiatrist Hans Gerhard Creutzfeldt

(1885-1964) and the German neurologist Alfons Maria Jakob (1884-1931).

CRH (physiology/ biochemistry) An abbreviation of 'C'orticotropin-'R'eleasing 'H'ormone.

critical angle (optics) The smallest ANGLE OF INCIDENCE at which total internal REFLECTION occurs.

critical pressure (physics) PRESSURE necessary to condense a substance at its CRITICAL TEMPERATURE.

critical state (physics) Conditions of TEMPERATURE and PRESSURE at which the LIQUID and GAS phases become one PHASE, *i.e.* they have the same DENSITY.

critical temperature (1, 2 physics) 1 TEMPERATURE above which a GAS cannot be liquefied (no MATTER how high the PRESSURE). 2 TEMPERATURE at which a magnetic material loses its MAGNETISM. Also termed: Curie point.

critical volume (physics) VOLUME of one UNIT of MASS of a substance at its CRITICAL PRESSURE and CRITICAL TEMPERATURE.

CRO (equipment) An abbreviation of 'c'athode-'r'ay 'o'scilloscope.

cross linkage (chemistry) Cross-linking between chains within a POLYMER.

crossing over (genetics) Exchange of material between HOMOLOGOUS CHROMO-SOMES during MEIOSIS (CELL DIVISION). It is the mechanism that alters the pattern of genes in the chromosomes of offspring, giving the genetic VARIATION associated with SEXUAL REPRODUCTION.

CrP (physiology/ biochemistry) An abbreviation of 'Cr'eatinine 'P'hosphate.

CRT (physics) An abbreviation for 'C'athode 'R'ay 'T'ube.

cryogenics (physics) Branch of physics that involves low temperatures and their effects.

Crypto. (parasitology) An abbreviation of '*Cryto'sporidium.*

cryst. (chemistry) An abbreviation of 'cryst'al/ 'cryst'alline.

crystal lattice (crystallography) Regular arrangement of atoms or ions in a crystal.

crystalline (crystallography) Having the form of crystals, as opposed to being AMORPHOUS.

crystallization (crystallography) Process in which crystals form from a molten MASS or SOLUTION.

crystallog. (chemistry) An abbreviation of 'crystallog'raphy.

crystallography (chemistry) Study of crystals.

crystalloid (physics) Substance that is not a COLLOID and can therefore pass through a SEMIPERMEABLE MEMBRANE.

crystd (chemistry) An abbreviation of 'cryst'allise'd'.

crystn (chemistry) An abbreviation of 'cryst'allisatio'n'.

CS (physiology/ biochemistry) An abbreviation of 'C'onditioned 'S'timulus.

Cs (chemistry) CHEMICAL SYMBOL for CAESIUM (*USA*: cesium).

CSA (1 quality standards; 2 Immunology) 1 An abbreviation of 'C'anadian 'S'tandards 'A'ssociation. 2 An abbreviation of 'C'olony 'S'timulating 'A'ctivity.

CSF (1 anatomy; 2 physiology) 1 An abbreviation of 'C'erebro'S'pinal 'F'luid; 2 An abbreviation of 'C'olony-'S'timulating 'F'actor.

CSLT (society) An abbreviation of 'C'anadian 'S'ociety of 'L'aboratory 'T'echnologists.

CSM (medical) An abbreviation of 'C'erebro'S'pinal 'M'eningitis.

CSO (education) An abbreviation of 'C'hief 'S'cientific 'O'fficer.

CST (education) An abbreviation of 'C'ollege of 'S'cience and 'T'echnology.

C_{19} steroids (physiology/ biochemistry) A symbol for steroids containing 19 carbon atoms.

C_{21} steroids (physiology/ biochemistry) A symbol for steroids containing 21 carbon atoms.

CT (radiology) An abbreviation for 'C'omputerized 'T'omography.

CTA (society) An abbreviation of 'C'anadian 'T'uberculosis 'A'ssociation.

C terminal (physiology/ biochemistry) A term signifying an end to peptide or PROTEIN having a free -COOH group.

CTP (physiology/ biochemistry) Abbreviation of 'C'ytidine 'T'ri'P'hosphate.

Cu (chemistry) CHEMICAL SYMBOL for COPPER. [The symbol is derived from Latin, 'cuprum'.]

cu. (measurement) An abbreviation of 'cu'bic.

cu. ft (measurement) An abbreviation of 'cu'bic 'f'ee't'/ 'f'oo't'.

cu. in. (measurement) An abbreviation of 'cu'bic 'in'ch.

cubic (cu.) (measurement) Of three dimensions.

cupric (chemistry) BIVALENT COPPER. Also termed: COPPER(II).

cuprite (chemistry) Mineral form of COPPER(I) OXIDE.

cuprous (chemistry) MONOVALENT COPPER. Also termed: COPPER(I).

curie (Ci) (measurement) Measure of RADIOACTIVITY. 1 Ci = 3.700 x 10^{10} disintegrations per second. It was named after the Polish-born French scientist Marie Curie (1867-1934). It has been replaced in SI UNITS by the BECQUEREL.

curium Cm (chemistry) RADIOACTIVE ELEMENT in GROUP IIIA of the PERIODIC TABLE (one of the ACTINIDES), made by the alpha-PARTICLE bombardment of PLUTONIUM-239. It has several isotopes, with half-lives up to 1.7 x 10^7 years. At. no. 96; r.a.m. 247 (most STABLE ISOTOPE).

cusp (1 mathematics; 2 anatomy) 1 In CO-ORDINATE geometry, point on a curve where it crosses itself, the two branches being on opposite sides of a common tangent. 2 The pointed part of a TOOTH.

CV (1 measurement; 2 medical; 3 physiology) 1 Abbreviation of 'C'alorific 'V'alue. 2 An abbreviation of 'C'ardio'V'ascular. 3 An abbreviation of 'C'losing 'V'olume.

CVA (medical) An abbreviation of 'C'erebro-'V'ascular 'A'ccident.

CVR (physiology) An abbreviation of 'C'erebral 'V'ascular 'R'esistance.

cw (general terminology) An abbreviation of 'c'lock'w'ise.

CY (chemistry) An abbreviation of 'CY'anide.

cy (general terminology) An abbreviation of 'c'apacit'y'.

cyanide (chemistry) COMPOUND containing the CYANIDE ION (CN-); a SALT of HYDROCYANIC ACID (HCN). All cyanides are highly poisonous.

cyanobacteria (microbiology) An alternative term for the CYANOPHYTA.

cyanoferrate (chemistry) *See* FERRICYANIDE; FERROCYANIDE.

cyanogen (chemistry) NCCN Colourless (*USA*: colorless) highly poisonous GAS made by the ACTION of acids on cyanides.

Cyanophyta (microbiology) DIVISION of single-celled, photosynthetic, PROKARYOTIC organisms. Cyanophytes sometimes join together in colonies, and are most commonly found in WATER. Also termed: BLUE-GREEN ALGAE; CYANOBACTERIA; Cyanophyceae.

cycle (physics) One of a repeating SERIES of similar changes. *e.g.* in a WAVE motion or vibration. One CYCLE is equal to the PERIOD of the motion; the number of cycles per UNIT time is its FREQUENCY. A FREQUENCY of 1 CYCLE per second = 1 hertz.

cyclic (chemistry) Describing the MOLECULE of any (usually organic) COMPOUND whose atoms form a ring. BENZENE and the cycloALKANES are simple CYCLIC compounds.

See also ACYCLIC COMPOUND; ALICYCLIC COMPOUNDS; CARBOCYCLIC; HETEROCYCLIC.)

cyclicAMP (physiology/ biochemistry) An abbreviation of 'cyclic' 'A'denosine 3',5'-'M'ono'P'hosphate.

cyclizine (pharmacology) An ANTIHISTAMINE drug which can be administered orally or by injection as an ANTINAUSEANT.

cycloalkane (chemistry) Saturated CYCLIC HYDROCARBON whose MOLECULE has a ring of CARBON atoms, GENERAL FORMULA C_nH_{2n}; *e.g.* cyclohexane, C_6H_{12}.

cyclophosphamide (pharmacology) A cytotoxic drug that acts by interfering with DNA and so preventing CELL replication. It is used as an ANTICANCER AGENT and also has uses as an immuno-suppressant.

cyclosporin (pharmacology) An immuno-suppressant drug that can be administered orally or by INTRAVENOUS infusion to limit tissue rejection during and following organ transplant surgery.

cyclopenthiazide (pharmacology) A DIURETIC of the THIAZIDE class which can be administered orally as a hypertensive, and in the treatment of OEDEMA (*USA*: edema).

cyproterone acetate (pharmacology) A sex HORMONE anAGONIST that reduces the effects of ANDROGENS that is administered as an ANTICANCER treatment for cancer of the prostate gland.

cysteine (biochemistry) $HSCH_2CH(NH_2)$-COOH AMINO ACID found in proteins.

cystic fibrosis (medical/ genetics) A hereditary disease in which a thick MUCUS is produced that obstructs intestinal GLANDS, PANCREAS and bronchi. Severe respiratory infections are a common complication. The GENE responsible was known by the early 1980s to be situated on CHROMOSOME 7, and was found, isolated and cloned in 1989. It differs from the equivalent NORMAL GENE in having a deletion of three BASE-pairs (*i.e.* one codon) so that one AMINO ACID is missing from the GENE PRODUCT. The fact that the GENE has been identified means that in most cases carriers of the GENE can now be identified, and prenatal diagnosis carried out.

cystine (biochemistry) $(SCH_2CH(NH_2)$-COOH$)_2$ Dimeric form of the AMINO ACID CYSTEINE, found in KERATIN.

cystinuria (biochemistry) The abnormal presence in the urine of the amino acid cystine, usually as a result of an inherited kidney tubule defect that allows some amino acids to pass into the urine from the blood.

cytochrome (biochemistry) RESPIRATORY PIGMENT found in organisms that use AEROBIC RESPIRATION.

cytochrome b (biochemistry) A microsomal CYTOCHROME involved in such metabolic activities as FATTY ACID desaturation.

cytochrome c (biochemistry) A respiratory chain enzyme having the same prosthetic group as haemoglobin (*USA*: hemoglobin).

cytochrome oxidase stain (histology) ENZYME histochemical staining technique.

cytochrome P450 (biochemistry) *See* P450.

cytogenetics (genetics) The scientific study of the number, BEHAVIOUR (*USA*: behavior) and MORPHOLOGY of chromosomes as a means of understanding the genetics of an organism.

cytokines (immunology) Substances, usually peptides or proteins, that act as GROWTH factors, *i.e.* affect the GROWTH, DIVISION or differentiation of CELLS. Examples include INTERFERON and PLATELET derived GROWTH FACTOR.

cytology (medical) The study of living CELLS, their ORIGIN, structure, FUNCTION and PATHOLOGY.

cytomegalovirus (CMV) (virology) One of a GROUP of' highly HOST-specific HERPES VIRUSES that affect humans and other animals. They generally produce mild flu-like symptoms but infections can be more severe and in the immunosuppressed it may cause pneumonia.

cytoplasm (cytology) PROTOPLASM of a CELL other than that of the NUCLEUS.

cytosine (biochemistry) Colourless (*USA*: colorless) CRYSTALLINE COMPOUND, derived from PYRIMIDINE. It is a major constituent of DNA and RNA. Also termed: 4-amino-2(H)-pyrimidinone.

cytosol (histology/ cytology) A watery material remaining when all the organelles and membranes have been removed from an homogenate of CELLS by centrifugation.

cytotoxic (1 toxicology; 2 pharmacology)
1 Poisonous to CELLS. 2 Describing a drug
that destroys or prevents the replication
of CELLS, used in CHEMOTHERAPY to treat
CANCER.

CZI (physiology/ biochemistry) An
abbreviation of 'C'rystalline 'Z'inc
'I'nsulin.

D

D (1 chemistry; 2 biochemistry) 1 CHEMICAL SYMBOL for DEUTERIUM. 2 Symbol for aspartic acid.

d (1 measurement; 2 physics; 3 medical; 4 general terminology) 1 An abbreviation of prefix 'd'eci, 10^{-1}. 2 An abbreviation of 'd'euteron. 3 An abbreviation of 'd'ied. 4 An abbreviation of 'd'ay.

D- (biochemistry) A symbol for the geometric isomer Of L- form of chemical compound.

Da (chemistry) CHEMICAL SYMBOL for davyum.

da (measurement) Prefix m eaning 10, used with units of measurement. Also termed deca.

dB (measurement) An abbreviation of 'd'eci'B'el.

DBP (physiology/ biochemistry) An abbreviation of 'Vitamin 'D'-'B'inding 'P'rotein.

dc (physics) An abbreviation of 'd'irect 'c'urrent.

dacryo (medical) Prefix denoting tears or the lacrimal system.

DAG (biochemistry) An abbreviation of 'D'i'A'cyl'G'lycerol.

dag (measurement) An abbreviation of 'd'ek'ag'ram (10 grams). Also termed decagram.

dalton (measurement) An alternative term for ATOMIC MASS UNIT.

Dalton's atomic theory (physics) Theory that states that MATTER consists of tiny particles (atoms), and that all the atoms of a particular ELEMENT are exactly alike, but different from the atoms of other elements in BEHAVIOUR (*USA*: behavior) and MASS. The theory also states that chemical ACTION takes place as a result of attraction between atoms, but it fails to account satisfactorily for the VOLUME relationships that exist between combining gases. It was proposed by the British scientist John Dalton (1766-1844).

Dalton's law of partial pressures (physics) In a MIXTURE of gases, the PRESSURE exerted by one of the COMPONENT gases is the same as if it alone occupied the total VOLUME.

damping (physics) REDUCTION in the AMPLITUDE of a waveform or oscillation.

danazol (pharmacology) A HORMONE ANTAGONIST which acts as an antioestrogen and antiprogesterone drug, that has weak ANDROGEN activity. It can be administered orally to inhibit the release of pituitary HORMONES, gonadotrophins, to treat a variety of conditions including endometriosis and menstrual disorders.

dander (immunology) Small scales of ANIMAL SKIN, HAIR or feathers. DANDER commonly cause allergic effects, especially asthma.

Daniell cell (physics) ELECTROLYTIC CELL that consists of a ZINC HALF-CELL and a COPPER HALF-CELL, usually arranged as a ZINC CATHODE and a COPPER ANODE dipping into an ELECTROLYTE of DILUTE SULPHURIC ACID (*USA*: sulfuric acid).

DAP&E (education) An abbreviation of 'D'iploma in 'A'pplied 'P'arasitology and 'E'ntomology.

Daphnia magna (toxicology) A standard INVERTEBRATE used for aquatic toxicology tests. The common name is 'water flea'.

DApp.Sc. (education) An abbreviation of 'D'octor of 'App'lied 'Sc'ience.

daraf (measurement) UNIT of the elastance of an electrical COMPONENT. It is the RECIPROCAL of CAPACITANCE (the word is farad backwards).

darwin (measurement/ genetics) A UNIT of evolutionary change. A darwin is equal to a change, increase or decrease, in any one CHARACTER by a FACTOR of 2.7 per million years. As this is a very fast rate of change, most evolutionary change is expressed in millidarwins.

Darwinism (biology) Theory of EVOLUTION which states that living organisms arise in their different forms by gradual change over many generations, and that this process is governed by NATURAL SELECTION. It was proposed by the British naturalist Charles Darwin (1809-82).

data (statistics) Collection of information, often referring to results of a statistical study or to information supplied to, processed by or provided by a COMPUTER. The plural of 'datum'.

data bank (computing) An alternative term for a DATA BASE.

data base (1, 2 computing) 1 Organized collection of DATA that is held on a COMPUTER, where it is regularly updated and can easily be accessed (often by many users). Also termed: DATA BANK. 2 APPLICATIONS PROGRAM that controls and makes use of a DATA BASE.

data base management system (DBMS) (computing) COMPUTER SOFTWARE designed to establish and maintain a DATA BASE.

data processing (DP) (computing) The process of inputting, storing, and manipulating large amounts of information, using a COMPUTER.

data transmission (computing) Transfer of DATA between outstations and a central COMPUTER or between different COMPUTER systems.

dative bond (chemistry) An alternative term for a CO-ORDINATE BOND.

daughter cell (cytology) One of the two CELLS produced when a CELL divides, *e.g.* as a result of MITOSIS.

daughter nucleus (cytology) One of the two nuclei produced when the NUCLEUS of a CELL divides.

db (measurement) An abbreviation of 'd'eci'b'el. Also termed dB.

dB (measurement) *See* db.

dbl (general terminology) An abbreviation of 'd'ou'bl'e.

DBMS (computing) An abbreviation of 'D'ata 'B'ase 'M'anagement 'S'ystem.

DC (physics) An abbreviation of 'D'irect 'C'urrent. Also termed: d.c.

D & C (medical) An abbreviation of 'D'ilatation 'and' 'C'urettage.

DCl. Sc. (education) An abbreviation of 'D'octor of 'Cl'inical 'Sc'ience.

dcm (measurement) An abbreviation of 'd'e'c'a'm'etre (*USA*: decameter).

DCP (education) An abbreviation of 'D'iploma of 'C'linical 'P'athology.

DCPath. (education) An abbreviation of 'D'iploma of the 'C'ollege of 'Path'ologists.

DCSO (governing body) An abbreviation of 'D'eputy 'C'hief 'S'cientific 'O'fficer.

DCTD (education) An abbreviation of 'D'iploma in 'C'hest and 'T'uberculous 'D'iseases.

DDAVP (biochemistry) An abbreviation of 1- 'D'eamino- 8- 'D'- 'A'rginine 'V'aso- 'P'ression.

DDR (education) An abbreviation of 'D'iploma in 'D'iagnostic 'R'adiology.

DEA (biochemistry) An abbreviation of 'D'ehydro'E'pi'A'ndrosterone.

dead (medical) Deceased.

deaminase (biochemistry) ENZYME that catalyses the removal of an AMINO GROUP ($-NH_2$) from an organic MOLECULE.

deamination (biochemistry) Enzymatic removal of an AMINO GROUP ($-NH_2$) from a COMPOUND. The process is important in the breakdown of AMINO ACIDS in the LIVER and KIDNEY. AMMONIA formed by DEAMINATION is converted to UREA and excreted.

DEAS (biochemistry) An abbreviation of 'D'ehydro'E'pi'A'ndrosterone 'S'ulphate (*USA*: Dehydroepiandrosterone sulfate).

debug (computing) To remove a fault in a COMPUTER PROGRAM; hence, by analogy, to correct any form of fault.

Debye-Hückel theory (physics) Theory that explains variations from the ideal BEHAVIOUR (*USA*: behavior) of electrolytes in terms of interionic attraction, and assumes that electrolytes in SOLUTION are completely dissociated into charged ions. It was named after the Dutch physicists Peter Debye (1884-1966) and Erich Hückel (1896 -1980).

dec. (1 medical; 2 measurement) 1 An abbreviation of 'dec'eased. 2 An abbreviation of 'dec'imetre (*USA*: decimeter).

deca (measurement) Prefix meaning 10 times, used with units of measurement. Also termed da; deka.

decalcification (1 biochemistry; 2 histology) 1 Loss of CALCIUM and other MINERAL SALTS from the normally mineralized tissues, BONE and TEETH. 2 A histological LABORATORY technique.

decant (chemistry) Carefully pour away the LIQUID above a PRECIPITATE, once it has settled.

decay (1 biology; 2 radiology) 1 Natural breakdown of an organic substance; DECOMPOSITION. 2 Breakdown, through RADIOACTIVITY, of a RADIOACTIVE substance. The rate of such DECAY is typically an EXPONENTIAL FUNCTION.

See also HALF-LIFE.

deceased (dec.) (medical) Pertaining to a person who has died.

deci (measurement) Prefix meaning one-tenth, used with units of measurements.

decibel (db or dB) (measurement) UNIT used for comparing POWER levels (on a LOGARITHMIC SCALE); one-tenth of a BEL. It is commonly used in comparisons of sound INTENSITY.

See also BEL.

decigram (dg) (measurement) One-tenth of a gram.

decim. (measurement) An abbreviation of 'decim'etre (*USA*: decimeter).

decimal system (mathematics) Number system that uses the BASE 10; *i.e.* it uses the digits 1 to 9 and 0.

See also BINARY NOTATION.

decimetre (dm; decim.) (measurement) One-tenth of a METRE (*USA*: meter). (*USA*: decimeter).

decomposer (microbiology) Saprophytic organism that breaks down organic materials into simple molecules, *e.g.* FUNGI.

decomposition (1 chemistry; 2 microbiology) 1 Breaking down of a chemical COMPOUND into its COMPONENT parts (elements or simpler substances), often brought about by HEAT, LIGHT or ELECTROLYSIS. *See also* DOUBLE DECOMPOSITION. 2 Rotting of a dead organism, often brought about by BACTERIA or FUNGI.

decubitus ulcers (medical) Bedsores. ulcers caused by unduly sustained SKIN PRESSURE.

defect (chemistry/ crystallography) An irregularity in the ordered arrangement of atoms, ions or electrons in a crystal.

deficiency disease (medical/ biochemistry) Disorder brought about by the lack of a certain food substance in the diet, *e.g.* a VITAMIN, mineral or AMINO ACID.

definite integral (mathematics) INTEGRAL that has exact limits.

deg. (measurement) An abbreviation of 'deg're e.

deglutition (physiology) Another term for swallowing.

degradation (1 chemistry; 2 physics) 1 The conversion of a MOLECULE into simpler components. 2 The irreversible loss of ENERGY available to do WORK.

degree (1, 2 measurement) 1 UNIT of difference in TEMPERATURE used in TEMPERATURE SCALES. 2 UNIT derived by dividing a circle into 360 segments, used to measure angles and describe direction. It is subdivided into minutes and seconds (of ARC). Both types of degrees have the symbol °.

degree of freedom (physics) One of several VARIABLE factors, *e.g.* TEMPERATURE, PRESSURE and CONCENTRATION, that must be made CONSTANT for the condition of a system at EQUILIBRIUM to be defined.

dehalogenation (biochemistry) The process of removal of HALOGEN substituents from organic chemicals.

dehydrating agent (chemistry) An alternative term for a DESICCANT.

dehydration (1 chemistry; 2 medical) 1 Elimination of WATER from a substance or organism. 2 Lack of WATER in the body.

dehydrogenase (biochemistry) An ENZYME that activates OXIDATION-REDUCTION RE-ACTIONS by the removal of a pair of HYDROGEN atoms from a MOLECULE.

deionization (chemistry) A method of purifying or otherwise altering the composition of a SOLUTION using ION EXCHANGE.

deka (measurement) Prefix meaning 10, used with units of measurement. Also termed da; deca.

deliquescence (chemistry) The gradual change undergone by certain substances that absorb WATER from the ATMOSPHERE to become first damp and then AQUEOUS SOLUTIONS.

deliquescent (chemistry) Describing a substance that exhibits DELIQUESCENCE.

delocalization (chemistry) Phenomenon that occurs in certain molecules, *e.g.* BENZENE. Some of the electrons involved in bonding the atoms are not restricted to one particular BOND, but are free to move between two or more bonds. The electrical CONDUCTIVITY of metals is due to the presence of delocalized electrons.

See also AROMATICITY.

delta ray (physics) ELECTRON that is ejected from an ATOM when it is struck by a high-ENERGY PARTICLE.

demise (medical) Death.

denature (chemistry) To unfold the structure of the POLYPEPTIDE chain of a PROTEIN by exposing it to TEMPERATURE or extremes of PH. This results in the loss of biological activity and a decrease in SOLUBILITY.

dendrite (1 biology; 2 crystallography) 1 An elongated process from a NERVE CELL that projects it towards another NERVE CELL. Also termed: DENDRON. 2 A branching crystal, such as occurs in some rocks and minerals.

dendron (1 biology; 2 crystallography) An alternative term for DENDRITE.

denitrification (microbiology) Process that occurs in organisms, *e.g.* BACTERIA in soil, which breaks down NITRATES and nitrites, with the liberation of NITROGEN.

denominator (mathematics) The lower number of a FRACTION (the upper number of the NUMERATOR); *e.g.* in the fractions 2/3, 7/12 and 83/100, the denominators are 3, 12 and 100.

See also COMMON DENOMINATOR.

dens. (physics) An abbreviation of 'dens'ity.

density (1 physics; 2 statistics) 1 MASS of a UNIT VOLUME of a substance. For an OBJECT of MASS m and VOLUME V, the DENSITY d is m/V. It is commonly expressed in units such as g cm^{-3} (although the SI UNIT is kg m^{-3}). 2 Number of items in a defined surface AREA (*e.g.* population DENSITY, CHARGE DENSITY).

DEnt. (education) An abbreviation of 'D'octor of 'Ent'omology.

dent. (medical) An abbreviation of 'dent'al.

dental formula (anatomy) Notation that shows the number of each kind of TOOTH possessed by a mammal. The number of TEETH in one side of the JAW is given, with the number in the upper JAW before that in the lower JAW, and in the ORDER incisors, canines, premolars, molars; *e.g.* the human FORMULA is 2/2 1/1 2/2 3/3.

dentine (histology) Layer that occurs under the ENAMEL of TEETH. It is similar to BONE, but harder, and is perforated by thin extensions from TOOTH-forming CELLS.

deoxyribonucleic acid (DNA) (molecular biology) NUCLEIC ACID that is usually referred to by its abbreviation. The long thread-like MOLECULE consists of a double HELIX of polynucleotides held together by HYDROGEN BONDS. DNA is found chiefly in chromosomes, and is the material that carries the hereditary information of all living organisms (although most, but not all, VIRUSES have only RIBONUCLEIC ACID, RNA).

deoxyribonucleotides (molecular biology) Compounds that are the FUNDAMENTAL UNITS of DNA. Each nuelcotide contains a nitrogenous BASE, a PENTOSE SUGAR and phosphoric ACID. The four bases CHARACTERISTIC of DEOXYRIBONUCLEOTIDES are ADENINE, GUANINE, CYTOSINE and THYMINE.

See also DEOXYRIBONUCLEIC ACID.

deoxyribose (biochemistry) The SUGAR that forms part of the structure of DNA.

dependence (1 medical; 2 statistics) 1 A condition that is said to exist when equivalent or increasing doses of a drug are necessary to avoid WITHDRAWAL SYMPTOMS. 2 Changes in one VARIABLE occurring systematically with changes in another.

depolarization (physics/ chemistry) Removal or prevention of electrical POLARITY or POLARIZATION.

depression of freezing point (physics) REDUCTION of the FREEZING POINT of a LIQUID when a SOLID is dissolved in it. At CONSTANT PRESSURE and for DILUTE solutions of a non-VOLATILE SOLVENT, the depression of the FREEZING POINT is directly proportional to the CONCENTRATION of the solutes.

derivative (1 chemistry; 2 mathematics) 1 A COMPOUND, usually organic, obtained from another COMPOUND. 2 A COEFFICIENT representing the rate of change of one quantity.

dermal (medical) Pertaining to the SKIN.

dermatitis (medical) INFLAMMATION of the SKIN.

dermis (histology) Layer of SKIN that is the innermost of the two main layers. It is composed of CONNECTIVE TISSUE and contains BLOOD, LYMPH vessels, sensory NERVES, HAIR follicles, SWEAT GLANDS and some MUSCLE CELLS.

See also EPIDERMIS.

DES (pharmacology) An abbreviation of 'D'i'E'thyl'S'tilbestrol.

desiccant (chemistry) Substance that absorbs WATER and can therefore be used as a drying agent or to prevent DELIQUESCENCE (*e.g.* ANHYDROUS CALCIUM CHLORIDE, SILICA GEL), often used in a DESICCATOR. Also termed: DEHYDRATING AGENT.

desiccator (laboratory equipment) Apparatus used for drying substances or preventing DELIQUESCENCE, *e.g.* a closed GLASS VESSEL containing a DESICCANT.

desk top publishing (DTP) (computing) Technique that uses a microcomputer linked to a WORD PROCESSOR, with access to various type founts and justification programs, and a LASER PRINTER to produce multiple copies of a document that rivals conventional printing in quality. The addition of a SCANNER allows the introduction of graphics or illustrations.

desorption (1, 2 chemistry) 1 Reverse process to ADSORPTION. 2 Removal of an adsorbate from an ADSORBENT in CHROMATOGRAPHY.

detergent (chemistry) SURFACTANT that is used as a cleaning agent. Detergents are particularly useful for cleaning because they lower SURFACE TENSION and emulsify FATS AND OILS (allowing them to go into SOLUTION with WATER without forming a scum with any of the substances that cause HARDNESS OF WATER). Soaps act in a similar way, but form an INSOLUBLE scum in hard WATER.

determinant (1 immunology; 2 biology; 3 mathematics) 1 Region or regions of an ANTIGEN MOLECULE required for its recognition (binding) by a PARTICLE or ANTIBODY. The selective nature of this molecular INTERACTION confers specificity on the immune REACTION of the ANTIBODY-producer. 2 FACTOR that transmits inherited characteristics, *e.g.* a GENE. 3 Quantity obtained by adding products of elements of a square MATRIX according to certain rules.

deuterated compound (chemistry) Substance in which ordinary HYDROGEN has been replaced by DEUTERIUM.

deuterium D$_2$ (chemistry) One of the three isotopes of HYDROGEN, having one NEUTRON and one PROTON in its NUCLEUS. R.a.m. 2.0141. Also termed: heavy HYDROGEN.

See also TRITIUM.

deuterium oxide (chemistry) D$_2$O Chemical name of heavy WATER.

deuteron (chemistry) Positively charged PARTICLE that is composed of one NEUTRON and one PROTON; it is the NUCLEUS of a DEUTERIUM ATOM.

deviation (mathematics) The amount by which one value in a SET of values differs from the ARITHMETIC MEAN.

See also STANDARD DEVIATION.

devitrification (optics) Loss of transparency, *e.g.* in GLASS, caused by CRYSTALLIZATION.

dexamethasone (pharmacology) A corticosteroid and ANTI-INFLAMMATORY drug that, administered orally, topically or by injection, can be used for a variety of purposes including the suppression of allergic and inflammatory conditions.

dextrin (chemistry) POLYSACCHARIDE of INTERMEDIATE chain length produced from the ACTION of AMYLASES on STARCH.

dextromoethorphan hydrobromide (pharmacology) A drug that is used to suppress coughing which is used in a variety of linctuses and syrups.

dextronic acid (chemistry) An alternative term for gluconic ACID.

dextrorotatory (chemistry) Describing an OPTICALLY ACTIVE COMPOUND that causes the plane of POLARIZED LIGHT to rotate in a clockwise direction. It is indicated by the prefix (+)- or *d-*.

dextrose (chemistry) An alternative term for GLUCOSE.

df (statistics) An abbreviation for 'd'egrees of 'f'reedom.

DFP (biochemistry) An abbreviation of 'D'iisopropyl 'F'luoro'P'hosphate.

dg (measurement) An abbreviation of 'd'eci'g'ram.

DHEW (governing body) An abbreviation of 'D'epartment of 'H'ealth, 'E'ducation and 'W'elfare.

DHHS (governing body) An abbreviation of 'D'epartment of 'H'ealth and 'H'uman 'S'ervices.

DHP (education) An abbreviation of *'D'iplome en 'H'ygiene 'P'ublique.* [French, meaning 'Diploma in Public Health'.]

DHS (education) An abbreviation of 'D'octor of 'H'ealth 'S'ciences.

DHT (biochemistry) An abbreviation of 'D'i'H'ydro'T'estosterone.

diabetes (medical/ biochemistry) *See* DIABETES MELLITUS.

diabetes mellitus (medical/ biochemistry) A disease in which the supply of insulin is insufficient for the body's needs. Type 1 diabetes results from destruction of the insulin-producing cells in the pancreas by an auto-immune process probably triggered by a virus infection. Type 2 diabetes is due to a relative insufficiency

of INSULIN along with impaired sensitivity to the actions of insulin.

diag. (1 medical; 2, 3 general terminology) 1 An abbreviation of 'diag'nose. 2 An abbreviation of 'diag'onal. 3 An abbreviation of 'diag'ram.

diakinesis (cytology) PHASE of CELL DIVISION that occurs at the final stage of PROPHASE of the first DIVISION in MEIOSIS. During this PHASE the chromosomes become short and thick, forming more chiasmata, the nucleoli and NUCLEAR MEMBRANE disappear, and the spindle appears for the process of DIVISION,

Dial. (chemistry/ pharmacology) An abbreviation of 'dial'lyl-BARBITURIC ACID.

dialysed iron (chemistry) Colloidal SOLUTION of IRON(III) HYDROXIDE, $Fe(OH)_3$. It is a red LIQUID, used in medicine.

dialysis (biochemistry) Separation of colloids from crystalloids using selective DIFFUSION through a SEMIPERMEABLE MEMBRANE. It is the process by which globular proteins can be separated from low-MOLECULAR WEIGHT solutes, as in filtering ('purifying') BLOOD in an artificial KIDNEY machine: the MEMBRANE retains PROTEIN molecules and allows small SOLUTE molecules and WATER to pass through.

diam. (measurement) An abbreviation of 'diam'eter. Also termed dia.

diameter (dia. or diam.) (measurement) The length of a line segment intersecting the circle's centre (*USA*: center) between two points on the circle.

diamorphine hydrochloride (pharmacology) The chemical name of heroin hydrochloride which, administered orally or by injection, is a powerful, additive narcotic ANALGESIC.

diaph. (anatomy) An abbreviation of 'diaph'ragm.

diaphragm (1 anatomy; 2 medical) 1 A sheet of MUSCLE present in mammals, located below the lungs attached to the body wall at the sides and separating the THORAX from the ABDOMEN. During RESPIRATION it forms an important part of the mechanism for filling and expelling AIR from the lungs. 2 A birth-control device fitted over the entrance to the UTERUS to prevent the entry of SPERM. Also termed: Dutch cap.

diarrhoea (medical) The result of too rapid a transit of the BOWEL contents so that there is insufficient time for reabsorption of water from the FAECES (*USA*: FECES). Consequently, the stools are loose, liquid and are passed more frequently than normal. (*USA*: diarrhea).

diastase (biochemistry) An alternative term for AMYLASE.

diastole (physiology) PHASE of the HEARTBEAT in which the HEART undergoes relaxation and refills with BLOOD from the veins. The term also applies to a CONTRACTILE VACUOLE in a CELL when it refills with FLUID.

See also SYSTOLE.

diatomic (chemistry) Describing a MOLECULE that is composed of two identical atoms, *e.g.* O_2, H_2 and Cl_2.

See also ATOMICITY.

diazepam (pharmacology) A benzodiazepine drug which can be administered orally, through suppositories or by injection, as an ANXIOLYTIC, hypnotic, ANTICONVULSANT, sedative, skeletal muscle relaxant and ANTI-EPILEPTIC. It is used in a variety of treatments including the treatment of anxiety and epilepsy.

diazo compound (chemistry) ORGANIC COMPOUND that contains two adjacent NITROGEN atoms, but only one attached to a CARBON ATOM. Formed by DIAZOTIZATION, DIAZO COMPOUNDS are very important in SYNTHESIS, being the starting point of various dyes and drugs.

diazonium compound (chemistry) An ORGANIC COMPOUND of the type $RN_2{}^+X^-$, where R is an ARYL GROUP. The compounds are colourless (*USA*: colorless) solids, extremely SOLUBLE in WATER, used for making AZO DYES. Many of them (particularly the NITRATES) are explosive in the SOLID state.

diazotization (chemistry) Formation of a DIAZO COMPOUND by the INTERACTION of SODIUM NITRITE, an inORGANIC ACID, and a primary aromatic AMINE at low temperatures.

dibasic (chemistry) Describing an ACID that contains two replaceable HYDROGEN atoms in its molecules. *e.g.* CARBONIC ACID, H_2CO_3, SULPHURIC ACID (*USA*: sulfuric acid), H_2SO_4. A DIBASIC ACID can form two types of salts: a NORMAL SALT, in which both HYDROGEN atoms are replaced by a METAL or its equivalent (*e.g.* SODIUM CARBONATE, Na_2CO_3), and an acidic SALT, in which only one HYDROGEN ATOM is replaced, *e.g.* SODIUM HYDROGENSULPHATE (*USA*: sodium hydrogen sulfate) (BISULPHATE [*USA*: bisulfate]), $NaHSO_4$.

dicarboxylic acid (chemistry) ORGANIC ACID that contains two CARBOXYL GROUPS.

dichroism (chemistry) Property of some substances that makes them transmit some colours (*USA*: colors) and reflect others, or which DISPLAY certain colours when viewed from one angle and different colours when viewed from another.

dichromate (chemistry) SALT containing the DICHROMATE(VI) ION ($Cr_2O_7^{2-}$), an OXIDIZING AGENT; *e.g.* POTASSIUM DICHROMATE, $K_2Cr_2O_7$. Also termed: BICHROMATE.

diclofenac sodium (pharmacology) A non-steroidal ANTI-INFLAMMATORY drug (NSAID) which, administered orally, topically as suppositories or by injection, is used as a non-narcotic ANALGESIC and ANTIRHEUMATIC to treat pain and inflammation in rheumatic disease and other musculo-skeletal conditions.

dielectric constant (physics) An alternative term for RELATIVE PERMITTIVITY.

dielectric (physics) Nonconductor of ELECTRICITY in which an ELECTRIC FIELD persists in the presence of an inducing FIELD (but opposes it). A DIELECTRIC is the insulating material in a CAPACITOR.

dielectric strength (physics) Property of an INSULATOR that enables it to withstand electric STRESS without breaking down.

dielectrophoresis (physics) Movement of electrically polarized particles in a VARIABLE ELECTRIC FIELD.

1,1-diethoxyethane (chemistry) An alternative term for acetal.

differential calculus (mathematics) Branch of mathematics that deals with continuously varying quantities. It uses differentiation for calculating rates of change, slopes of curves, maximum and minimum values, etc.

differentiation (mathematics) Method used in CALCULUS to determine the DERIVATIVE f' of a FUNCTION f. If $f'(x) = Ax^n$, $f'(x) = nAx^{n-1}$.

diffraction (physics) Bending of the path of a beam (*e.g.* of LIGHT or electrons) at the edge of an OBJECT.

diffraction grating (optics) Optical device that is used for producing spectra. It consists of a sheet of GLASS or plastic marked with closely spaced parallel lines (as many as 10,000 per centimetre). The spectra are produced by a COMBINATION of DIFFRACTION and INTERFERENCE.

diffusion (chemistry) The process by which a gas or a substance in solution expands, because of the motion of its particles, to fill all of the available volume. *Contrast* ACTIVE TRANSPORT.

diffusion of gases (chemistry) Phenomenon by which gases mix together, reducing any CONCENTRATION GRADIENT to zero. *e.g.* in GAS EXCHANGE between plant leaves and AIR.

See also ACTIVE TRANSPORT.

diffusion of light (physics) Spreading or SCATTERING OF LIGHT.

diffusion of solutions (chemistry) Free movement of molecules or ions of a dissolved substance through a SOLVENT, resulting in complete mixing.

See also OSMOSIS.

diffusion pump (laboratory equipment) Apparatus used to produce a high VACUUM. The PUMP employs MERCURY or oil at low VAPOUR PRESSURE which carries along in its flow molecules of a GAS from a low PRESSURE established by a backing PUMP. Also termed: CONDENSATION PUMP; VACUUM PUMP.

diflunisal (pharmacology) A non-steroidal ANTI-INFLAMMATORY drug (NSAID) which, administered orally, is used as a non-narcotic ANALGESIC and ANTIRHEUMATIC to treat pain and inflammation in rheumatic disease and other musculoskeletal conditions.

di-form (chemistry) Term indicating that a MIXTURE contains the DEXTROROTATORY and the LAEVOROTATORY forms of an OPTICALLY ACTIVE COMPOUND in equal molecular proportions.

digestion (physiology) Breakdown of complex substances in food by ENZYMES in the ALIMENTARY CANAL to produce simpler SOLUBLE compounds, which pass into the body by ABSORPTION and ASSIMILATION. Ultimately carbohydrates (*e.g.* STARCH, SUGAR) are broken down to GLUCOSE, proteins to AMINO ACIDS, and fats to FATTY ACIDS and GLYCEROL.

digit (1 mathematics/ computing; 2 anatomy) 1 A single NUMERAL; an INTEGER under 10. 2 A finger or toe.

digital computer (computing) COMPUTER that operates on DATA supplied and stored in digital or number form.

digital display (equipment) DISPLAY that shows readings of a measuring machine, clock, etc. by displaying NUMERALS.

digitalis (pharmacology) Potent ALKALOID that is extracted from plants of the GENUS *DIGITALIS* (foxgloves). It is used in medicine as a HEART stimulant.

digital/ analog converter (computing) Device that converts digital signals into continuously VARIABLE electrical signals for use by an ANALOG COMPUTER.

digitoxin (pharmacology) A cardiac glycoside derived from the leaf of the *Digitalis* foxglove, which administered orally acts as a cardiac stimulant increasing the force of contraction of the HEART in congestive HEART FAILURE, and as an ANTI-ARRHYTHMIC.

digoxin (pharmacology) A cardiac glycoside, similar to DIGITOXIN, derived from the leaf of the *Digitalis* foxglove, which administered orally or by injection acts as a cardiac stimulant increasing the force of contraction of the HEART in congestive HEART FAILURE, and as an ANTI-ARRHYTHMIC.

dihydrate (chemistry) Chemical (a HYDRATE) whose molecules have two associated molecules of WATER OF CRYSTALLIZATION; *e.g.* SODIUM DICHROMATE, $Na_2Cr_2O_7.2H_2O$.

2,3-dihydroxybutanedioic acid (chemistry) An alternative term for TARTARIC ACID.

Dihydroxyphenylalanine (dopa) (pharmacology) AMINO ACID DERIVATIVE that is a PRECURSOR in the SYNTHESIS of DOPAMINE and has laevorotation (L-DOPA). Found particularly in the ADRENAL GLAND and in some types of beans, it is used in the TREATMENT of PARKINSON'S DISEASE.

dihydroxypurine (chemistry) An alternative term for XANTHINE.

dihydroxysuccinic acid (chemistry) An alternative term for TARTARIC ACID.

dilate (physiology) To widen; to produce DILATION.

113

dilation (physiology) The widening or expansion of an ORGAN, opening, passage or VESSEL. An alternative term: dilatation.

diltiazem hydrochloride (pharmacology) A calcium-channel blocker drug used as an orally administered ANTI-ANGINA drug in the prevention of attacks and as an ANTIHYPERTENSIVE treatment.

diluent (chemistry) SOLVENT used to reduce the strength of a SOLUTION.

dilute (1, 2 chemistry) 1 To reduce the strength of a SOLUTION by adding WATER or other SOLVENT. 2 Describing a SOLUTION in which the amount of SOLUTE is small compared to that of the SOLVENT.

dilution (chemistry) Process that involves the lowering of CONCENTRATION.

dim. (general terminology) An abbreviation of 'dim'ension.

dimenhydrinate (pharmacology) An ANTIHISTAMINE drug which can be administered orally as an ANTINAUSEANT in the treatment of nausea, motion sickness etc.

dimension (mathematics) POWER to which a fundamental UNIT is raised in a derived UNIT; *e.g.* ACCELERATION has the dimensions [LT^{-2}], *i.e.* + 1 for length and - 2 for time, equivalent to length divided by the square of time.

dimensional analysis (mathematics) Prediction of the relationship of quantities. If an equation is correct the dimensions of the quantities on each side must be identical. It is an important way of checking the VALIDITY of an equation.

dimer (chemistry) Chemical formed from two similar MONOMER molecules.

dimethylbenzene (chemistry) An alternative term for XYLENE.

dinitrogen oxide N_2O (chemistry/ medical) Colourless (*USA*: colorless) GAS made by heating AMMONIUM NITRATE and used as an ANAESTHETIC (*USA*: anesthetic). Also termed: NITROGEN OXIDE; NITROUS OXIDE; dental GAS; laughing GAS.

dinoprostone (pharmacology) The prostaglandin E_2, which administered orally, topically as pessaries or by injection causes contractions in the muscular walls of the uterus. It can be used to induce labour or to assist in termination of PREGNANCY.

diode (1, 2 physics) 1 ELECTRON TUBE (VALVE) containing two electrodes, an ANODE and a CATHODE. 2 RECTIFIER made up of a semiconducting crystal with two terminals.

diol (chemistry) ORGANIC COMPOUND containing two HYDROXYL GROUPS and having the GENERAL FORMULA $C_nH_{2n}(OH)_2$. Diols are thick liquids or CRYSTALLINE solids, and some have a sweet TASTE. ETHANE-1,2-DIOL (ETHYLENE GLYCOL) is the simplest DIOL, widely used as a SOLVENT and as an antifreeze agent. Also termed: dihydric ALCOHOL; GLYCOL.

dioptre (measurement) UNIT that is used to express the POWER of a LENS. It is the RECIPROCAL of the FOCAL LENGTH of the LENS in metres. The POWER of a convergent LENS with a FOCAL LENGTH of one METRE is said to be + 1 dioptre. The POWER of a divergent LENS is given a negative value.

dioxan (chemistry) $(CH_2)_2O_2$ Colourless (*USA*: colorless) LIQUID CYCLIC ETHER. It is INERT to many reagents and frequently used in mixtures with WATER to increase the SOLUBILITY of ORGANIC COMPOUNDs such as ALKYL HALIDEs. Also termed: 1,4-DIOXAN.

dioxin (chemistry) $C_{12}H_4Cl_4O_2$ BY-PRODUCT of organic SYNTHESIS (*e.g.* of the disinfectant trichlorophenol) which can cause allergic SKIN reactions. Also termed: 2,3,7,8-tetrachlorodibenzo-*p*-DIOXIN.

dip. (education) An abbreviation of 'dip'loma.

Dip. Pharm (education) An abbreviation of 'Dip'loma in 'Pharm'acy.

Dip.App.Sc. (education) An abbreviation of 'Dip'loma of 'App'lied 'Sc'ience.

Dip.Bac. (education) An abbreviation of 'Dip'loma in 'Bac'teriology.

Dip.BMS (education) An abbreviation of 'Dip'loma in 'B'asic 'M'edical 'S'ciences.

diphenhydramine hydrochloride (pharmacology) An ANTIHISTAMINE drug which can be administered orally for the symptomatic relief of allergic symptoms and as a sedative for relief of occassional insomnia.

diphenoxylate hydrochloride (pharmacology) An opiod anti-diarrhoeal (*USA*: anti-diarrheal) drug used to treat chronic DIARRHOEA (*USA*: diarrhea).

diploid (genetics) In a CELL or organism, describing the existence of chromosomes in HOMOLOGOUS pairs, *i.e.* twice the HAPLOID number (2*n*). Apart from gametes, it is CHARACTERISTIC of all ANIMAL CELLS.

diplotene (genetics) In MEIOSIS, the stage in late PROPHASE when the pairs of chromatids begin to separate from the TETRAD formed by the association of HOMOLOGOUS CHROMOSOMES. Chiasmata can be seen at this stage.

dipole (physics) Pair of equal and opposite ELECTRIC CHARGEs at a (short) distance from each other. Some asymmetric molecules act as dipoles.

dipole moment (physics) PRODUCT of one CHARGE of a DIPOLE and the distance between the charges.

dipso. (medical) An abbreviation of 'dipso'maniac.

dipyridamole (pharmacology) An anti-thrombotic drug administered orally or by injection that prevents blood-clot formation, but does not have the usual action of an ANTICOAGULANT. It acts by preventing platelets sticking together or to surgically inserted objects such as tubes or valves.

dir. (governing body) An abbreviation of 'dir'ector.

direct current (d.c.) (physics) ELECTRIC CURRENT that always flows in the same direction (as opposed to ALTERNATING CURRENT). Also termed: DC.

direct dye (chemistry) Dye that does not require a mordant.

director (dir.) (governing body) The HEAD of a department or institution.

dis. (medical) An abbreviation of 'dis'CHARGE. Also termed disch.

disab. (medical) An abbreviation of 'disab'ility. Also termed disabl.

disaccharide (chemistry) One of the CLASS of common sugars, including LACTOSE and SUCROSE, that can be broken down by HYDROLYSIS, under the ACTION of ENZYMES, to yield two monosaccharides.

disch. (medical) *See* dis.

discharge (1, 2 physics) 1 High-VOLTAGE 'spark' (CURRENT flow) between points of large POTENTIAL difference (*e.g.* lightning); 2 Removal of the CHARGE between the plates of a CAPACITOR by allowing CURRENT to flow out of it; 3 Removal of ENERGY from an ELECTROLYTIC CELL (BATTERY or ACCUMULATOR) by allowing CURRENT to flow out of it. 4. In ELECTROCHEMISTRY, the process by which ions are converted to NEUTRAL atoms at an ELECTRODE during ELECTROLYSIS (by GAIN or loss of electrons).

discriminant (mathematics) Quantity $b^2 - 4ac$, derived from the coefficients of a QUADRATIC EQUATION of GENERAL FORMULA $ax^2 + bx + c = 0$.

disintegration (radiology) Break-up of an atomic NUCLEUS either through bombardment by SUBATOMIC PARTICLES or through RADIOACTIVE DECAY.

disintegration constant (radiology) Probability of a RADIOACTIVE DECAY of an atomic NUCLEUS per UNIT time. Also termed: DECAY CONSTANT; TRANSFORMATION CONSTANT.

disk (computing) Magnetic disc used to RECORD DATA in computers.

See also FLOPPY DISK, HARD DISK.

diskette (computing) An alternative term for a FLOPPY DISK.

dislocation (crystallography) Imperfection in a CRYSTAL LATTICE.

disodium oxide (chemistry) An alternative term for SODIUM monoxide.

disodium tetraborate (chemistry) An alternative term for BORAX.

disp. (pharmacology) An abbreviation of 'disp'ensary.

dispensary (pharmacology) A department of a hospital or clinic supplying drugs and other medical supplies on demand.

dispersion (physics) Splitting of an ELECTROMAGNETIC RADIATION (*e.g.* VISIBLE LIGHT) into its COMPONENT wavelengths when it passes through a medium (because different wavelengths undergo different degrees of DIFFRACTION or REFRACTION).

displacement (mathematics) Position of one point relative to another, including both the distance between the two points and the direction of the first point from the second point.

displacement reaction (chemistry) An alternative term for SUBSTITUTION REACTION.

display (equipment) Short name for a LIQUID-CRYSTAL DISPLAY (LCD) or a visual DISPLAY UNIT (VDU).

dissociation constant (chemistry) EQUILIBRIUM CONSTANT of a DISSOCIATION REACTION, and therefore a measure of the AFFINITY of atoms or molecules in a COMPOUND.

dissociation (chemistry) The temporary reversible chemical DECOMPOSITION of a substance into its COMPONENT atoms or molecules, which often take the form of ions, *e.g.* it occurs when most ionic compounds dissolve in WATER.

distillate (chemistry) Condensed LIQUID obtained by DISTILLATION.

distillation (chemistry) Method for purification or separation of liquids by heating to the BOILING POINT, condensing the VAPOUR, and collecting the DISTILLATE. Formerly, the method was used to produce DISTILLED WATER for chemical experiments and processes that required WATER to be much purer than that in the mains WATER supply. In this application DISTILLATION has been largely superseded by ION EXCHANGE.

distilled water (chemistry) *See* DISTIL-LATION.

distortion (physics) Change from the ideal shape of an OBJECT or IMAGE, or in the form of a WAVE pattern (*e.g.* an electrical signal).

disulphuric acid (chemistry) An alternative term for olcum. (*USA*: disulfuric acid).

DIT (biochemistry) An abbreviation of 'D'i'I'odo'T'yrosine.

dithionate (chemistry) SALT derived from DITHIONIC ACID ($H_2S_2O_6$). Also termed: hyposulphate (*USA*: hyposulfate).

dithionic acid (chemistry) $H_2S_2O_6$ STRONG ACID that decomposes slowly in concentrated solutions and when heated. Also termed: HYPOSULPHURIC ACID (*USA*: hyposulfuric acid).

dithionite (chemistry) Name that is given to any of the salts of DITHIONOUS ACID, all of which are strong REDUCING AGENTS.

dithionous acid (chemistry) $H_2S_2O_4$ Strong but unstable ACID that is found only in SOLUTION.

diuresis (pharmacology) An unusually or abnormally large output of URINE.

diuretics (pharmacology) Drugs used to reduce fluid in the body by increasing the excretion of water and mineral salts by the KIDNEY, so increasing URINE production. DIURETICS are divided into a number of distinct classes in relation to their specific actions and uses: OSMOTIC DIURETICS, LOOP DIURETICS, POTASSIUM-SPARING DIURETICS, CARBONIC ANHYDRASE INHIBITORS, ALDOSTERONE ANTAGONISTS and THIAZIDE and THIAZIDE-LIKE DIURETICS.

diurnal (physiology/ pharmacology) Pertaining to a day, in the sense of occurring every 24 hours.

divalent (chemistry) Capable of combining with two atoms of HYDROGEN or their equivalent. Also termed: BIVALENT.

diverging lens (optics) LENS that spreads out a beam of LIGHT passing through it, often a CONCAVE LENS.

dividend (mathematics) Number to be divided by another one (the DIVISOR). The result of the DIVISION is the QUOTIENT.

division (1, 2 biology; 3 mathematics) 1 In biological CLASSIFICATION, one of the major groups into which the plant KINGDOM is divided. The members of the GROUP, although often quite different in form and structure, share certain common features, *e.g.* bryophytes include the mosses and liverworts. Divisions are divided into classes, often with an INTERMEDIATE subdivision. The equivalent of a DIVISION in the ANIMAL KINGDOM is a PHYLUM. 2 In biology, the formation of a pair of DAUGHTER CELLS from a parent CELL. *See* CELL DIVISION. 3 In mathematics, the inverse of multiplication, in which a DIVIDEND is divided by a DIVISOR to give a QUOTIENT.

divisor (mathematics) Number that is divided into another one (the DIVIDEND). The result of the DIVISION is the QUOTIENT.

D-lines (physics) Pair of CHARACTERISTIC lines in the yellow region of the SPECTRUM of SODIUM, used as standards in SPECTROSCOPY.

dm (measurement) An abbreviation of 'd'eci'm'etre (*USA*: decimeter).

DMed. (education) An abbreviation of 'D'octor of 'Med'icine.

dmg. (general terminology) An abbreviation of 'd'a'm'a'g'e.

DMLT (education) An abbreviation of 'D'iploma in 'M'edical 'L'aboratory 'T'echnology.

DMPB (education) An abbreviation of 'D'iploma in 'M'edical 'P'athology and 'B'acteriology.

DMR (education) An abbreviation of 'D'iploma in 'M'edical 'R'adiology; 'D'iploma in 'M'edical 'R'adiodiagnostics.

DMR(T) (education) An abbreviation of 'D'iploma in 'M'edical 'R'adio 'T'herapy.

DMRD (education) An abbreviation of 'D'iploma in 'M'edical 'R'adio'D'iagnosis.

DMRE (education) An abbreviation of 'D'iploma in 'M'edical 'R'adiology and 'E'lectrology.

DMS (1 computing; 2 education; 3 chemistry) 1 An abbreviation of 'D'ata 'M'anagement 'S'ystem. 2 An abbreviation of 'D'octor of 'M'edical 'S'cience. 3 An abbreviation of 'D'ocumentation of 'M'olecular 'S'pectroscopy.

DMSO (chemistry) An abbreviation of 'D'i'M'ethyl 'S'ulph'O'xide (*USA*: dimethyl sulfoxide).

DMT (biochemistry) An abbreviation of N,N-'D'i'M'ethyl'T'ryptamine.

DNA (molecular biology) An abbreviation of 'D'eoxyribo'N'ucleic 'A'cid.

DNA hybridization (molecular biology) Technique in which DNA from one SPECIES is induced to undergo base pairing with DNA or RNA from another SPECIES to produce a HYBRID DNA (a process known as ANNEALING).

D/N ratio (physiology/ biochemistry) An abbreviation of 'D'extrose to 'N'itrogen 'ratio' in the URINE.

D$_2$O (biochemistry) Symbol for Deuterium oxide (heavy water).

DOA (1 medical; 2 chemistry) 1 An abbreviation of 'D'ead 'O'n 'A'rrival. 2 An abbreviation of 'D'issolved 'O'xygen 'A'nalyser.

dob (statistics) An abbreviation of 'd'ate 'o'f 'b'irth.

dobutamine hydrochloride (pharmacology) A cardiac stimulant drug with sympathomimetic and beta-receptor stimulant properties which administered by infusion increases the HEART's force of contraction and can be used to treat various serious HEART disorders.

DOCA (biochemistry) An abbreviation of 'D'es'O'xy'C'orticosterone 'A'cetate.

dod (1 statistics; 2 medical) 1 An abbreviation of 'd'ate 'o'f 'd'eath. 2 An abbreviation of 'd'ied 'o'f 'd'isease.

dodecanoic acid (chemistry) An alternative term for LAURIC ACID.

dodecylbenzene (chemistry) $C_6H_5(CH_2)_{11}$-CH_3 HYDROCARBON of the BENZENE FAMILY, important in the manufacture of detergents.

DOM (biochemistry) Abbreviation of 2,5-D'imeth'O'xy-4-'M'ethyl-amphetamine.

DOMA (biochemistry) An abbreviation of 3,4-'D'ihydr'O'xy'M'andelic 'A'cid.

dominant (genetics) In a HETEROZYGOUS organism, describing the GENE that prevents the expression of a RECESSIVE ALLELE in a pair of HOMOLOGOUS CHROMOSOMES. Thus the PHENOTYPE of an organism with a COMBINATION of DOMINANT and RECESSIVE genes is similar to that with two DOMINANT ALLELES.

donor (1 medical; 2 chemistry; 3 physics) 1 Person or ANIMAL that donates BLOOD, TISSUE or organs for use by another person or ANIMAL. 2 ATOM that donates both electrons to form a CO-ORDINATE BOND. 3 An ELEMENT that donates electrons to form an n-type semiconductor; e.g. ANTIMONY or ARSENIC may be DONOR elements for GERMANIUM or SILICON.

Dopa (biochemistry) An abbreviation of 'D'IHYDR'O'XY'P'HENYL'A'LANINE.

DOPAC (biochemistry) An abbreviation of 3,4-'D'ihydr'O'xy'P'henylacetic 'AC'id.

dopamine (biochemistry) PRECURSOR in the SYNTHESIS of ADRENALINE (*USA*: epinephrine) and NORADRENALINE (*USA*: norepinephrine) in animals. It is found in highest CONCENTRATION in the corpus striatum of the BRAIN, where it functions as a NEUROTRANSMITTER. Low levels are associated with Parkinson's disease in human beings.

DOPEG (biochemistry) An abbreviation of 3,4-'D'ihydr'O'xy'P'h'E'nyl'G'lycol.

DOPET (biochemistry) An abbreviation of 3,4-'D'ihydr'O'xy'P'henyl 'ET'hanol.

dormancy (physiology) PERIOD of minimal metabolic activity of an organism or reproductive body. It is a means of surviving a PERIOD of adverse environmental conditions, *e.g.* cold or drought. Examples of some dormant structures are spores, cysts and perennating organs of plants. Environmental factors such as day length and TEMPERATURE control both the onset and ending of DORMANCY. DORMANCY may also be prompted and terminated by the ACTION of HORMONES, *e.g.* abscinic ACID and gibberellins, respectively.

dorsal (anatomy) Describing the upper surface of an organism. In vertebrates this is the surface nearest to the BACKBONE. In plants a DORSAL surface is considered to be one facing away from the main stem or ROOT.

DOS (computing) An abbreviation of 'D'isk 'O'perating 'S'ystem.

dosimeter (radiology) Instrument that measures the dose of RADIATION received by an individual or an AREA.

double bond (chemistry) COVALENT BOND that is formed by sharing two pairs of electrons between two atoms.

double decomposition (chemistry) RE-ACTION between two dissolved ionic substances (usually salts) in which the reactants 'change partners' to form a new SOLUBLE SALT and an INSOLUBLE one, which is precipitated *e.g.* solutions of SODIUM CHLORIDE (NaCl) and SILVER NITRATE ($AgNO_3$) react to form a SOLUTION of SODIUM NITRATE ($NaNO_3$) and a PRECIPITATE of SILVER CHLORIDE (AgCl).

double recessive (genetics) HOMOZYGOTE condition in which two RECESSIVE ALLELES of a particular GENE are at the same LOCUS on a pair of HOMOLOGOUS CHROMOSOMES, so that the RECESSIVE form of the GENE is expressed in the PHENOTYPE.

double refraction (crystallography) Phenomenon shown by certain crystals (*e.g.* calcite) that split an incident RAY of LIGHT into two refracted rays (termed ordinary and extraordinary rays) polarized at right-angles to each other. Also termed: birefringence.

Down's syndrome (medical/ genetics) ABNORMAL chromosomal condition caused by the presence of an extra autosomal CHROMOSOME 21. It is characterized by ABNORMAL physical development and mental retardation. Also termed: MONGOLISM; TRISOMY 21.

DP (computing) An abbreviation of 'D'ata 'P'rocessing.

DPath. (education) An abbreviation of 'D'iploma in 'Path'ology.

DPG (biochemistry) An abbreviation of 2,3-'D'i'P'hospho'G'lycerate.

DPH (education) An abbreviation of 'D'epartment/ 'D'iploma/ 'D'octor of 'P'ublic 'H'ealth.

DPhil. (education) An abbreviation of 'D'octor of 'Phil'osophy.

DPL (biochemistry) An abbreviation of 'D'i'P'almitoyl 'L'ecithin.

DPN (biochemistry) An abbreviation of 'D'i'P'hosphopyridine 'N'ucleotide.

DPPC (biochemistry) An abbreviation of 'D'i'P'almitoyl'P'hosphatidyl'C'holine.

DPT (immunology) An abbreviation of 'D'iphtheria, 'P'ertussis, 'T'etanus (VAC-CINE).

DR (education) An abbreviation of 'D'iploma in 'R'adiology.

Dr (education) An abbreviation of 'D'octo'r'.

Dr Med. (education) An abbreviation of 'D'octo'r' of 'Med'icine.

Dr PH (education) An abbreviation of 'D'octor of 'P'ublic 'H'ealth.

DRCPath (education) An abbreviation of 'D'iploma of the 'R'oyal 'C'ollege of 'Path'ologists.

dry cell (physics) ELECTROLYTIC CELL containing no free LIQUID ELECTROLYTE. A moist paste of AMMONIUM CHLORIDE (NH_4Cl) often acts as the ELECTROLYTE. DRY CELLS are used in batteries for torches, portable radios, etc.

dry ice (chemistry) SOLID CARBON DIOXIDE.

DS (education) An abbreviation of 'D'octor of 'S'cience. Also termed DSc.

DSc. (education) *See* ds.

DSc.-(PH) (education) An abbreviation of 'D'octor of 'Sc'ience –('P'ublic 'H'ealth).

DSc.-(Tech.) (education) An abbreviation of 'D'octor of 'Sc'ience -('Tech'nical).

DTCD (education) An abbreviation of 'D'iploma in 'T'uberculosis and 'C'hest 'D'iseases.

DTCH (education) An abbreviation of 'D'iploma in 'T'ropical 'C'hild 'H'ealth.

DTD (education) An abbreviation of 'D'iploma in 'T'uberculosis/ 'T'uberculous 'D'iseases.

DTech. (education) An abbreviation of 'D'octor of 'Tech'nology.

DTH (education) An abbreviation of 'D'iploma in 'T'ropical 'H'ygiene.

DTM (education) An abbreviation of 'D'iploma in 'T'ropical 'M'edicine.

DTM&H (education) An abbreviation of 'D'iploma in 'T'ropical 'M'edicine and 'H'ygiene.

DTP (computing) An abbreviation of 'D'esk 'T'op 'P'ublishing.

DTPH (education) An abbreviation of 'D'iploma in 'T'ropical 'P'ublic 'H'ealth.

DTR (education) An abbreviation of 'D'iploma in 'T'herapeutic 'R'adiology.

DT's (medical) An abbreviation of 'D'elirium 'T'remens.

ductless gland (anatomy) An alternative term for ENDOCRINE GLAND

duodecimal system (mathematics) Number system that uses the BASE 12, which requires two additional numbers in addition to 1 to 9 (to represent ten and eleven), usually called A and B.

duodenum (anatomy) First SECTION of the SMALL INTESTINE which is mainly secretory in FUNCTION, producing digestive ENZYMES. It also receives pancreatic juice from the PANCREAS and BILE from the GALL BLADDER.

dv (medical) An abbreviation of 'd'ouble 'v'ision.

DXR (radiology) An abbreviation of 'D'eep 'X'-'R'ay.

Dy (chemistry) The CHEMICAL SYMBOL for DYSPROSIUM.

dynamic isomerism (chemistry) An alternative term for TAUTOMERISM.

dyne (measurement) FORCE that gives an OBJECT of MASS 1 gram an ACCELERATION of 1 cm s^{-2}. The SI UNIT of FORCE is the NEWTON, equal to 10^5 dynes.

dysprosium Dy (chemistry) Silvery metallic ELEMENT in GROUP IIIB of the PERIODIC TABLE (one of the LANTHANIDES), used to make magnets and nuclear REACTOR control rods. At. no. 66; r.a.m. 162.50.

E

E (biochemistry) A symbol for glutamic acid.

E_1 (biochemistry) A symbol for estrone.

E_2 (biochemistry) A symbol for estradiol.

e (1 mathematics; 2 physics) 1 Fundamental mathematical CONSTANT and the BASE of natural (Napierian) logarithms. It is an IRRATIONAL NUMBER, the limiting value of the SERIES $(1 + l/n)^n$ as n tends to INFINITY, approximately equal to 2.71828. It is the CONSTANT in an EXPONENTIAL FUNCTION or SERIES. 2 An abbreviation of 'e'lectron.

EACA (biochemistry) An abbreviation of 'E'psilon-'A'mino'C'aproic 'A'cid.

ear (anatomy) One of a pair of hearing and BALANCE sensory organs situated on each side of the HEAD of vertebrates. In mammals it consists of three parts: the outer, middle and INNER EAR.

ear drum (anatomy) MEMBRANE at the inner end of the AUDITORY CANAL of the OUTER EAR which transmits sound vibrations to the EAR OSSICLES of the MIDDLE EAR. Also termed: tympanum.

ear ossicle (anatomy) Small BONE found in the MIDDLE EAR of vertebrates. In mammals there are three, which transmit sound waves from the EAR DRUM to the hearing sensory CELLS in the COCHLEA of the INNER EAR. The three mammalian OSSICLES are the mailcus, INCUS and stapes. Amphibians, reptiles and birds have only one EAR OSSICLE, the columella auris.

earth (physics) In electric circuits, a connection to a piece of METAL that is in turn linked to the EARTH. It has the effect of preventing any earthed apparatus from retaining an ELECTRIC CHARGE.

EB virus (virology) See EBV.

EBV (virology) An abbreviation of 'E'pstein-'B'arr 'V'irus. Also termed EB VIRUS.

ec (literary terminology) An abbreviation of 'e'xempli 'c'ausa. [Latin, meaning, 'for example'.]

E cells (physiology) A symbol for expiratory neurons.

ECF (histology) An abbreviation of 'E'xtra'C'ellular 'F'luid.

ECG (physiology) An abbreviation of 'E'lectro'C'ardio'G'ram.

eCG (biochemistry) An abbreviation of 'e'quine 'C'horionic 'G'onadotrophin (USA: equine Chorionic Gonadotropin).

echovirus (virology) Any of a subgroup of human enteroviruses associated with neurological disorders. There are 34 serovars, each designated by an Arabic NUMERAL; ECHOVIRUS 1, ECHOVIRUS 2, etc. [From 'e'nteric 'c'ytopathic 'o'rphan 'VIRUS'.]

ECoG (physiology) An abbreviation of 'E'lectro'Co'rtico'G'ram.

ecological niche (biology) Position that a particular SPECIES occupies within an ECOSYSTEM. The term both describes the FUNCTION of a SPECIES in terms of interactions with other SPECIES, *e.g.* feeding BEHAVIOUR (*USA*: behavior), and defines the physical boundaries of the ENVIRONMENT occupied by the SPECIES, *e.g.* bats are said to occupy an airborne NICHE.

ecology (biology) Study of INTERACTION of organisms between themselves and with their physical ENVIRONMENT.

ecosystem (biology) Natural UNIT that contains living and non-living components (*e.g.* a community and its ENVIRONMENT) interacting and exchanging materials, and generally balanced as a STABLE system; *e.g.* grassland or rainforest.

ECT (medical) An abbreviation of 'e'lectro-'c'onvulsant 't'herapy.

ectoderm (histology) Outermost GERM LAYER of the EMBRYO of a metazoan which develops into tissues of the EPIDERMIS, *e.g.* SKIN, HAIR, SENSE ORGANS. Also termed: EPIBLAST.

ectoparasite (parasitology) PARASITE that lives on the outside of its HOST; *e.g.* flea.

ectoplasm (cytology) Non-granulated jelly-like outer layer of CYTOPLASM that is located below the PLASMA MEMBRANE. It is CHARACTERISTIC of most amoeboid ANIMAL CELLS, in which at its boundary with PLASMASOL it aids cytoplasmic streaming, and thus movement; *e.g.* in amoeboid PROTOZOA and LEUCOCYTES.

ED (pharmacology) An abbreviation of 'E'ffective 'D'ose.

Ed. in Ch. (literary terminology) An abbreviation of 'Ed'itor in 'Ch'ief.

eddy current (physics) ELECTRIC CURRENT within a CONDUCTOR caused by ELECTROMAGNETIC INDUCTION. Such currents result in losses of ENERGY in electrical machines (*e.g.* a transformer, in which they are overcome by laminating the CORE), but are utilized in INDUCTION HEATING and some braking systems.

Edison accumulator (physics) An alternative term for NICKEL-IRON ACCUMULATOR.

EDRF (physiology) An abbreviation of 'E'ndothelium-'D'erived 'R'elaxing 'F'actor.

EDTA (biochemistry/ pharmacology) An abbreviation of 'E'thylene'D'iamine-'T'etracetic 'A'cid. It is a white CRYSTALLINE ORGANIC COMPOUND, used generally as its SODIUM SALT as an analytical REAGENT and ANTIDOTE for heavy-METAL poisoning, when it forms chelates.

EEG (physiology) An abbreviation of 'E'lectro'E'ncephalo'G'ram.

EET (biochemistry) An abbreviation of 'E'poxy'E'icosa'T'etraenoic acid.

effective resistance (physics) Total ALTERNATING CURRENT resistance of a CONDUCTOR of ELECTRICITY.

effector (physiology) TISSUE or ORGAN that responds to a nervous STIMULUS (*e.g.* ENDOCRINE GLAND, MUSCLE).

efferent (anatomy) Leading away from, as applied to vessels, fibres (*USA*: fibers) and ducts leading from organs.

See also AFFERENT.

effervescence (chemistry) EVOLUTION of bubbles of a GAS from a LIQUID.

efflorescence (chemistry) Property of certain CRYSTALLINE salts that lose WATER OF CRYSTALLIZATION on exposure to AIR and become powdery; *e.g.* SODIUM CARBONATE decahydrate (WASHING SODA), $Na_2CO_3.10H_2O$. It is the opposite of DELIQUESCENCE.

effort (physics) In a simple machine (*e.g.* lever, pulley) the FORCE that is applied to move a load. The ratio of the load to the EFFORT is the mechanical advantage (FORCE RATIO).

effusion (physics) Passage of gases under PRESSURE through small holes.

e.g. (literary terminology) An abbreviation of *'e'xempli 'g'ratia*. [Latin, meaning, 'for example'.]

EGA (computing) An abbreviation of 'E'nhanced 'G'raphics 'A'dapter.

EGF (histology) An abbreviation of 'E'pidermal 'G'rowth 'F'actor.

egg membrane (histology) Thin protective MEMBRANE that surrounds the fertilized OVUM of animals. It is secreted by the OOCYTE and the FOLLICLE CELLS.

See also CHORION.

egg (cytology) *See* OVUM.

ego (medical) Psychological term for the aspect of personality concerned with rationality and common sense.

See also id.

EHF (physics) An abbreviation of 'E'xtremely 'H'igh 'F'requency.

Einstein equation (physics) Equation deduced from Einstein's special theory of RELATIVITY: $E = mc^2$, where E is ENERGY, m is MASS and c is the velocity of LIGHT. It is named after the German-born American physicist Albert Einstein (1879-1955).

einsteinium Es (chemistry) RADIOACTIVE metallic ELEMENT in GROUP IIIB of the PERIODIC TABLE (one of the LANTHANIDES). It has several isotopes, with half-lives of up to 2 years. At. no. 99; r.a.m. 254 (most STABLE ISOTOPE).

EJP (physiology) An abbreviation of 'E'xcitatory 'J'unction 'P'otential.

elastic Van Gieson stain (histology) A histological technique that may be used for staining elastic and CONNECTIVE TISSUE.

electrical conductivity (measurement) Measure of the ability of a substance to conduct ELECTRICITY, the RECIPROCAL of resistivity. It is measured in ohms^{-1} m^{-1}.

See also CONDUCTANCE.

electric charge (physics) Excess or deficiency of electrons in an OBJECT, giving rise to an overall POSITIVE or negative ELECTRIC CHARGE respectively.

electric constant (physics) An alternative term for the absolute permittivity of free space.

See also RELATIVE PERMITTIVITY.

electric current (physics) Flow of electrons through a CONDUCTOR in the same direction, usually because there is a POTENTIAL DIFFERENCE across it.

electric displacement (physics) ELECTRIC CHARGE per UNIT AREA, in coulombs persquare METRE ($C\ m^{-2}$). Also termed: ELECTRIC FLUX DENSITY.

electric field (physics) Region surrounding an ELECTRIC CHARGE in which a charged PARTICLE is subjected to a FORCE.

electric flux (physics) Lines of FORCE that make up an ELECTRIC FIELD.

electric motor (physics) Device that converts electrical ENERGY into mechanical ENERGY. A simple ELECTRIC MOTOR consists of a CURRENT-carrying coil that rotates in the MAGNETIC FIELD between the poles of a permanent MAGNET.

electric polarization (physics) Difference between the DISPLACEMENT of CHARGE and the ELECTRIC FIELD strength in a DIELECTRIC.

electrical condenser (physics) An alternative term for CAPACITOR.

electrical line of force (physics) Line radiating from an ELECTRIC FIELD.

electrical relay (physics) Electromagnetic switching device that brings about changes in an independent CIRCUIT.

electrical resistance (physics) Property of an electrical CONDUCTOR that makes it oppose the flow of CURRENT through it. It is measured in ohms.

electricity (physics) Branch of science that is concerned with all phenomena caused by static or dynamic ELECTRIC CHARGES.

electrocardiogram (ECG) (physiology) RECORD of the electrical activity of the HEART produced by an electrocardiograph machine. Also termed: CARDIOGRAM.

electrocardiograph (physiology) Machine that uses electrodes taped to the body to produce electrocardiograms.

electrochemical series (chemistry) List of metals arranged in ORDER of their ELECTRODE POTENTIALS. A METAL will displace from their salts metals lower down in the SERIES. Also termed: ELECTROMOTIVE SERIES.

electrochemistry (chemistry) Branch of science that is concerned with the study of electrical chemical ENERGY, such as the effects of ELECTRIC CURRENT on chemicals (particularly electrolytes) and the generation of ELECTRICITY by chemical ACTION (as in an ELECTROLYTIC CELL).

electrode (1, 2 chemistry) 1 Conducting plate (ANODE or CATHODE) that collects or emits electrons from an ELECTROLYTE during ELECTROLYSIS. 2 Conducting plate in an ELECTROLYTIC CELL (BATTERY), DISCHARGE tube or VACUUM tube.

electrode potential (chemistry) POTENTIAL developed by a substance in EQUILIBRIUM with a SOLUTION of its ions.

electrodeposition (chemistry) Deposition of a substance from an ELECTROLYTE on to an ELECTRODE, as in electroplating.

electrodialysis (chemistry) Removal of salts from a SOLUTION (often a COLLOID) by placing the SOLUTION between two SEMIPERMEABLE MEMBRANES, outside which are electrodes in pure SOLVENT.

electrodynamics (physics) Study of moving ELECTRIC CHARGES, especially in electric or MAGNETIC FIELDS, which has important applications in the design of generators and motors.

electroencephalogram (EEG) (physiology) RECORD of the electrical activity of the BRAIN produced by an ELECTROEN-CEPHALOGRAPH machine.

electroencephalograph (physiology) Machine that uses electrodes taped to the SKULL to produce electroencephalograms.

electrokinetic potential (physics) An alternative term for ZETA POTENTIAL.

electrokinetics (physics) Branch of science concerned with the study of ELECTRIC CHARGEs in motion.

electrolysis (chemistry) Conduction of ELECTRICITY between two electrodes, through a SOLUTION of a substance (or a substance in its molten state) containing ions and accompanied by chemical changes at the electrodes.

electrolyte (chemistry) Substance that in its molten state or in SOLUTION can conduct an ELECTRIC CURRENT.

electrolytic capacitor (physics) ELEC-TROLYTIC CELL in which a thin FILM of nonconducting substance has been deposited on one of the electrodes by an ELECTRIC CURRENT.

electrolytic cell (physics) Apparatus that consists of electrodes immersed in an ELECTROLYTE.

electrolytic dissociation (chemistry) The partial or complete reversible DECOM-POSITION of a substance in SOLUTION or the

molten state into electrically charged ions.

electrolytic rectifier (physics) RECTIFIER that consists of two electrodes and an ELECTROLYTE in which the CURRENT flows in one direction only.

electrolytic separation (chemistry) A method of separating metals from a SOLUTION by varying the applied POTENTIAL according to the ELECTRODE POTENTIALs of the metals.

electromagnet (physics) A temporary MAGNET consisting of a CURRENT-carrying coil of wire WOUND on a ferromagnetic core. It is the basis of many items of electrical equipment, *e.g.* electric bells, solenoids and lifting magnets.

electromagnetic induction (physics) The ELECTROMOTIVE FORCE (emf) produced in a CONDUCTOR when it is moved in a MAGNETIC FIELD. It is the WORKING principle of an electrical generator (*e.g.* dynamo). It can give rise to a BACK EMF and EDDY CURRENTs.

electromagnetic interaction (physics) INTERACTION between electrically charged ELEMENTARY PARTICLES.

electromagnetic radiation (physics) The ENERGY that results from moving ELECTRIC CHARGEs and travels in association with electric and MAGNETIC FIELDs, *e.g.* radio waves, HEAT rays, LIGHT and X-RAYS, which form part of the ELECTROMAGNETIC SPECTRUM.

electromagnetic spectrum (physics) The range of frequencies over which ELECTROMAGNETIC RADIATION is propagated. In ORDER of increasing FREQUENCY (decreasing WAVELENGTH) it consists of radio waves, microwaves, INFRA-RED

RADIATION, VISIBLE LIGHT, ULTRAVIOLET RADIATION, X-RAYS and gamma-rays.

electromagnetic wave (physics) WAVE formed by electric and MAGNETIC FIELDS, *i.e.* of ELECTROMAGNETIC RADIATION. Such waves do not require a medium in which to propagate, and will travel in a VACUUM.

electromagnetism (physics) COMBINATION of an ELECTRIC FIELD and a MAGNETIC FIELD, their INTERACTION with stationary or moving ELECTRIC CHARGEs, and their study and application. It therefore applies to LIGHT and other forms of ELECTROMAGNETIC RADIATION, as well as to devices such as electromagnets, ELECTRIC MOTORS and generators.

electromotive force (emf) (physics) POTENTIAL DIFFERENCE of a source of ELECTRIC CURRENT, such as an ELECTROLYTIC CELL (BATTERY) or generator. Often it can be measured only at EQUILIBRIUM (when there is no CURRENT flow). An alternative term: VOLTAGE.

electromotive series (chemistry) An alternative term for ELECTROCHEMICAL SERIES.

electron (physics) A fundamental negatively-charged SUBATOMIC PARTICLE (RADIUS 2.81777×10^{-15} m; rest MASS 9.10908×10^{-31} kg; CHARGE 1.602102×10^{-19} coulombs). Every NEUTRAL ATOM has as many orbiting electrons as there are protons in its NUCLEUS. A flow of electrons constitutes an ELECTRIC CURRENT.

electron affinity (physics) ENERGY liberated when an ELECTRON is acquired by a NEUTRAL ATOM.

electron capture (1,2 physics) 1 Formation of a negative ION through the capture of an ELECTRON by a substance. 2

TRANSFORMATION of a PROTON into a NEUTRON in the NUCLEUS of an ATOM (accompanied by the emission of X-RAYS) through the capture of an ORBITAL ELECTRON, so converting the ELEMENT into another with an ATOMIC NUMBER one less.

electron charge (e) (measurement) Fundamental physical CONSTANT, equal to 1.602102×10^{-19} coulombs.

electron configuration (physics) *See* CONFIGURATION.

electron density (physics) DENSITY of ELECTRIC CHARGE.

electron diffraction (physics) Method of determining the arrangement of the atoms in a SOLID, and hence its crystal structure, by the DIFFRACTION of a beam of electrons.

electron donor (chemistry) An alternative term for REDUCING AGENT.

electron gun (physics) ELECTRODE assembly for producing a narrow beam of electrons, as used, *e.g.* in CATHODE-RAY TUBES.

electron lens (physics) Arrangement of electrodes or of permanent magnets or electromagnets used to FOCUS or divert beams of electrons in the same way as an optical LENS modifies a beam of LIGHT, as in, *e.g.* an ELECTRON MICROSCOPE.

electron microscope (microscopy) An instrument that uses a beam of electrons from an ELECTRON GUN to produce magnified images of extremely small objects, beyond the range of an optical MICROSCOPE.

electron multiplier (physics) An alternative term for PHOTOMULTIPLIER.

electron octet (chemistry) *See* OCTET.

electron optics (physics) Study of the control of FREE ELECTRONS by curved electric and MAGNET fields, particularly the use of such fields to FOCUS and deflect beams of electrons.

electron probe microanalysts (EPM) (physics) QUANTITATIVE ANALYSIS of small amounts of substances by FOCUSING a beam of electrons on to a point on the surface of the SAMPLE so that CHARACTERISTIC X-RAY intensifies are produced.

electron radius (r_e) (measurement) A fundamental physical CONSTANT, which is equal to 2.81777×10^{-15} m.

electron rest mass (m_e) (measurement) Fundamental physical CONSTANT, equal to 9.10908×10^{-31} kg.

electron transport (physiology) Process found mainly in AEROBIC RESPIRATION and PHOTOSYNTHESIS that provides a source of ENERGY in the form of ATP. HYDROGEN atoms are used in this system and taken up by a HYDROGEN CARRIER, *e.g.* fad; the electrons of the HYDROGEN pass along a chain of carriers which are in turn reduced and oxidized. This is coupled to the formation of ATP. The HYDROGEN atoms together with OXYGEN eventually form WATER.

electron tube (physics) An alternative term for a VALVE.

electron volt (eV) (measurement) General UNIT of ENERGY equal to WORK done on an ELECTRON when it passes through POTENTIAL GRADIENT of 1 VOLT.

electron-deficient compound (chemistry) A COMPOUND in which there are insufficient electrons to form two-

ELECTRON COVALENT BONDs between all the adjacent atoms (*e.g.* boranes).

electronegativity (chemistry) POWER of an ATOM in a MOLECULE to attract electrons. For elements arranged in the PERIODIC TABLE, it increases up a GROUP and across a PERIOD.

electronics (physics) Branch of science concerned with the study of ELECTRICITY in a VACUUM, in gases and in semiconductors.

electron-spin resonance (ESR) (physics) Branch of MICROWAVE SPECTROSCOPY in which RADIATION of measurable FREQUENCY and WAVELENGTH is used to supply ENERGY to protons.

electrophile (chemistry) An ELECTRON-deficient ION or MOLECULE that attacks molecules of high ELECTRON DENSITY.

See also NUCLEOPHILE.

electrophilic addition (chemistry) A CHEMICAL REACTION that involves the addition of a MOLECULE to an UNSATURATED ORGANIC COMPOUND across a double or TRIPLE BOND.

electrophilic reagent (chemistry) REAGENT that attacks molecules of high ELECTRON DENSITY.

electrophilic substitution (chemistry) A REACTION that involves the substitution of an ATOM or GROUP of atoms in an ORGANIC COMPOUND. An ELECTROPHILE is the attacking SUBSTITUENT.

electrophoresis (physics) Movement of charged COLLOID particles in a SOLUTION placed in an ELECTRIC FIELD.

electrophorus (physics) A device for producing charges by electrostatic INDUCTION; an electrostatic generator.

electropositive (physics) Tending to form POSITIVE ions; having a deficiency of electrons.

electrostatic field (physics) ELECTRIC FIELD associated with stationary ELECTRIC CHARGES.

electrostatic units (ESU) (measurement) System of electrical units based on the FORCE exerted between two ELECTRIC CHARGES.

electrostatics (physics) The branch of ELECTRICITY concerned with the study of electrical charges at rest.

electrostriction (physics) Change in the dimensions of a DIELECTRIC that is caused by the reorientation of molecules when an ELECTRIC FIELD is applied.

electrovalent bond (chemistry) An alternative term for IONIC BOND.

electrovalent crystal (crystallography) Crystal in which the ions are linked by a BOND resulting from electrostatic attraction between their charges. Also termed: IONIC CRYSTAL.

element (1 chemistry; 2 mathematics; 3 physics) 1 Substance consisting of similar atoms of the same ATOMIC NUMBER. It cannot be decomposed by chemical ACTION to a simpler substance. Also termed: chemical ELEMENT. *See also* ISOTOPE; PERIODIC TABLE. 2 In mathematics, one of the members of a SET. 3 In physics, one of several lenses in a COMPOUND LENS, or one of several components in an electrical CIRCUIT.

elementary particle (physics) SUBATOMIC PARTICLE not known to be made up of simpler particles.

elevation of boiling point (physics) Rise in the BOILING POINT of a LIQUID caused by dissolving a substance in the LIQUID.

ELF (physics) An abbreviation of 'E'xtremely 'L'ow 'F'requency.

eluate (chemistry) SOLUTION obtained from ELUTION.

eluent (chemistry) SOLVENT used for ELUTION, the mobile PHASE.

elution (chemistry) Removal of an adsorbed substance by washing the ADSORBENT with a SOLVENT (ELUENT). The technique is used in some forms of CHROMATOGRAPHY.

EM (microscopy) An abbreviation of 'E'lectron 'M'icroscope.

em (physics) An abbreviation of 'e'lectro'm'agnetic.

e-mail (computing) An abbreviation of 'e'lectronic 'mail'.

EMBO (society) An abbreviation of 'E'uropean 'M'olecular 'B'iology 'O'rganisation.

embryo (biology) Organism formed after CLEAVAGE of the ZYGOTE before birth. A maturing EMBRYO is often termed a FOETUS (*USA*: fetus).

embryogenesis (medical) The development of the EMBRYO.

embryol. (medical) An abbreviation of 'embryol'ogy.

embryology (biology) Study of embryos, their formation and development.

EMC virus (virology) An abbreviation of 'E'ncephalo'M'yo'C'arditis 'VIRUS'.

emer. (general terminology) An abbreviation of 'emer'gency.

emergency room (ER) (medical) The part of a hospital that provides immediate care.

emesis (medical) The act of vomiting.

emetics (medical) Drugs which cause vomiting.

emf (physics) An abbreviation of 'e'lectro'm'otive 'f'orce.

EMG (physiology) An abbreviation of 'E'lectro'M'yo'G'ram.

emission spectrum (physics) SPECTRUM obtained when the LIGHT from a luminous source undergoes DISPERSION and is observed directly.

EMK (physics) An abbreviation of 'E'lektro-'M'otorische 'K'raft. [German, meaning 'ELECTROMOTIVE FORCE'.]

empirical formula (chemistry) CHEMICAL FORMULA that shows the simplest ratio between atoms of a MOLECULE e.g. GLUCOSE, MOLECULAR FORMULA $C_6H_{12}O_6$, and acetic (ethanoic) ACID, $C_2H_4O_2$, both have the same EMPIRICAL FORMULA, CH_2O.

See also MOLECULAR FORMULA; STRUCTURAL FORMULA.

EMSA (society) An abbreviation of 'E'lectron 'M'icroscope 'S'ociety of 'A'merica.

EMTD (toxicology) An abbreviation of 'E'stimated 'M'aximum 'T'olerated 'D'ose.

emulsion (chemistry) Colloidal SUSPENSION of one LIQUID dispersed in another.

enamel (histology) White protective calcified outer coating of the crown of the TOOTH of a VERTEBRATE. It is produced by epidermal CELLS, the ameloblasts, and it consists almost entirely of CALCIUM salts bound together by KERATIN fibres (USA: keratin fibers).

enatiomer (chemistry) MOLECULE that is a mirror IMAGE of another, and which cannot be superimposed on it. Both molecules are OPTICALLY ACTIVE, but differ in the direction in which they rotate the plane of POLARIZED LIGHT.

encephalin (biochemistry) One of two peptides which are natural ANALGESICS, produced in the BRAIN and released after injury. The encephalins have properties similar to MORPHINE. Also termed: ENDORPHIN; enkephalin.

end point (chemistry) Point at which a CHEMICAL REACTION is complete, such as the end of a TITRATION.

See also VOLUMETRIC ANALYSIS.

endemic (EPIDEMIOLOGY) Describing a disease that continually occurs among people or animals in a particular region.

See also EPIDEMIC; PANDEMIC.

endocrine gland (anatomy) Ductless ORGAN or discrete GROUP of CELLS that synthesize HORMONES and secrete them directly into the bloodstream. Such GLANDS include the PITUITARY, pineal, THYROID, PARATHYROID and ADRENAL

GLANDS, the GONADS and PLACENTA (in mammals), ISLETS OF LANGERHANS (in the PANCREAS) and parts of the ALIMENTARY CANAL. Their FUNCTION is parallel to the NERVOUS SYSTEM, that of regulation of responses in animals. Also termed: DUCTLESS GLAND.

endocrinology (histology/ biochemistry) Study of structure and FUNCTION of ENDOCRINE GLANDS and the roles of their HORMONES as the chemical messengers of the body.

endogenous (biology) Produced or originating within an organism.

endolymph (anatomy) FLUID that fills the cavity of the middle, inner and the SEMICIRCULAR CANALS of the EAR.

endoparasite (parasitology) PARASITE that lives inside the body of its HOST, *e.g.* FLUKE, MALARIA PARASITE, TAPEWORM.

endoplasm (cytology) Central portion of CYTOPLASM, surrounded by the ECTOPLASM and containing organelles. Also termed: PLASMASOL.

endoplasmic reticulum (ER) (cytology) Structure that occurs in most EUKARYOTIC CELLS in the form of a flattened MEMBRANE-bound sac of CELL organelles, continuous with the outer NUCLEAR MEMBRANE. When covered with ribosomes it is termed rough ER, in their absence smooth ER. Its main FUNCTION is the SYNTHESIS of proteins and their transport within or to the outside of the CELL. In LIVER CELLS ER is involved in detoxification processes and in LIPID and CHOLESTEROL METABOLISM. In association with the GOLGI APPARATUS, ER is involved in LYSOSOME production.

endorphin (biochemistry) One of a GROUP of peptides that are produced by the PITUITARY GLAND and which act as painkillers in the body.

endoscope (optics) A tubular optical device, perhaps using FIBRE OPTICS (*USA*: fiber optics), that is inserted into a natural orifice or a surgical incision to study organs and tissues inside the body.

endospore (1, 2 biology) 1 Innermost layer of the wall of a SPORE. 2 Tough ASEXUAL SPORE that is formed by some BACTERIA to resist adverse conditions.

endothelium (histology) TISSUE formed from a single layer of CELLS found lining spaces and tubes within the body, *e.g.* lining the HEART in vertebrates.

See also EPITHELIUM.

endothermic (chemistry) Describing a process in which HEAT is taken in; *e.g.* in many CHEMICAL REACTIONS.

See also EXOTHERMIC.

energy (physics) CAPACITY for doing WORK, measured in joules. ENERGY takes various forms: *e.g.* KINETIC ENERGY, POTENTIAL ENERGY, electrical ENERGY, chemical ENERGY, HEAT, LIGHT and sound. All forms of ENERGY can be regarded as being aspects of kinetic or POTENTIAL ENERGY; *e.g.* HEAT ENERGY in a substance is the KINETIC ENERGY of that substance's molecules.

energy level (physics) The ENERGY of electrons in an ATOM is not continuously VARIABLE, but has a discrete SET of values, *i.e.* ENERGY LEVELS. At any instant the ENERGY of a given ELECTRON can correspond to only one of these levels.

enflurane (pharmacology) An inhalant general anaesthetic drug, which is similar to halothane. It is often used along with nitrous oxide-oxygen mixtures for the induction and maintenance of anaesthesia during major surgery.

enol (chemistry) ORGANIC COMPOUND that contains the GROUP $C = CH(OH)$; the ALCOHOLic form of a KETONE.

enrichment (microbiology) ISOLATION of a particular type of organism by enhancing its GROWTH over other organisms in a mixed population.

ENT (medical) An abbreviation of 'E'ar, 'N'ose and 'T'hroat.

Ent. (parasitology) An abbreviation of 'Ent'omology.

enthalpy (*H*) (physics) Amount of HEAT ENERGY a substance possesses, measurable in terms of the HEAT change that accompanies a CHEMICAL REACTION carried out at CONSTANT PRESSURE. In any system, $H = U + pV$, where U is the INTERNAL ENERGY, p the PRESSURE and V the VOLUME.

entropy (S) (physics) In THERMODYNAMICS, quantity that is a measure of a system's disorder, or the unavailability of its ENERGY to do WORK. In a REVERSIBLE PROCESS the change in ENTROPY is equal to the amount of ENERGY adsorbed divided by the ABSOLUTE TEMPERATURE at which it is taken up.

envelope (mathematics) Curve that touches every one of a whole FAMILY of curves.

environment (biology) All the conditions in which an organism lives, including the amount of LIGHT, TEMPERATURE, WATER supply and presence of other (competing) organisms.

enzyme (biochemistry) PROTEIN that acts as a CATALYST for the CHEMICAL REACTIONS that occur in living systems. Without such a CATALYST most of the reactions of METABOLISM would not occur under the conditions that prevail. Most ENZYMES are specific to a particular SUBSTRATE (and therefore a particular REACTION) and act by activating the SUBSTRATE and binding to it.

EP (physiology/ biochemistry) An abbreviation of 'E'ndogenous 'P'yrogen.

EPI (biochemistry/ pharmacology) An abbreviation for 'EPI'nephrine. (*UK*: ADRENALINE).

epiblast (biology) An alternative term for ECTODERM.

epidemic (epidemiology) Describing a disease that, for a limited time, affects many people or animals in a particular region.

See also ENDEMIC; PANDEMIC.

epidemiology (epidemiology) Study of diseases as they affect the population, including their INCIDENCE and prevention.

epidermis (histology) Layer of CELLS at the surface of a plant or ANIMAL. In plants and some invertebrates, it forms a single protective layer, often overlaid by a cuticle which is IMPERMEABLE to WATER. In vertebrates, it forms the SKIN and is composed of several layers of CELLS, the outermost becoming keratinized. *See* KERATINIZATION.

epididymis (anatomy) Long coiled tube in the TESTES of some vertebrates through which SPERM from the seminiferous tubules pass, before going into the VAS DEFERENS and to the exterior.

epiglottis (anatomy) VALVE-like flap of CARTILAGE in mammals that closes the opening into the LARYNX, the GLOTTIS, during swallowing.

epinephrine (biochemistry) An alternative term for ADRENALINE.

epiphysis (1, 2 anatomy) 1 Growing end of a BONE, at which CARTILAGE is converted to SOLID BONE. 2 An alternative term for PINEAL GLAND.

epithelium (histology) ANIMAL lining TISSUE of varying complexity, whose main FUNCTION is protective. It may be specialized for lining a particular ORGAN. e.g. SQUAMOUS EPITHELIUM lines capillaries and is PERMEABLE to molecules in SOLUTION, glandular EPITHELIUM contains CELLS that are secretory.

epithermal neutron (physics) NEUTRON that has ENERGY of between 10^{-2} and 10^2 ELECTRON volts (eV); a NEUTRON having ENERGY greater than that associated with thermal agitation.

epoxide (chemistry) ORGANIC COMPOUND whose molecules include a three-membered OXYGEN ring (a CYCLIC ETHER).

epoxy resin (chemistry) SYNTHETIC polymeric thermosetting RESIN with EPOXIDE groups (e.g. polyethers). Such resins are used in surface coatings and as adhesives and electrical insulators. Also termed: EPOXIDE RESIN.

EPP (haematology) An abbreviation of 'E'rythrocyte 'P'roto'P'orphyrin.

EPP (physiology) An abbreviation of 'e'nd 'p'late 'p'otential.

Epsom salt (pharmacology) $MgSO_4.7H_2O$ White CRYSTALLINE SALT, used in mineral waters, as a laxative. Also termed: epsomite; MAGNESIUM SULPHATE (*USA*: magnesium sulfate).

EPSP (physiology) An abbreviation for 'e'xcitatory 'p'ost's'ynaptic 'p'otential.

eq (chemistry) An abbreviation of 'eq'uivalent(s).

equation of state (physics) Any FORMULA that connects the VOLUME, PRESSURE and TEMPERATURE of a given system, e.g. van der Waals' equation.

equilibrium (1, 2 physics) 1 An OBJECT is in EQUILIBRIUM when the forces acting on it are such that there is no tendency for the OBJECT to move. 2 State in which no change occurs in a system if no change occurs in the surrounding ENVIRONMENT (e.g. CHEMICAL EQUILIBRIUM).

equilibrium constant (K_c) (chemistry) CONCENTRATION of the products of a CHEMICAL REACTION divided by the CONCENTRATION of the reactants, in accordance with the CHEMICAL EQUATION, at a given TEMPERATURE.

equimolecular mixture (chemistry) A MIXTURE of substances in equal molecular proportions.

equivalence point (chemistry) Theoretical END POINT of a TITRATION.

See also VOLUMETRIC ANALYSIS.

equivalent fraction (mathematics) One of two or more fractions that represent the same number; *e.g.* the fractions 2/3, 4/6, 14/21 and 40/60 are equivalent.

equivalent weight (chemistry) Number of parts by MASS of an ELEMENT that can combine with or displace one part by MASS of HYDROGEN.

Er (chemistry) The CHEMICAL SYMBOL for ERBIUM.

ER (medical) An abbreviation of 'E'mergency 'R'oom.

erbium Er (chemistry) Metallic ELEMENT in GROUP IIIB of the PERIODIC TABLE (one of the LANTHANIDEs), used in making lasers for medical applications. Its pink OXIDE is used as a PIGMENT in ceramics. At. no. 68; r.a.m. 167.26.

ERG (physiology) An abbreviation of 'E'lectro'R'etino'G'ram.

erg (measurement) ENERGY transferred when a FORCE of 1 dyne moves through 1 cm, equivalent to 10^{-7} joules.

ergosterol (biochemistry) White CRYSTAL-LINE STEROL. It occurs in ANIMAL fat and in some MICRO-ORGANISMS. In animals it is converted to VITAMIN D_2 by ULTRAVIOLET RADIATION.

erogenous (biology) Originating outside an organism, ORGAN or CELL. The term may refer to such things as substances (*e.g.* nutrients) or stimuli (*e.g.* LIGHT).

ERPF (physiology) An abbreviation of 'E'ffective 'R'enal 'P'lasma 'F'low.

erythrocyte (haematology) RED BLOOD CELL. It contains HAEMOGLOBIN (*USA*: hemaglobin) and carries OXYGEN around the body. In mammals, ERYTHROCYTES have no nuclei.

See also LEUCOCYTE.

Es (chemistry) The CHEMICAL SYMBOL for EINSTEINIUM.

ES (society) An abbreviation of 'E'ntomological 'S'ociety.

ESA (society) An abbreviation of 'E'cological/ 'E'ntomological/ 'S'ociety of 'A'merica.

ESB (medical) An abbreviation of 'E'lectrical 'S'timulation of the 'B'rain.

ESC (society) An abbreviation of 'E'ntomological 'S'ociety of 'C'anada.

Escherichia coli (bacteriology) A member of the bacterial family Enterobacteriacae. A gram negative non-motile rod and a natural inhabitant of the intestinal tract in man; usually non-pathogenic, but pathogenic strains frequently cause urinary tract infections, enteritis, peritonitis, cystitis, and wound infections.

ESH (society) An abbreviation of 'E'uropean 'S'ociety of 'H'aematology.

esl (statistics) An abbreviation of 'e'xpected 's'ignificance 'l'evel.

esn (general terminology) An abbreviation of 'es'se'n'tial. Also termed esntl.

ESNZ (society) An abbreviation of 'E'ntomological 'S'ociety of 'N'ew 'Z'ealand.

esp. (general terminology) An abbreviation of 'esp'ecially.

ESR (1 haematology; 2 physics) 1 An abbreviation of 'E'rythrocyte 'S'edimentation 'R'ate. 2 An abbreviation of 'E'lectron 'S'pin 'R'esonance.

ESRA (governing body) An abbreviation of 'E'uropean 'S'ociety of 'R'egulatory 'A'ffairs.

essential amino acid (biochemistry) Any AMINO ACID that cannot be manufactured in some vertebrates, including human beings. These acids must therefore be obtained from the diet. They are as follows: ARGININE, HISTIDINE, ISOLEUCINE, LEUCINE, LYSINE, METHIONINE, PHENYLALANINE, THREONINE, TRYPTOPHAN and VALINE.

essential fatty acid (biochemistry) Any FATTY ACID that is required in the diet of mammals because it cannot be synthesized. They include linOLEIC ACID and γ-linolenic ACID, obtained from plant sources.

essential oil (chemistry) VOLATILE oil with a pleasant odour (USA: odor), obtained from various plants. Such oils are widely used in perfumery.

est. (general termino'ogy) An abbreviation of 'est'imated.

ester (chemistry) COMPOUND formed when the HYDROGEN ATOM of the hydroxy GROUP in an OXYGEN-containing ACID is replaced by an ALKYL GROUP. Most important esters are derived from CARBOXYLIC ACIDs.

esterification (chemistry) Formation of an ESTER, generally by REACTION between an ACID and an ALCOHOL.

estimated (est.) (general terminology) An approximation.

estn (general terminology) An abbreviation of 'est'imatio'n'.

et al. (literary terminology) An abbreviation of 'et' 'al'ii. [Latin, meaning, 'and others'.]

etc. (literary terminology) An abbreviation of 'et' 'c'etera. [Latin, meaning, 'and so forth'.]

ethanal (chemistry) An alternative term for ACETALDEHYDE.

ethanal trimer (chemistry) An alternative term for PARALDEHYDE,

ethane (chemistry) C_2H_6 Gaseous ALKANE which occurs with methane in natural GAS.

ethanedioic acid (chemistry) An alternative term for OXALIC ACID.

ethanoate (chemistry) An alternative term for ACETATE.

ethanoic acid (chemistry) An alternative term for acetic ACID.

ethanol (chemistry) C_2H_5OH Colourless (USA: colorless) LIQUID ALCOHOL. It is the active constituent of ALCOHOLic drinks (in which it is produced by FERMENTATION); it is also used as a fuel and in the preparation of esters, ethers and other ORGANIC COMPOUNDS. Also termed: ETHYL ALCOHOL; ALCOHOL.

ethanoyl chloride (chemistry) An alternative term for ACETYL CHLORIDE.

ethene (chemistry) $CH_2=CH_2$ Colourless (USA: colorless) GAS with a sweetish SMELL, important in chemical SYNTHESIS. Also termed: ETHYLENE.

ether (chemistry) Member of a GROUP of ORGANIC COMPOUNDS that have the GENERAL FORMULA ROR', where R and R' are ALKYL GROUPs. The commonest, diethyl OXIDE (diethyl ETHER, or simply ETHER), $(C_2H_5)O_2$, is a useful VOLATILE SOLVENT formerly used as an ANAESTHETIC (USA: anesthetic).

ethology (biology) Scientific study of ANIMAL BEHAVIOUR (*USA*: behavior) in the wild.

ethyl (chemistry) C_2H_5- Common ALKYL GROUP derived from ETHANE.

ethyl acetate (chemistry) An alternative term for ETHYL ETHANOATE.

ethyl alcohol (chemistry) An alternative term for ETHANOL.

ethyl carbamate (chemistry) An alternative term URETHANE.

ethyl ethanoate (chemistry) $CH_3COOC_2H_5$ Colourless (*USA*: colorless) LIQUID ESTER with a fruity SMELL, produced by the REACTION between ETHANOL (ETHYL ALCOHOL) and ethanoic (acetic) ACID, used as a SOLVENT and in medicine. Also termed: ETHYL ACETATE.

ethylbenzene (chemistry) An alternative term for styrene.

ethylene (chemistry) An alternative term for ETHENE.

ethylene dibromide (chemistry) An alternative term for dibromoethane.

ethylene glycol (chemistry) An alternative term for ethanediol.

ethylene tetrachloride (chemistry) An alternative term for TETRACHLOROETHENE.

ethyne (chemistry) An alternative term for ACETYLENE.

ETP (physiology) An abbreviation of 'E'lectron 'T'ransport 'P'article.

Eu (chemistry) The CHEMICAL SYMBOL for EUROPIUM.

EUA (medical) An abbreviation of 'E'xamination 'U'nder 'A'naesthetic (*USA*: examination under anesthetic).

eubacteria (bacteriology) The largest GROUP of BACTERIA, containing the most commonly encountered forms that inhabit soil and WATER. The GROUP contains gram POSITIVE BACTERIA and green photosynthetic BACTERIA.

eugenics (biology) Theory and practice of improving the human RACE through genetic principles. This can range from the generally discredited idea of selective breeding programmes to counselling of parents who may be carriers of harmful genes.

eukaryote (cytology) CELL with a certain LEVEL of complexity. Eukaryotes have a NUCLEUS separated from the CYTOPLASM by a NUCLEAR MEMBRANE. Genetic material is carried on chromosomes consisting of DNA associated with PROTEIN. The CELL contains MEMBRANE-bounded organelles, *e.g.* mitochrondria and chloroplasts. All organisms are EUKARYOTIC except for BACTERIA and cyanophytes, which are prokaryotes. Also termed: eucaryote.

eukaryotic (cytology) Describing or relating to a EUKARYOTE.

europium Eu (chemistry) Silvery-white metallic ELEMENT in GROUP IIIB of the PERIODIC TABLE (one of the LANTHANIDES), used in nuclear REACTOR control rods. At. no. 63; r.a.m. 151.96.

Eustachian tube (anatomy) Channel that connects the MIDDLE EAR with the PHARYNX at the back of the THROAT in mammals and some other vertebrates. It ensures that the AIR PRESSURE on each side of the EAR DRUM is equal. It is named after the

Italian anatomist Bartolomeo Eustachio (1520-74). (*USA*: eustachian tube).

eutectic mixture (chemistry) MIXTURE of substances in such proportions that no other MIXTURE of the same substances has a lower FREEZING POINT.

eV (measurement) An abbreviation of 'e'lectron 'V'olt.

evaporation (physics) Process by which a LIQUID changes to its VAPOUR. It can occur (slowly) at a TEMPERATURE below the BOILING POINT, but is faster if the LIQUID is heated and fastest when the LIQUID is boiling.

even-odd nucleus (chemistry) Atomic NUCLEUS with an even number of protons and an odd number of neutrons.

evolution (biology) Successive altering of SPECIES through time. Evolutionary theory states that the ORIGIN of all SPECIES is through EVOLUTION, and thus they are related by descent.

See also DARWINISM; NATURAL SELECTION.

ex. (literary terminology) An abbreviation of 'ex'ample. Also termed *e.g.*

exch. (chemistry) An abbreviation of 'exch'ange.

excitation (physics) Addition of ENERGY to a system, such as an ATOM or NUCLEUS, causing it to transfer from its GROUND STATE to one of higher ENERGY.

excitation energy (physics) ENERGY required for EXCITATION.

excited state (physics) ENERGY state of an ATOM or MOLECULE that is higher than the GROUND STATE, resulting from EXCITATION. *See also* ENERGY LEVEL.

exclusion principle (physics) An alternative term for the Pauli EXCLUSION PRINCIPLE.

excretion (physiology) Removal of waste products of METABOLISM, carried out by elimination from the body or STORAGE in INSOLUBLE form. Products of PROTEIN METABOLISM are the main substances liberated. The chief organs of EXCRETION in vertebrates are the kidneys.

exocrine gland (anatomy) GLAND that discharges secretions into ducts, *e.g.* salivary GLANDS.

See also ENDOCRINE GLAND.

exogamy (biology) Outbreeding as distinct from INBREEDING. *See* INBREEDING.

exothermic (chemistry) Describing a process in which HEAT is evolved.

exp. (1-7 general terminology) An abbreviation of 1 'exp'eriment. 2 'exp'ires. 3 'exp'onential. 4 'exp'eriment 5 'exp'erimental. 6 'exp'iration. 7 'exp'ire.

expansion of gas (physics) Increase in VOLUME of an ideal GAS is at the rate of 1/273 of its VOLUME at 0°C for each DEGREE rise in TEMPERATURE. *See* CHARLES'S LAW.

See also KINETIC THEORY.

exponent (mathematics) Number that indicates the POWER to which a quantity (the BASE) is to be raised, usually written as a superior number or symbol after the quantity, *e.g.* in 2^3, 2^x, the exponents are 3 and x.

exponential growth (microbiology) The GROWTH that occurs, *e.g.* in cultures of MICRO-ORGANISMS, in which a population of CELLS increases in numbers logarithmically.

exponential series (mathematics) A mathematical SERIES of functions of x that converges to e^x.

extracellular (histology) External to a CELL; in a MULTICELLULAR organism, EXTRACELLULAR TISSUE may still be within the organism.

See also INTRACELLULAR.

extrafusal fibres (histology) The large contractile fibres (*USA*: fibers) contained in MUSCLE; their movement causes MUSCLE contraction. They consist of longitudinally arranged filaments of two kinds: MYOSIN and ACTIN. (*USA*: extrafusal fibers).

extrapolation (statistics) Estimation of a value outside the range of those already known, usually by graphical methods.

eye (anatomy) ORGAN for detecting LIGHT.

eye tooth (anatomy) An alternative term for CANINE TOOTH.

F

F (1 measurement; 2 general terminolgy; 3 chemistry; 4 biochemistry) An abbreviation of 1 'F'ahrenheit. Also termed Fahr. 2 'F'emale. 3 The CHEMICAL SYMBOL for FLUORINE. 4 A symbol for phenylalanine.

F_1 (genetics) The offspring of any two parents. *Compare* F_2.

F_2 (genetics) The offspring of two F_1 parents (*i.e.* the third generation). *Compare* F_1.

f (microscopy) An abbreviation of 'f'ocal length.

fa (chemistry) An abbreviation of 'f'atty 'a'cid/ 'f'olic 'a'cid.

FAAAS (society) An abbreviation of 'F'ellow of the 'A'merican 'A'ssociation for the 'A'dvancement of 'S'cience.

FACA (education) An abbreviation of 'F'ellow of the 'A'merican 'C'ollege of 'A'llergists.

face-centred cube (crystallography) Crystal structure that is CUBIC with an ATOM or ION at the centre of each of the six faces of the cube in addition to the eight at its corners. (*USA*: face-centered cube).

FACG (education) An abbreviation of 'F'ellow of the 'A'merican 'C'ollege of 'G'astroenterology.

facilitated diffusion (biochemistry) MODE of transport through a MEMBRANE that involves CARRIER molecules in the MEMBRANE, which eases the transport of a specific substance but does not involve the use of ENERGY; *e.g.* the uptake of GLUCOSE by ERYTHROCYTES (RED BLOOD CELLS). The transport system can become saturated with the transported substance, in contrast to simple DIFFUSION.

FACR (education) An abbreviation of 'F'ellow of the 'A'merican 'C'ollege of 'R'adiology.

facs. (general terminology) An abbreviation of 'facs'imile. Also termed fs, and facsim.

facsim. (general terminology) *See* facs.

factor (1 general; 2, 3 statistics; 4 mathematics) 1 Anything having a causal influence on something, usually where there are several different causal influences. 2 A discrete VARIABLE used to classify DATA (*e.g.* an INDEPENDENT VARIABLE) *Compare* LEVEL. 3 Any of the INTERVENING VARIABLES discovered through FACTOR ANALYSIS that accounts for a significant proportion of the VARIANCE of the DATA. 4 A number that divides into another number without remainder.

factor analysis (statistics) A GENERIC term for techniques whose OBJECTIVE is to discover whether the correlations or covariances between a SET of observed variables can be accounted for in terms of their relationships to a small number of unobservable or INTERVENING VARIABLES *i.e.* the factors. Essentially FACTOR ANALYSIS postulates a LINEAR relation between the observed variables and the underlying factors, which may be ESTIMATED by a VARIETY of methods. At its simplest, FACTOR ANALYSIS is a method for DATA REDUCTION, reducing a large number of intercorrelated variables to a smaller number of INTERVENING VARIABLES which account for as much of the VARIANCE as possible.

factor axes (statistics) In FACTOR ANALYSIS the axes representing the relations of the factors to one another; they may be orthogonal or oblique.

factor (mathematics) One of the numbers that will divide exactly into another given number (*e.g.* 2 and 3 are factors of 6), or which is one of the polynomials that will divide exactly into another POLYNOMIAL (*e.g.* $(x + 2)$ and $(x - 5)$ are factors of $x^2 - 3x - 10$).

factor loading (statistics) In FACTOR ANALYSIS the correlation between a test item and a FACTOR, *i.e.* the extent to which the score on an item is determined by a FACTOR.

factor matrix (statistics) A table showing the FACTOR LOADING of each test item with each FACTOR.

factor VIII concentrate (medical/haematology) A concentrated preparation of FACTOR VIII that is used in the TREATMENT of those with HAEMOPHILIA A (*USA*: hemophilia A).

factorial (mathematics) PRODUCT of all the whole numbers from a given whole number *n* down to 1, written as *n*!; *e.g.* the FACTORIAL of 6 (written 6!) is 6 x 5 x 4 x 3 x 2 x 1 = 720.

factorial design (statistics) An experimental design in which each value (LEVEL) of each INDEPENDENT VARIABLE (FACTOR) is combined with each value (LEVEL) of every other INDEPENDENT VARIABLE (FACTOR); *e.g.* if there are two factors (A and B) each with two levels (1 and 2) the following combinations would be used: A1B1, A1B2, A2BI, A2B2.

factorial validity (statistics) The extent to which scores on different tests purporting to measure the same thing are correlated.

facultative anaerobe (microbiology) MICRO-ORGANISM that grows under either ANAEROBIC or AEROBIC conditions.

FAD (biochemistry) An abbreviation of 'F'lavin 'A'denine 'D'inucleotide.

faeces (medical) The waste products from the intestines, a third of which consists of dead or living BACTERIA. The remainder being made up of food which has not been digested, mostly CELLULOSE and FIBRE (*USA*: fiber), dead CELLS from the lining of the INTESTINE, WATER, MUCUS, and the whole coloured (*USA*: colored) by BILE pigments. (*USA*: feces).

Fahr. (measurement) An abbreviation of 'fahr'enheit.

Fahrenheit (F) (measurement) A UNIT of DEGREE of TEMPERATURE. The FREEZING POINT of WATER is 32^0 F; the BOILING POINT of WATER is 212^0 F under standard atmospheric PRESSURE. Named after the German physicist Gabriel Daniel Fahrenheit (1686-1736).

FAIC (education) An abbreviation of 'F'ellow of the 'A'merican 'I'nstitute of 'C'hemists.

Fajans' rules (chemistry) SET of rules that state when IONIC BONDS are likely in a chemical COMPOUND (as opposed to COVALENT BONDS). They were named after the Polish chemist Kasimir Fajans (1887-1975).

Fallopian tube (anatomy) Tube that in female mammals conducts ova (eggs) from an OVARY to the UTERUS (womb) by ciliary ACTION. FERTILIZATION can occur when SPERM meet eggs in the tube. It was named after the Italian anatomist Gabriel Fallopius (1523-62). Also termed: OVIDUCT. (*USA*: fallopian tube).

false negative (general terminology) Failure of a test to demonstrate the disease or condition when present. *Contrast* FALSE POSITIVE.

false positive (general terminology) A POSITIVE test result caused by a disease or condition other than the disease for which the test is designed, or in the absence of disease altogether.

false pregnancy (medical) An alternative term for PSEUDOPREGNANCY.

family (biology) In biological CLASSIFI-CATION, one of the groups into which an ORDER is divided, and which is itself divided into GENERA. *See* TAXONOMY.

FAMS (education) An abbreviation of 'F'ellow of the 'I'ndian 'A'cademy of 'M'edical 'S'ciences.

FANZAAS (education) An abbreviation of 'F'ellow of 'A'ustralian and 'N'ew 'Z'ealand 'A'ssociation for 'A'dvance-ment of 'S'cience.

FAPHA (education) An abbreviation of 'F'ellow of the 'A'merican 'P'ublic 'H'ealth 'A'ssociation.

FAPT (education) An abbreviation of 'F'ellow of the 'A'ssociation of 'P'hotographic 'T'echnicians.

farad (F) (measurement) SI UNIT of electrical CAPACITANCE, defined as the CAPACITANCE that, when charged by a POTENTIAL DIFFERENCE of 1 VOLT, carries a CHARGE of 1 coulomb. It was named after the British scientist Michael Faraday (1791-1867).

faraday (F) (measurement) UNIT of ELECTRIC CHARGE, equal to the quantity of CHARGE that during ELECTROLYSIS liberates one gram EQUIVALENT WEIGHT of an ELEMENT. It has the value 9.6487×10^4 coulombs per gram-equivalent.

See also FARAD; FARADAY CONSTANT.

Faraday constant (F) (physics) Funda-mental physical CONSTANT, the ELECTRIC CHARGE carried by one mole of singly-charged ions or electrons, equal to 9.6487×10^4 coulombs per mole. It is the PRODUCT of the AVOGADRO CONSTANT and the ELECTRON CHARGE.

Faraday effect (physics) Rotation of the plane of vibration of a beam of POLARIZED LIGHT passing through a substance such as GLASS, in the direction of an applied MAGNETIC FIELD.

Faraday's laws of electrolysis (1, 2 chemistry) 1 The amount of chemical DECOMPOSITION that takes place during ELECTROLYSIS is proportional to the ELECTRIC CURRENT passed. 2 The amounts of substances liberated during ELEC-TROLYSIS are proportional to their chemical EQUIVALENT WEIGHTs.

Faraday's laws of electromagnetic induction (1, 2 physics) 1 An induced ELECTROMOTIVE FORCE is established in an

141

electric CIRCUIT whenever the MAGNETIC FIELD linking that CIRCUIT changes. 2 The magnitude of the induced ELECTROMOTIVE FORCE in any CIRCUIT is proportional to the rate of change of the MAGNETIC FLUX linking the CIRCUIT.

farina (1, 2 biology) 1 STARCH or flour. 2 An alternative term for POLLEN.

farmer's lung (medical/ mycology/ immunology) A type of extrinsic allergic alveolitis sometimes called HYPERSENSITIVITY pneumonitis. It is caused by the inhalation of dust from mouldy (*USA*: moldy) hay or straw containing spores of the organisms *Micropolyspora faeni and Thermoactinomyces vulgaris*, which infect the hay when it is damp and warm, and are released when it has dried out. These, in those sensitive, sets up an allergic REACTION in the lungs, causing symptoms which include a FEVER, dry cough and shortness of breath. The disease may become CHRONIC with continued exposure and result in FIBROSIS of the LUNG.

FAS (1 medical/ biochemistry; 2 society) 1 An abbreviation of 'F'oetal 'A'lcohol 'S'yndrome. (*USA*: Fetal ALCOHOL SYNDROME). 2 An abbreviation of 'F'ederation of 'A'merican 'S'cientists.

fascia (histology) FIBROUS TISSUE organised to form sheets which lie just under the SKIN (superficial FASCIA), and round muscles (deep FASCIA). The superficial FASCIA contains fat and the NERVES and BLOOD VESSELS running to the SKIN. The deep FASCIA forms dense fibrous sheaths for the muscles and compartments in which groups of muscles lie together.

fascicle (histology) A slender bundle of NERVE FIBRES (*USA*: nerve fibers). Also termed fasciculus.

FASEB (society) An abbreviation of 'F'ederation of 'A'merican 'S'ocieties for 'E'xperimental 'B'iology.

fasting (general terminology) A length of time without food and WATER. BASE levels are often obtained after the patient has fasted where the intake of food may influence the LEVEL of the FACTOR under investigation, as is the case for instance with BLOOD GLUCOSE levels.

fat embolism (medical) Following serious BONE injuries fat globules may be released into the bloodstream and cause an embolism.

fate map (genetics) A map of the CELLS or tissues in the fertilized EGG or early EMBRYO that shows where they will end up in the adult organism. The DATA can be collected by staining specific CELLS in the EMBRYO with a non-diffusible dye; artificial chimaeras can also be used.

fats and oils (biochemistry) Naturally occurring esters (of GLYCEROL and FATTY ACIDS) that are used as ENERGY-STORAGE compounds. They are HYDROCARBONS and members of a larger CLASS of naturally occurring compounds called LIPIDS.

fatty acid (chemistry) A monobasic CARBOXYLIC ACID, an essential constituent of FATS AND OILS. The simplest FATTY ACIDS are formic (methanoic) ACID, HCOOH, and acetic (ethanoic) ACID, CH_3COOH.

fatty degeneration (histology) Disease of TISSUE caused by poisoning or lack of OXYGEN, in which droplets of fat form within CELLS.

fauces (anatomy) The opening between the mouth and the THROAT, bounded above by the SOFT PALATE, below by the TONGUE, and on each side by the tonsils.

The two folds of MUCOUS MEMBRANE containing MUSCLE fibres (*USA:* muscle fibers) before and behind the tonsils are called the pillars of the FAUCES.

FBP (physics) An abbreviation of 'F'inal 'B'oiling 'P'oint.

FCAP (education) An abbreviation of 'F'ellow of the 'C'ollege of 'A'merican 'P'athologists.

FCRA (education) An abbreviation of 'F'ellow of the 'C'ollege of 'R'adiologists of 'A'ustralasia.

FCS (education) An abbreviation of 'F'ellow of the 'C'hemical 'S'ociety.

FCST (governing body) An abbreviation of 'F'ederal 'C'ouncil for 'S'cience and 'T'echnology.

FD (microscopy) An abbreviation of 'F'ocal 'D'istance.

FDA (governing body) An abbreviation of 'F'ood and 'D'rug 'A'dministration.

F distribution (statistics) The theoretical distribution of the F RATIO. It is the distribution of the ratio of the variances of two independent samples drawn from NORMAL populations. It is used when testing the HYPOTHESIS that the samples yielding the F RATIO have been drawn from the same population. It plays a part in numerous tests including ANALYSIS OF VARIANCE and those used in regression ANALYSIS.

FDP (physiology/ biochemistry) An abbreviation of 'F'ibrinogen 'D'egradation 'P'roducts.

Fe (chemistry) The CHEMICAL SYMBOL for IRON. Derived from Latin, 'ferrum'.

feedback (cybernetics) The influencing of the BEHAVIOUR (*USA:* behavior) of a system by signals received about the effects of its output. In negative FEEDBACK (the most common kind) the activity of the system is reduced by FEEDBACK (a thermostat turns off the boiler when the external TEMPERATURE has risen enough). Most drives involve negative FEEDBACK. In POSITIVE feed-back the signals fed back increase the activity of the system, producing a runaway process.

feedback inhibition (genetics) End-PRODUCT INHIBITION. A GENETIC ENGINEERING control system in which the PRODUCT, *e.g.* an ENZYME, inhibits further production of itself.

feedback loop (cybernetics) The channel through which the output of a system is fed back to it. *See* FEEDBACK.

feeder cells (immunology) CELLS whose FUNCTION is to maintain the GROWTH of other CELLS, usually by secreting GROWTH factors.

Fehling's solution (biochemistry) Test REAGENT consisting of two parts: a SOLUTION of COPPER(II) SULPHATE (*USA:* copper(II) sulfate), and a SOLUTION of POTASSIUM SODIUM TARTRATE and SODIUM HYDROXIDE. When the two solutions are mixed, an ALKALINE SOLUTION of a SOLUBLE COPPER(II) complex is formed. In the presence of an ALDEHYDE or REDUCING SUGAR, a pink-red PRECIPITATE of COPPER(I) OXIDE forms. It was named after the German chemist Hermann Fehling (1812-85).

See also FEHLING'S TEST.

Fehling's test (biochemistry) Test for an ALDEHYDE GROUP or REDUCING SUGAR, indicated by the formation of COPPER(I)

OXIDE as a pink-red PRECIPITATE with FEHLING'S SOLUTION.

FEL (toxicology) An abbreviation of 'F'rank 'E'ffect 'L'evel.

FELASA (society) An abbreviation of 'F'ederation of 'E'uropean 'L'aboratory 'A'nimal 'S'cience 'A'ssociation.

felon (medical/ microbiology) An INFECTION and ABSCESS of the pulp of the finger.

fem. (general terminology) An abbreviation of 'fem'ale/ 'fem'inine.

femur (anatomy) The thigh BONE.

fermentation (chemistry/ microbiology) ENERGY-producing breakdown of ORGANIC COMPOUNDS by MICRO-ORGANISMS (in the absence of OXYGEN); *e.g.* the breakdown of SUGAR by yeasts into ETHANOL, CARBON DIOXIDE and ORGANIC ACIDS. FERMENTATION is a type of ANAEROBIC RESPIRATION.

fermium Fm (chemistry) RADIOACTIVE ELEMENT in GROUP IIIB of the PERIODIC TABLE (one of the ACTINIDES). It has several isotopes, with half-lives of up to 95 days. At. no. 100; r.a.m. (most STABLE ISOTOPE) 257.

ferric (chemistry) TRIVALENT IRON. Also termed: IRON(III).

ferricyanide (chemistry) $[Fe(CN)_6]^{3-}$ Very STABLE COMPLEX ION of IRON(III). A SOLUTION of the POTASSIUM SALT gives a deep blue PRECIPITATE (Prussian blue) in the presence of IRON(II) (FERROUS) ions. Also termed: hexacyanoferrate(III).

ferrimagnetism (physics) Property of certain compounds in which the magnetic moments of neighbouring ions align in anti-parallel fashion.

ferrite (chemistry) Non-conducting ceramic material that exhibits FERRI-MAGNETISM; GENERAL FORMULA MFe_2O_4, where M is a DIVALENT METAL of the TRANSITION ELEMENTS. Ferrites are used to make powerful magnets in radars and other high-FREQUENCY electronic apparatus, such as COMPUTER memories.

ferrocene (chemistry) $C_{10}H_{10}Fe$ Orange ORGAOMETALLIC COMPOUND, whose molecules consist of an IRON ATOM 'sandwiched' between two molecules of cyclopentadiene. Also termed: dicyclopentadienyliron.

ferrocyanide (chemistry) $[Fe(CN)_6]^{4-}$ Very STABLE COMPLEX ION of IRON(II). Also termed: hexacyanoferrate(II).

ferromagnetism (physics) Property of certain substances that in a magnetizing FIELD have INDUCED MAGNETISM, which persists when the FIELD is removed and they become permanent magnets. Examples include IRON, COBALT and their ALLOYS.

ferrous (chemistry) BIVALENT IRON. Also termed: IRON(II).

fertility drug (pharmacology) A drug given to a female to stimulate the OVARY to produce ripe eggs. A COMPOUND that stimulates the body's own production of the FOLLICLE-STIMULATING HORMONE (FSH) is used for this in the course of TREATMENT for infertility, when it is often responsible for the woman becoming pregnant with more than one baby.

fertilization (biology) FUSION of specialized SEX CELLS or gametes which are HAPLOID to form a single CELL, a DIPLOID ZYGOTE. It occurs in SEXUAL REPRODUCTION; *e.g.* in vertebrates the OVUM (female GAMETE) is fertilized by the SPERM (male GAMETE).

FES (education) An abbreviation of 'F'ellow of the 'E'ntomological 'S'ociety.

Feulgen reaction for DNA (histology) Histological staining technique for NUCLEIC ACIDS. Feulgen REAGENT which contains fuchsin and SULPHURIC ACID (*USA*: sulfuric acid) is named after the German physiologist and chemist, R. Feulgen (1884-1955).

FEV (physiology) An abbreviation of 'F'orced 'E'xpiratory 'V'olume - in first second of forced expiration after maximum inspiration.

fever (physiology) A condition in which the body TEMPERATURE is above NORMAL, *i.e.* 37°C. Body TEMPERATURE is controlled by a centre (*USA*: center) in the BRAIN which maintains a BALANCE between HEAT production and its loss from the surface of the body. INFECTION by BACTERIA or VIRUSES, excite the MACROPHAGE CELLS of the reticulo-endothelial system to produce pyrogens, substances which make the TEMPERATURE rise. A great number of conditions can produce FEVER, and when the cause of the FEVER is not known it is referred to as pyrexia of unknown (PUO).

FFA (biochemistry) An abbreviation of unesterified 'F'ree 'F'atty 'A'cid.

FGF (physiology) An abbreviation of 'F'ibroblast 'G'rowth 'F'actor.

FHR (medical) An abbreviation of 'F'oetal 'H'eart 'R'ate. (*USA*: Fetal HEART Rate).

fi (general terminology) An abbreviation of 'f'or 'i'nstance.

FIBiol (education) An abbreviation of 'F'ellow of the 'I'nstitute of 'Biol'ogy.

FIBMS (education) An abbreviation of 'F'ellow of the 'I'nstitute of 'B'io'-M'edical 'S'ciences.

fibre (anatomy) Any long thread-like structure in the body. (*USA*: fiber).

fibre optics (optics) Branch of OPTICS that uses bundles of pure GLASS fibres (*USA*: glass fibers) within straight or curved 'pipes' or cables, along which LIGHT travels as it is internally reflected. A modulated LIGHT signal in such a cable can carry much more DATA (*e.g.* COMPUTER DATA, telephone signals, television channels) than a wire of similar dimensions. FIBRE-OPTIC cables are also used for making endoscopes. Also termed: OPTICAL FIBRES (*USA*: optical fibers).

fibrescope (medical) An ENDOSCOPE using GLASS or plastic fibres (*USA*: fibers) to carry images and LIGHT, which means that the instrument is flexible and more readily introduced into the body cavity that is being examined than the older endoscopes which were rigid. (*USA*: fiberscope).

fibrillation (medical) MUSCLE fibres (*USA*: muscle fibers) normally contract in an orderly and co-ordinated fashion. In FIBRILLATION, the fibres contract independently and spontaneously.

fibrin (haematology) A PROTEIN substance which forms the framework of BLOOD clots. It is precipitated from the BLOOD by the ACTION of the ENZYME THROMBIN or FIBRINOGEN, which creates a BLOOD clot in a WOUND where BLOOD is exposed to AIR.

fibrinogen (haematology) SOLUBLE PLASMA PROTEIN found in BLOOD which, after triggering of chemical factors (*e.g.* caused by a WOUND), is converted to

FIBRIN as part of the BLOOD-clotting mechanism.

fibro-adenoma (histology) A BENIGN TUMOUR (*USA*: tumor) which is commonly found in the breast, consisting of glandular and FIBROUS TISSUE.

fibroblast (cytology) Long flat CELL found in CONNECTIVE TISSUE which secretes PROTEIN; *e.g.* COLLAGEN and elastic fibres (*USA*: elastic fibers).

fibrocystic disease (medical) *See* CYSTIC FIBROSIS.

fibroid (histology) A common BENIGN TUMOUR (*USA*: benign tumor) consisting of MUSCLE and FIBROUS TISSUE enclosed within a CAPSULE found in the UTERUS, usually in women over thirty years of age. There is often more than one, and symptoms may include pain, heavy menstrual PERIODS, and the size of the TUMOUR (*USA*: tumor) may interfere with the BLADDER and cause d'fficulty in passing URINE.

fibroma (histology) A BENIGN TUMOUR (*USA*: benign tumor) composed of FIBROUS TISSUE, usually small and unimportant.

fibrosarcoma (histology) A MALIGNANT TUMOUR (*USA*: malignant tumor) of FIBROUS TISSUE which grows relatively slowly, often in muscles near the surface of the body. It invades neighbouring tissues but is slow to spread to other parts; if it does so, it may metastasise to the lungs.

fibrosis (histology) Formation of FIBROUS TISSUE or scar TISSUE usually in repair or replacement of cellular elements destroyed by injury, INFECTION or deficient BLOOD supply.

fibrous tissue (histology) Scar TISSUE. A simple, strong structural or repair TISSUE comprising of two proteins, COLLAGEN and elastin, laid down by CELLS called fibroblasts.

fibula (anatomy) Leg BONE, located below the knee and outside the TIBIA (shin BONE) in the hind-limb of a tetrapod VERTEBRATE.

FIC (education) An abbreviation of 'F'ellow of the 'I'nstitute of 'C'hemistry.

fiche (general terminology) An abbreviation of micro'fiche'.

field (1 physics; 2 optics; 3 computing) 1 In physics, region in which one OBJECT exerts a FORCE on another OBJECT; *e.g.* ELECTRIC FIELD, GRAVITATIONal FIELD, MAGNETIC FIELD. 2 In OPTICS, AREA that is visible through an optical instrument. 3 In computing, specific part of a RECORD, or a GROUP of characters that make up one piece of information.

field-emission microscope (microscopy) MICROSCOPE used for the observation of the positions of atoms in a surface.

fig. (literary terminology) An abbreviation of 'fig'ure.

figure **(fig.)** (literary terminology) Referring to a chart or table within a text.

FIH (education) An abbreviation of 'F'ellow of the 'I'nstitute of 'H'ygiene.

filament (1 physics; 2, 3 biology) 1 In electrical apparatus, a fine wire of high resistance which is heated by passing an ELECTRIC CURRENT directly through it. Filaments are used in electric fires and incandescent lamps, and as heaters in thermionic valves. 2 HYPHA of a FUNGUS.

3 String of CELLS that make up certain ALGAE.

filariasis (medical/ parasitology) Infestation with *Filaria*, a genus of parasitic thread-like worms, found mainly in the tropics and subtropics. The adults of *Filaria bancrofti* and *Filaria malayi* live in lymphatics, connective tissues or mesentery, where they may cause obstruction, but the embryos migrate to the blood stream. Completion of the life cycle is dependent upon passage through a mosquito.

film (1 physics; 2 PHOTOGRAPHY) 1 Thin layer of one substance on the surface of another substance, *e.g.* oil floating on WATER. Thin films can sometimes diffract LIGHT and produce rainbow colours (*USA*: colors). *See* DIFFRACTION. 2 Plastic strip carrying a LIGHT-sensitive EMULSION that is used in PHOTOGRAPHY.

filter (1 physics; 2 OPTICS) 1 Porous material through which a LIQUID is passed to remove suspended MATTER. 2 In OPTICS, LIGHT-absorbing semi-TRANSPARENT material that passes only certain wavelengths (colours [*USA*: colors]). 3. In ELECTRONICS, device that passes only certain a.c. frequencies.

filter pump (laboratory equipment) Simple VACUUM PUMP in which a jet of WATER draws AIR molecules from the system. It can produce only low pressures and is commonly used to increase the speed of FILTRATION by drawing through the FILTRATE.

filtrate (chemistry) LIQUID obtained after FILTRATION.

filtration (chemistry) Method of separating a suspended SOLID from a LIQUID by passing the MIXTURE through a porous medium, *e.g.* FILTER paper or GLASS WOOL, through which only the LIQUID passes.

fine chemical (chemistry) Chemical produced in pure form and in small quantities.

fine structure (physics) Splitting of certain lines in a line SPECTRUM into a number of further discrete lines, which are observable only when high resolution is employed.

FInst. P (education) An abbreviation of 'F'ellow of the 'Inst'itute of 'P'hysics.

firing (physiology) The initiation of a NERVE IMPULSE.

Fisher's exact probability test (statistics) A test of independence in two-by-two contingency tables giving exact probability levels for all SAMPLE sizes.

Fisher's z-test (statistics) A test to determine the significance of a correlation COEFFICIENT employing FISHER'S Z-TRANSFORMATION.

Fisher's z-transformation (statistics) A TRANSFORMATION of the PRODUCT-moment correlation which yields an approximately NORMAL DISTRIBUTION. It is useful in constructing tests of the significance of correlations and their differences.

fission (1 physics; 2 biology) Splitting. 1 In atomic physics, DISINTEGRATION of an ATOM into two parts, usually with the release of ENERGY and one or more neutrons. 2 In biology, DIVISION of a CELL or single-celled organism into two. *See* MEIOSIS; MITOSIS.

fissure (anatomy) A groove in a surface, particularly a comparatively large groove in the surface of the CORTEX. The term sulcus is used of smaller grooves in the CORTEX, but in practice the terms are often interchangeable.

fistula (medical) An opening either into the interior of the body or in an internal ORGAN, such as can be produced by a WOUND, or by surgery (*e.g.* a tube implanted through the wall of the STOMACH). The term is used both for the opening in the TISSUE and for any tube that is passed through it.

fixation of nitrogen (biology) Part of the NITROGEN CYCLE that involves the conversion and eventual incorporation of atmospheric NITROGEN into compounds that contain NITROGEN. NITROGEN FIXATION in nature is carried out by nitrifying soil BACTERIA or BLUE-GREEN ALGAe (CYANO-PHYTA) in the sea. Soil BACTERIA may exist symbiotically in the ROOT nodules of leguminous plants or they may be free-living. Small amounts of NITROGEN are also fixed, as NITRIC OXIDE, by the ACTION of lightning. *See* SYMBIOSIS.

fixed point (physics) Standard TEM-PERATURE chosen to define a TEMPERATURE SCALE or at which properties are measured, *e.g.* the ICE POINT (0°C) and the steam point (100°C). Also termed: fixed TEMPERATURE.

fl.rt (general terminology) An abbreviation of 'fl'ow 'r'a't'e.

flagellate (microbiology) Single-celled protozoan ANIMAL that moves by beating flagella. *See* FLAGELLUM.

flagellum (microbiology) Long HAIR-like ORGANELLE whose beating movement causes locomotion or the movement of FLUID over a CELL. Flagella are present in most MOTILE gametes and UNICELLULAR plants or animals (*e.g.* PROTOZOA), in which they occur singly or in small clusters. In some MULTICELLULAR organisms (*e.g.* sponges and hydra) they are used for circulation of WATER containing food and respiratory gases.

See also CILIUM.

flame test (chemistry) QUALITATIVE chemical test in which an ELEMENT in a substance is identified by the CHARAC-TERISTIC COLOUR (*USA*: color) it imparts to a BUNSEN burner flame.

flash point (chemistry) Lowest TEM-PERATURE at which a substance or a MIXTURE gives off sufficient VAPOUR to produce a flash on the application of a flame.

flavin adenine dinucleotide (FAD) (chemistry) Co-ENZYME that functions in the OXIDATION-REDUCTION REactions of ENZYMES, *e.g.* the oxidative DEGRADATION of PYRUVATE, FATTY ACIDS and AMINO ACIDS, and in ELECTRON TRANSPORT. Also termed: flavine.

flavonoid (chemistry) Aromatic, OXYGEN-containing HETEROCYCLIC ORGANIC COM-POUND. Many natural pigments are flavonoids.

flavoprotein (chemistry) Member of a GROUP of CONJUGATED proteins in which the PROSTHETIC GROUP constitutes a DERIVATIVE of RIBOFLAVIN (*e.g.* FAD or FMN). FLAVOPROTEIN dehydrogenases (ENZYMES) are involved in the ELECTRON TRANSPORT chain of AEROBIC RESPIRATION.

flocculation (chemistry) COAGULATION of a finely divided PRECIPITATE into larger particles.

floppy disk (computing) Flexible, portable MAGNETIC DISK that provides DATA and PROGRAM STORAGE for microcomputers. The DISK may be enclosed in a flexible or a rigid casing. Also termed: DISKETTE.

See also HARD DISK.

fluid (physics) Form of MATTER that can flow; thus both gases and liquids are fluids. Fluids can offer no permanent resistance to changes of shape. Resistance to flow is manifest as VISCOSITY.

fluid balance (physiology) On AVERAGE the loss of FLUID through URINE, between 1200 ml and 1500 ml a day, and from perspiration and in the breath, up to 1000 ml, requires to be balanced by the intake of about two or three LITRES of FLUID a day. Additional loss through vomiting or DIARRHOEA (*USA*: diarrhea), which also results in a loss of essential electrolyes, requires additional intake of FLUID and electrolyes. *See* DEHYDRATION.

fluid ounce (measurement) Measure of the VOLUME of liquids. 1 fl oz = 28.41 cm^3.

fluid retention (medical) A condition in which URINE DISCHARGE from the urinary tract is drastically reduced. The most common cause is impaired KIDNEY FUNCTION. FLUID RETENTION can have important consequences on both WATER and ELECTROLYTE BALANCE and is treated symptomatically during maintenance THERAPY.

fluidity (physics) Property of flowing easily; the opposite of VISCOSITY.

flukes (TREMATODES) (parasitology) A large GROUP of parasitic flatworms which can infest the intestines, LIVER, lungs and the BLOOD. Some such as *Chlonorchis sinensis*, the LIVER FLUKE, parasitises humans and causes disease.

fluor. (1 physics; 2 chemistry) 1 An abbreviation of 'fluor'escent. 2 An abbreviation of 'fluor'ide.

fluorescein (chemistry) $C_{20}H_{12}O_5$ A dark orange-red dye which dissolves in ALKALIS (*USA*: alkalies) to give a solution with a green FLUORESCENCE. It is used as a chemical marker and for dyeing textiles. Also termed: resorcinolphthalein.

fluorescence (chemistry) Emission of RADIATION (generally VISIBLE LIGHT) after ABSORPTION of RADIATION of another WAVELENGTH (usually ULTRAVIOLET RADIATION or near-ULTRAVIOLET RADIATION) or electrons; it ceases when the stimulating source is removed.

See also LUMINESCENCE; PHOSPHORESCENCE.

fluorescent lamp (laboratory equipment) MERCURY-VAPOUR DISCHARGE LAMP that uses phosphors to produce LIGHT by FLUORESCENCE.

fluoridation (chemistry) Addition of inorganic fluorides to drinking WATER to combat dental DECAY.

fluoride (chemistry) COMPOUND containing FLUORINE; SALT of HYDROFLUORIC ACID (HF).

fluorination (chemistry) Replacement of atoms, usually HYDROGEN, in an ORGANIC COMPOUND by FLUORINE.

fluorine F (chemistry) Gaseous nonmetallic ELEMENT in GROUP VIIA of the PERIODIC TABLE (the HALOGENS). A pale green-yellow poisonous GAS, it is highly reactive and the most electronegative ELEMENT, occurring in FLUORIDE minerals such as

149

FLUORSPAR. It is used, as the gaseous URANIUM(VI) FLUORIDE (UF_6), in the separation by DIFFUSION of URANIUM isotopes and in making fluorocarbons. Inorganic fluorides are added to WATER supplies to combat TOOTH DECAY. At. no. 9; r.a.m. 18.9984.

fluorite (chemistry) An alternative term for FLUORSPAR.

fluorocarbon (chemistry) Very STABLE ORGANIC COMPOUND in which some or all of the HYDROGEN atoms have been replaced by FLUORINE. Fluorocarbons are used as solvents, AEROSOL propellants and refrigerants. Their use is being limited because they have been implicated in damage to the OZONE layer of the ATMOSPHERE.

See also FREON.

fluoroscope (radiology) FLUORESCENT screen that allows direct observation of X-RAY images, often connected to a camera. It is used in medicine (RADI-OGRAPHY) and industrial X-RAY applications.

fluorspar (chemistry) CaF_2 Naturally occurring CALCIUM FLUORIDE, used as a flux in GLASS and as a COMPONENT of certain cements. Also termed: FLUORITE.

Fm (chemistry) The CHEMICAL SYMBOL for FERMIUM.

FMN (biochemistry) An abbreviation of 'F'lavin 'M'ono'N'ucleotide.

fn. (literary terminology) An abbreviation of 'f'oot'n'ote.

f-number (photography) Method of denoting the DIAMETER of a LENS APERTURE in a camera. For a simple LENS it is the FOCAL LENGTH divided by the DIAMETER of the APERTURE. The smaller the f-number, the larger the APERTURE. In the usual sequence *f*22, *f*11, *f*8, *f*5.6, *f*4 etc., each APERTURE has twice the AREA, and therefore admits twice the amount of LIGHT as the preceding one in the series.

FNZ1C (education) An abbreviation of 'F'ellow of the 'N'ew 'Z'ealand 'I'nstitute of 'C'hemistry.

foam (physics) *See* FROTH.

focal distance (FD) (microscopy) Distance from the OPTICAL CENTRE (*USA*: center) of a LENS to the point where LIGHT rays from a distant OBJECT converge. Also known as FOCAL LENGTH.

focal length (optics) Distance from the centre (*USA*: center) of a LENS or curved mirror to its FOCUS. Also termed: FOCAL DISTANCE.

focal plane (microscopy) A plane perpendicular to the OPTICAL AXIS of a LENS and passing through the FOCAL POINT.

focal point (microscopy) The point on the OPTICAL AXIS of a LENS at which parallel rays converge.

focus (1, 2 microscopy) 1 The point or plane at which LIGHT rays, or other electromagnetic rays, converge after passing through an optical system. An IMAGE on this plane is said to be 'in FOCUS' and will have the minimum amount of blur. 2 An alternative term for FOCAL LENGTH.

focusing (microsopy) Adjusting a LENS or optical system so that LIGHT rays from points at a given distance converge to form an IMAGE in a particular plane.

foetal abnormalities (toxicology) The results of teratogenic effects on the FOETUS (*USA*: fetus). These differ from those that occur on exposure of the EMBRYO. Characteristically they are GROWTH retardation and functional deficits rather than anatomical birth defects. (*USA*: fetal abnormalities).

foetal stage (medical) The stage of prenatal existence that follows the embryonic stage; it lasts from about the eighth week after conception until birth. (*USA*: fetal stage).

foetus (biology) The unborn mammalian EMBRYO from the time that it has the recognisable features of its final form *i.e.* from the end of the second month after conception. (pl. foetuses). (*USA*: fetus. pl. fetuses). *See* EMBRYOGENESIS.

folic acid (haematology/ biochemistry) A WATER SOLUBLE VITAMIN of the B complex which acts as a COENZYME in various processes involing the METABOLISM of purines and pyrimidines and which is essential for the formation of NORMAL RED BLOOD CELLS. Insufficient FOLIC ACID in the diet, available in green leafy vegetables and YEAST, or impaired ABSORPTION because of intestinal disease leads to deficiency of this VITAMIN. Deficiency may result in a REDUCTION of RED BLOOD CELLS and those that are present may be larger than they should be, a state called megaloblastic ANAEMIA (*USA*: megaloblastic anemia). Deficiency of FOLIC ACID may also be caused by CHRONIC ALCOHOLISM and as the result of taking certain drugs such as phenytoin.

follicle (histology) A very small secreting GLAND, or cyst.

follicle stimulating hormone (FSH) (biochemistry) Member of a GROUP of HORMONES that are secreted by the ANTERIOR LOBE of the PITUITARY GLAND in vertebrates. It stimulates the GROWTH and maturation of OVARIAN FOLLICLES and the GROWTH only of oocytes, which are matured under the ACTION of LUTEINIZING HORMONE. In males FSH stimulates SPERM formation in the TESTES.

follicular phase (physiology) The PHASE of the OESTROUS CYCLE (*USA*: estrous cycle) in which the OVUM matures in women, roughly the first 14 days of the CYCLE.

fomites (EPIDEMIOLOGY) Articles that have been in contact with an infected person such as clothes, bedding, toys, books, etc; that might be capable of becoming contaminated and of spreading the INFECTION.

Fontana stain (histology) Histological staining technique for MELANIN.

fontanelle (anatomy) The hole covered by a MEMBRANE in the infant's SKULL where the bones are not yet fully closed.

Food and Drug Administration (FDA) (governing body) A US government agency within the Department of Health and Human Services that monitors the purity and safety of food, cosmetics, and drugs; truth in packaging and labelling information; and sanitary practices in restaurants and other food-handling establishments.

food poisoning (medical/ microbiology/ toxicology) Food poisoning can be due to toxic chemicals contaminating the food, to eating poisonous plants or, in most cases, to BACTERIAL INFECTION. The commonest organisms are *Campylobacter jejuni*, *Salmonella sp.*, *Staphylococcus aureus*, and *Clostridium perfringens* and very rarely *Clostridium botulinum*.

Occasionally *Bacillus cereus* is the cause. *See* DIARRHOEA.

foot (measurement) UNIT of length in the IMPERIAL SYSTEM, corresponding to 12 inches or 1/3 of a YARD, and equal to 30.48 centimetres.

foot-pound (measurement) WORK done when a MASS of 1 pound is lifted 1 foot against the FORCE of gravity, equivalent to 1.3558 joules. Also termed: foot-pound-FORCE.

footprinting (molecular biology) Technique for finding DNA sequences that have a PROTEIN bound to them which protects them from being cut by endonucleases. Two samples of the whole DNA MOLECULE are prepared, one with the PROTEIN and one without. Both are digested with a restriction endonuclease and the resulting fragments are run on an electrophoretic GEL. When the two gels are compared, the bands that have resisted cutting by the ENZYME, because of being protected by the PROTEIN, will be distinguishable because they do not match the bands on the other GEL. In this way, DNA sequences that bind proteins, such as regulatory sequences, promoters, and so on, can be identified.

for. (1 general terminology; 2 medical) 1 An abbreviation of 'for'eign. 2 An abbreviation of 'for'ensic.

force (physics) Influence that can make a stationary OBJECT move, or a moving OBJECT change speed or direction, *i.e.* that changes the OBJECT's momentum. It is equal to MASS multiplied by ACCELERATION. The SI UNIT of FORCE is the NEWTON.

force ratio (physics) An alternative term for mechanical advantage.

forebrain (anatomy) Largest and topmost portion of the VERTEBRATE BRAIN that comprises the CEREBRAL HEMISPHERES and the BASAL NUCLEUS.

forensic medicine (medical) That part of medicine concerned with the LAW.

formal saline (histology) A 10 per cent SOLUTION of FORMAL SALINE is used as a fixative preparation.

formaldehyde (chemistry) HCHO Colourless (*USA*: colorless) pungent organic GAS, an ALDEHYDE, which is readily SOLUBLE in WATER. It is used as a disinfectant and in the manufacture of plastics. Also termed: METHANAL.

formalin (histology) A 40 per cent SOLUTION of the GAS FORMALDEHYDE, used for fixing and preserving tissues, and in DILUTION as an ANTISEPTIC.

formic acid (chemistry) HCOOH Simplest CARBOXYLIC ACID, made commercially by the catalytic COMBINATION of CARBON MONOXIDE and SUPERHEATED STEAM. It occurs naturally in the stings of certain insects such as ants, bees and wasps. Also termed: METHANOIC ACID.

formula (1 mathematics; 2 chemistry) 1 Mathematical expression that shows the relationship between various quantities; *e.g.* the FORMULA for the AREA of a circle of RADIUS r is $A = \pi r^2$. 2 Chemical composition of a substance indicated by the symbols of each ELEMENT present in it and subscripts that show the number of each type of ATOM involved; *e.g.* the FORMULA for WATER is H_2O, that for POTASSIUM DICHROMATE is $K_2Cr_2O_7.2H_2O$. Also termed: CHEMICAL FORMULA.

Fortin barometer (physics) MERCURY BAROMETER, used for the accurate measurement of ATMOSPHERIC PRESSURE. It was named after the French physicist Jean Fortin (1750-1831).

FORTRAN (computing) An abbreviation of 'FOR'mula 'TRAN'slation. A COMPUTER programming language designed for mathematical and scientific use.

forward mutation (genetics) A change from the NORMAL, or wild-type, version of an ALLELE to a MUTANT form. The vast majority of MUTATIONS are of this type. *Contrast* back MUTATION.

fossa (anatomy) A depressed or hollow AREA.

Fouchet stain (histology) Histological staining technique for BILE pigments.

Fourier analysis (mathematics) Mathematical method of expressing a complex FUNCTION that represents a WAVE as a SERIES of simpler SINE WAVES. It was named after the French mathematical physicist Jean Fourier (1768-1830).

fovea (histology) Part of the RETINA of the EYE that has a CONCENTRATION of cones (but no rods), which comes into play when ACUTE vision is required. Also termed: YELLOW SPOT.

foxglove (pharmacology) A plant, *DIGITALIS purpurea* in the FAMILY Scrophulariaceae, that contains the cardioactive agent DIGITALIS.

See also DIGITALIS.

fp (1 general terminology; 2, 3 physics; 4 literary terminology) 1 Abbreviation of 'f'lame'p'roof. 2 Abbreviation of 'f'lash'-p'oint. 3 An Abbreviation of 'f'reezing'-p'oint. 4 Abbreviation of 'f'rontis'p'iece.

FPAS (education) An abbreviation of 'F'ellow of the 'P'akistan 'A'cademy of 'S'ciences.

FPharmS (education) An abbreviation of 'F'ellow of the 'Pharm'aceutical 'S'ociety of Great Britain.

Fr (chemistry) The CHEMICAL SYMBOL for FRANCIUM.

FRACI (education) An abbreviation of 'F'ellow of the 'R'oyal 'A'ustralian 'C'hemical 'I'nstitute.

fraction (mathematics) Part of a whole, represented mathematically by a pair of numbers. The upper NUMERATOR is written above the lower DENOMINATOR and separated from it by a horizontal or diagonal line; *e.g.* 1/2, 3/4, 7/10. Fractions of a hundred may be given as percentages; *e.g.* 65/100 = 65 per cent (sometimes written 65%). In decimal fractions, the denominators are powers of 10 (10, 100, 1,000, etc.), usually written using a decimal point and place values as for whole numbers, for instance 27/1,000 = 0.027.

See also COMMON DENOMINATOR.

fractional crystallization (chemistry) Separation of mixtures of substances by the repeated CRYSTALLIZATION of a SOLUTION, each time at a lower TEMPERATURE.

fractional distillation (chemistry) Separation of a number of liquids with different BOILING POINTS by DISTILLATION and collecting separately the liquids that come off at different temperatures. Also termed: FRACTIONATION.

fractionating column (chemistry) Long vertical tube containing bubble-caps, sieve plates, or various irregular packing materials, used for industrial FRACTIONAL DISTILLATION.

fractionation (chemistry) An alternative term for FRACTIONAL DISTILLATION.

fragile x syndrome (genetics) A genetic disorder causing mental retardation in males. It is the result of a MUTATION in the region at the very end of the X CHROMOSOME, which is particularly liable to lose pieces - hence the name 'fragile X'. Some female carriers are also slightly affected.

fragilitas ossium (medical/ genetics) A rare inherited disease in which the bones are abnormally fragile. Also termed osteogenesis imperfecta.

framboesia (bacteriology) *See* YAWS.

frameshift mutation (genetics) A MUTATION in which one or more BASE-pairs are inserted into or deleted from a GENE, so that the reading frame of every codon after that point is shifted along. For example, if the original code was UCU-CAA-AGG-UUA, and the MUTATION put an extra U at the beginning, the message would be read as UUC-UCA-AAG and so on.

francium Fr (chemistry) RADIOACTIVE metallic ELEMENT in GROUP IA of the PERIODIC TABLE (the ALKALI METALS), made by PROTON bombardment of THORIUM. It has several isotopes with half-lives of up to 22 min. At. no. 87; r.a.m. 223 (most STABLE ISOTOPE).

frank effect level (FEL) (toxicology) A LEVEL of exposure to a chemical or MIXTURE that provides an ACUTE, unequivocal deleterious effect.

F ratio (statistics) The ratio of the variances of two independent samples from NORMAL populations. It is used in ANALYSIS OF VARIANCE. *See* F DISTRIBUTION.

FRCPath. (education) An abbreviation of 'F'ellow of the 'R'oyal 'C'ollege of 'Path'ologists.

FRCR (education) An abbreviation of 'F'ellow of the 'R'oyal 'C'ollege of 'R'adiologists.

free electron (physics) An eLECTRON free to move from one ATOM or MOLECULE to another under the influence of an ELECTRIC FIELD. The movement of free electrons enables a CONDUCTOR to carry an ELECTRIC CURRENT.

free energy (physics) Measure of the ability of a system to perform WORK.

free erythrocyte protoporphyrin (FEP) (haematology) An indirect measure of LEAD levels in BLOOD. Protoporphyrin is formed in the MITOCHONDRION during the differentiation of the ERYTHROCYTE in the BONE MARROW. The conversion to haem (*USA*: heme) requires the INSERTION of IRON into the protoporphyrin ring. There is an exponential increase in INHIBITION of porphobilinogen synthase (aminolevulinic ACID dehydratase, ALAD) as BLOOD levels of LEAD increases. The result is a decreased production of porphobilinogen (protoporphyrin PRECURSOR) and inhibition of ferrochelatase, which causes accumulation of inactive HAEMOGLOBIN (*USA*: hemaglobin) molecules which contain ZINC protoporphyrin (ZPP) instead of haem (*USA*: heme). The FEP ANALYSIS, based on the FLUORESCENCE of ZPP, is technically much simpler than the measurement of LEAD in BLOOD.

See also LEAD.

free radical (chemistry) INTERMEDIATE and highly reactive MOLECULE that has an unpaired ELECTRON and so easily forms a CHEMICAL BOND.

freeze drying (chemistry) Method of drying HEAT-sensitive substances such as BLOOD PLASMA or food by FREEZING them below 0°C and then removing the frozen WATER by volatilization in a VACUUM.

freezing (physics) Solidification of a LIQUID that occurs when it is cooled sufficiently (to below its FREEZING POINT).

freezing mixture (chemistry) MIXTURE of two substances that absorbs HEAT and can be used to produce a TEMPERATURE below 0°C.

See also EUTECTIC MIXTURE.

freezing point (physics) TEMPERATURE at which a LIQUID solidifies. Also termed: solidification point.

FREnt.S (education) An abbreviation of 'F'ellow of the 'R'oyal 'Ent'omological 'S'ociety.

free energy (physics) Measure of the ability of a system to perform WORK.

free erythrocyte protoporphyrin (FEP) (haematology) An indirect measure of LEAD levels in BLOOD. Protoporphyrin is formed in the MITOCHONDRION during the differentiation of the ERYTHROCYTE in the BONE MARROW. The conversion to haem (*USA*: heme) requires the INSERTION of

freon (chemistry) Trade name for certain fluorocarbons and chlorofluorocarbons derived from methane and ETHANE. They are used as refrigerants.

freq. (general terminology) An abbreviation of 'freq'uency.

frequency (freq.) (1 physics; 2 statistics) 1 Rate of recurrence of WAVE, *i.e.* number of cycles, oscillations or vibrations in UNIT time, usually one second. The FREQUENCY of a WAVE is inversely proportional to the WAVELENGTH. The SI UNIT of FREQUENCY is the hertz (which corresponds to 1 CYCLE per second). 2 The number of times a given phenomenon occurs.

frequency curve (statistics) A curve in which the FREQUENCY of occurrence of each of a SET of consecutive values, or of values grouped in intervals, is plotted on the vertical AXIS and the values on the horizontal AXIS.

frequency distribution (statistics) The FREQUENCY with which the members of a SAMPLE or of a population take one of a SET of consecutive values, or values grouped in intervals, or with which they are distributed among different categories.

FRES (education) An abbreviation of 'F'ellow of the 'R'oyal 'E'ntomological 'S'ociety of London.

FRIC (education) An abbreviation of 'F'ellow of the 'R'oyal 'I'nstitute of 'C'hemistry.

Friedman test (statistics) A non-parametric test applicable to DATA in which there are more than two MATCHED SAMPLES. It is based on ranking the scores within each SAMPLE. *Compare* Wilcoxon test.

FRIPHH (education) An abbreviation of 'F'ellow of the 'R'oyal 'I'nstitute of 'P'ublic 'H'ealth and 'H'ygiene.

FRMS (education) An abbreviation of 'F'ellow of the 'R'oyal 'M'icroscopical 'S'ociety.

frontal (anatomy) Towards the front of the body or of an ORGAN.

froth (physics) Collection of fairly STABLE small bubbles in a LIQUID produced by shaking, aeration or addition of a foaming agent, *e.g* a DETERGENT. Also termed: foam.

frozen section (histology) A process in which a BIOPSY is taken, frozen and cut into sections for the pathologist to examine under the MICROSCOPE and provide a rapid answer as to whether a TISSUE is MALIGNANT or not.

FRS (education) An abbreviation of 'F'ellow of the 'R'oyal 'S'ociety.

FRSSI (education) An abbreviation of 'F'ellow of the 'R'oyal 'S'tatistical 'S'ociety of 'I'reland.

FRSSS (education) An abbreviation of 'F'ellow of the 'R'oyal 'S'tatistical 'S'ociety of 'S'cotland.

FRSTM & H (education) An abbreviation of 'F'ellow of the 'R'oyal 'S'ociety of 'T'ropical 'M'edicine and 'H'ygiene.

fructose (chemistry) $C_6H_{12}O_6$ Fruit SUGAR, a MONOSACCHARIDE CARBOHYDRATE (HEXOSE) found in sweet fruits and honey. Also termed: LAEVULOSE.

fs (general terminology) *See* FACS.

FSH (biochemistry) An abbreviation of 'F'ollicle-'S'timulating 'H'ormone.

FSH-RH (physiology/ biochemistry) Abbreviation of 'FSH'-'R'eleasing 'H'ormone

F test (statistics) A statistical test based on the F RATIO and F DISTRIBUTION. It is used in anova and in testing whether two variances are equal.

fulminant (medical) Severe.

fumigation (microbiology/ parasitology) The process of burning or volatilising substances in ORDER to produce vapours which destroy infective organisms and vermin. It is now rarely employed.

function (1 general terminology; 2 mathematics; 3 computing) 1 The natural use to which anything can be put, its role or purpose. 2 Mathematical expression that involves one or more variables. 3 Any operation performed by a PROGRAM, a use similar to the term's mathematical meaning.

functional group (chemistry) ATOM or GROUP of atoms that cause a chemical COMPOUND to behave in a particular way; *e.g.* the FUNCTIONAL GROUP in ALCOHOLs is the -OH (hydroxyl) GROUP.

fundamental units (measurements) Units of length, MASS and time that form the basis of most systems of units. *See* SI UNITS.

fungi (mycology) One of the five kingdoms of living things, containing a number of GENERA that are medically important such as Candida SPECIES and Aspergillus SPECIES, and others of economical importance such as the YEAST *Saccharomyces*. Much genetic research has been done on other FUNGI, including the moulds (*USA*: molds) *Aspergillus* and *Neurospora*. Although they are plants, FUNGI are unable to photosynthesize (*i.e.* utilize ENERGY from sunlight to synthesize ORGANIC COMPOUNDS), so they have to obtain their food by living off other plants or animals, alive or dead. FUNGI can reproduce either by CELL DIVISION (equal or unequal, the latter including either BUDDING or the production of spores) or by SEXUAL REPRODUCTION, in which case they have alternation of generations, with HAPLOID and DIPLOID forms.

See also CLASSIFICATION.

fungicides (pharmacology/ mycology) Substance that kills FUNGI. A diverse GROUP of chemicals drawn from several different classes, produced for the control of PATHOGENIC FUNGI, primarily those affecting food and ornamental plants, although a few drugs are available to treat fungal diseases of humans and animals.

fungus (mycology) Mainly terrestrial plant-like organism, different from other plants because of its lack of chlorophyll. Most FUNGI are saprophytic or parasitic organisms *e.g.* moulds (*USA*: molds) whose walls consists of CHITIN, although a few produce CELLULOSE as well. They are classified as the plant DIVISION (PHYLUM) Mycota, although some authorities put them in a KINGDOM of their own.

furanose (chemistry) Any of a GROUP of MONOSACCHARIDE sugars (pentoses) whose molecules have a five-membered HETERO-CYCLIC ring of four CARBON atoms and one OXYGEN ATOM.

See also PYRANOSE.

furuncle (medical) A boil.

fuse (physics) Device used for protecting against an excess ELECTRIC CURRENT passing through a CIRCUIT. It consists of a piece of METAL, connected into the CIRCUIT, that heats and melts (thereby breaking the CIRCUIT) when the CURRENT exceeds a certain value.

fusiform (microbiology) Spindle shaped, as in the ANAEROBE *Fusobacterium nucleatum*.

fusiform cell (cytology) A type of stellate CELL in the CORTEX that has two short vertical projections which divide into many long processes running upwards or downwards from the CELL BODY.

fusiform layer (histology/ cytology) The innermost layer of NERVE CELLS in the CEREBRAL CORTEX, containing mostly FUSIFORM CELLS.

fusion (1 cytology; 2 physics) 1 The intimate mixing of CELLS to produce a HYBRID CELL. 2 Act of melting or joining together.

fusion gene (genetics) A GENE resulting from the accidental mixing of parts of two different genes. This may happen as the result of a small deletion occurring between two genes, leaving their ends joined up. FUSION GENES can also be made *in vitro* using RECOMBINANT DNA technology.

G

G (1 measurement; 2 computing; 3 physics; 4 biochemistry) 1 An abbreviation of 'G'iga-. 2 An abbreviation of 'G'igabyte. 3 An abbreviation of 'G'ravitational CONSTANT. 4 A symbol for glycine.

g (measurement) An abbreviation of 'g'ram. Also termed gm.

Ga (chemistry) The CHEMICAL SYMBOL for GALLIUM.

GABA (biochemistry) An abbreviation for 'G'amma-'A'mino'B'utyric 'A'cid.

GABA-T (biochemistry) An abbreviation of 'GABA' 'T'ransaminase.

GAD (biochemistry) An abbreviation of 'G'lut'A'mate 'D'ecarboxylase.

gadolinium Gd (chemistry) Silvery-white metallic ELEMENT in GROUP IIIB of the PERIODIC TABLE (one of the LANTHANIDES), which becomes strongly magnetic at low temperatures. At. no. 64; r.a.m. 157.25.

gain (physics) The DEGREE to which a signal is amplified (POSITIVE GAIN) or reduced (negative GAIN) when it passes through a system or from one system to another.

galactosaemic (biochemistry) A genetically determined disease in which the LIVER degenerates from early infancy owing to the inability to metabolize the SUGAR GALACTOSE; there is also serious mental deterioration. If the condition is diagnosed at birth, the baby can be put on a GALACTOSE-free (*i.e.* nonmilk) diet, in which case there are no ill effects. This diet can be relaxed after the age of five. The genetic cause is an autosomal RECESSIVE, and about 1 in 50,000 babies is affected. HETEROZYGOTES (*i.e.* carriers) among the siblings of an affected child can be identified by biochemical tests. (*USA*: galactosemic).

galactose (chemistry) $C_6H_{12}O_6$ MONO-SACCHARIDE SUGAR that occurs in milk and in certain gums and seaweeds as the POLYSACCHARIDE galactan.

gall (biochemistry) An alternative term for BILE.

gall bladder (anatomy) STORAGE ORGAN in some vertebrates that, stimulated by HORMONES, releases BILE (along the BILE DUCT) to the DUODENUM during DIGESTION.

gallium Ga (chemistry) Blue-grey metallic ELEMENT in GROUP IIIa of the PERIODIC TABLE, used in low-MELTING POINT ALLOYS and thermometers. At. no. 31; r.a.m. 69.72.

gallon (measurement) UNIT of LIQUID and dry CAPACITY, equal to four quarts or eight pints. One Imperial gallon is the VOLUME occupied by ten pounds of DISTILLED WATER. One Imperial gallon = 4.54609 LITRES. One US gallon = 5/6 Imperial gallons, or 3.7854 LITRES.

gallstone (biochemistry) Accretion, usually of CHOLESTEROL or CALCIUM salts, that occurs in the GALL BLADDER or its ducts. Also termed: BILIARY CALCULUS.

gallyas technique (histology) A staining technique that may be used to show neurofibrillary changes in CNS.

GALT (histology) An abbreviation of 'G'ut 'A'ssociated 'L'ymphoid 'T'issue.

galvanic (physics) Pertaining to DIRECT CURRENT, as opposed to ALTERNATING CURRENT.

galvanic cell (physics) An alternative term for a VOLTAIC CELL.

galvanic skin response (GSR) (physiology) A decrease in the ELECTRICAL RESISTANCE of the SKIN, occurring in a state of arousal, whether pleasant or unpleasant; it is produced by activity of the SWEAT GLANDS. The resistance change is often measured in ORDER to detect arousal.

galvanometer (physics) Device that detects or measures small ELECTRIC CURRENTs passing through it.

gamete (cytology) Specialized SEX CELL (*e.g.* an OVUM or a SPERM), which is usually HAPLOID (containing half the NORMAL number of chromosomes). Gametes are customarily produced by a male and a female, and they combine at FERTILIZATION to form a ZYGOTE that develops into a new organism (with the NORMAL, DIPLOID, CHROMOSOME number). Also termed: GERM CELL.

See also PARTHENOGENESIS.

gamma globulin (immunology) An alternative term for IMMUNOGLOBULIN.

gamma radiation (radiology) Penetrating form of ELECTROMAGNETIC RADIATION of shorter WAVELENGTH than X-RAYS, produced, *e.g.* during the DECAY of certain RADIO-ISOTOPES. It is used to sterilize food, to make industrial radiographs and in medicine (RADIO-THERAPY).

gamma rays (radiology) High-ENERGY photons that make up GAMMA RADIATION.

gamma-aminobutyric acid (GABA) (biochemistry) An AMINO ACID that is an inhibitory NEUROTRANSMITTER; it is found in the CORTEX, basal ganglia, and elsewhere in the CENTRAL NERVOUS SYSTEM.

ganglion (1, 2, medical) 1 A collection of NERVE CELLS in the course of a NERVE or a NETWORK of NERVE FIBRES (*USA*: nerve fibers) outside the CENTRAL NERVOUS SYSTEM. *Compare* NUCLEUS. 2 A cystic swelling found in relation to a TENDON.

ganglion cell (cytology) A CELL with a large roughly spherical body. They are found, *e.g.* as the third-ORDER retinal CELLS (whose axons enter the OPTIC NERVE) and as the first-ORDER AUDITORY CELLS, as well as in other sensory systems.

gangrene (medical/ microbiology) Death of a part or TISSUE due to failure of BLOOD supply, disease, or injury.

gap junction (physiology) A SYNAPSE at which the gap between the presynaptic and postsynaptic CELLS is only about 2 nm wide and is bridged by channels of membranous particles. Ions and other small molecules can pass through it from one CELL to the other. GAP JUNCTIONs are the basis of the electrical SYNAPSE.

gas (chemistry) Form (PHASE) of MATTER in which the atoms and molecules move randomly with high speeds, occupy all the space available, and are comparatively far apart; a VAPOUR. A LIQUID heated above its BOILING POINT changes into a GAS.

gas chromatography (biochemistry) A method of analysing mixtures of substances. The SAMPLE is volatilized and then introduced into a column containing the stationary PHASE (a SOLID or a non-VOLATILE LIQUID on an INERT support), and an INERT CARRIER GAS (*e.g.* ARGON) is passed through the column. Components of the MIXTURE are removed from the column by the CARRIER GAS at different rates. A detector measures the electrical CONDUCTIVITY of the GAS leaving the column, which is recorded on a chart as a SERIES of peaks corresponding to each of the components. The chart is calibrated by passing samples of known composition through the machine.

gas constant (R or R₀) (physics) A CONSTANT in the GAS EQUATION, value 8.31434 j mol^{-1} K^{-1}. Also termed: universal molar gas constant.

gas equation (physics) For n moles of a GAS, $pV = nRT$, where p = PRESSURE, V = VOLUME, n = number of moles, R = the GAS CONSTANT and T ABSOLUTE TEMPERATURE.

gas exchange (physiology) Part of RESPIRATION in which organisms exchange gases (CARBON DIOXIDE and OXYGEN) with their ENVIRONMENT: AIR for terrestrial plants and animals, WATER for aquatic ones. It may involve the use of lungs (mammals, birds, adult amphibians and reptiles), gills (larval amphibians, fish and other aquatic animals), spiracles (insects and other terrestrial arthropods) or stomata (green plants). In other organisms (*e.g.* aquatic plants, FUNGI) GAS EXCHANGE takes place directly between CELLS and the ENVIRONMENT.

gas laws (physics) Relationships between PRESSURE, VOLUME and TEMPERATURE of a GAS. The COMBINATION of Boyle's, CHARLES'S and Gay-Lussac's laws is the GAS EQUATION.

gas thermometer (physics) THERMOMETER based on the VARIATION in PRESSURE or VOLUME of a GAS. Also termed: CONSTANT-VOLUME GAS THERMOMETER.

gas-liquid chromatography (physics/chemistry) (GLC) Type of GAS CHROMATOGRAPHY in which the column contains a non-VOLATILE LIQUID on an INERT support.

gastric (medical) Pertaining to the STOMACH or DIGESTION.

gastric juice (biochemistry) FLUID secreted by GLANDS in the STOMACH wall during DIGESTION; it contains two principal ENZYMES, PEPSIN and RENNIN, and HYDROCHLORIC ACID.

gastric lavage (medical) The washing of the STOMACH usually with SALINE solutions via a lavage tube. It is used as a rapid method to remove STOMACH contents in poisoning cases, particularly in cases in which EMESIS is not recommended.

gastric ulcer (medical) *See* PEPTIC ULCER.

gastritis (medical) INFLAMMATION of the STOMACH.

gastrointestinal (anatomy) Pertaining to the digestive tract. In humans, this consists of the BUCCAL CAVITY, OESOPHAGUS (*USA*: esophagus), STOMACH, SMALL INTESTINE (DUODENUM, JEJUNUM and ILEUM), LARGE INTESTINE (COLON and RECTUM), with various associated GLANDS and accessory structures.

gastroscope (medical) An ENDOSCOPE for viewing the interior of the STOMACH. No ANAESTHETIC (*USA*: anesthetic) is needed for the examination, which is perhaps uncomfortable but safe.

gastrostomy (medical) An operation on the STOMACH in which an opening is made between the STOMACH and the overlying abdominal wall, used in cases in which the OESOPHAGUS (*USA*: esophagus) is blocked or the patient is unable to swallow. A self-retaining catheter or tube is introduced into the opening through which the patient is fed.

gate (computing) An electronic CIRCUIT (switch) that produces a single output signal from two or more input signals. Also termed: LOGIC ELEMENT.

Gay-Lussac's law of volume (physics) When gases react their volumes are in a simple ratio to each other and to the VOLUME of products, at the same TEMPERATURE and PRESSURE. It was named after the French chemist and physicist Joseph Gay-Lussac (1778-1850).

GBG (biochemistry) An abbreviation of 'G'onadal steroid-'B'inding 'G'lobulin.

G-CSF (physiology) An abbreviation of 'G'ranulocyte - 'C'olony 'S'timulating 'F'actor.

Gd (chemistry) The CHEMICAL SYMBOL for GADOLINIUM.

Ge (chemistry) The CHEMICAL SYMBOL for GERMANIUM.

Geiger counter (radiology) Instrument for detecting atomic and sub-atomic particles (*e.g.* ALPHA PARTICLES and BETA PARTICLES), used for RADIOACTIVITY measurements. It was named after the

German physicist Hans Geiger (1882-1945). Also termed: Geiger-Müller COUNTER.

See also COUNTER.

Geiger-Nuttal law (physics) Empirical LAW for calculating the distance that an ALPHA PARTICLE can travel once it is emitted from a RADIOACTIVE substance.

gel filtration chromatography (biochemistry) *See* CHROMATOGRAPHY, GEL FILTRATION.

gel filtration (chemistry) A type of CHROMATOGRAPHY in which compounds are separated according to their molecular size. Molecules of the components of a MIXTURE penetrate the surface of an INERT porous material in proportion to their size. Also termed: gel permeation.

gel. (chemistry) An abbreviation of 'GEL'ATIN.

gelatin (chemistry) A colourless (*USA*: colorless) and TRANSPARENT substance made from the COLLAGEN of the CONNECTIVE TISSUE of animals. It has the consistency of jelly.

See COLLOID.

gen. (1, 2 classification; 3 genetics; 4 anatomy) 1 An abbreviation of 'gen'eric. 2 An abbreviation of 'gen'us. 3 An abbreviation of 'gen'etic. 4 An abbreviation of 'gen'ital.

gene (genetics) The BASIC UNIT of HEREDITY. A GENE is a sequence of DNA, occupying its own place, or LOCUS, on a CHROMOSOME. Most genes are structural, *i.e.* they code for a particular PROTEIN; these genes are divided into housekeeping and LUXURY GENES. Other genes code for the RNA molecules that are necessary for PROTEIN SYNTHESIS, and others again provide recognition markers for the polymerase ENZYMES involved in GENE REGULATION. A GENE may exist in two or more alternative forms, called ALLELES. Genes do not change except in the very rare event of MUTATION. There are many genes in the human GENOME that have been passed unchanged down the generations for millions of years.

See also MUTATION.

gene amplification (genetics) The process by which extra copies of a GENE that is needed temporarily are made. This can occur naturally, *e.g.* in *Drosophila* females who when required multiply ten fold the genes that code for the proteins that compose the membranes of their eggs. Gene amplification can also be artificially induced, and has been observed in mice, who respond to a sub-lethal dose of CADMIUM by multiplying copies of the genes coding for the PROTEIN metallothioncin that neutralizes the POISON.

gene cloning (genetics) The technique of taking a complete GENE from an organism's GENOME and inserting it, via a plasmid, into a HOST BACTERIAL CELL. To make sure that the GENE will be expressed by the BACTERIAL CELL, regulatory regions as well as the coding sequence of the GENE must be included. This technique, perhaps the most BASIC one in GENETIC ENGINEERING, can be used to produce large amounts of the PRODUCT of any GENE that has been isolated. Human genes have been cloned in *ESCHERICHIA COLI* to produce once scarce proteins for TREATMENT of people whose own GENE is defective; these proteins include GROWTH HORMONE and INSULIN.

gene divergence (genetics) The process by which a sequence of related genes arises from an original single GENE that has been duplicated a number of times and then undergone divergent changes in the different copies.

gene dosage (genetics) The number of times that a GENE is represented in an organism's CELLS, or total GENOME. It can range from as low as one, if there is a single-copy GENE on the X CHROMOSOME in animals, to many thousands for a highly duplicated GENE.

gene expression (genetics) The production of RNA and cellular proteins.

gene flow (genetics) The movement of genes from one population into a neighbouring one. It may happen by interbreeding or migration or both.

gene frequency (genetics) The FREQUENCY with which a particular ALLELE occurs at a given LOCUS. It is expressed as a decimal: if there are only two ALLELES, the GENE frequencies could be, for example, 0.1 and 0.9 (the total must add up to 1). EVOLUTION is really a matter of changing GENE frequencies: the old ALLELE gets rarer as the new one comes in, and finally the new one may become fixed, so that there is a complete change in the genetic constitution of the population in respect of that LOCUS. Taken over a sufficient number of loci (which could perhaps be rather few), this gives rise to a new SPECIES. Changes in GENE FREQUENCY are brought about by NATURAL SELECTION, GENE FLOW, founder effect and GENETIC DRIFT.

gene library (genetics) A collection of the genes from a SPECIES, maintained as GENE clones. It is different from a DNA library in that the items stored are whole genes, not DNA fragments.

gene pool (genetics) The total number of ALLELEs in an interbreeding population.

gene product (genetics) The MOLECULE that is made from the information in a single GENE. In the majority of cases it is a PROTEIN or POLYPEPTIDE, but some genes code for a sequence of RNA. *See* PROTEIN SYNTHESIS.

gene regulation (genetics) The various systems by which genes that are not constitutive *i.e.* in use all the time, are switched on and off. GENE REGULATION is the means by which CELLS specialize into the very many different CELL types found in even quite simple organisms, and by which organisms respond moment by moment to changes in their external and internal ENVIRONMENT. Most of what is known about regulation has been discovered in prokaryotes, and EUKARYOTE GENE REGULATION is still hardly understood. The key feature in prokaryotes is the OPERON, a sequence of DNA in which the regulatory genes and the several structural genes *e.g.* for a metabolic process, are in a line, one next to the other. Some operons are inducible, that is they are not transcribed until they are switched on by the presence of some MOLECULE within the CELL. Others are repressible, *i.e.* they are normally transcribed until they are switched off by some MOLECULE within the CELL.

gene splicing (genetics) *See* RECOMBINANT DNA.

gene switch (genetics) The moment when a developing organism changes over from one GENE, or SET of genes, to another related one. A classic example is the change in humans from foetal HAEMOGLOBIN (*USA*: fetal hemaglobin) to the adult equivalent. The SERIES of 'choices' made by GENE SWITCHing are irreversible.

gene therapy (medical/ genetics) The TREATMENT of disorders by altering the genetic material in a CELL, *e.g.* by microinjection of favourable genes into a GERM CELL. Genetic disorders that could possibly be suitable for this approach Include HAEMOPHILIA (*USA*: hemophilia), severe combined immune deficiency, sickle-CELL ANAEMIA (*USA*: sickle-cell anemia), and THALASSAEMIA (*USA*: thalassemia).

genera (biology) Plural of GENUS.

general formula (chemistry) Expression representing the common CHEMICAL FORMULA of a GROUP of compounds *e.g.* C_nH_{2n+2} is the GENERAL FORMULA for an ALKANE. A SERIES of compounds of the same GENERAL FORMULA constitute an HOMOLOGOUS SERIES.

generally regarded as safe (GRAS) (toxigenicity) Term used by the Food and Drug Administration applied to substances that are not known to cause harm when used as directed.

generation time (1 genetics; 2 microbiology) 1 The AVERAGE time in a SPECIES between the birth of an individual and its production of offspring. 2 The time within a population of CELLS (*e.g.* MICROORGANISMS) that it takes for them to undergo DIVISION to form pairs of DAUGHTER CELLS; *i.e.* the doubling time.

generic (classification) The official name of a drug is the generic name, as opposed to the brand name given it by the manufacturer.

genet (genetics) An organism raised clonally from a single ZYGOTE. *See* CLONE.

See also ORTET.

genetic code (genetics) A code which consists of three NUCLEOTIDE bases occurring in a DNA or RNA MOLECULE. It determines which AMINO ACID is incorporated into a PROTEIN at a given point in the sequence. The code thus contains instructions for all ENZYMES produced in the CELL, and consequently the characteristics of the organism.

genetic death (genetics) The death of a GENE, in the sense that the individual who carried it failed to reproduce. This may have been because the individual itself died as a result of carrying the GENE, but not necessarily. From the genetical point of view, it is the fact that fertility was reduced to zero that counts.

genetic distance (genetics) A measure of the amount of relatedness of two individuals or populations, in terms of the probability of their possessing the same ALLELES at a LOCUS or loci.

genetic drift (genetics) Random fluctuation in the FREQUENCY of particular genes in a population. It becomes an important effect in small populations when drift can cause the loss of an ALLELE from the GENE POOL even though it was a useful one.

genetic engineering (genetics) Manipulation of genetic material such as DNA for practical use, *e.g.* the introduction of foreign genes into MICRO-ORGANISMS for the production of a useful PROTEIN (such as human INSULIN). The DNA so produced is called RECOMBINANT DNA, and the term 'RECOMBINANT DNA technology' is often

used. The technique is also used in the study of genetic material.

genetic fingerprinting (genetics) A technique which distinguishes the individuality of an individuals DNA. Devised by the British geneticist Alec Jeffreys (1950-), GENETIC FINGERPRINTING is the ANALYSIS of the Alu sequence that is present in many repeats in the human GENOME. The number of repeats, their position in the GENOME and their exact sequence differs from one person to another. The repeats are digested with restriction endonucleases and identified by SOUTHERN BLOTTING. The technique has been used in forensic science in two ways. First it can identify with certainty whether a SAMPLE of BLOOD, SALIVA or SEMEN came from a particular individual. Second, it can establish whether a child is or is not the offspring of an alleged mother or father, given that the genetic fingerprint of the other parent is available.

genetic load (genetics) The hidden burden on a population of deleterious RECESSIVE MUTATIONS. While these ALLELES are in the HETEROZYGOUS state, they do no harm, but once they meet in the HOMOZYGOUS state, they damage the individual and therefore the population.

genetic map (genetics) A diagram that shows the position on a CHROMOSOME of the various genes that are known to be on it. A method has been devised using the FREQUENCY of crossing-over between two genes as a measure of how far apart they are on a CHROMOSOME: two genes exactly next to each other will very seldom have a cross-over between them, but genes at opposite ends of a CHROMOSOME will be separated by any cross-over along the length of the CHROMOSOME. The BASIC technique of mapping is therefore to make large numbers of crosses involving two or more loci at which there are distinguishable variant ALLELES, and to RECORD the number of times that RECOMBINATION of the original types has taken place. The FREQUENCY of the crossovers is expressed as a PERCENTAGE, and one PERCENTAGE point is known as a MAP UNIT. When three or more loci are mapped in this way, the MAP UNITS add up as they should. For example, if LOCUS A and LOCUS B have a 7 per cent cross-over FREQUENCY between them, and LOCUS B and LOCUS C have 10 per cent, loci A and C have crossovers in 17 per cent of instances. Other methods of locating genes on chromosomes include deletion mapping, and restriction mapping.

genetic screening (genetics) There are two different types of GENETIC SCREENING. The first is the search within a well-defined population or community for carriers of a deleterious RECESSIVE GENE, in ORDER to advise them of the risk of having an affected child. This can only be done if (a) the community can be identified as having a significantly HIGH FREQUENCY of the MUTANT GENE; (b) there is a simple and cheap test to identify carriers; (c) there is a prenatal test to be used for pregnancies at risk; and (d) the procedure is acceptable to the community. Given these conditions, GENETIC SCREENING can be successful in reducing the number of babies born with a particular DEFECT. The second type of GENETIC SCREENING is the genetic inspection of persons for employment, insurance assessment and other commercial transactions. This is more a problem for the future than for the present, as genetic factors affecting employment (*e.g.* susceptibilities to particular workplace hazards) are not, at present, understood. The ethical issue

will have to be confronted, as to whether it is justifiable to exclude a person from a job or benefit because of his or her GENOTYPE. On the face of it, there does not seem to be much difference between GENETIC SCREENING and ordinary medical screening, where the civil rights of the person not to be discriminated against has to be weighed against the civil rights of other people who may be put at risk by that person's medical condition.

genetic variance (genetics) The proportion of the total VARIANCE of a trait that is due to genes. It may have several components, due to the ADDITIVE EFFECTS of separate genes, or dominance, or INTERACTION. The rest of the VARIANCE is environmentally produced. The relative contribution of genetic factors to VARIANCE is not a fixed feature of any trait. *See* HERITABILITY.

genetics (genetics) Study of inheritable characteristics of organisms; *i.e.* HEREDITY.

genito-urinary (GU) (anatomy) Pertaining to both the reproductive structures and the urinary tract.

genocopy (genetics) A genetically determined CHARACTER that mimics the appearance of another genetically determined CHARACTER, though caused by an ALLELE at a different LOCUS.

genome (genetics) The total amount of genetic information that an organism possesses; the sum of its genes. In eukaryotes, this means the entire SET of genes in a HAPLOID SET of chromosomes. The GENOME of a VIRUS may be made up of either DNA (single or double stranded) or RNA; it can be as small as 3500 BASE-pairs and may contain as few as three genes.The GENOME of a PROKARYOTE

(BACTERIA, etc.) is contained in a doublestranded DNA MOLECULE (not strictly a CHROMOSOME), and contains from about 750,000 to 4,500,000 BASE-pairs, comprising up to about 1500 genes. This MOLECULE is extremely compact. The eukaryotes have even larger genomes, and in general, the higher up the evolutionary scale, the larger the GENOME (but with exceptions: some SPECIES of amphibians and fish have genomes nearly 40 times larger than the AVERAGE for mammals). The size of the GENOME bears no simple relationship to the number of chromosomes: closely related SPECIES may have either a large number of small chromosomes or vice versa, for roughly the same-sized GENOME. Humans have a GENOME of about 2900 million basepairs of DNA, which, if it were all in one DNA MOLECULE, would be 1 METRE long. (This is the HAPLOID total; each of our body CELLS has twice this amount.) It would be physically possible for there to be as many as one million genes encoded in that much DNA, but in common with other eukaryotes, humans have many instances of repetitive sequences of DNA that do not seem to have any meaning, and the actual number of WORKING genes is probably much lower. There are also many genes that are present in multiple copies.

genotype (genetics) Genetic constitution of an organism, *i.e.* the characteristics specified by its ALLELES. It is the outward appearance of the organism, as opposed to the way its genes are expressed (which is the PHENOTYPE).

gentian violet (chemistry) An ANILINE dye used by microscopists as a stain. As crystal violet it may be used on unbroken SKIN as an ANTISEPTIC.

genus (gen.) (taxonomy) In biological CLASSIFICATION, one of the groups into which a FAMILY is divided, and which is itself divided into SPECIES.

See also BINOMIAL NOMENCLATURE.

geometric isomerism (chemistry) Form of stercoisomerism that results from there being no free rotation about a BOND between two atoms. Groups attached to each ATOM may be on the same side of the BOND (the *cis*-ISOMER) or on opposite sides (the *trans*-ISOMER). Also termed: cistrans isomerism.

geometric mean (statistics) A measure of central tendency, arrived at by taking the nth ROOT of the PRODUCT of all scores, where n is the number of scores. *Contrast* ARITHMETIC MEAN.

geometric progression (statistics) Sequence of numbers whose sucessive members differ by a CONSTANT multiplier. *E.g.* for the geometric progression, 2, 8, 32, 128, ... the common multiplier is 4.

See also ARITHMETIC PROGRESSION.

geometric series (statistics) SERIES whose terms form a GEOMETRIC PROGRESSION.

germ cell (genetics) *See* GAMETE.

germ (microbiology) Imprecise term for a MICRO-ORGANISM that can cause disease; a PATHOGEN. GERMS include BACTERIA; PROTOZOA; VIRUSES.

germ layer (histology) Layer of CELLS present in an EMBRYO. In triploblastic organisms the layers consist of ECTODERM, MESODERM and endoderm, which each give rise to particular tissues.

german measles (medical/ virology) *See* RUBELLA.

germanium Ge (chemistry) Grey-white semi-metallic ELEMENT in GROUP IVA of the PERIODIC TABLE, which occurs in some SILVER ores. It is an important semiconductor, used for making solid-state diodes and transistors. Its OXIDE is used in optical instruments and INFRA-RED cameras. At. no. 32; r.a.m. 72.59.

germinal stage (physiology) The first stage of embryonic development, which lasts about two weeks, during which there is little cellular differentiation in the human EMBRYO.

gerontology (physiology) The study of aging.

gestation (physiology) The process of carrying the EMBRYO and fetus from conception to birth. The duration of PREGNANCY.

gestational diabetes (biochemistry) ABNORMAL GLUCOSE TOLERANCE during PREGNANCY with return to NORMAL after delivery.

GeV (measurement) An abbreviation of 'G'iga-'e'lectron-'V'olt, which is 10^9 ELECTRON volts.

GFR (physiology) An abbreviation of 'G'lomerular 'F'iltration 'R'ate.

gg (immunology) An abbreviation of 'g'amma 'g'lobulin.

GH (biochemistry) An abbreviation for 'G'rowth 'H'ormone.

GI (anatomy) An abbreviation of 'G'astro'I'ntestinal.

giant pyramidal cell (cytology) *See* BETZ CELL.

giardiasis (parasitology) A protozoan INFECTION with *Giardia lamblia*, a PARASITE with flagellae found in the SMALL INTESTINE. It produces cysts, which are passed in the FAECES (*USA*: FECES) and spread by contaminated food and WATER. The organism is found worldwide, but is most common in the hotter countries. It causes ACUTE or CHRONIC DIARRHOEA (*USA*: chronic diarrhea), and is a cause of TRAVELLER'S DIARRHOEA (*USA*: traveller's diarrhea) in some cases. It is also liable to infect those with immune deficiency syndromes. The condition is treated with metronidazole or tinidazole; cases of cyst carriers who have no symptoms may also be treated with these drugs.

GIBiol. (education) An abbreviation of 'G'raduate of the 'I'nstitute of 'Biol'ogy.

Giemsa for helicobacter pylori (histology) A histological staining technique that may be used to make *helicobacter pylori* visible under the MICROSCOPE.

Giemsa stain (histology) A histological staining technique that may be used to make BLOOD CELLS and PARASITES visible under the MICROSCOPE.

GIFT (medical) An abbreviation of 'G'amete 'I'ntra-'F'allopian 'T'ransfer. A form of assisted REPRODUCTION in which EGG and SEMEN are deposited in the FALLOPIAN TUBE via the laparoscope.

giga- (G) (measurement) A prefix meaning 1,000,000,000 [one BILLION], used with units of measurement.

gigabyte (G) (computing) A COMPUTER term denoting one BILLION bytes or 1,000 megabytes of information or STORAGE space.

gigantism (medical/ biochemistry) The state of having abnormally large bones, caused by an excess of GROWTH HORMONE.

GIH (physiology/ biochemistry) An abbreviation of 'G'rowth HORMONE-'I'nhibiting 'H'ormone.

Gimenez stain (histology) A histological staining technique that may be used to make *helicobacter pylori* visible under the MICROSCOPE.

gingivitis (medical) INFLAMMATION of the gums.

GIP (physiology/ biochemistry) An abbreviation of 'G'astric 'I'nhibitory 'P'eptide.

GIU (biochemistry) An abbreviation of 'G'lucose 'I'n the 'U'rine. *See* DIABETES MELLITUS.

g/ l (measurement) grams per LITRE.

Gla (biochemistry) A symbol for gamma-carboxyglutamic acid.

glabrous (microbiology) Smooth.

glacial (chemistry) Describing a COMPOUND of ICE-like CRYSTALLINE form, especially that of the SOLID form of a LIQUID. *e.g.* GLACIAL ACETIC (ethanoic) ACID.

glacial acetic acid (chemistry) CRYS-TALLINE form of acetic (ethanoic) ACID below its FREEZING POINT.

gland (anatomy) In animals, ORGAN that synthesizes and secretes specific chemicals, either directly into the bloodstream (ENDOCRINE GLAND) or through a duct (EXOCRINE GLAND) into tubular organs or onto the body surface.

glanders (bacteriology) A disease of horses, donkeys and mules, which is due to INFECTION by the BACTERIUM *Pseudomonas mallei*, which has virtually been eliminated in the Western world. It can be passed on to man, and the disease is almost invariably fatal.

glands (histology) A specialised GROUP of CELLS which secrete or excrete substances which are not the same as those needed for their own METABOLISM, and which act on other tissues and in places other than the GLAND itself. GLANDS are 'exocrine', when the SECRETION is removed through a duct, or 'endocrine', when it passes into the bloodstream. The word is also used to MEAN a LYMPH NODE.

glandular fever (virology) *See* infective mononucleosis.

glass electrode (laboratory equipment) GLASS MEMBRANE ELECTRODE used to measure HYDROGEN ION CONCENTRATION or PH.

glass (chemistry) Hard brittle AMORPHOUS MIXTURE of the silicates of SODIUM and CALCIUM, or of POTASSIUM and CALCIUM. In some particularly strong or HEAT-resistant forms of GLASS, BORON replaces some of the atoms of SILICON. GLASS is usually TRANSPARENT or TRANSLUCENT.

glass wool (chemistry) Material that consists of fine GLASS fibres (*USA*: glass fibers), used in filters, as a thermal INSULATOR and for making fibreglass (*USA*: fiberglass).

Glauber's salt (chemistry) An alternative term for SODIUM SULPHATE (*USA*: sodium sulfate), named after the German physician Johann Glauber (1603-68).

glaucoma (medical) a disease of the EYE occurring usually after middle age, in which the PRESSURE of the FLUID inside the EYE rises and damages the OPTIC NERVE and the RETINA because the NORMAL drainage passages at the margin of the IRIS are blocked and the AQUEOUS HUMOUR cannot escape.

GLC (chemistry) An abbreviation of 'G'as-'L'iquid 'C'hromatography. *See* CHROMATOGRAPHY.

gleo (medical/ bacteriology) A slight watery penile DISCHARGE typical of CHRONIC GONORRHOEA.

GLI (biochemistry) An abbreviation of 'GLI'centin.

glia (medical) An abbreviation of neuro'glia'.

glioma (histology) A TUMOUR (*USA:* tumor) of the BRAIN or SPINAL CORD arising from neuroglial TISSUE.

Gln (biochemistry) An abbreviation of 'Gl'utami'n'e.

globins (biochemistry) A GROUP of proteins involved in the transport of OXYGEN in BLOOD, muscles, etc. *See* HAEMOGLOBIN.

globulin (chemistry) WATER-INSOLUBLE PROTEIN that is SOLUBLE in AQUEOUS SOLUTIONS of certain salts. Globulins generally contain glycin and are coagulated by HEAT; *e.g.* IMMUNOGLOBULIN.

glomerulonephritis (medical) A disease of the kidneys affecting the glomeruli,

formerly known as BRIGHT'S DISEASE. *See* KIDNEY.

glomerulus (anatomy) Ball of capillaries located in the BOWMAN'S CAPSULE of the KIDNEY.

glomus tumour (histology) there are normally in the fingertips, and other parts of the body such as the ears and the face, communications between small arteries and veins which when open allow the BLOOD to bypass the CAPILLARY vessels. These are called glomus bodies and are concerned with the regulation of SKIN TEMPERATURE. Occasionally they form very small pink tumours, which are extremely tender and painful; they may occur under the NAIL, and only respond to surgical removal. (*USA:* glomus tumor).

gloss. (literary terminology) An abbreviation of 'gloss'ary.

glossina (parasitology) The TSETSE FLY, a biting fly which transmits the trypanosomes of African sleeping sickness.

glossitis (medical) INFLAMMATION of the TONGUE.

glottis (anatomy) Front opening of the LARYNX, through which AIR passes from the PHARYNX to the TRACHEA (windpipe) of vertebrates.

glove box (laboratory equipment) Closed box that has gloves fixed into holes in the walls, and in which operations involving hazardous substances, such as RADIOACTIVE materials or toxic chemicals, may be carried out safely. Also termed: dry box.

GLP (quality standards) An abbreviation of 'G'ood 'L'aboratory 'P'ractice.

GLP-1 (biochemistry) An abbreviation of 'G'lucagon'L'ike 'P'olypeptide-1.

GLP-2 (biochemistry) An abbreviation of 'G'lucagon'L'ike 'P'olypeptide-2.

Glu (biochemistry) An abbreviation of 'Glu'tamic acid.

glucagon (biochemistry) A pancreatic HORMONE that increases BLOOD SUGAR LEVEL. A POLYPEPTIDE HORMONE that, like INSULIN, is synthesized and secreted by the ISLETS OF LANGERHANS in the PANCREAS. Produced in RESPONSE to low BLOOD PRESSURE, it stimulates GLYCOGEN breakdown in the LIVER, with release of GLUCOSE into the bloodstream. Its ACTION is therefore opposite to that of INSULIN (which reduces BLOOD GLUCOSE levels).

glucocorticoids (biochemistry) STEROID HORMONES (*e.g.* HYDROCORTISONE) secreted by the ADRENAL CORTEX that promote the conversion of fats and proteins to GLYCOGEN and GLUCOSE.

glucoreceptor (biochemistry) A hypothetical RECEPTOR sensitive to the LEVEL of GLUCOSE in the BLOOD, thought to exist in the HYPOTHALAMUS.

glucose (chemistry) $C_6H_{12}O_6$ MONO-SACCHARIDE CARBOHYDRATE, a SOLUBLE colourless (*USA*: colorless) CRYSTALLINE SUGAR (HEXOSE). It is the substance into which all higher carbohydrates are converted in the body; it is the-main source of ENERGY when it is broken down into WATER and CARBON DIOXIDE. It is absorbed without having to be digested. Also termed: DEXTROSE; grape SUGAR.

glucose-6-phosphate dehydrogenase deficiency (G6PD deficiency) (genetics/ biochemistry) A hereditary lack of an ENZYME involved in the METABOLISM of carbohydrates. Inability to produce this ENZYME is inherited as an X-linked RECESSIVE. Under NORMAL circumstances, people with this GENE show no ill effects, but when they eat broad beans (also known as fava beans), they suffer a severe bout of haemolytic ANAEMIA (*USA*: hemolytic anemia) (ANAEMIA caused by the destruction of RED BLOOD CELLS). The GENE causing G6PD deficiency is found at frequencies of up to 30 per cent in countries around the Mediterranean (Sardinia, Greece, Israel), in parts of Africa (especially the Congo Basin) and in India, and it seems likely that its distribution is connected with that of MALARIA, because the trait gives some resistance to malarial INFECTION (as do the genes for sickle-CELL ANAEMIA [*USA*: sicle cell anemia] and THALASSAEMIA [*USA*: thalassemia]).

glucoside (chemistry) *See* GLYCOSIDE.

glucostatic theory (biochemistry) The theory that eating is regulated by the BRAIN's monitoring of the rate at which GLUCOSE is removed from the BLOOD (as measured by the difference in GLUCOSE levels between arteries and veins): the lower the rate the more the ANIMAL eats. Low use of GLUCOSE indicates that the BLOOD levels are low and are being replaced by GLUCOSE derived from fats.

glue ear (medical) Secretory otitis media, found in children between six months and 10 years old. A FACTOR in the development of this condition is CHRONIC blockage of the EUSTACHIAN TUBE, and another is INFECTION of the middle ear, which may have been successfully treated. The symptom is deafness, for the MIDDLE EAR becomes full of a sticky thick material which interferes with the movement of the ear-drum and the ossides. Many mild cases resolve spontaneously, but it may be necessary to insert a small hollow plastic tube called a grommet into the ear-drum to allow ventilation of the middle ear. This small operation may be accompanied by removal of the ADENOIDS.

glue sniffing (medical) The practice of inhaling the vapors of glue, presumably for their CNS effects. Although there may be multiple solvents in glue, the alkylbenzene TOLUENE is usually a major constituent. Even at low concentrations, TOLUENE produces fatigue, weakness and confusion. ACIDOSIS, potentially due to acidic metabolises of TOLUENE, has been reported in humans abusing glue solvents. Inhalation of the vapors of glue containing BENZENE or HEXANE may result in hematological effects or PERIPHERAL neuropathies.

See also TOLUENE.

glutamate (MONOSODIUM GLUTAMATE, MSG) (biochemistry) An excitatory AMINO ACID NEUROTRANSMITTER. It has been demonstrated that NEONATAL animals are sensitive to large doses of GLUTAMATE, which cause permanent lesions of the HYPOTHALAMUS, resulting in profound neuroendocrine deficits. Toxicity presumably involves increased availability of GLUTAMATE due to an immaturity of the BLOOD-BRAIN barrier or removal mechanisms, followed by death of neurons due to prolonged excitatory stimulation. Infantile mice are also reported to have retinopathies after large doses of GLUTAMATE. Some humans are sensitive to ingestion of large amounts of GLUTAMATE added as a food flavour enhancer (*USA*: flavor enhancer) and experience headaches or 'CHINESE RESTAURANT SYNDROME'.

See also CHINESE RESTAURANT SYNDROME.

GLUT (physiology/ biochemistry) An abbreviation of 'GLU'cose 'T'ransporter.

glutamic acid (biochemistry) An AMINO ACID that is the PRECURSOR of GABA. It is thought to be a NEUROTRANSMITTER.

gluten (chemistry) PROTEIN that occurs in cereals, particularly wheat flour. People with coeliac disease cannot tolerate GLUTEN, and have to eat a GLUTEN-free diet.

Gly (biochemistry) An abbreviation of 'Gly'cine.

glyceride (chemistry) ESTER of GLYCEROL with an ORGANIC ACID. The most important glycerides are FATS AND OILS.

glycerol (chemistry) $HOCH_2CH(OH)CH_2OH$ Colourless (*USA*: colorless) sweet syrupy LIQUID, a trihydric ALCOHOL that occurs as a constituent of FATS AND OILS (from which it is obtained). It is used in foodstuffs, medicines and in the preparation of alkyd resins and nitroglycerine (glyceryl trinitrate). Also termed: glycerin; glycerine; propan-1,2,3-triol.

glycine (biochemistry) $CH_2(NH_2)CO_2H$ Simplest AMINO ACID, found in many proteins and certain ANIMAL excretions. It is a PRECURSOR in the biological SYNTHESIS of purines, porphyrins and CREATINE. It is also a COMPONENT of glutathione and the BILE SALT glycocholate. It acts as a NEUROTRANSMITTER at inhibitory NERVE synapses in vertebrates. Also termed: aminoacetic ACID; aminoETHANOIC ACID.

glycogen (biochemistry) A POLYSACCHARIDE stored in the LIVER, which when required can be broken down into GLUCOSE for release into the BLOOD stream under the control of ADRENALINE (*USA*:

epinephrine). AMYLASE ENZYMES convert it to GLUCOSE, for use in METABOLISM.

glycol (chemistry) An alternative term for any DIOL or, specifically, ETHYLENE GLYCOL (ethanediol).

glycol ethers (chemistry) A CLASS of ALIPHATIC COMPOUNDS containing both a HYDROXYL GROUP (-OH) and an ETHER (-C-O-C-) LINKAGE (*e.g.* ETHYLENE GLYCOL monomethyl ETHER, HOCH,CH,OCH,). Widely used as solvents, they are MISCIBLE with WATER and organic solvents. GLYCOL ETHERS are not toxic ACUTEly, but toxicity of some members of the SERIES has been noted in both humans and animals.

glycolipid (biochemistry) Member of a FAMILY of compounds that contain a SUGAR linked to FATTY ACIDs. Glycolipids are present in higher plants and NEURAL TISSUE in animals. Also termed: glycosyl-acylglycerol; glycosyldiacylglycerol.

glycolysis (biochemistry) Conversion of glucose to lactic or PYRUVIC ACID with the release of ENERGY in the form of ADENOSINE TRIPHOSPHATE (ATP). In animals it may occur during short bursts of muscular activity.

glycoproteins (biochemistry) Proteins with CARBOHYDRATE groups attached at specific locations. They include BLOOD GLYCOPROTEINS, some HORMONES and ENZYMES.

glycoside (chemistry) COMPOUND formed from a MONOSACCHARIDE in which an alcoholic or phenolic GROUP replaces the first HYDROXYL GROUP. If the MONOSACCHARIDE is GLUCOSE, it is termed a GLUCOSIDE.

glycosuria (biochemistry) An excess of GLUCOSE in the URINE indicating that the BLOOD levels of GLUCOSE have risen, usually above 10 mmol/ l.

glycosylase (biochemistry) An ENZYME which recognizes and removes physically or chemically modified bases (*e.g.* alkyl purines) from the SUGAR phosphate DNA chain leaving behind a hole (an abasic site).

glycosylation (biochemistry) The attachment of a CARBOHYDRATE MOLECULE to another MOLECULE such as a PROTEIN.

gm (measurement) An abbreviation of 'g'ra'm'. Also termed gramme; g.

gm mol; g.mol. (measurement) gram-MOLECULE, MOLECULAR WEIGHT in grams.

GM tube (radiology/ physics) An abbreviation of 'G'eiger 'M'üller tube.

GMAG (governing body) An abbreviation of 'G'enetic 'M'anipulation 'A'dvisory 'G'roup.

GM-CSF (physiology) An abbreviation of 'G'ranulocyte-'M'acrophage 'C'olony-'S'timulating 'F'actor.

GnRH (physiology/ biochemistry) An abbreviation of 'G'o'n'adotropin-'R'eleasing 'H'ormone.

goblet cell (cytology) MUCUS-secreting CELL in MUCOUS MEMBRANES.

goitre (medical/ biochemistry) A swelling of the THYROID gland in the neck. Goitres may be associated with under or over-activity of the gland, or a deficiency of iodine in the diet.

gold Au (chemistry) Soft yellow metallic ELEMENT in GROUP IB of the PERIODIC TABLE. It occurs as the free METAL in lodes and placer deposits. Most gold is held in currency reserve stocks, although some is used, usually as an ALLOY in dentistry and in electroplating electronic circuits and components. At. no. 79; r.a.m. 196.9665.

Golgi apparatus (cytology) Organale that occurs in most EUKARYOTIC CELLS as stacks of flattened MEMBRANE-bounded sacs. It is involved in the formation of ZYMOGEN granules, SYNTHESIS and transport of secretory POLYSACCHARIDES (*e.g.* CELLULOSE in CELL plate or SECONDARY CELL wall formation) and formation of MUCUS in GOBLET CELLS; assembly of GLYCOPROTEINS; packing of HORMONES in NERVE CELLS that carry out neurosecretion; formation of lysosomes.3 and probably production of the PLASMA MEMBRANE. The synaptic vesicles and their contents are manufactured in the GOLGI APPARATUS. It was named after the Italian histologist Camillo Golgi (1843-1926). Also termed: Golgi body; Golgi complex.

Golgi cell (cytology) A large interneuron found in the CEREBELLUM. Activated by mossy fibres (*USA*: mossey fibers), climbing fibres (*USA*: climbing fibers), and parallel fibres (*USA*: parallel fibers), they inhibit the GRANULE CELLS.

Golgi stain (histology) A histological staining technique that may be used to make NERVE CELLS visible under the MICROSCOPE. It is a SILVER stain which percolates to all parts of a living NERVE CELL.

gomori trichrome (histology) CONNECTIVE TISSUE stain for MUSCLE BIOPSY.

gonad (anatomy) Reproductive ORGAN of an ANIMAL, *e.g.* OVARY or TESTIS, in which ova (eggs) and SPERM are formed respectively. GONADS may also FUNCTION as ENDOCRINE GLANDS, secreting SEX HORMONES.

gonadal (anatomy) Pertaining to the GONADS.

See also GONAD.

gonadotrophic hormone (biochemistry) The ANTERIOR PITUITARY HORMONES that promote GROWTH or activity of the GONADS, controlling the initiation of puberty, the MENSTRUAL CYCLE and LACTATION in females and SPERM-formation in males. It is produced by the PITUITARY GLAND. It is also used for the TREATMENT of infertility in women. Also termed: GONADOTROPHIN.

gonadotrophin (biochemistry) *See* GONADOTROPHIC HORMONE.

gonadotrophin releasing hormone (GNRH) (physiology/ biochemistry) An hypothalamic HORMONE that acts on the pituitary gland to release the gonadotrophins, i.e. luteinizing HORMONE, LH and follicle-stimulating HORMONE, FSH.

gonads (anatomy) The organs that produce spermatozoa and ova, *i.e.* the TESTIS and OVARY.

goniometer (crystallography) Instrument for measuring angles, particularly the angles between the faces of crystals.

gonococcus (bacteriology) The Gram-negative BACTERIUM, *Neisseria gonorrhoeae*, that causes gonorrhea and is often found in pairs (diplococcus) within WHITE BLOOD CELLS.

gonorrhoea (medical) A common SEXUALLY TRANSMITTED DISEASE, caused by the GONOCOCCUS *Neisseria gonorrhoeae*. In the male, a DISCHARGE from the PENIS with pain on passing water begins between two and ten days after INFECTION. The DISCHARGE is thick and yellow. If it is left untreated, the DISCHARGE turns clear and sticky; the EPIDIDYMIS of the testicle may become inflamed, and lymphatic GLANDS draining the AREA are enlarged and painful. Most importantly a stricture may develop in the URETHRA, causing later difficulty in passing WATER. In women there is a DISCHARGE from the URETHRA and VAGINA, but these are not infrequently unnoticed; in children, usually the victims of sexual assault, the external genitalia may show signs of INFLAMMATION. The most important complication in women is pelvic inflammation involving the FALLOPIAN TUBEs, for this leads to pain, possibly an ABSCESS, CHRONIC INFLAMMATION and infertility. Because the symptoms of the original INFECTION may be overlooked it is important that the slightest suspicion of exposure should call for medical attention. It is uncommon now for newborn infants to acquire INFECTION of the eyes from the mother, but once ths was a cause of blindness. TREATMENT has been revolutionised by antibiotics: ampicillin or amoxycillin, in one large dose of 3.5 g together with probenecid, which reduces the EXCRETION of PENICILLIN, is effective except in cases where the organism is PENICILLIN-resistant, when spectinomycin or cefuroxime may be used. Prophylactic EYE-drops are used on newborn babies.

good laboratory practices (GLP) (quality standards) Regulations governing good LABORATORY practices are in effect in the UK, USA and OECD, covering all phases of LABORATORY testing, including facilities, personnel training, DATA gathering, laboratory inspections, ANIMAL health and welfare, chemical ANALYSIS and SAMPLE preparation.

goodness of fit (statistics) The extent to which DATA points match theoretical expectations.

Gordon & Sweets stain (histology) A histological staining technique that may be used to make reticulin visible under the MICROSCOPE.

gout (medical) A disease associated with a high LEVEL of URIC ACID in the BLOOD, causing painful INFLAMMATION usually of one joint, the first JOINT of the great toe, which suddenly becomes red, swollen and ACUTEly painful. The disease is commonest in men, the first attack occurring between the ages of 30 and 60 but it is not found in boys before the age of puberty, nor in women until after the MENOPAUSE. Other joints may be affected such as the ankle, elbow, knee and wrist, but only one at a time. It may be associated with stones in the KIDNEY, and sufferers are usually overweight.

GP (1, 2 medical; 3 education) 1 An abbreviation of 'G'eneral 'P'aralysis. 2 An abbreviation of 'G'eneral 'P'ractitioner. 3 An abbreviation of 'G'raduate in 'P'harmacy. Also termed G PH.

G6PD (biochemistry) An abbreviation of 'G'lucose '6'-'P'hosphate 'D'ehydrogenase.

gpl (measurement) An abbreviation of 'g'rams 'p'er 'l'itre.

GRA (physiology/ biochemistry) Abbreviation of 'G'lucocorticoid-'R'emediable 'A'ldosteronism.

Graafian follicle (histology) FLUID-filled ball of CELLS in the mammalian OVARY inside which an OOCYTE develops. It matures periodically and then bursts at the surface of the OVARY (at OVULATION) to release an OVUM (EGG). The FOLLICLE then temporarily becomes a SOLID body, the CORPUS LUTEUM. It was named after the Dutch anatomist Regnier de Graaf (1641-73). Also termed: OVARIAN FOLLICLE.

gradient (1, 2 mathematics) 1 Amount of inclination of a line (or a curve at a particular point) to the horizontal; its slope. 2 Rate of rise or fall of a VARIABLE quantity such as TEMPERATURE or PRESSURE.

graft (medical) Transplantation of an ORGAN or TISSUE from one organism into the body of another or from one position on or in the body to another. A HOMOGRAFT is a GRAFT where the RECIPIENT and the DONOR are of the same SPECIES; a HETEROGRAFT is one carried out between two different SPECIES.

Graham's law (physics) Velocity of DIFFUSION of a GAS is inversely proportional to the SQUARE ROOT of its DENSITY. It was named after the British chemist Thomas Graham (1805-69).

grain (1, 2 measurement) 1 Small WEIGHT in apothecaries' and troy WEIGHT (in which it equals 1/5760 lb), and in AVOIRDUPOIS WEIGHT (in which it equals 1/7000 lb). It is equivalent to 0.0648 grams. 2 One-quarter of a (metric) carat, equal to 0.050 grams.

gram (g or gm) (measurement) The BASIC UNIT of WEIGHT in the METRIC SYSTEM, defined as the MASS of 1 CUBIC millilitre (*USA*: milliliter) of WATER at 4°C [39°F]. 1000 g = 1 kg. 1oz. = 28.35 gm.

gram molecule (measurement) MOLECULAR WEIGHT of a substance in grams; 1 mole.

gram (measurement) UNIT of MASS in the METRIC SYSTEM, a fundamental UNIT in the *e.g.*s. system and equal to 1/1000 kg. Also termed: gramme. *See* SI UNITS.

Gram/ Twort stain (histology) A histological staining technique that may be used to make BACTERIA visible under the MICROSCOPE.

Gram's stain (bacteriology) A staining technique that may be used to make BACTERIA visible under the MICROSCOPE. The staining method is to use crystal violet, then IODINE SOLUTION, then ETHANOL or ETHANOL-acetone, and then COUNTER-stain. The BACTERIA which are stained purple are called Gram-POSITIVE, those which have been decolourised (*USA*: decolorized) and have taken up the COUNTER-stain Gram-negative. The different uptake of stain is due to differences in cell-wall structure. This method of staining separates BACTERIA into two large groups, Gram-POSITIVE and Gram-negative. Named after the Danish physician, H. Gram (1853-1938).

grand mal (medical) A major epileptic seizure with both tonic and clonic convulsions and loss of consciousness. *Contrast* PETIT MAL.

granisetron (pharmacology) An ANTI-EMETIC and ANTINAUSEANT drug which, administered orally, by injection or infusion, acts by blocking the action of the natural mediator SEROTONIN.

granular layer (1, 2 histology) 1 Either of two layers of NERVE CELLS in the CEREBRAL CORTEX; numbered from the surface inwards, the external GRANULAR LAYER is the second layer and the internal

GRANULAR LAYER is the fourth layer; the name derives from the large number of golgi type 11 CELLS or GRANULE CELLS in these layers. 2 The innermost of the three layers of the CEREBELLUM, which contains GRANULE CELLS and receives an input from the mossy fibres (*USA*: mossy fibers).

granulation tissue (histology) the TISSUE formed by fibroblasts and endothelial CELLS which grows over a raw surface in the process of healing.

granule cell (cytology) A small stellate CELL; the name 'granule' is used because these CELLS look granular under a MICROSCOPE. The expression 'GRANULE CELL' is preferred to 'stellate CELL' for the GRANULE CELLS in the GRANULAR LAYERs of the CORTEX and CEREBELLUM.

granuloma (histology) Aggregation and proliferation of MACROPHAGES to form small (usually microscopic) nodules.

grape sugar (chemistry) An alternative term for GLUCOSE.

graph (statistics) Mathematical diagram that shows how one quantity varies in relation to another.

See also BAR CHART; HISTOGRAM; PIE CHART.

GRAS (toxicology) An abbreviation of 'G'enerally 'R'ecognised 'A's 'S'afe.

Grave's disease (medical) *See* HYPER-THYROIDISM.

gravid (medical) Pregnant; primigravida, one who is in her first PREGNANCY.

gravidity (medical) The number of pregnancies. Includes the CURRENT one if the woman is pregnant.

gravimetric analysis (chemistry) QUANTI-TATIVE chemical ANALYSIS made ultimately by weighing substances.

gravitation (physics) An alternative term for the FORCE of gravity.

gray (Gy) (chemistry) Amount of absorbed RADIATION dose in SI UNITS, equal to supplying 1 JOULE of ENERGY per kg. It is equivalent to 100 rad (the UNIT it superseded).

Greco latin square (statistics) A latin square in which there are two conditions each with the same number of values, and in which each COMBINATION of values appears once in each row and once in each column.

green vitriol (chemistry) Old name for IRON(II) SULPHATE (*USA*: iron(II) sulfate) (FERROUS SULPHATE [*USA*: ferrous sulfate]).

grey matter (anatomy) Any region of the CENTRAL NERVOUS SYSTEM containing many CELL bodies and their processes, and having unmyelinated axons. All parts of a CELL look grey except for a myelinated AXON. The expression usually refers to the layers of the CEREBRAL CORTEX, but GREY MATTER also exists in the cerebellar CORTEX and SPINAL CORD.

GRH (physiology/ biochemistry) An abbreviation of 'G'rowth HORMONE-'R'eleasing 'H'ormone.

Grimelius stain (histology) A histological staining technique that may be used to make argyrophil CELLS visible under the MICROSCOPE.

griseofulvin (pharmacology) An ANTIBIOTIC active against FUNGUS INFECTION when given by mouth. It is concentrated in KERATIN, and is therefore useful for infections involving the SKIN and nails. It is used in intractable or widespread infections, and TREATMENT has to be continued for a month or more. It should not be taken during PREGNANCY.

Grocott hexamine silver stain (histology) A histological staining technique that may be used to make FUNGI visible under the MICROSCOPE.

GRP (physiology/ biochemistry) Abbreviation of 'G'astrin-'R'eleasing 'P'olypeptide.

GRPP (biochemistry) An abbreviation of 'G'licentin-'R'elated 'P'oly'P'eptide.

gross weight (gr wt) (measurement) The entire WEIGHT of a PRODUCT, including its container. Found on packaging and labelling.

ground state (physics) Lowest ENERGY state of an ATOM or MOLECULE, from which it can be raised to a higher ENERGY state by EXCITATION.

See also ENERGY LEVEL.

group (chemistry) Column, or vertical row, of elements in the PERIODIC TABLE (horizontal rows are PERIODS). The GROUP number (I to VIII and 0) indicates the number of electrons in the ATOM's outermost shell.

grouping (statistics) Assigning DATA to CLASS intervals.

grouping error (statistics) Any statistical error introduced by the way in which DATA are grouped, *e.g.* by GROUPING in such a way that the distribution of scores within a GROUP is not NORMAL.

growth (genetics) Increase in size of an organism, either by an increase in CELL size or, much more usually, by an increase in CELL number. Most organisms have a SPECIES-typical GROWTH rate and final size, both of which are, to some extent, genetically controlled, as is shown by the fact that they can be changed by artificial selection, but are also much influenced by environmental factors. Some fishes and reptiles grow all their lives.

growth hormone (biochemistry) A PROTEIN HORMONE produced by the PITUITARY GLAND in the BASE of the SKULL that controls GROWTH and differentiation in animals. Either deficiency of it or excess production can be genetically determined, the former causing a form of dwarfism and the latter GIGANTISM (excess GROWTH in childhood) and ACROMEGALY (enlargement of the JAW, hands and feet in adult life). The dwarfism can be treated with human GROWTH HORMONE, which formerly had to be obtained from human cadavers but can now be made by GENE CLONING. Also termed: SOMATOTROPHIN.

Grp (general terminology) An abbreviation of 'Gr'ou'p'.

GTP (biochemistry) An abbreviation of 'G'uanosine 'T'ri'P'hosphate.

GU (medical) An abbreviation of 'G'enito-'U'rinary.

guanethidine monosulphate (pharmacology) An ADRENERGIC neurone blocker, which is an ANTISYMPATHETIC class of drug that prevents release of NORADRENALINE from sympathetic nerves. Administered orally or by injection it is used as an ANTIHYPERTENSIVE.

guanine (molecular biology) $C_5H_5N_5O$ Colourless (*USA*: colorless) CRYSTALLINE

ORGANIC BASE (a PURINE DERIVATIVE) that occurs in DNA.

gumma (medical/ bacteriology) A hard granulomatous swelling occurring in the third stage of syphilis anywhere in the body. It develops anything between one and ten years after the primary INFECTION.

gust (measurement) A UNIT used in scales of TASTE; one GUST is produced by a 1 per cent SUCROSE SOLUTION.

gustation (physiology) The sense of TASTE.

gustometer (measurement) A device for measuring TASTE thresholds. It consists of a U-tube with a small hole at the bottom; the tube is placed upright on a particular part of the TONGUE, and a SOLUTION is poured through it: the TONGUE is thus exposed to a CONSTANT amount of SOLUTION.

gut (anatomy) An alternative term for ALIMENTARY CANAL.

gyn. (1, 2 medical) An abbreviation of 1 'gyn'aecology (*USA*: gynecology). Also termed gynae.; gynacol. 2 'gyn'aecologist (*USA*: gynecologist).

gynaecologist (medical) A medical doctor specialising in GYNAECOLOGY (*USA*: gynecology). (*USA*: gynecologist).

gynaecology (gyn.; gynac.; gynacol) (medical) That branch of medicine dealing with the diseases of women, especially concerning the reproductive system of women. (*USA*: gynecology).

gypsum (chemistry) $CaSO_4.2H_2O$ Very soft CALCIUM mineral, a form of CALCIUM SULPHATE (*USA*: calcium sulfate), used in making cement and plasters. Also termed: CALCIUM SULPHATE DIHYDRATE (*USA*: calcium sulfate dihydrate).

gyromagnetic ratio (physics) Ratio of the magnetic moment of an ATOM or NUCLEUS to its angular momentum.

gyrus (anatomy) One of the convolutions on the surface of the BRAIN.

H

H (1 chemistry; 2 biochemistry) 1 The CHEMICAL SYMBOL for HYDROGEN. 2 An abbreviation of 'H'istidine.

h (1 measurement; 2 physics) 1 An abbreviation of 'h'our. 2 Symbol for PLANCK'S CONSTANT.

HA (biochemistry) General symbol for an acid.

habituation (physiology) Process by which the NERVOUS SYSTEM becomes accustomed to a particular STIMULUS and after a time is no longer irritated by it; *e.g.* the feel of one's clothes or the background noise of machinery.

haem. (1, 2 haematology) An abbreviation of 1'haem'oglobin (*USA*: HEMO-GLOBIN); 2 'haem'orrhage (USA: hemorrhage). (*USA*: hem).

haem (chemistry) IRON-containing GROUP of atoms attached to a POLYPEPTIDE chain; *e.g.* in HAEMOGLOBIN (*USA*: hemaglobin) and MYOGLOBIN. (*USA*: heme).

haemagglutination (haematology/ immunology) The AGGLUTINATION of RED BLOOD CELLS caused by certain antibodies, VIRUS particles, or high MOLECULAR WEIGHT POLYSACCHARIDES. (*USA*: hemagglutination).

haemangioma (histology) A TUMOUR (*USA*: tumor) composed of BLOOD VESSELS. (*USA*: hemANGIOMA). *See* ANGIOMA.

haematogenous (microbiology) Disseminated by the bloodstream. (*USA*: hematogenous).

haematology (haematology) The branch of medicine which deals with the BLOOD and its disorders. (*USA*: hematology).

haematoma (medical) A swelling containing BLOOD effused into the tissues, usually as the result of injury. (*USA*: hematoma).

haematopoietic STEM CELLS (cytology) (*USA*: hematopoietic stem cells). *See* STEM CELLS.

haematoxylin & eosin (H&E) (histology/ haematology) A MIXTURE of HAEMATOXYLIN (*USA*: hematoxylin) in DISTILLED WATER and an AQUEOUS eosin SOLUTION; a stain used routinely for examination of tissues. (*USA*: hematoxylin & eosin).

haematoxylin (histology) An ACID colouring (*USA*: coloring) MATTER from the heartwood. A histological stain that may be used to make CELL nuclei visible under the MICROSCOPE. (*USA*: hematoxylin).

haematuria (medical) The presence of BLOOD in the URINE. (*USA*: hematuria).

haemocyanin (haematology) The BLOOD PIGMENT that contains COPPER as its PROSTHETIC GROUP for the transport of OXYGEN. It is confined to lower animals. *e.g.* molluscs. (*USA*: hemocyanin).

haemocytometer (haematology) Apparatus for counting BLOOD CELLS. (*USA*: hemocytometer).

haemodialysis (medical) *See* DIALYSIS.

haemoglobin (Hb) (medical) The OXYGEN carrying PIGMENT of the RED BLOOD CELLS (ERYTHROCYTES). It is a CONJUGATED PROTEIN containing four haem groups (*USA*: heme groups) and GLOBIN. A MOLECULE of HAEMOGLOBIN contains 4 GLOBIN POLYPEPTIDE chains - designated alpha, beta, gamma and delta. In the adult, haemoglobin A predominates (alpha2, beta2). (*USA*: hemoglobin).

haemoglobinuria (haematology) Appearance of HAEMOGLOBIN (*USA*: hemaglobin) in the URINE. (*USA*: hemoglobinuria).

haemolysis (haematology) Breakdown of RED BLOOD CELLS (ERYTHROCYTES) which results in the release of HAEMOGLOBIN (*USA*: hemaglobin) from the red CELLS and its appearance in PLASMA. (*USA*: hemolysis).

haemophilia (medical/ haematology) A hereditary bleeding disorder caused by a deficiency in the ability to synthesise one or more of the BLOOD COAGULATION proteins, *e.g.* FACTOR VIII (HAEMOPHILIA A) (*USA*: hemophilia A) or FACTOR IX (HAEMOPHILIA B) (USA: hemophilia B). Sufferers are at CONSTANT risk of bleeding excessively from even minor injuries. (*USA*: hemophilia).

haemoptysis (medical) The spitting of BLOOD or BLOOD-stained sputum. (*USA*: hemoptysis).

haemorrhage (medical) Bleeding, which may be internal or external, arterial, venous or CAPILLARY. In arterial bleeding the BLOOD is bright red, and may spurt out with the beat of the HEART; venous BLOOD is darker and escapes in a steady stream; CAPILLARY BLOOD oozes from the damaged tissues. (*USA*: hemorrhage).

haemostasis (medical) The process of stopping BLOOD flow. (*USA*: hemostasis).

haemothorax (medical) BLOOD in the PLEURAL cavity, the space between the chest wall and the LUNG. It may he the result of a penetrating WOUND or injury, or the presence of a MALIGNANT TUMOUR (*USA*: malignant tumor). (*USA*: hemothorax).

hafnium Hf (chemistry) Silvery metallic ELEMENT in GROUP IVB of the PERIODIC TABLE (a TRANSITION ELEMENT), used to make control rods for nuclear reactors. At. no. 72; r.a.m. 178.49.

Haga-Yamagchi methenamine silver stain (histology) A histological staining technique that may be used to make senile plaques visible under the MICROSCOPE.

hahnium Ha (chemistry) ELEMENT no. 105 (a post-ACTINIDE). It is a RADIOACTIVE METAL with short-lived isotopes, made in very small quantities by bombardment of an ACTINIDE with atoms of an ELEMENT such as CARBON or OXYGEN.

hair (1, 2 anatomy) 1 DERIVATIVE of ECTODERM composed of INSOLUBLE proteins or keratins. Its role in mammals includes assisting regulation of body temperature. 2 In plants, any of various outgrowths from the EPIDERMIS, *e.g.* ROOT HAIRS, which absorb WATER. Also termed: trichome.

half-cell (physics) Half of an ELECTROLYTIC CELL, consisting of an ELECTRODE immersed in an ELECTROLYTE.

half-life (1, 2 measurement/ radiology) 1 Time taken for something whose DECAY is exponential to reduce to half its value. 2 More specifically, time taken for half the nuclei of a RADIOACTIVE substance to DECAY spontaneously. The HALF-LIFE of some unstable substances is only a few seconds or less, whereas for other substances it may be thousands of years; *e.g.* LAWRENCIUM has a HALF-LIFE of 8 seconds, and the ISOTOPE PLUTONIUM-239 has a HALF-LIFE of 24,400 years.

halide (chemistry) A BINARY COMPOUND containing a HALOGEN: a FLUORIDE, CHLORIDE, BROMIDE or IODIDE.

halite (chemistry) Naturally occurring form of SODIUM CHLORIDE. Also termed: COMMON SALT; ROCK SALT.

Hall effect (physics) Production of a VOLTAGE in a semiconductor or METAL carrying an ELECTRIC CURRENT in a strong transverse MAGNETIC FIELD. It was named after the American physicist Edwin Hall (1855-1938).

haloalkane (chemistry) An alternative term for HALOGENOALKANE.

haloform (chemistry) An ORGANIC COMPOUND of the type CHX_3, where X is a HALOGEN (CHLORINE, BROMINE or IODINE); *e.g.* CHLOROFORM (TRICHLOROMETHANE), IODOFORM (TRIIODOMETHANE). The compounds are prepared by the ACTION of the HALOGEN on heating with ETHANOL in the presence of SODIUM HYDROXIDE.

halogen (chemistry) ELEMENT in GROUP VIIA of the PERIODIC TABLE: FLUORINE, CHLORINE, BROMINE, IODINE or ASTATINE.

halogenation (chemistry) A CHEMICAL REACTION that involves the addition of a HALOGEN to a substance.

halogenoalkane (chemistry) A HALOGEN DERIVATIVE of an ALKANE, GENERAL FORMULA $C_nH_{2n\ +\ 1}X$, where X is a HALOGEN (FLUORINE, CHLORINE, BROMINE or IODINE). Also termed: HALOALKANE; monohalogenoALKANE.

halophilic (biology) Exhibiting a preference for an ENVIRONMENT containing SALT (*e.g.* sea-WATER). The term is usually applied to BACTERIA.

halothane (pharmacology) An inhalant general anaesthetic drug, which is used for induction and maintenance of anaesthesia during surgery.

haploid (cytology) Having half the number of chromosomes of the organism in the CELL NUCLEUS. The HAPLOID state is found in gametes (resulting from MEIOSIS), the gametophyte generation and spores. It occurs after MEIOSIS or REDUCTION DIVISION.

See also DIPLOID.

hard copy (computing) Document that people can read (*e.g.* a PRINT-OUT in plain language).

hard disk (computing) Rigid MAGNETIC DISK that provides DATA and PROGRAM STORAGE for computers, including microcomputers. HARD DISKS can hold a high DENSITY of DATA. Also termed: DISKETTE.

See also FLOPPY DISK.

hardness of water (chemistry) Property of water that prevents it forming a lather with soap because of the presence of dissolved compounds of calcium or magnesium.

See also SOFT WATER

hardware (computing) Electronic, electrical, magnetic and mechanical parts that make up a COMPUTER system.

See also SOFTWARE.

harmonic progression (mathematics) SERIES of numbers whose reciprocals have a CONSTANT difference (form an ARITHMETIC PROGRESSION). *e.g.* $1/1 + 1/2 + 1/3 + 1/4$.

Haversian canal (anatomy) Any of the numerous channels that occur in BONE TISSUE, containing BLOOD VESSELS and NERVES. An organic MATRIX is laid down in layers encircling each Haversian canal. It was named after the English physician Clopton Havers (1650 - 1702).

Hb (haematology) An abbreviation of 'H'aemo'g'lobin (*USA*: HEMOGLOBIN).

hb (general terminology) An abbreviation of 'h'uman 'b'eing.

HBE (physiology) An abbreviation of 'H'is 'B'undle 'E'lectrogram.

HbO₂ (physiology/ biochemistry) A symbol for Oxyhemoglobin.

HBV (virology) An abbreviation of 'H'epatitis 'B' 'V'irus.

HCC (biochemistry) An abbreviation of 25-'H'ydroxy'C'hole'C'alciferol.

hCG (physiology/ biochemistry) An abbreviation of 'h'uman 'C'horionic 'G'onadotropin.

hCS (physiology/ biochemistry) An abbreviation of 'h'uman 'C'horionic 'S'omatomammotropin.

Hct (haematology) An abbreviation of 'H'aemato'c'ri't' (*USA*: Hematocrit).

HDL (biochemistry) An abbreviation of 'H'igh-'D'ensity 'L'ipoPROTEIN.

H & E (histology/ haematology) An abbreviation of 'h'aematoxylin & 'e'osin.

He (chemistry) The CHEMICAL SYMBOL for HELIUM.

head (computing) In a tape recorder, video recorder, record player or COMPUTER input/ output device, an electromagnetic COMPONENT that can read, erase or write signals off or onto tapes and disks.

Health and Safety at Work Act (legislation) Important UK legislation of 1974, resulting from the recommendations of the Robens committee in July 1972, that covers all aspects of safety at the workplace including the POTENTIAL exposure of workers to toxic and infectious substances.

Health and Safety Commission (governing body) A commission, consisting of employers' and union representatives, that was established under the UK Health and Safety at WORK Act. The Commission, which is advised by various advisory committees on health hazards in the workplace from toxic chemicals and infectious agents, and related hazards to the public, has overall powers to propose health and safety regulations and to approve codes of practice. It is directly responsible to the Secretary of State for Employment. *See* HEALTH AND SAFETY AT WORK ACT.

Health and Safety Executive (governing body) The body that enforces the statutory duties laid down in the UK Health and Safety at WORK Act. The

Executive is responsible to the Health and Safety Commission.

heart (anatomy) An ORGAN chiefly consisting of CARDIAC MUSCLE that in vertebrates is responsible for pumping BLOOD into a system of arteries. BLOOD returns to the heart from the tissues via veins, and is passed to the lungs to become reoxygenated. The mammalian HEART is divided into four chambers, the right and left atria (auricles) and right and left ventricles, so that deoxygenated and oxygenated BLOOD remain separate. It demonstrates inherent rhythmicity of contraction because of the presence of PACEMAKER TISSUE, such as the sinoatrial NODE. The NEUROTRANSMITTER ACETYLCHOLINE slows the heart and reduces the FORCE of contraction, whereas NORADRENALINE (USA: norepinephrine) quickens the heart and increases the FORCE. Drugs and toxicants affecting cholinergic and ADRENERGIC transmission can therefore affect CARDIAC FUNCTION and subsequently BLOOD PRESSURE. Atherosclerotic agents affect coronary arteries and can result in HYPERTENSION and heart attacks.

heartbeat (physiology) The alternate contraction and relaxation of the HEART, corresponding to DIASTOLE and SYSTOLE.

heartburn (medical) A burning pain felt behind the BREASTBONE extending into the THROAT. It is associated with conditions that allow REFLUX of the ACIDcontents of the STOMACH into the lower OESOPHAGUS (USA: esophagus), such as HIATUS HERNIA. It is relieved by ALKALIS (USA: alkalies), e.g. ALUMINIUM HYDROXIDE or MAGNESIUM CARBONATE.

heart failure (medical) Failure of the HEART to carry out its function properly because of congenital or acquired disease. Failure may be mainly of the right or left side, the latter being the most common, following disease of the mitral or aortic valves, coronary insufficiency or high BLOOD PRESSURE.

heat (physics) Form of ENERGY, the ENERGY of motion (KINETIC ENERGY) possessed by the atoms or molecules of all substances at temperatures above ABSOLUTE ZERO.

heat capacity (physics) Quantity of HEAT required to produce UNIT rise of TEMPERATURE in an OBJECT.

heat of activation (physics) Difference between the values of the thermodynamic functions for the activated complex and the reactants for a CHEMICAL REACTION (all the substances being in their STANDARD STATES).

heat of atomization (measurement) Amount of HEAT that is required to convert 1 mole of an ELEMENT into the gaseous state.

heat of combustion (measurement) HEAT change that accompanies the complete COMBUSTION of 1 mole of a substance.

heat of formation (measurement) HEAT change that occurs when 1 mole of a COMPOUND is formed from its elements, in their NORMAL states.

heat of neutralization (measurement) HEAT change that occurs when 1 mole of AQUEOUS HYDROGEN IONS are neutralized by a BASE in DILUTE SOLUTION.

heat of reaction (measurement) HEAT change that occurs when the MOLAR quantities (lowest possible multiples of 1 mole) of reactants as stated in a CHEMICAL EQUATION react together.

heat of solution (measurement) HEAT change that occurs when 1 mole of a substance is dissolved in so much WATER that further DILUTION with WATER produces no further HEAT change.

Heberden's nodes (medical) Small hard swellings on the finger joints which occurs in some cases of osteoarthritis. Named after the English physician, W. Heberden (1767-1845).

hecto- (measurement) Metric prefix for a multiple of 10^2; denotes 100 times.

height (ht or hgt) (measurement) The LINEAR measurement of an OBJECT from top to bottom.

Heinz bodies (haematology) Dark-staining bodies found in ERYTHROCYTES that lie on the inner surface.

Heisenberg uncertainty principle (physics) The precise position and momentum of an ELECTRON cannot be determined simultaneously. It was named after the German physicist Werner Heisenberg (1901-1976).

Hela cells (cytology) A line of human CANCER CELLS that has been maintained in culture since 1951 and has been much used in CANCER research. It is named after the patient from whom the CELLS were taken, Henrietta Lacks in 1951, who had CANCER of the CERVIX. *See* TISUUE CULTURE.

heliotherapy (medical) TREATMENT by exposure to natural sunlight. Once popular but now confined to cases of psoriasis for which it can be greatly benificial.

helium He (chemistry) Gaseous ELEMENT in GROUP 0 of the PERIODIC TABLE (the RARE GASes), which occurs in some natural GAS deposits. It is INERT and noninflammable, used to fill airships and balloons (in preference to inflammable HYDROGEN) and in HELIUM-OXYGEN 'AIR' mixtures for divers (in preference to the NITROGEN-OXYGEN MIXTURE of real AIR, which can cause the bends). It is also used in GAS lasers. LIQUID HELIUM is employed as a COOLANT in CRYOGENICS. At. no. 2; r.a.m. 4.0026.

helix (molecular biology) A spiral shape. The shape of the thread of a bolt or screw. It occurs in nature as the three-dimensional structure of DNA, which is a double HELIX. The alpha HELIX, described by Linus Pauling, is the secondary structure of many proteins, *i.e.* they are twisted threads that are subsequently folded into a particular three-dimensional shape.

'HELLP' syndrome (medical) Variant of pre-eclampsia typified by HAEMOLYSIS (*USA*: hemolysis) (H), elevated LIVER (EL) ENZYMES, and low platelets (LP).

helminths (parasitology) Parasitic WORMS. *See* WORMS.

hemianaesthesia (medical) The loss of sensation on one side of the body; it is caused by UNILATERAL damage to the somaesthetic system (*USA*: hemianesthesia).

hemianopia (medical) Loss of vision in the right or left half of the visual FIELD of one or both eyes. It is caused by UNILATERAL damage to the visual CORTEX, OPTIC radiations, or OPTIC chiasm. Also termed hemiopia.

hemihydrate (chemistry) COMPOUND containing one WATER MOLECULE for every two molecules of the COMPOUND; *e.g.* $CaSO_4.1/2H_2O$.

hemiopia (medical) *See* HEMIANOPIA.

hemiplegia (medical) Paralysis of one side of the body; it is caused by UNILATERAL damage to part of the motor system, usually caused by a STROKE.

hemoglobin (haematology) *See* HAEMO-GLOBIN.

hemp plant (toxicology) *Cannabis sativa* or *Cannabis indica*, the plant from which hashish and MARIJUANA are derived.

henry (H) (measurement) SI UNIT of electrical INDUCTANCE, defined as the INDUCTANCE that produces an induced ELECTROMOTIVE FORCE of 1 VOLT for a CURRENT change of 1 AMPERE per second. It was named after the American physicist Joseph Henry (1797-1878).

Henry's law (physics) WEIGHT of GAS dissolved by a LIQUID is proportional to the GAS PRESSURE. It was named after the British chemist William Henry (1774-1836).

heparin (haematology) A substance found in many tissues of the body, but mostly in the LIVER, which prevents the clotting of BLOOD by interfering with the formation of THROMBIN from prothrombin. It is used in medicine to prevent clotting, and acts quickly; but the ACTION is shortlived, and it has to be given by injection, either into the veins or under the SKIN. It is particularly useful in CARDIAC surgery and renal DIALYSIS. If HAEMORRHAGE (*USA*: hemorrhage) should be provoked, the ANTIDOTE is protamine SULPHATE (*USA*: protamine sulfate). *See* COAGULATION of the BLOOD.

hepatic portal system (physiology) In vertebrates, system of BLOOD capillaries into which dissolved foods (except for FATTY ACIDS and GLYCEROL) pass from the INTESTINE lining for transport to the LIVER.

hepatic (anatomy) Relating to the LIVER.

hepatitis (medical/ virology) INFLAMMATION of the LIVER, caused by VIRUS INFECTION, many drugs, and various chemicals including ALCOHOL. VIRUSES causing HEPATITIS are described as A, B, C, D, E, non-A and non-B.

hepatoma (histology) A MALIGNANT tumor of the LIVER.

hepatomegaly (medical) Enlargement of the LIVER.

hepatosplenomegaly (medical) Enlargement of the LIVER and SPLEEN.

hepatotoxicants (toxicology) Chemicals that cause adverse effects on the LIVER.

See also HEPATOTOXICITY.

hepatotoxicity (toxicology) Adverse effects on the LIVER. The LIVER is particularly susceptible to chemical injury because of its anatomical relationship to the most important portal of entry, the GASTROINTESTINAL tract, and its high CONCENTRATION of XENOBIOTIC metabolizing enyzmes. Many of these ENZYMES, particularly the CYTOCHROME P450-dependent monooxygenase system, metabolize xenobiotics to produce reactive intermediates that can react with ENDOGENOUS macromolecules such as proteins and DNA to produce adverse effects.

heptane (chemistry) C_7H_{16} LIQUID ALKANE HYDROCARBON, the seventh member of the methane SERIES, present in petrol.

heptavalent (chemistry) With a VALENCY of seven. Also termed: SEPTIVALENT.

heredity (genetics) The process by which characteristics are genetically transmitted from one generation to the next. *See* GENETICS.

heritability (genetics) The proportion of the VARIABILITY of the PHENOTYPE of a trait that is attributable to genetic factors. HERITABILITY is not a fixed property of the genes concerned but depends in each situation on how much VARIATION there is both in genotypes and in the ENVIRONMENT.

hermaphrodite (genetics) An ANIMAL that has the reproductive organs of both sexes. Animals that are normally hermaphroditic include flatworms, LEECHES, land snails, some fish and some flies. They are capable of self-FERTILIZATION, unless they are sequential hermaphrodites (*i.e.* they have first one SET of sex organs, then the other). Hermaphrodites do not have SEX CHROMOSOMES. In humans, hermaphroditism is a rare abnormality. The person has both ovarian and testicular TISSUE, which may occur as (a) one OVARY plus one TESTIS, (b) two ovotestes or (c) one ovotestis plus either an OVARY or a TESTIS; the external genitalia are ambiguous. The condition is the result of a single OVUM being fertilized simultaneously by an X and a Y SPERM, so that the person is a CHIMAERA of XX and XY CELLS. *See* SEX DETERMINATION.

hernia (medical) The ABNORMAL protrusion of one structure through another. The commonest type is protrusion of part of the abdominal contents through the abdominal wall.

heroin (H) (toxicology/ pharmacology) Diamorphine, a highly addictive opiate derived from MORPHINE.

herpes (medical) INFLAMMATION of the SKIN characterized by clusters of small vesicles (*e.g.* HERPES simplex).

herpes gestationis (medical) SKIN disease of PREGNANCY.

herpes simplex virus 1 (HSV-I) (virology) A VIRUS that results in cold sores or FEVER blisters, most often on the mouth or around the eyes. Like all HERPES VIRUSES, it may lie dormant for months or years in NERVE tissues and flare up in times of STRESS, TRAUMA, INFECTION or IMMUNOSUPPRESSION. It may also cause a mild form of MENINGITIS, or a much more dangerous encephalitis which follows a first INFECTION, and is not likely to affect those with cold sores or other types of HERPES.

herpes simplex virus 11 (HSV-11) (virology) A VIRUS that causes painful sores on the genitals or ANUS. It is one of the most common SEXUALLY TRANSMITTED DISEASES in the United States.

herpes varicella zoster virus (HVZ) (virology) The VARICELLA VIRUS causes chicken pox in children and may reappear in adulthood as herpes zoster. Herpes zoster, also called SHINGLES, is characterized by small, painful blisters on the SKIN along NERVE pathways. The most dangerous AREA for the disease to appear is in the face and forehead, for the EYE may be involved and this may LEAD to complications.

herpes virus (virology) Any of a GROUP of ANIMAL DNA VIRUSES responsible for various diseases; *e.g.* chickenpox (VARIOLA) and HERPES simplex (coldsore), and HERPES ZOSTER (SHINGLES). Their GENOME is double-stranded DNA.

See also HERPES SIMPLEX VIRUS 1 (HSV-I); HERPES SIMPLEX VIRUS 11 (HSV-11); HERPES VARICELLA ZOSTER VIRUS (HVZ).

hertz (Hz) (measurement) SI UNIT of FREQUENCY. 1 Hz = 1 CYCLE per second. It was named after the German physicist Heinrich Hertz (1858-94).

Hess's law (chemistry) Total ENERGY change resulting from a CHEMICAL REACTION is dependent only on the initial and final states, and is independent of the REACTION route. It was named after the Austrian-born American physicist Victor Hess (1883-1964).

heterarchy (computing) The CHARAC-TERISTIC of a COMPUTER PROGRAM that does not process DATA merely through successively higher levels, but can call many different routines to help in the processing of the DATA at each LEVEL, including routines from higher levels.

hetero- (biology) Prefix denoting other or different.

See also HOMO-.

heterochromatic flicker photometer (physics) *See* PHOTOMETER.

heterochromatin (molecular biology) CHROMATIN, the substance of which chromosomes are made, that is in a highly condensed state because the DNA, not being actively transcribed, can be packed densely around the HISTONES. Examples are the DNA in the centromeres and in Barr bodies. Because of its more condensed state, HETEROCHROMATIN is more intensely coloured (*USA*: colored)

when stained than ordinary CHROMATIN (euchromatin).

heterochrony (measurment) A difference in the rate or timing of events.

heterocyclic (chemistry) Describing a CYCLIC ORGANIC COMPOUND that contains atoms other than CARBON in the ring, *e.g.* PYRIDINE.

See also HOMOCYCLIC;

heteroduplex (molecular biology) A NUCLEIC ACIDmolecule that consists of two strands of different genetic origins. It can be either a double-stranded DNA MOLECULE or a DNA-RNA COMBINATION. Where the sequences are HOMOLOGOUS, the two strands will link; non-HOMOLOGOUS sequences can then be seen under the ELECTRON MICROSCOPE looking like bubbles. Examination of a HET-ERODUPLEX made from DNA strands from wild-type and MUTANT-type DNA will show where there are deletions or insertions; this is called 'HETERODUPLEX mapping'.

heterogametic (genetics) Describing an organism that produces two kinds of gametes, each possessing a different SEX CHROMOSOME. These are usually produced by the male; *e.g.* in human males half the sperms contain an X-CHROMOSOME and half a Y-CHROMOSOME. The opposite is HOMOGAMETIC.

heterogeneous nuclear RNA (genetics) The RNA MOLECULE that reads the DNA code in eukaryotes. *See* MESSENGER RNA.

heterogeneous Relating to more than one PHASE, *e.g.* describing a CHEMICAL REACTION that involves one or more solids in addition to a GAS or a LIQUID PHASE.

See also HOMOGENEOUS.

heterograft (medical) *See* GRAFT.

heterokaryon (genetics) A CELL or individual that contains two nuclei, each of different genetic ORIGIN. It can happen naturally when CELLS of two different FUNGI FUSE, and it can be artificially induced by mixing the CELLS of higher organisms *in vitro.*

heterolytic fission (chemistry) Breaking of a TWO-ELECTRON COVALENT BOND to give two fragments, with one fragment retaining both electrons. Also termed: heterolytic CLEAVAGE.

See also HOMOLYTIC FISSION.

heterosis (genetics) The technical term for the phenomenon more generally known as HYBRID VIGOUR.

heterosome (genetics) The X or Y CHROMOSOME, each of which, unlike the other chromosomes can pair with a different CHROMOSOME. *Compare* AUTOSOME.

heterotroph (microbiology) Organism that requires an organic CARBON source.

heterotrophism (physiology) MODE of nutrition exhibited by most animals, FUNGI, BACTERIA and some flowering plants. It involves the intake of organic substances from the ENVIRONMENT due to the inability of the organism to synthesize them from inorganic materials.

See also AUTOTROPHISM.

heterozygote (genetics) An organism having two different ALLELES at the same LOCUS on a pair of chromosomes. The term 'double HETEROZYGOTE' refers to an individual who, at two given loci, has unlike ALLELES. *Contrast* HOMOZYGOTE.

heterozygous advantage (genetics) the situation where an organism that is HETEROZYGOUS at a given LOCUS has greater genetic fitness than either of the two homozygotes. It is one way in which two different ALLELES can be maintained within a population at STABLE frequencies: neither is better on its own, but the two in COMBINATION are the most successful GENOTYPE, and therefore neither ALLELE is lost from the population. The classic example of this is sickle-CELL ANAEMIA (*USA*: sickle-cell anemia) in humans, in which homozygotes for the MUTANT ALLELE have severe ANAEMIA (*USA*: anemia), homozygotes for the NORMAL ALLELE are liable to get MALARIA, but HETEROZYGOTES are neither anaemic (*USA*: anemic) nor subject to MALARIA. In a more general sense, organisms that are HETEROZYGOUS at many loci are at an advantage over more HOMOZYGOUS ones; this is known as HYBRID VIGOUR. *See* POLYMORPHISM.

heterozygous (genetics) Describing an organism that possesses two dissimilar ALLELES in a pair of chromosomes. A DOMINANT ALLELE can be expressed in the HETEROZYGOUS or HOMOZYGOUS state, but a RECESSIVE ALLELE can be expressed only in the HOMOZYGOUS state.

heuristic (philosophy) Describing an approach to problem-solving that is based on trial and error rather than theory. The term is sometimes used to describe COMPUTER programs that can 'learn' from their mistakes.

hexadecimal (computing) Describing a number system based on 16 (its digits are 1-9, A, B, C, D, E, F), commonly used in DIGITAL COMPUTERS.

hexamine (chemistry) $C_6H_{12}N_4$ ORGANIC COMPOUND made by condensing METHANAL (FORMALDEHYDE) with AMMONIA, used as a camping fuel and ANTISEPTIC drug. It can be nitrated to make the high explosive cyclonite. Also termed: hexamethylenetetramine.

hexane (chemistry) C_6H_{14} Colourless (*USA*: colorless) LIQUID ALKANE, used as a SOLVENT.

hexanedioic acid (chemistry) An alternative term for adipic ACID.

hexose (chemistry) MONOSACCHARIDE CARBOHYDRATE (SUGAR) that contains six CARBON atoms and has the GENERAL FORMULA $C_6H_{12}O_6$; *e.g.* GLUCOSE and FRUCTOSE.

Hf (chemistry) The CHEMICAL SYMBOL for HAFNIUM.

hf (physics) An abbreviation of 'h'igh 'f'requency.

HFG (physics) An abbreviation of 'H'igh 'F'requency 'G'as.

Hg (chemistry) The CHEMICAL SYMBOL for MERCURY. The symbol is derived from Latin hydragyrum, meaning MERCURY.

hg (measurement) An abbreviation of 'h'ecto'g'ram.

HGH (biochemistry) An abbreviation of 'H'uman 'G'rowth 'H'ormone.

hgt (measurement) An abbreviation of 'h'ei'g'h't'. Also termed ht.

hi temp (measurement) An abbreviation of 'hi'gh 'temp'erature.

5-HIAA (biochemistry) An abbreviation of 5-'H'ydroxy'I'ndole'A'cetic 'A'cid.

hiatus hernia (medical) Protrusion of the upper part of the STOMACH through the diaphram MUSCLE through which the OESOPHAGUS (*USA*: esophagus) passes. (*USA*: hiatal HERNIA).

high blood pressure (medical) *See* HYPERTENSION.

high frequency (HF) (1, 2 physics) 1 A radio FREQUENCY with a range of 3 to 30 megahertz. 2 Rapidly alternating ELECTRIC CURRENT or WAVE.

high iron diamine stain (histology) A histological staining technique that may be used to make sulphomucins (*USA*: sulfomucins) visible under the MICROSCOPE.

highest common factor (HCF) (mathematics) Of two or more numbers is the largest number that divides exactly into each of them; *e.g.* the HCF of 21, 35 and 63 is 7.

Highmans congo red stain (histology) A histological staining technique that may be used to make amyloid visible under the MICROSCOPE.

high-pass filter (physics) A FILTER that transmits from a waveform only the frequencies higher than a specified FREQUENCY.

high-risk behaviour (epidemiology) A term used to describe certain activities that increase the risk of disease exposure. (*USA*: high-risk behavior).

high-risk groups (epidemiology) Those groups of people that show a behavioural risk for exposure to a disease or condition.

high voltage (HV) (physics) Marked on wires carrying a high load of ELECTRICITY to indicate danger of electrocution.

HIOMT (biochemistry) An abbreviation of 'H'ydroxy'I'ndole-'O'-'M'ethyl'T'ransferase.

H-ion (chemistry) An abbreviation of 'H'ydrogen 'ION'.

hip joint (anatomy) The ball-and-socket JOINT between the ballshaped HEAD of the FEMUR, the thigh-BONE, and the acetabulum, a cup-shaped hollow in the side of the PELVIS.

hippocampus (histology) Structure of NERVE TISSUE within the VERTEBRATE BRAIN. It is implicated in emotions and also possibly in MEMORY, since bilateral removal in humans produces severe and permanent anterograde deficits in MEMORY.

Hirschaprung's disease (medical) See MEGACOLON.

hirsutism (medical) The GROWTH of superfluous HAIR, especially in women. It is due to androgenic HORMONES, and commonly starts soon after the onset of the MENSES. If the PERIODS are NORMAL, there is very little likelihood of underlying disease, but if they cease or are very irregular there may be some cause such as a polycystic OVARY.

Hirudinea (biology) CLASS of annelids consisting of the LEECHES, some of which are BLOOD-sucking.

His. (biochemistry) An abbreviation of 'His'tidine.

histamine (biochemistry) ORGANIC COMPOUND that is released from CELLS in CONNECTIVE TISSUE during an allergic REACTION. It causes DILATION of capillaries and constriction of bronchi. See ALLERGY.

histamine N-methyltransferase (biochemistry) See n-METHYLATION.

histidine (His.) (chemistry) $(C_3H_3N_2)$-$CH_2CH(NH_2)COOH$ CRYSTALLINE SOLUBLE SOLID, an OPTICALLY ACTIVE BASIC ESSENTIAL AMINO ACID. Also termed: 2-amino-3-imidazolylPROPANOIC ACID.

histocompatibility (histology) See T CELLS.

histocompatibility complex (genetics) The system whereby the body recognizes as foreign any TISSUE other than its own. It is medically important in that differences between DONOR and RECIPIENT LEAD to the rejection of *transplants*. Each of the individual's own CELLS has on its surface a number of specific proteins, the histocompatibility antigens (also known as HLA, HUMAN LEUCOCYTE ANTIGENS), of which there are six different types, each with dozens of allelic variants. The probability of any two people other than identical twins having exactly the same COMBINATION is correspondingly remote.

histogram (statistics) A chart containing adjacent parallel bars, usually vertical, whose lengths represent the FREQUENCY DISTRIBUTION on a continuous DIMENSION.

histology (histology) The study of the structure of TISSUE particularly at the microscopic LEVEL.

histone (biochemistry) One of a GROUP of small proteins with a large proportion of BASIC AMINO ACIDS, *e.g.* ARGININE or lycine. Histones are found in combination with

NUCLEIC ACID in the CHROMATIN of EUKARYOTIC CELLS.

histoplasmosis (mycology) A FUNGUS INFECTION by the organism *Histoplasma capsulatum.* The FUNGUS is found in the soil where bird excreta are present, and if it is inhaled affects the lungs, but may spread throughout the body. Symptoms usually include FEVER, shortness of breath, cough, WEIGHT loss and physical exhaustion.

hit (computing) The detection of a signal when it is there.

HIV (virology) An abbreviation of 'H'uman 'I'mmunodeficiency 'V'irus.

hives (immunology) NETTLE RASH or URTICARIA.

HIV-positive (virology) Presence of the human immunodeficiency VIRUS in the body.

HLA (haematology) An abbreviation of 'H'uman 'L'eucocyte 'A'ntigen.

HLA system (immunology) An abbreviation of 'h'uman 'l'eucocyte 'a'ntigen system.

HMG-CoA reductase (biochemistry) An abbreviation of 3-'H'ydroxy-3-'M'ethyl-'G'lutaryl 'Co'enzyme 'A' 'reductase'.

HMO (medical) An abbreviation of 'H'ealth 'M'aintenance 'O'rganisation.

HNC (education) An abbreviation of 'H'igher 'N'ational "C'ertificate.

HND (education) An abbreviation of 'H'igher 'N'ational 'D'iploma.

hndbk (general terminology) An abbreviation of 'h'a'n'd'b'oo'k'.

hnRNA (genetics) An abbreviation of 'h'eterogeneous 'n'uclear 'RNA'.

Ho (chemistry) The CHEMICAL SYMBOL for HOLMIUM.

HOC (chemistry) An abbreviation of 'H'eavy 'O'rganic 'C'hemical.

Hodgkin's disease (medical/ histology) A disease of the reticular and lymphatic tissues of the body. It causes painless enlargement of the LYMPH GLANDS and may be accompanied by a FEVER and night sweats. As the disease spreads LYMPH GLANDS become enlarged, and the SPLEEN and later the LIVER may also become enlarged. Named after the English physician, T. Hodgkin (1798-1866).

holandric (genetics) Occurring only in males, *i.e.* a GENE that is on the Y CHROMOSOME.

holmium Ho (chemistry) Silvery metallic ELEMENT in GROUP IIIB of the PERIODIC TABLE (one of the LANTHANIDES). At. no. 67; r.a.m. 164.9303.

holoenzyme (biochemistry) ENZYME that forms from the COMBINATION of a COENZYME and an APOENZYME. The former determines the nature and the latter the specificity of a REACTION.

homatropine (pharmacology) An ALKALOID derived from ATROPINE, used to DILATE the pupil of the EYE.

homeo. (medical) An abbreviation of 'homeo'pathic.

homeostasis (physiology) The tendency of a physiological system to maintain itself in BALANCE, whatever the changes in the internal or external ENVIRONMENT. From the Greek 'homoio', meaning 'equal', and 'stasis', meaning 'state'. HOMEOSTASIS is an evolved mechanism, operated by the switching off and on of many genes. An example is maintenance of body TEMPERATURE or the BALANCE of salts in the BLOOD.

homeotic mutation (genetics) A MUTATION that replaces a NORMAL structure with another structure that is also NORMAL but is in the wrong place.

homo- (biology) Prefix denoting the same or similar.

See also HETERO-.

homo sapiens (genetics) The SPECIES to which all human beings alive belong. *Homo sapiens* has 22 pairs of autosomal chromosomes plus two SEX CHROMOSOMES (XX or XY); the amount of DNA in each human SOMATIC CELL is about 6 picograms, and if fully extended would be about 1.9 metres long. The number of genes is ESTIMATED at somewhere in the region of 100,000.

homocyclic (chemistry) Describing a chemical COMPOUND that contains one or more closed rings comprising CARBON and HYDROGEN atoms only, *e.g.* BENZENE. Also termed: CARBOCYCLIC.

See also HETEROCYCLIC.

homoeopathy (medical) System of ALTERNATIVE MEDICINE that treats disorders by introducing substances into the body that provoke similar symptoms and so encourage the body's own defences. Medical opinion on the value of HOMOEOPATHY is divided. Also termed: homeopathy.

homogametic (genetics) Describing an organism with HOMOLOGOUS SEX CHROMOSOMES (*e.g.* XX). This sex can only produce one type of GAMETE, with a single X CHROMOSOME, and therefore does not determine the sex of the offspring. In humans the female is the HOMOGAMETIC sex. *See* HETEROGAMETIC; BARR BODY.

homogeneity of variance (statistics) Similarity of VARIANCE, *i.e.* lack of a significant difference in VARIANCE. Most parametric tests are only valid if the samples being compared are from populations with the same VARIANCE.

homogeneous (1 biology; 2 chemistry; 3 mathematics) 1 In biology, describing similar structures found in different SPECIES that are thought to have originated from a common ancestor. 2 In chemistry, relating to a single PHASE (*e.g.* describing a CHEMICAL REACTION in which all the reactants are solids, or liquids or gases); describing a system of uniform composition. 3 In mathematics, describing a POLYNOMIAL whose terms all have the same DEGREE; *e.g.* $2x^3 - 3x^2y + xy^2 + 5y^3$ is HOMOGENEOUS (of DEGREE 3).

See also HETEROGENEOUS.

homograft (medical) A GRAFT taken from another individual of the same SPECIES. Also called an allograft.

homoiothermic (physiology) Describing animals that maintain a more-or-less CONSTANT body TEMPERATURE (*e.g.* mammals, birds). Also termed: WARM-BLOODED.

homologous (biology) Describing things with common ORIGIN, but not necessarily the same appearance or FUNCTION (*e.g.* the arms of a human and the wings of a bat).

See also ANALOGOUS.

homologous chromosomes (genetics) the members of a pair of chromosomes that carry the same genes but not always the same ALLELES for a given CHARACTER as the other member of the pair. All the AUTOSOMES come in HOMOLOGOUS pairs. In the case of the SEX CHROMOSOMES, the X and the Y are not HOMOLOGOUS as they do not carry the same GENE sequence, but two X CHROMOSOMES are HOMOLOGOUS with each other. *See* MEIOSIS.

homologous series (chemistry) FAMILY of organic chemical compounds with the same GENERAL FORMULA; *e.g.* ALKANES, ALKENES and alkynes.

homologue (1 chemistry; 2 biology) 1 A member of a HOMOLOGOUS SERIES. 2 A HOMOLOGOUS CHROMOSOME.

homolytic fission (chemistry) Breaking of a two-ELECTRON COVALENT BOND in such a way that each fragment retains one ELECTRON of the BOND. Also termed: homolytic CLEAVAGE.

See also HETEROLYTIC FISSION.

homozygote (genetics) An organism having two identical ALLELES at the same site on a pair of chromosomes.

homozygous (genetics) Having the same two ALLELES for a given GENE. Two organisms that are HOMOZYGOUS for the same ALLELES breed true for the CHARACTER in question, thus producing progeny which are HOMOZYGOUS and identical to the parent with respect to that GENE.

See also HETEROZYGOUS.

hookworm infestation (parasitology) Ancylostomiasis. Parasitisation by one of the roundworms (nematodes) *Ancylostoma duodenale* or *Necator americanus*.

horizontal cells of Cajal (cytology) FUSIFORM CELLS in the plexiform layer of the CORTEX whose dendrites spread horizontally in opposite directions.

horizontal transmission (genetics) The transmission of DNA by viral INFECTION into CELLS. NORMAL genetic transmission is VERTICAL TRANSMISSION. *See* TRANSDUCTION.

hormone (biochemistry) A chemical released by an ENDOCRINE GLAND and carried round in the bloodstream to alter the BEHAVIOUR (*USA*: behavior) of other specific target CELLS or tissues. STEROID HORMONES are small LIPID molecules that enter the target CELLS; they include the SEX HORMONES. Other HORMONES are polypeptides (chains of AMINO ACIDS shorter than proteins) which bind on to the outside of the target CELL; they include GROWTH HORMONE and INSULIN. Many HORMONES can be synthesised to provide TREATMENT for patients with a deficiency; some can now also be produced by GENE CLONING.

hormone replacement therapy (HRT) (pharmacology) A drug treatment, which may be administered orally, or topically, for women to supplement the diminished production of the sex HORMONE OESTROGEN during the MENOPAUSE.

horseradish peroxidase (biochemistry) An ENZYME that is taken up by NERVE CELLS and that flows in a retrograde direction from AXON terminals to the CELL BODY and dendrites; after being made RADIOACTIVE, it can be used to identify the location of CELL bodies whose axonal terminals are elsewhere.

hosp. (medical) An abbreviation of 'hosp'ital.

host (1, 2 biology) 1 The RECIPIENT of a GRAFT or transplant. 2 The CELL, organism or person that is infected by some PATHOGEN or PARASITE, *e.g.* a BACTERIUM invaded by a VIRUS. *See* PARASITISM.

hot spot (molecular biology) A site in a DNA MOLECULE where MUTATIONS or recombinations occur with much higher FREQUENCY than elsewhere.

housekeeping genes (genetics) A GENE that has a PRODUCT essential for the NORMAL metabolic requirements of any CELL. These genes are active in most or all CELLS, in contrast to the CELL-specific LUXURY GENES. The parts of the CHROMOSOME where they are situated show up as LIGHT-staining interbands.

hPL (physiology/ biochemistry) An abbreviation of 'h'uman 'P'lacental 'L'actogen.

HPLC (biochemistry) An abbreviation of 'H'igh 'P'erformance 'L'iquid 'C'hromatography.

HPRT (immunology) An abbreviation of 'H'ypoxanthine 'P'hospho 'R'ibosyl 'T'ransferase.

HSC (governing body) An abbreviation of 'H'ealth and 'S'afety 'C'ommission.

HS-CoA (physiology/ biochemistry) A symbol for reduced coenzyme A.

HSS (society) An abbreviation of 'H'istory of 'S'cience 'S'ociety.

ht (measurement) An abbreviation of 'h'eigh't'. Also termed hgt.

H-T, HT (measurement) An abbreviation of 'H'igh-'T'emperature.

HTLV (virology) An abbreviation of 'H'uman 'T'-CELL 'L'eukaemia (*USA*: leukemia) 'V'irus.

HTRF (biochemistry) An abbreviation for 'H'ypo-'T'halamic-'R'eleasing 'F'actors.

human equivalent dose (pharmacology/ toxicology) A dose which, when administered to humans, produces an effect equal to that produced by a given dose in another ANIMAL.

human leucocyte antigens (HLA) (haematology) PROTEIN markers of self used in histocompatibility testing. It plays a most important part in determining whether transplanted tissues will be rejected by the RECIPIENT, and some HLA types also correlate with certain AUTO-IMMUNE DISEASES. For example, ANKYLOSING SPONDYLITIS is 120 times more likely to occur in people with ALLELE B27.

human t-cell leukaemia virus (HTLV) (virology) Any of several retroviruses that infect T-CELLS, causing a rare strain of LEUKAEMIA (*USA*: leukemia) to develop. (*USA*: human T-cell leukemia virus).

humerus (anatomy) Upper BONE in the forelimb of a tetrapod VERTEBRATE; in human beings, the upper arm BONE.

humi. (physics) An abbreviation of 'humi'dity.

humidity (physics) Measure of the amount of WATER VAPOUR in a GAS, *e.g.* the AIR, usually expressed as a PER-CENTAGE. RELATIVE HUMIDITY is the amount of VAPOUR divided by the maximum amount of VAPOUR the GAS will hold (at a particular TEMPERATURE).

humoral immunity (immunology) The production of antibodies for defense against INFECTION or disease.

hundredweight (cwt) (measurement) UNIT of MASS equal to 112 lb or 50.85 kg (USA: equal to 100 lb or 45.40 kg).

Hunterian chancre (medical) The primary sore of syphilis, which has an ulcerated hard BASE. The DISCHARGE is thin and watery. Named after the London surgeon, J. Hunter (1728-93).

Hunter's syndrome (genetics) A human disease caused by an X-linked RECESSIVE ALLELE. The biochemical problem (as with HURLER'S SYNDROME) is that the patient is unable to break down mucopolysaccharides, large compounds of sugars that combine with proteins and are important in NERVE CELL function. A build-up of these molecules leads to mental deterioration and deafness, as well as various disfiguring symptoms. Women in families where the disease has occurred can be tested to see whether they are carriers; and prenatal diagnosis is reliable.

Huntingtons chorea (medical/ genetics) A human disease caused by a single DOMINANT ALLELE. The underlying mechanism is not known, but the disease is a distressing one consisting of involuntary movements and mental deterioration.

Hurler's syndrome (genetics) A human disease caused by a RECESSIVE ALLELE. The biochemical problem is the same as in HUNTER'S SYNDROME, but the effects are worse, with dwarfism and HEART problems leading to death at the age of 8-10. CARRIER females can be identified biochemically, as can affected foetuses (*USA*: fetuses). About 1 in 100,000 babies has Hurler's syndrome.

HV (physics) An abbreviation of 'H'igh 'V'oltage.

HVA (biochemistry) An abbreviation of 'Homo'V'anillic 'A'cid.

hyaluronidase (biochemistry) A naturally occurring ENZYME which has the property of breaking down hyaluronic ACID.

hybrid (genetics) The offspring of parents that are genetically unlike, particularly of parents of different SPECIES or of different varieties within a SPECIES.

hybrid DNA (molecular biology) DNA that is artificially made *in vitro* by mixing two strands of DNA (or one of DNA and one of RNA) of different genetic origins. It is not the same as RECOMBINANT DNA.

hybrid vigour (genetics) The phenomenon in which the HYBRID is more vigorous than either of its parental strains resulting from an increase in genetical VARIATION.

hybridization (1, 2 genetics) 1 Crossing of animals or plants to produce a HYBRID. 2 COMBINATION of ATOMIC ORBITALS to produce HYBRID orbitals.

hybridoma (immunology/ genetics) An artificially produced HYBRID CELL, combining a NORMAL lymphocyte and a myeloma (cancerous) LYMPH CELL, and used in the preparation of MONOCLONAL antibodies.

hydatid disease (parasitology) INFECTION with the dog TAPEWORM, *Echinococcus granulosus*.

hydatidiform mole (medical) A disease of the superficial layer of the CHORION, the outer of the two membranous layers covering the FOETUS (*USA*: fetus) in the UTERUS, in which the UTERUS becomes full of vesicles like grapes; it results from ABNORMAL development of the fertilized OVUM.

hydrargyrum (chemistry) MERCURY.

hydrate (chemistry) Chemical COMPOUND that contains WATER OF CRYSTALLIZATION.

hydrated (1, 2 chemistry) 1 Describing a substance after TREATMENT with WATER. 2 Describing a COMPOUND that contains chemically bonded WATER, a HYDRATE.

hydrated lime (chemistry) An alternative term for CALCIUM HYDROXIDE.

hydration (chemistry) Attachment of WATER to the particles (particularly ions) of a SOLUTE during the dissolving process.

hydrazine (chemistry) NH_2NH_2 Colourless (*USA*: colorless) LIQUID, a powerful REDUCING AGENT used in organic SYNTHESIS.

hydrazone (chemistry) Member of a FAMILY of ORGANIC COMPOUNDS that contain the GROUP $-C=NNH_2$. Hydrazones are formed by the ACTION of HYDRAZINE on an ALDEHYDE or KETONE, and are used in identifying them.

hydride (chemistry) COMPOUND formed between HYDROGEN and another ELEMENT (*e.g.* CALCIUM HYDRIDE, CaH_2).

hydro- (biology) Prefix denoting WATER.

hydrobromic acid HBr (chemistry) Colourless (*USA*: colorless) acidic AQUEOUS SOLUTION of HYDROGEN BROMIDE; its salts are bromides.

hydrocarbon (chemistry) ORGANIC COMPOUND that contains only CARBON and HYDROGEN. The chief naturally occurring HYDROCARBONS are bitumen, coal, methane, natural GAS and petroleum. Most of these, and HYDROCARBONS derived from them, are used as fuels. The ALIPHATIC COMPOUNDS form three HOMOLOGOUS SERIES: ALKANES, ALKENES and alkynes. Aromatic HYDROCARBONS are CYCLIC compounds. *See* AROMATIC COMPOUNDS.

hydrocephalus (medical) An ABNORMAL amount of CEREBROSPINAL FLUID within the ventricles of the BRAIN, eventually leading to malformation of BRAIN TISSUE.

hydrochloric acid (chemistry) HCl Colourless (*USA*: colorless) acidic AQUEOUS SOLUTION of HYDROGEN CHLORIDE, a STRONG ACID that dissolves most metals with the release of HYDROGEN; its salts are chlorides. It is contained in NORMAL STOMACH juices in a diluted form.

hydrocortisone A STEROID HORMONE secreted by the ADRENAL CORTEX. It may be used to treat rheumatism and inflammatory and allergic conditions.

hydrocyanic acid HCN (chemistry) Very poisonous SOLUTION of HYDROGEN CYANIDE in WATER. Its salts are cyanides. Also termed: prussic ACID.

hydrofluoric acid HF (chemistry) Colourless (*USA*: colorless) corrosive AQUEOUS SOLUTION of HYDROGEN FLUORIDE; its salts are fluorides. It is used for etching GLASS (and must be stored in plastic bottles).

hydrogen H (chemistry) Gaseous ELEMENT usually given its own place at the beginning of the PERIODIC TABLE, but sometimes assigned to GROUP IA, colourless (*USA*: colorless), odourless

(*USA*: odorless) and highly inflammable, it is the lightest GAS known and occurs abundantly in COMBINATION in WATER (H_2O), coal and petroleum (mainly as HYDROCARBONS) and living things (mainly as carbohydrates). In addition to the common form (sometimes called protium, r.a.m. 1.00797) there are two other isotopes: DEUTERIUM or heavy HYDROGEN (r.a.m. 2.01410) and the RADIOACTIVE TRITIUM (r.a.m. 3.0221). At. no. 1; r.a.m. (of the naturally occurring MIXTURE of isotopes) 1.0080.

hydrogen bond (chemistry) Strong CHEMICAL BOND that holds together some molecules that contain HYDROGEN, *e.g.* WATER molecules, which become associated as a result. A HYDROGEN ATOM bonded to an electronegative ATOM interacts with a (non-bonding) lone pair of electrons on another electronegative ATOM.

hydrogen bromide HBr (chemistry) Pale yellow GAS which dissolves in WATER to form HYDROBROMIC ACID.

hydrogen chloride HCl (chemistry) Colourless (*USA*: colorless) GAS which dissolves readily in WATER to form HYDROCHLORIC ACID. It is made by treating a CHLORIDE with concentrated SULPHURIC ACID (*USA*: sulfuric acid) or produced as a BY-PRODUCT of electrolytic processes involving chlorides.

hydrogen cyanide HCN (chemistry) Colourless (*USA*: colorless) poisonous GAS, which dissolves in WATER to form HYDROCYANIC ACID (prussic acid). It has a CHARACTERISTIC SMELL of bitter almonds.

hydrogen electrode (physics) HALF-CELL that consists of HYDROGEN GAS bubbling around a PLATINUM ELECTRODE, covered in PLATINUM black (very finely divided

PLATINUM). It is immersed in a MOLAR ACID solution and used for determining STANDARD ELECTRODE POTENTIALS. Also termed: HYDROGEN HALF-CELL.

hydrogen fluoride HF (chemistry) Colourless (*USA*: colorless) fuming LIQUID, which is extremely corrosive and dissolves in WATER to form HYDROFLUORIC ACID.

hydrogen half-cell (physics) An alternative term for HYDROGEN ELECTRODE.

hydrogen halide (chemistry) COMPOUND of HYDROGEN and a HALOGEN; *e.g.* HYDROGEN FLUORIDE, HF.

hydrogen ion H^+ (chemistry) Positively-charged HYDROGEN ATOM; a PROTON. A CHARACTERISTIC of an ACID is the production of HYDROGEN IONS, which in AQUEOUS SOLUTION are HYDRATED to HYDROXONIUM IONS, H_3O^+. HYDROGEN ION CONCENTRATION is a measure of acidity, usually expressed on the PH SCALE.

hydrogen peroxide (chemistry) H_2O_2 Colourless (*USA*: colorless) syrupy LIQUID with strong oxidizing powers, SOLUBLE in WATER in all proportions. DILUTE solutions are used as an OXIDIZING AGENT, disinfectant and BLEACH.

hydrogen spectrum (physics) SPECTRUM produced when an electric DISCHARGE is passed through HYDROGEN GAS. The HYDROGEN molecules dissociate and the atoms emit LIGHT at a SERIES of CHARACTERISTIC frequencies.

See also BALMER SERIES.

hydrogen sulphide H_2S (chemistry) Colourless (*USA*: colorless) poisonous GAS with a CHARACTERISTIC SMELL (when impure) of bad eggs. It is formed by rotting SULPHUR (*USA*: sulfur) containing organic MATTER and the ACTION of acids on sulphides (*USA*: sulfides).

hydrogenation (chemistry) Method of chemical SYNTHESIS by adding HYDROGEN to a substance. It forms the basis of many important industrial processes, such as the conversion of LIQUID oils to SOLID fats.

hydrogencarbonate (chemistry) Acidic SALT containing the ION HCO_3^-. Also termed: BICARBONATE.

hydrogen sulphate (chemistry) Acidic SALT containing the ION HSO_4^-. Also termed: BISULPHATE (*USA*: bisulfate). (*USA*: hydrogen sulfate).

hydrogen sulphite (chemistry) Acidic SALT containing the ION HSO_3^-. Also termed: BISULPHITE (*USA*: bisulfite). (*USA*: hydrogen sulfite).

hydrolysis (biochemistry) CLEAVAGE of a MOLECULE by the addition of WATER, with a HYDROXYL GROUP (-OH) from the WATER taking part in the REACTION; *e.g.* esters hydrolyse to form ALCOHOLs and acids.

hydrolytic enzymes (biochemistry) Any ENZYME capable of splitting a MOLECULE into components by inserting WATER. HYDROLYTIC ENZYMES include lysosomal ACID hydrolases and a number of the ENZYMES in PROTEIN, CARBOHYDRATE, LIPID and NUCLEIC ACID CATABOLISM.

hydrometer (physics) Instrument for measuring the DENSITY of a LIQUID. It consists of a weighted GLASS bulb with a long graduated stem, which floats in the LIQUID being tested.

hydrophilic (biochemistry) Possessing an AFFINITY for WATER. Refers to chemicals that are WATER-SOLUBLE or to the regions of chemicals that are polar and therefore attracted to WATER. HYDROPHILIC compounds do not diffuse easily through membranes.

hydrophobia (virology) Popular name for RABIES, though it in fact only refers to one of the symptoms, the irrational fear of WATER.

hydrophobic (chemistry) WATER-repellent; having no attraction for WATER.

hydrophobic binding (biochemistry) When two non-polar groups come together they exclude the WATER between them, and this mutual exclusion of WATER results in a HYDROPHOBIC interaction. In the aggregate they present the least possible disruption of interactions among polar WATER molecules, and thus can LEAD to STABLE complexes. Some authorities consider this a special case involving VAN DER WAALS' FORCES. The minimization of thermodynamically unfavourable (*USA*: unfavorable) contact of a polar GROUPING with WATER molecules provides the major stabilizing effect in HYDROPHOBIC interactions.

hydrops fetalis (medical) Accumulation of FLUID in the body cavities and SUBCUTANEOUS TISSUEs of the fetus. Causes include Rhesus disease.

hydrosol (chemistry) AQUEOUS SOLUTION of a COLLOID.

hydrous (chemistry) Containing WATER.

hydroxide (chemistry) COMPOUND of a METAL that contains the HYDROXYL GROUP (-OH) or the HYDROXIDE ION (OH⁻). Many METAL hydroxides are bases.

hydroxonium ion (chemistry) HYDRATED HYDROGEN ION, H_3O^+.

hydroxybenzene (chemistry) An alternative term for PHENOL.

hydroxybenzoic acid (chemistry) An alternative term for SALICYLLIC ACID.

hydroxyl group (-OH) (chemistry) GROUP containing OXYGEN and HYDROGEN, characteristics of ALCOHOLs and some hydroxides.

hydroxypropionic acid (chemistry) An alternative term for LACTIC ACID.

hygrometer (physics) Instrument for measuring the HUMIDITY of AIR, the amount of WATER VAPOUR in the ATMOS-PHERE.

hygroscope (physics) Instrument for indicating the HUMIDITY of AIR.

hygroscopic (chemistry) Having the tendency to absorb moisture from the ATMOSPHERE.

Hyl (biochemistry) An abbreviation of 'Hy'droxy'l'ysine.

Hyp (biochemistry) An abbreviation of 4-'Hy'droxy'p'roline.

hyperaemia (haematology) Congestion of a part with BLOOD. (*USA*: hyperemia).

hyperchlorhydria (biochemistry) Excess of HYDROCHLORIC ACID in the STOMACH.

hypermetropia (medical) Longsighted-ness, a VISUAL DEFECT in which the eyeball is too short (front to back) so that LIGHT rays entering the EYE from nearby objects would be brought to a FOCUS at a point behind the RETINA. It can be corrected by

spectacles or contact lenses made from converging (CONVEX) lenses. Also termed: hyperopia.

See also MYOPIA.

hyperphoshataemia (haematology/ bio-chemistry) Elevated levels of phosphates in the blood. (*USA*: hyperphoshatemia).

hypersensitivity (immunology) Over-REACTION by the IMMUNE SYSTEM. It involves the mounting of a large-scale immunological defence against antigens that are in low CONCENTRATION and are possibly not harmful to the organism in that low CONCENTRATION though they would be at a higher one. *See* ALLERGY.

hypertension (medical) High arterial BLOOD PRESSURE.

hyperthyroidism (biochemistry) *See* THYROID.

hypertrophy (histology) Increased size of an ORGAN due to enlargement of individual CELLS.

hypha` (mycology) Microscopic hollow FILAMENT CHARACTERISTIC of FUNGI. Hyphae form a NETWORK called a MYCELIUM.

hypo (chemistry) Popular name for SODIUM THIOSULPHATE (*USA*: sodium thiosulfate).

hypocalcaemia (biochemistry) A low LEVEL of CALCIUM in the BLOOD.

hypochlorite (chemistry) SALT of HYPO-CHLOROUS ACID (containing the ION ClO^-). Hypochlorites are used as bleaches and disinfectants.

hypochlorous acid (chemistry) (HOCl) A weak LIQUID ACID stable only in SOLUTION, used as an OXIDIZING AGENT and BLEACH. Its salts are hypochlorites. Also termed: chloric(I) ACID.

hypoglycaemia (biochemistry) A low LEVEL of GLUCOSE in the BLOOD and symptoms are likely to appear if the LEVEL falls below 2.5 mmol/1. By far the most common cause of this is failure in a diabetic to cover the dose of INSULIN or similar drug with food, although there are a number of rare conditions that can lower the BLOOD SUGAR. (*USA*: hypoglycemia).

hypokalaemia (biochemistry) Abnormally low LEVEL of POTASSIUM in the BLOOD. (*USA*: hypokalemia).

hyponatraemia (biochemistry) Abnormally low LEVEL of SODIUM in the BLOOD. (*USA*: hyponatremia).

hypophysis (anatomy) An alternative term for PITUITARY.

hypoplasia (histology) Underdevelopment of a TISSUE or ORGAN.

hyposulphuric acid (chemistry) An alternative term for DITHIONIC ACID. (*USA*: hyposulfuric acid).

hypotension (medical) Abnormally low BLOOD PRESSURE.

hypoth. (biology) An abbreviation of 'hypoth'esis.

hypothalamic-releasing factors (HTRF) (biochemistry) HORMONES produced by NERVE CELLS in the HYPOTHALAMUS that selectively promote the release of five PITUITARY HORMONES: ADRENOCORTICO-TROPHIN, LUTEINIZING HORMONE, THYRO-TROPHIN, FOLLICLE-STIMULATING HORMONE, and GROWTH HORMONE.

hypothalamus (anatomy) Floor and sides of the VERTEBRATE FOREBRAIN, which is concerned with physiological co-ordination of the body; *e.g.* regulation of body TEMPERATURE, HEART rate, BREATHING rate, BLOOD PRESSURE, sleep pattern as well as drinking, eating, WATER EXCRETION and other metabolic functions.

hypothermia (medical) Abnormally low body TEMPERATURE.

hypothesis (philosophy) A provisional scientific explanation that is unproved, but either thought of as probably true or used as a basis for further investigation.

hypothyroidism (biochemistry) *See* THYROID.

hypotonic (biochemistry) Having a lower CONCENTRATION of a SOLUTE, used of one SOLUTION with reference to another. *Compare* hypertonic.

hypotrophy (medical) *See* ATROPHY.

hypovolaemia (medical) A decrease in the VOLUME of FLUID in the EXTRACELLULAR spaces, which can be caused by lack of WATER or severe bleeding and which produces volumetric thirst. (*USA*: hypovolemia).

hypoxaemia (medical) Deficiency of OXYGEN in the BLOOD. (*USA*: hypoxemia).

hysterectomy (medical) Surgical removal of the UTERUS.

hysterosalpingogram (radiology) X-RAY examination to outline the cavity of the UTERUS and lumina of the FALLOPIAN TUBES by the injection of RADIO-OPAQUE dye.

hysteroscopy (medical) Inspection of the uterine cavity through a fibreoptic (*USA*: fiberoptic) scope.

Hz (measurement) An abbreviation of 'H'ert'z'.

I

I (1 measurement; 2 biochemistry) 1 An abbreviation for 'I'ntensity. 2 A symbol for Isoleucine.

I Biol (society) Institute of Biology.

I (chemistry) The CHEMICAL SYMBOL for IODINE.

IAMS (society) An abbreviation of 'I'nternational 'A'ssociation of 'M'icro-biological 'S'ocieties/ 'S'tudies.

IAP (education) An abbreviation of 'I'nternational 'A'cademy of 'P'athology.

IARC (education) An abbreviation of 'I'nternational 'A'gency for 'R'esearch on 'C'ancer.

iatrogenic (medical) Caused by medical TREATMENT or mistreatment.

IB (medical) An abbreviation of 'I'nfectious 'B'ronchitis.

IBC (education) An abbreviation of 'I'nternational 'B'iotoxicological 'C'entre.

ibid (literary terminology) Latin, meaning, 'in the same place'. Refers to the source most recently cited. Found in footnotes and text of dissertations, theses, papers, and the like.

ibp (physics) An abbreviation for 'i'nitial 'b'oiling 'p'oint.

ICD (taxonomy) An abbreviation for 'I'nternational 'C'lassification of 'D'iseases.

ice (chemistry) WATER in its SOLID state (*i.e.* below its FREEZING POINT, 0°C). It is less dense than WATER, because HYDROGEN BONDS give its crystals an open structure, and it therefore floats on WATER. This also means that WATER expands on FREEZING.

ice point (measurement) FREEZING POINT of WATER, 0°C, used as a FIXED POINT on TEMPERATURE SCALES.

Iceland spar (chemistry) Very pure TRANSPARENT form of calcite (CALCIUM CARBONATE), noted for the property of DOUBLE REFRACTION.

I cells (physiology) A symbol for Inspir-atory neurons.

ICRO (education) An abbreviation of 'I'nternational 'C'ell 'R'esearch 'O'rganiz-ation.

ICSH (biochemistry) An abbreviation of 'I'nterstitial 'C'ell-'S'timulating 'H'or-mone.

ICU (medical) An abbreviation of 'I'ntensive 'C'are 'U'nit.

id (measurement) An abbreviation of 'i'nner 'd'iameter.

IDAV (virology) An abbreviation of 'I'mmune 'D'eficiency-'A'ssociated 'V'irus.

IDDM (medical/ biochemistry) An abbreviation of 'I'nsulin-'D'ependent 'D'iabetes 'M'ellitus.

idiogram (genetics) A formal representation of all the chromosomes in an individual's KARYOTYPE, usually consisting of photographed chromosomes from a single CELL-DIVISION, which have been cut out and arranged in ORDER. Preparation of an IDIOGRAM is an essential step in diagnosing CHROMOSOME abnormalities.

idiopathic (medical) A term applied to diseases when their cause is unknown, or of spontaneous ORIGIN.

idiotypes (immunology) The unique and CHARACTERISTIC parts of an ANTIBODY'S VARIABLE REGION, which can themselves serve as antigens.

IDL (biochemistry) An abbreviation of 'I'ntermediate-'D'ensity 'L'ipoPROTEIN.

IDU (medical) An abbreviation of 'I'njection 'D'rug 'U'ser.

i.e. (literary terminology) An abbreviation of 'i'd 'e'st. Latin, meaning 'that is'. Used to clarify or restate what has been said or written.

IF (immunology) An abbreviation of 'I'nter'F'eron. Also termed: IFN.

IFEMS (society) An abbreviation of 'I'nternational 'F'ederation of 'E'lectron 'M'icroscope 'S'ocieties.

IFN (physiology/ biochemistry) An abbreviation of 'I'nter'F'ero'N'. Also termed IF.

IGF-I, IGF-II (physiology/ biochemistry) An abbreviation of 'I'nsulin-like 'G'rowth 'F'actors I and II.

^{123}I-IMP (biochemistry) An abbreviation of '^{123}I'-labeled 'I'odoa'MP'hetamine.

IJP (physiology) An abbreviation of 'I'nhibitory 'J'unction 'P'otential.

IL (physiology/ biochemistry) Abbreviation of 'I'nter'L'eukin.

Ile (biochemistry) An abbreviation of 'I'so'le'ucine.

ileitis (medical) INFLAMMATION of the ILEUM. It occurs in a localised AREA in the last part of the ILEUM, which forms the last three-fifths of the SMALL INTESTINE, and may extend into the COLON. Named after the American surgeon, B. B. Crohn (1874-1983), it is often called Crohn's disease.

ileum (anatomy) Last SECTION of the SMALL INTESTINE continuous with the JEJUNUM above and the COLON below, where both DIGESTION and ABSORPTION take place.

See also DUODENUM; JEJUNUM.

illuminance (physics) The amount of LIGHT falling per UNIT AREA on a surface as measured by PHOTOMETRY; the standard UNIT of measurement is the LUX.

illuminometer (physics) A device for measuring LUMINANCE by matching a comparison FIELD of known brightness to the standard.

ILT (medical) An abbreviation of 'I'nfectious 'L'aryngo-'T'racheitis.

image (optics) Point from which rays of LIGHT entering the EYE appear to have originated. A REAL IMAGE, *e.g.* one formed by a CONVERGING LENS, can be focused on a screen; a virtual IMAGE, *e.g.* one formed in a plane mirror, can be seen only by the eyes of the observer and has no physical existence.

image converter (physics) ELECTRON TUBE for converting INFRA-RED or other invisible images into visible images.

IMI (medical) An abbreviation of 'I'ntra'M'uscular 'I'njection.

imidazole amines (biochemistry) A CLASS of biogenic amines containing an IMIDAZOLE ring, *e.g.* HISTAMINE.

imidazole (biochemistry) $C_3H_4N_2$ An aromatic HETEROCYCLIC COMPOUND whose ring contains three CARBON atoms and two NITROGEN atoms. Also termed: glyoxaline.

imide (chemistry) ORGANIC COMPOUND derived from an ACID ANHYDRIDE, GENERAL FORMULA R-CONHCO-R', where R and R' are organic radicals. Also termed: IMIDO COMPOUND.

imido compound (chemistry) An alternative term for IMIDE.

imido-urea (chemistry) An alternative term for guanidine.

imine (chemistry) Secondary AMINE, an ORGANIC COMPOUND derived from AMMONIA, GENERAL FORMULA RNHR', where R and R' are organic radicals. Also termed: IMINO COMPOUND.

imino compound (chemistry) An alternative term for IMINE.

IML (physiology) An abbreviation of 'I'nter'M'edio'L'ateral gray column.

immiscible (chemistry) Describing two or more liquids that will not mix (when shaken together they separate into layers); *e.g.* oil and WATER.

immun. (immunology) An abbreviation of 'immun'ity/ 'immun'isation/ 'immun'ology.

immune complex (immunology) A cluster of interlocking antigens and antibodies.

immune response (immunology) The REACTION of the IMMUNE SYSTEM to invasion by a foreign substance (ANTIGEN). It involves the production of specific ANTIBODY molecules, which combine with the ANTIGEN to form an ANTIGEN-ANTIBODY complex. Antibodies may be present in body fluids or carried by LYMPHOCYTES.

immune status (immunology) The state of the body's natural defense to diseases. It is influenced by HEREDITY, age, past illness history, diet and physical and mental health. It includes production of circulating and local antibodies and their mechanism of ACTION.

immune system (immunology) The system by which the body overcomes infections and other invasions by foreign bodies. 'Natural', or 'non-specific', IMMUNITY works by PHAGOCYTOSIS and by the ACTION of the PROTEIN INTERFERON. 'Specific IMMUNITY', *i.e.* a RESPONSE to one particular infective agent (all of which, whether VIRUSES, BACTERIA, PARASITES, or non-living particles are known as antigens in this context), is most highly developed in vertebrates, including humans. It is of two kinds: 'HUMORAL IMMUNITY', in which ANTIBODY molecules circulate in the LYMPH and BLOOD; and 'CELL-mediated' IMMUNITY, in which LYMPH CELLS directly bind to the antigens. In HUMORAL IMMUNITY, the arrival of the ANTIGEN stimulates the appropriate line of B LYMPHOCYTES in the BONE MARROW; these CELLS, and their descendants in the LYMPH NODES and SPLEEN, produce the specific

ANTIBODY molecules which bind on to the antigens, either making them incapable of infective ACTION or holding them in lumps so that they can be easily engulfed and dissolved by the large MACROPHAGE CELLS (this is facilitated by a GROUP of proteins collectively known as complement, activated by the ANTIBODY-ANTIGEN complex). CELL-mediated IMMUNITY is similar, with the ANTIGEN binding being done by T LYMPHOCYTES which originate in the THYMUS GLAND. The HUMORAL IMMUNITY produced by circulating ANTIBODY is most effective against infections by BACTERIA and VIRUSES while they are outside the CELLS; CELL-mediated IMMUNITY is better against VIRUSES inside CELLS, PARASITES, CANCER CELLS and foreign TISSUE. *See* AUTO-IMMUNE DISEASES; IMMUNISATION.

immunisation (immunology) The technique of artificially creating ACTIVE IMMUNITY by injecting the patient with non-virulent antigens that resemble the disease-causing pathogens. A specific ANTIBODY or IMMUNOGLOBULIN is formed in RESPONSE and may persist in the body, preventing further INFECTION by the same organism. Some diseases have a more lasting IMMUNITY than others: the acquired IMMUNITY to MEASLES and mumps is generally lifelong, but in some cases (*e.g.* flu) it is very shortlived. This is probably because of changes in the VIRUS responsible, which affect its antigenic properties.The term is also used for giving passive IMMUNITY by the injection of ANTISERUM. IMMUNISATION can also MEAN any experimental process in which animals are injected with some substance to which they acquire IMMUNITY.

immunity (immunology) Protection by an organism against INFECTION. Defence may be divided into passive and active mechanisms. Passive processes prevent the entry of foreign invasion, *e.g.* SKIN,

MUCOUS MEMBRANES. Active mechanisms include PHAGOCYTOSIS by LEUCOCYTES and the IMMUNE RESPONSE in animals. Plants can have IMMUNITY, *e.g.* by means of phytoalexins.

immunoassay (immunology) Any of a number of assays based on the binding of ANTIBODY to ANTIGEN. Often the ANTIBODY is linked to a marker such as a FLUORESCENT MOLECULE, a RADIOACTIVE MOLECULE or an ENZYME. Immunoassays include RADIAL IMMUNODIFFUSION and immunoelectrophoresis, both of which utilise ANTIBODY incorporated into a uniform GEL; radioimmunoassay where the ANTIBODY is linked to a RADIOACTIVE TRACER; and ENZYME-linked immunosorbent assay (elisa) where the ANTIBODY is linked to an ENZYME.

immunocompetent (immunology) Capable of developing an IMMUNE RESPONSE

immunofluorescence technique (immunology) A method of locating targets by linking them to ANTIBODY tagged with FLUORESCENT dyes so that they can be made visible under a FLUORESCENT-MICROSCOPE.

immunoglobulin (biochemistry) Large globular proteins found in the body fluids. The BASIC UNIT of IMMUNOGLOBULIN structure consists of four POLYPEPTIDE chains, two identical LIGHT chains and two identical heavy chains, which are disulphide bonded (*USA*: disulfide bonded) to form two identical ANTIGEN-binding (VARIABLE) regions. Humans possess five distinct classes of IMMUNOGLOBULIN (IgG, IgA, IgM, IgD, IgE) distinguishable by differences in the carboxy-terminal portion of the heavy chain. IMMUNOGLOBULIN is a GENERIC term. Immunoglobulins known to bind specifically with a particular ANTIGEN are referred to as antibodies.

See also ANTIBODY.

immunol. (immunology) An abbreviation of 'immunol'ogy.

immunology (immunol.) (immunology) The scientific study of IMMUNITY, antigens and antibodies and their role in immune mechanisms and INFECTION.

immunostimulants (immunology) Agents that boost the natural IMMUNE RESPONSE. Therapeutic IMMUNOSTIMULANTS have been used in CANCER treatments to restore or augment the antitumor RESPONSE.

immunosuppression (immunology) The state of an altered IMMUNE SYSTEM that may LEAD to impaired immune FUNCTION. Drugs such as CYTOTOXIC drugs that inhibit CELL DIVISION are powerful immunosuppressants and depression of immune FUNCTION can LEAD to increased susceptibility to BACTERIAL, viral and parasitic infections, and possibly increased INCIDENCE of NEOPLASM.

immunosuppressive (pharmocology) Describing a drug that suppresses the IMMUNE RESPONSE, given to recipients of transplanted organs to minimize that chance of rejection.

immunosuppressor (immunology) A CELL or SOLUBLE mediator that suppresses IMMUNE RESPONSES. Immunosuppressors may FUNCTION to regulate IMMUNE RESPONSES, preventing excessive, potentially TISSUE-damaging responses.

impedance (Z) (physics) Property of an electric CIRCUIT or CIRCUIT COMPONENT that opposes the passage of a CURRENT. For DIRECT CURRENT (d.c.) it is equal to the resistance (R). For ALTERNATING CURRENT (a.c.) the reactance (X) also has an effect, such that $Z^2 = R^2 + X^2$, or $Z = R + iX$, where $i^2 = -1$.

imperial system (measurement) Comprehensive system of weights and measures (feet and inches, AVOIRDUPOIS weights, pints and gallons, etc.) that was formerly used throughout the British Empire. SI UNITS have replaced the IMPERIAL SYSTEM for scientific measurement.

impermeable (physics) Describing a substance that will not allow a FLUID (GAS or LIQUID) to pass through it (*e.g.* granite is IMPERMEABLE to WATER).

impetigo (medical) An INFECTION of the SKIN, particularly of the face, with streptococci or staphylococci, which is found in children and is very contagious.

implantation (physiology) Process in which a fertilized OVUM (EGG) or EMBRYO becomes attached to the lining of the UTERUS (womb) of a mammal. It is the beginning of PREGNANCY.

implicit function (mathematics) VARIABLE x is an IMPLICIT FUNCTION of y when x and y are connected by a FUNCTION that is not explicit (*i.e.* in which x is not directly expressed in terms of y).

improper fraction (mathematics) FRACTION whose upper part (NUMERATOR) is larger than the lower part (DENOMINATOR) *e.g.* 7/3, 11/4, 3/25. It is always greater than 1, as can be seen by converting it to a mixed number (the previous examples become 2 1/3, 2 3/4, 1 7/25).

impulse (1 biology; 2 physics) 1 In biology, transmission of a message along a NERVE FIBRE (*USA*: nerve fiber). The NERVE IMPULSE is an electrical phenomenon which results in DEPOLARIZATION of the NERVE MEMBRANE. This ACTION POTENTIAL lasts for a millisecond before the RESTING POTENTIAL is restored. *See also* ALL-OR-NONE RESPONSE. 2 In physics, when two objects collide, over the PERIOD of impact there is a large reactionary FORCE between them whose time INTEGRAL is the IMPULSE of the FORCE (equal to either OBJECT's change of momentum).

IMR (statistics) An abbreviation of 'I'nfant 'M'ortality 'R'ate.

IMS (chemistry) An abbreviation of 'I'ndustrial 'M'ethylated 'S'pirit.

In. (biochemistry) An abbreviation of 'In'ulin.

inborn errors of metabolism (genetics/biochemistry) A GROUP of disorders in which the BASIC cause is the lack of an ENZYME involved in NORMAL METABOLISM. These disorders are almost always inherited as recessives. For example, if the NORMAL GENE coding for the ENZYME is T, and the MUTANT GENE is t, a HETEROZYGOUS person Tt will be healthy because the T GENE can produce sufficient quantities of the ENZYME; whereas the person with GENOTYPE tt will be without the genetic means to produce the ENZYME and will therefore have a block in a metabolic pathway. Most patients with these disorders can be treated with diets that avoid taking in the substance that cannot be metabolized. *See* ALKAPTONURIA; CYSTINURIA; PHENYLKETONURIA.

inbreeding (biology) REPRODUCTION between closely related organisms of a SPECIES.

incandescence (physics) LIGHT emission that results from the high TEMPERATURE of a substance; *e.g.* the FILAMENT in an electric lamp is incandescent.

See also LUMINESCENCE.

inch (measurement) UNIT of length equal to 1/12 of a foot; 1 in = 25.4 mm.

incid. (general terminology) An abbreviation of 'incid'ental.

incidence (epidemiology) The rate of occurrence of new cases of a disorder over a given PERIOD of time, usually expressed as the number of new cases per 100,000 members of the population.

incisor (anatomy) Chisel-shaped cutting TOOTH of mammals located at the front of the upper and lower JAWS; human beings have eight incisors. They grow continually in rodents, which use them for gnawing.

inclusion bodies (virology) Microscopic bodies, usually within body CELLS, thought to be VIRUS particles in morphogenesis.

incompatibility (haematology) Mismatching of biochemical components, *e.g.* between BLOOD GROUPS or between a transplanted DONOR ORGAN and its RECIPIENT or between a scion and the plant on which it is grafted. With an ORGAN transplant it can LEAD to immunological rejection (counteracted by IMMUNOSUPPRESSIVE drugs).

incomplete dominance (genetics) The condition in which neither of a pair of ALLELES completely masks the presence of the other phenotypically.

See also PHENOTYPE; DOMINANT.

incr. (general terminology) An abbreviation of 'incr'ease.

incubation period (1 medical; 2 microbiology) 1 The time elapsing between INFECTION with the organisms of a disease and the appearance of symptoms. In any given disease it is relatively CONSTANT. People who have been exposed to an INFECTIOUS DISEASE and may be incubating it and who may become infectious, are known as contacts. 2 The time PERIOD that AGAR plates, TISSUE CULTUREs etc are held in incubators before being examined.

incus (anatomy) One of the EAR OSSICLES. An alternative term: anvil.

independent assortment (genetics) The second of MENDEL'S LAWS, which states that genes are transmitted independently from parents to offspring and assort freely. Thus there is an equal chance of any particular GENE being transmitted to the gametes. It does not apply to genes that exhibit LINKAGE.

independent variable (mathematics) If y is a FUNCTION of x, i.e. $y = f(x)$, x is the INDEPENDENT VARIABLE of the FUNCTION (and y is the dependent one).

index (mathematics) An EXPONENT or POWER; e.g. in the terms 5^4 and $x^{-1/2}$, 4 and 1/2 are indices. Multiplication is achieved by adding indices (e.g. $x^3 \times x^2 = x^{3+2} = x^5$); DIVISION by subtracting indices (e.g. $x^3 B x^2 = x^{3-2} = x$).

indicator (1 chemistry; 2 biology) 1 In chemistry, substance that changes COLOUR (USA: color) to indicate the end of a CHEMICAL REACTION or the pH of a SOLUTION; e.g. LITMUS. Indicators are commonly used in titrations in VOLUMETRIC ANALYSIS. 2 In biology, organism that survives only in certain environments; its presence gives information about the ENVIRONMENT e.g. the presence in WATER of certain BACTERIA that normally live in FAECES (USA: FECES) indicates that the WATER is polluted with sewage.

indigenous flora (microbiology) NORMAL or resident flora.

indigo (chemistry) $C_{16}H_{10}N_2O_2$ A blue organic dye, a DERIVATIVE of INDOLE, that occurs as a GLUCOSIDE in plants of the GENUS Indigofera.

indirect peroxidase technique (histology) Immunohistochemical technique for visualising material from FROZEN SECTION.

indirect-transmission (epidemiology) The transmission of a disease to a susceptible person by means of vectors or by airborne route.

indium In (chemistry) Silvery-white metallic ELEMENT of GROUP IIIA of the PERIODIC TABLE, used in making mirrors and semiconductors. At. no. 49; r.a.m. 114.82.

indole (biochemistry) C_8H_7N Colourless (USA: colorless) organic SOLID, a HETEROCYCLIC AROMATIC COMPOUND consisting of fused BENZENE and PYRROLE rings, normally found in FAECES (USA: FECES) which is in part responsible for the CHARACTERISTIC SMELL. Also termed: BENZPYRROLE.

indole amines (biochemistry) A CLASS of biogenic AMINE formed by the COMBINATION of INDOLE with an AMINE GROUP. They are NEUROTRANSMITTERS and include SEROTONIN.

induced magnetism (physics) Creation of a MAGNET by aligning the MAGNETIC DOMAINS in a ferromagnetic substance by placing it in the MAGNETIC FIELD of a permanent MAGNET or ELECTROMAGNET.

induced radioactivity (physics) An alternative term for ARTIFICIAL RADIOACTIVITY.

inducer (molecular biology) A MOLECULE that binds to a repressor to turn on the TRANSCRIPTION of an inducible OPERON. The INDUCER is usually a small MOLECULE, smaller than the repressor, a PROTEIN, but able to alter the latter's CONFIGURATION so that it dissociates from the OPERATOR region and allows TRANSCRIPTION to proceed. The INDUCER is often the SUBSTRATE of the ENZYME whose production is being induced. *See* GENE REGULATION.

inducible enzyme (molecular biology) An ENZYME which is produced only when its SUBSTRATE is present to act as INDUCER. The opposite is a repressible ENZYME. *See* OPERON; GENE REGULATION.

inductance (1 physics; 2 measurement) 1 Property of a CURRENT-carrying electric CIRCUIT or CIRCUIT COMPONENT that causes it to form a MAGNETIC FIELD and store magnetic ENERGY. 2 Measurement of ELECTROMAGNETIC INDUCTION.

induction (medical) Setting in motion or beginning, used mostly of anaesthesia (*USA*: anesthesia) or LABOUR (*USA*: labor).

induction coil (physics) Type of transformer for producing high-VOLTAGE ALTERNATING CURRENT from a low-VOLTAGE source. INDUCTION COILS can be used to produce a HIGH VOLTAGE PULSE, *e.g.* for FIRING spark plugs in a petrol engine.

induction (1, 2 physics) MAGNETIZATION or electrification produced in an OBJECT.

1 ELECTROMAGNETIC INDUCTION is the production of an ELECTRIC CURRENT in a CONDUCTOR by means of a varying MAGNETIC FIELD near it. 2 MAGNETIC INDUCTION is the production of a MAGNETIC FIELD in an unmagnetized METAL by a nearby MAGNETIC FIELD. 3 Electrostatic INDUCTION is the production of an ELECTRIC CHARGE on an OBJECT by a charged OBJECT brought near it.

induction heating (physics) Heating effect that arises from the ELECTRIC CURRENT induced in a conducting material by an alternating MAGNETIC FIELD.

inductor (1 chemistry; 2 physics) 1 Substance that accelerates a CHEMICAL REACTION between two other substances by reacting rapidly with one of them. 2 Any COMPONENT of an electrical CIRCUIT that possesses significant INDUCTANCE. Also termed: choke; coil.

induration (histology) ABNORMAL hardness of a TISSUE or part resulting from HYPERAEMIA (*USA*: hyperemia) or INFLAMMATION, as in a reactive tuberculin SKIN test.

inert (chemistry) Chemically nonreactive, *e.g.* GOLD is INERT in AIR at NORMAL temperatures.

inert gas (chemistry) Member of GROUP 0 of the PERIODIC TABLE; the unreactive elements HELIUM, NEON, ARGON, KRYPTON, XENON and RADON. Also termed: NOBLE GAS; RARE GAS.

inertia (physics) Resistance offered by an OBJECT to a change in its state of rest or motion. INERTIA is a property of the MASS of an OBJECT.

infarction (medical) When an ARTERY is suddenly blocked by THROMBOSIS or by an embolus and there is no alternative circulation to keep the tissues nourished.

infection (microbiology) Invasion by and multiplication of MICRO-ORGANISMS in body TISSUE which may or may not result in overt disease. The organisms concerned are called pathogens, and include BACTERIA, VIRUSES, PROTOZOA, WORMS, and FUNGI.

infectious disease (microbiology) A disease which is caused by MICRO-ORGANISMS or VIRUSES living in or on the body as PARASITES. *See* INFECTION.

infective endocarditis (medical) INFECTION of the lining of the HEART, which may be ACUTE or subACUTE.

inferential statistics (statistics) The branch of statistics that enables one to assess the VALIDITY of a conclusion drawn from the DATA, *e.g.* whether two means are significantly different from one another, or whether there is a significant correlation between two variables. *Contrast* DESCRIPTIVE STATISTICS.

inferior (anatomy) Towards the lower part of the body, the BRAIN or any other ORGAN. *Contrast* superior.

infestation (parasitology) The presence on or in the body of PARASITES mites and fleas, or other MULTICELLULAR organisms, such as TICKS.

infinity (∞) (mathematics) Quantity that is larger than any quantified concept. It may be considered as the RECIPROCAL of zero.

infl. (general terminology) Inflammable.

inflammation (medical) Localised protective response elicited by injury or destruction of tissues, which serves to destroy, dilute, or wall off both the injurious agent and the injured tissue.

inflammatory response (immunology) Redness, warmth and swelling in RESPONSE to injury or INFECTION; the result of increased BLOOD flow and a gathering of immune CELLS and secretions. It involves DILATION of BLOOD VESSELS, migration of LEUCOCYTES to the site of injury, and movement of FLUID and PLASMA PROTEINS into the inflamed TISSUE.

inflection (optics) Point on a curve where it changes from being CONCAVE to CONVEX (or CONVEX to CONCAVE).

influenza (virology) ACUTE INFECTION with the respiratory VIRUS influenza A, B or C. The INCIDENCE of the disease is seasonal.

info. (general terminology) information.

information retrieval (computing) Science of storing and accessing DATA, which may use microfilm, microfiche, magnetic tape and COMPUTER STORAGE DEVICES.

informed consent (biology) Agreement to take part in an experiment or medical trial, or to receive a medical procedure, with sufficient knowledge of the protocol and risks to reach a rational decision.

infradian rhythm (biology) Any biological rhythm with cycles longer than a day, *e.g.* the MENSTRUAL CYCLE.

infra-red radiation (physics) ELECTRO-MAGNETIC RADIATION in the WAVELENGTH range from 0.75 μm to 1 mm approximately; between the visible and MICROWAVE regions of the ELECTRO-MAGNETIC SPECTRUM. It is emitted by all objects at temperatures above ABSOLUTE ZERO, as HEAT (thermal) RADIATION.

infrasound (physics) Sound waves with a FREQUENCY below the THRESHOLD of human hearing, *i.e.* less than about 20 Hz.

inheritance (genetics) The acquisition of a CHARACTERISTIC through genetic factors or the characteristics so acquired.

inhibition (biology) The prevention of life or deactivation of a process.

inj (1, 2 medical) 1 An abbreviation of 'inj'ection. 2 An abbreviation of 'inj'ury.

injection drug user (IDU) (medical) Someone who uses drugs that are injected into the body.

innate (genetics) Genetically caused; INNATE characteristics sometimes only appear quite late in life.

inner diameter (id) (measurement) The distance from the centre (*USA*: center) of the opening of a tube to the inside edge of the material the tube is made from.

inner ear (anatomy) FLUID-filled part of the EAR that contains both the organs that convert sound to NERVE IMPULSES and the organs of BALANCE.

innocent (histology) A term sometimes used of BENIGN as opposed to MALIGNANT tumours (*USA*: maglignant tumors).

inoculation (medical) Accidental or intentional introduction of foreign MATTER into a living organism or culture medium. Used of the injection of vaccines to prevent disease. *See* VACCINE.

inorganic chemistry (chemistry) Study of non-CARBON based compounds and their reactions.

See also ORGANIC CHEMISTRY.

inorganic compound (chemistry) A COMPOUND that does not contain CARBON, with the exception of CARBON's oxides, metallic carbides, carbonates and hydrogencarbonates.

See also ORGANIC COMPOUNDS.

input device (computing) Part of a COMPUTER that feeds in with DATA and PROGRAM instructions. The many types of INPUT DEVICES include a KEYBOARD, punched CARD READER, paper tape reader, OPTICAL CHARACTER RECOGNITION, LIGHT pen (with a VDU) and various types of devices equipped with a read HEAD to input magnetically recorded DATA (*e.g.* on MAGNETIC DISK, tape or drum).

insecticide (parasitology) Substance used to kill insects of agricultural or public health importance. There are two main types: those that are eaten (with food) or inhaled by insects, and those that kill by contact. Important classes of insecticides include: chlorinated HYDROCARBONS (including DDT analogs, chlorinated ALICYCLIC COMPOUNDS, cyclodicnes and chlorinated terpenes); organophosphates; carbamates; thiocyanates; dinitrophenols; botanicals (including pyrethroids, rotenoids and nicotinoids); JUVENILE HORMONE analogs; GROWTH regulators; and inorganics (including arsenicals and fluorides). Non-biodegradable insecticides may persist for a long time and become concentrated in food chains, where they have a damaging ecological effect.

insemination (medical) The transfer of SEMEN into the VAGINA naturally or artificially.

insertion (molecular biology) The addition of one or more BASE-pairs into a DNA sequence. The effect of a small INSERTION may be a FRAMESHIFT MUTATION, but a larger INSERTION can upset GENE REGULATION around it, either by activating genes that should be inactive or vice versa. *See* INSERTIONAL INACTIVATION.

insertional inactivation (genetics) A technique used in GENETIC ENGINEERING to prevent expression of a GENE by inserting a foreign DNA sequence adjacent to it or in its coding region.

in situ (biology) In the NORMAL or natural location.

insoluble (chemistry) Describing a substance that does not dissolve in a given SOLVENT; not capable of forming a SOLUTION.

Inst. (education) An abbreviation of 'Inst'itute/ 'Inst'itution.

insulation (physics) Layer of material (an INSULATOR) used to prevent the flow of ELECTRICITY or HEAT.

insulator (physics) Substance that is a poor CONDUCTOR of ELECTRICITY or HEAT; a non-CONDUCTOR. Most non-metallic elements (except CARBON) and polymers are good insulators. The presence of entrapped AIR (as in a foam plastic or woollen garment) increases the effectiveness of a thermal INSULATOR.

insulin (biochemistry) A HORMONE secreted in the PANCREAS that is responsible for increasing the PERME-ABILITY of CELLS to GLUCOSE, thereby reducing BLOOD GLUCOSE. A PROTEIN isulin is produced by the beta-CELLS of the pancreatic ISLETS OF LANGERHANS and consists of two PEPTIDE chains. A deficiency of INSULIN results in the disorder DIABETES MELLITUS, whose symptoms include excessive thirst and high levels of GLUCOSE in the BLOOD and URINE.

integer (mathematics) Whole number; it may be POSITIVE or negative.

integral (1, 2 mathematics) 1 Value that results from the process of INTEGRATION. 2 Describing a whole number value.

integration (mathematics) In CALCULUS, the process of summation of the SERIES of infinitely small quantities that make up the difference between two values of a given FUNCTION. It is the inverse of differentiation and is used in the SOLUTION of such problems as finding the AREA enclosed by a given curve or the VOLUME enclosed by a given surface.

intensity (physics) POWER of sound, LIGHT or other WAVE-form (*e.g.* the loudness of a sound or the brightness of LIGHT), determined by the AMPLITUDE of the WAVE.

Intensive Care Unit (ICU) (medical) The SECTION of a hospital where critically ill patients are monitored around the clock.

interaction (1 general; 2 physics) 1 The effect which two or more substances, such as drugs, have on each other. 2 In atomic physics, exchange of ENERGY between a PARTICLE and a second one or ELECTROMAGNETIC RADIATION.

interaction variance (statistics) The proportion of the total VARIANCE caused by the INTERACTION of the INDEPENDENT VARIABLES.

intercellular (biology) Between CELLS; *e.g.* INTERCELLULAR FLUID surrounds CELLS, maintaining a CONSTANT internal ENVIRONMENT.

See also INTRACELLULAR.

intercostal muscle (histology) Any of the muscles between a mammal's ribs, which are important in BREATHING movements.

intercross (genetics) a cross between two individuals or strains that are themselves HYBRID. *See* F_2.

intercurrent (medical) Term applied to a second disease or INFECTION occurring during the course of the original disease.

interface (1 physics; 2 computing) 1 In physics, boundary of contact (the common surface) of two adjacent phases, either or both of which may be SOLID, LIQUID or a GAS. 2 The point at which two systems, or two parts of one system, interact.

interference (physics) INTERAction between two or more waves of the same FREQUENCY emitted from coherent sources. The waves may reinforce each other or tend to cancel each other; the resultant WAVE is the ALGEBRAic sum of the COMPONENT waves. The phenomenon occurs with ELECTROMAGNETIC WAVES and sound.

interferon (IF) (immunology) A PROTEIN produced by the body to counteract a viral INFECTION by slowing or stopping the VIRUS from replicating. Its ACTION is not specific to any particular GROUP of VIRUSES. Genes for human interferons have been cloned so the proteins can be produced in bulk.

interkrometer (physics) Instrument that makes use of INTERFERENCE for measuring such things as wavelengths and other small distances.

intermediate (1, 2 chemistry) 1 In industrial chemistry, COMPOUND to be subjected to further chemical TREATMENT to produce finished products such as dyes and pharmaceuticals. 2 Short-lived SPECIES in a complex CHEMICAL REACTION.

intermediate compound (chemistry) COMPOUND of two or more metals that are present in definite proportion although they frequently do not follow NORMAL VALENCE rules.

intermediate host (parasitology) Required HOST in the LIFE CYCLE in which essential larval development must occur before a PARASITE is infective to its definitive HOST or to additional INTERMEDIATE HOSTs.

intermolecular force (physics) FORCE that binds one MOLECULE to another. INTERMOLECULAR FORCES are much weaker than the bonding forces holding together the atoms of a MOLECULE.

See also VAN DER WAALS' FORCE.

internal conversion (physics) Effect on the NUCLEUS of an ATOM produced by a gamma-RAY PHOTON emerging from it and giving up its ENERGY on meeting an ELECTRON of the same ATOM.

internal energy (physics) Total quantity of ENERGY in a substance, the sum of its KINETIC ENERGY and POTENTIAL ENERGY.

internal friction (physics) *See* VISCOSITY.

internal resistance (physics) ELECTRICAL RESISTANCE in a CIRCUIT of the source of CURRENT, *e.g.* a CELL.

international candle (measurement) The former UNIT of LUMINOUS INTENSITY.

International Classification of Diseases (ICD) (governing body) A CLASSIFICATION, made by the World Health Organization, of diseases including mental disorders.

intereceptor (physiology) A RECEPTOR located in or on an internal ORGAN.

interphase (cytology) State of CELLS when not undergoing DIVISION. Preparation for DIVISION (MITOSIS) is carried out during this PHASE, including REPLICATION of DNA and CELL constituents.

interpolation (statistics) Inferring a value or values for points on a DIMENSION from the obtained values of points lying to each side. *Compare* EXTRA-POLATION.

interpose (genetics) The stage on the CELL CYCLE between divisions. This is the PHASE during which the chromosomes are active in synthesising proteins.

interpreter (computing) A PROGRAM that translates another PROGRAM written in a high-LEVEL language into MACHINE CODE and executes each instruction before translating the next. An INTERPRETER is slower in execution than a COMPILER and the user's PROGRAM must be translated afresh every time it is run.

interquartile range (IQR) (statistics) In a FREQUENCY DISTRIBUTION, the difference between the upper and lower quartiles; hence it contains the middle 50 per cent of cases.

intersegmental tracts (anatomy) Short tracts connecting different segments of the SPINAL CORD.

intersex (genetics) A broad term covering various conditions in which an individual does not have NORMAL reproductive organs but is not a HERMAPHRODITE. Male pseudohermaphroditism is the condition in which there are TESTES (probably internal) but the external genitalia appear more or less female; the cause can be CHROMOSOME abnormality, a single GENE (as in testicular feminization) or HORMONE imbalance in *utero*. Female pseudoher-maphroditism, in which there is a COMBINATION of NORMAL ovaries and more or less male external genitalia, is not caused by CHROMOSOME disorders, but by a SERIES of RECESSIVE ALLELES, with a combined FREQUENCY of about one in 7000 births. HORMONE imbalance in *utero* can also be responsible.

See also KLINEFELTER'S SYNDROME.

interstitial atom (chemistry) ATOM that is in a position other than a NORMAL LATTICE place.

interstitial cells (cytology) In mammals, CELLS present in the male and female GONADS. In males they are found between the TESTIS tubules and in females in the OVARIAN FOLLICLE. When stimulated by LUTEINIZING HORMONE, they produce ANDROGENS in males and OESTROGEN (*USA*: estrogen) in females.

interstitial cell-stimulating hormone (ICSH) (biochemistry) A gonadotropin from the ADENOHYPOPHYSIS that stimulates the testicular INTERSTITIAL CELLS to produce ANDROGENS. It is equivalent to LUTEINIZING HORMONE (LH) in the female. Its SECRETION is stimulated by hypothalamic gonadotropin releasing HORMONE (GnRH).

interstitial compound (chemistry) The chemical COMPOUND formed by penetra-tion of non-metallic atoms of small

DIAMETER between the atoms of a METAL (usually a TRANSITION ELEMENT).

intertrigo (medical) Erythematous SKIN eruption of adjacent SKIN parts.

interval scale (measurement) A scale having equal intervals, but no zero point *e.g.* Centigrade.

intervening variable (statistics) A VARIABLE operating within a theoretical model that mediates the effects of the INDEPENDENT VARIABLES on the dependent variables. There may be several INTERVENING VARIABLES all interacting with one another. The value of an INTERVENING VARIABLE is usually affected by more than one INDEPENDENT VARIABLE and it may in turn affect several dependent variables.

intestine (anatomy) The ALIMENTARY CANAL after it leaves the STOMACH. It is divided into small and LARGE INTESTINE; the SMALL INTESTINE is the longer, and is continuous with the STOMACH at the gastro-duodenal junction. The SMALL INTESTINE is concerned with the further DIGESTION of food and the ABSORPTION into the bloodstream of already digested AMINO ACIDS and monosaccharides. The LARGE INTESTINE is mainly concerned with the ABSORPTION of WATER from semi-SOLID indigestible remains, which form the FAECES (*USA*: FECES).

intracellular fluid (cytology) The FLUID contained within the CELL MEMBRANE.

intracellular (cytology) Occurring within the boundary of a CELL or CELLS.

See also INTERCELLULAR.

intrachromosomal recombination (genetics) Exchange of sequences of DNA between sister chromatids (*i.e.* two halves of the same CHROMOSOME) during MEIOSIS. Because the sister chromatids are identical, there is no genetic effect, unlike in the NORMAL process of RECOMBINATION, when non-sister chromatids from HOMOLOGOUS CHROMOSOMES exchange genetic material.

intracranial (medical) Inside the SKULL.

intradermal (medical) In the SKIN.

intramuscular (medical) Inside a MUSCLE.

intrauterine device (IUD) (medical) A birth control device consisting of a plastic coil placed in the UTERUS to prevent conception. An improperly fitted IUD can cause uterine bleeding.

intravenous (IV) (medical) Directly into a VEIN.

intubation (medical) The introduction of a tube into the body, used mostly of the process of inserting a tube into the TRACHEA to maintain an airway during the administration of an ANAESTHETIC (*USA*: anesthetic), or for the purpose of artificial RESPIRATION by a BREATHING machine.

in utero (biology) Within the UTERUS.

inverse function (mathematics) Mathematical FUNCTION of such a nature in respect to another operation, relation, etc. that the starting point of one FUNCTION is the conclusion of the other, and vice versa. A FUNCTION that is opposite in effect or nature, *e.g.* inverse hyperbolic functions and inverse trigonometrical functions.

inverse square law (physics) The LAW that the INTENSITY of a WAVE, *e.g.* LIGHT or ACOUSTIC waves, travelling in a homogenous medium decreases in proportion to the square of the distance from the source. For instance in OPTICS, the quantity of LIGHT from a given source on a surface of definite AREA is inversely proportional to the square of the distance between the source and the surface.

inversion (1 genetics; 2 chemistry) 1 A MUTATION consisting of the reversal of the ORDER of the genes in part of a CHROMOSOME. 2 Splitting of DEXTRO-ROTATORY higher sugars (*e.g.* SUCROSE) into equivalent amounts of LAEVORO-TATORY lower sugars (*e.g.* FRUCTOSE and GLUCOSE).

invert sugar (chemistry) A natural DISACCHARIDE SUGAR that consists of a MIXTURE of GLUCOSE and FRUCTOSE, found in many fruits.

invertebrate (biology) ANIMAL that does not possess a BACKBONE.

See also VERTEBRATE.

inverted-U curve (statistics) A curve that looks like a letter U upside-down, starting low, reaching a peak and then declining; when performance on a task is plotted against arousal LEVEL or drive strength such curves are frequently obtained.

in vitro (biology) From the Latin, meaning 'in GLASS'. A term for processes that happen in a controlled ENVIRONMENT outside of a living organism. It is strictly speaking an adverb but is often used adjectivally. *Contrast IN VIVO.*

in vitro **fertilization** (medical) The technique of fertilizing one or several ova with SPERM outside the body of the female, in a GLASS culture dish.

in vivo (biology) From the Latin, meaning 'in a living thing'. A term used for processes that happen in a living organism. It does not imply that the process described is as it occurs in natural conditions, because the word is applied to what happens in experiments; it is used solely in contrast to what happens *in vitro*. It is strictly speaking an adverb, but is often used adjectivally. *Contrast IN VITRO.*

involuntary muscle (histology) MUSCLE not under conscious control, located in internal organs and tissues, *e.g.* in the ALIMENTARY CANAL and BLOOD VESSELS. Also termed: SMOOTH MUSCLE.

See also VOLUNTARY MUSCLE.

involution forms (microbiology) Abnormally shaped BACTERIAL CELLS occurring in an aging culture population.

IOAT (society) An abbreviation of 'I'nternational 'O'rganisation 'A'gainst 'T'rachoma.

IoB (society) An abbreviation of 'I'nstitute 'o'f 'B'iology.

iodide (chemistry) COMPOUND of IODINE and another ELEMENT; SALT of hydriodic ACID (HI).

iodine I (chemistry) Non-metallic ELEMENT in GROUP VIIA of the PERIODIC TABLE (the halogens), extracted from Chile SALTPETRE (in which it occurs as an iodate impurity of SODIUM NITRATE) and certain seaweeds. It forms purple-black crystals that sublime on heating to produce a violet VAPOUR. It is essential for the SECRETION of the THYROID HORMONES THYROXINE and tri-iodothyronine, usually present in sufficient quantities in NORMAL diets. IODINE and its ORGANIC COMPOUNDS are used in medicine; SILVER IODIDE is used in

PHOTOGRAPHY. At. no. 53; r.a.m. 126.9044.

iodine number (chemistry) Number that indicates the amount of IODINE taken up by a substance, *e.g.* by fats or oils; it gives a measure of the number of UNSATURATED bonds present. Also termed: IODINE value; IODINE ABSORPTION.

iodoform (chemistry) An alternative term for TRIIODOMETHANE.

ion (chemistry) ATOM or MOLECULE that has POSITIVE or negative ELECTRIC CHARGE because of the loss or GAIN of one or more electrons. Many INORGANIC COMPOUNDS dissociate into ions when they dissolve in WATER. Ions are the ELECTRIC CURRENT-carriers in ELECTROLYSIS and in DISCHARGE tubes.

ion channels (physiology/ pharmacology) Channels or pores composed of PROTEINS that allows exchange of ions or water between the CYTOPLASM and the EXTRACELLULAR fluid. Ion channels are vital in the control of CELL volume and the activity of electrically excitable CELLS. Conformation changes within the PROTEIN channel lead to opening or closing of the pore. Some drugs bind to sites on the EXTRACELLULAR surface of the ion channel to influence channel opening or closing, other drugs influence channel opening following interaction with a G-PROTEIN coupled receptor.

ion exchange (chemistry) REACTION in which ions of a SOLUTION are retained by oppositely-charged groups covalently bonded to a SOLID support, such as ZEOLITE or a SYNTHETIC RESIN. The process is used in WATER softeners, desalination plants and for ISOTOPE separation.

ion pair (chemistry) Two charged fragments that result from simultaneous IONIZATION of two unchanged ones, a POSITIVE and a negative ION.

ion pump (physics) High-VACUUM PUMP for removing a GAS from a system by ionizing its atoms or molecules and adsorbing the resulting ions on a surface.

ionic bond (physics) Electrostatic attraction that occurs between two oppositely charged ions, *e.g.* proteins binding with METAL ions. The DEGREE of binding varies with the chemical nature of each COMPOUND and the net CHARGE. DISSOCIATION of IONIC BONDS usually occurs readily, but some members of the TRANSITION GROUP of metals exhibit high association constants (*i.e.* low Kd values) and exchange is slow. Also termed: ELECTROVALENT BOND.

See also COVALENT BOND.

ionic crystal (crystallography) Crystal composed of ions. Also termed: ELECTROVALENT CRYSTAL; POLAR CRYSTAL.

ionic product (chemistry) PRODUCT (in moles per LITRE) of the concentrations of the ions in a LIQUID or SOLUTION, *e.g.* in SODIUM CHLORIDE SOLUTION, the IONIC PRODUCT of SODIUM CHLORIDE is given by [Na^+] [Cl^-]. In a pure LIQUID, it results from the DISSOCIATION of molecules in the LIQUID.

ionic radius (crystallography) RADIUS of an ION in a crystal.

ionization (chemistry/ physics) Formation of ions. It is generally achieved by chemical or electrical processes, or by DISSOCIATION of ionic compounds in SOLUTION, although at extremely high temperatures (such as those in stars) HEAT can cause IONIZATION.

ionization chamber (physics) Apparatus consisting of a GAS-filled container with a pair of high-VOLTAGE electrodes. It is used to study the IONIZATION of gases or IONIZING RADIATION.

ionization potential (chemistry) ELECTRON bonding ENERGY, the ENERGY required to remove an ELECTRON from a NEUTRAL ATOM.

ionizing radiation (radiology) RADIATION of sufficiently high ENERGY to produce ions in the medium through which it passes, *e.g.* high-ENERGY (electrons, protons) or short-WAVE RADIATION (UV, X-RAYS).

IPA (chemistry) An abbreviation of 'I'so'P'ropyl 'A'lcohol, also termed ISOPROPANOL.

IPSP (physiology) An abbreviation of 'I'nhibitory 'P'ostS'ynaptic 'P'otential.

iridium Ir (chemistry) Steel-grey metallic ELEMENT in GROUP VIII of the PERIODIC TABLE (a TRANSITION ELEMENT). It is used (with PLATINUM or OSMIUM) in hard ALLOYS for bearings, surgical tools and crucibles. At. no. 77; r.a.m. 192.22.

iris (anatomy) Pigmented part of the human EYE that controls the amount of LIGHT entering the EYE.

See also IRIS DIAPHRAGM.

iris diaphragm (photography) Adjustable APERTURE in a camera or incorporated in a LENS to control the amount of LIGHT passing through the LENS.

iritis (medical) INFLAMMATION of the IRIS. The IRIS, CILIARY BODY and CHOROID make up the uveal tract, and they have the same BLOOD supply, so that INFECTION can easily spread from one to the other. There are a number of causes, including HERPES, syphilis and TOXOPLASMOSIS.

iron Fe (chemistry) SILVER-grey magnetic metallic ELEMENT in GROUP VIII of the PERIODIC TABLE (a TRANSITION ELEMENT). It is the fourth most abundant ELEMENT in the EARTH's crust and probably forms much of the CORE. It is also the most widely used METAL, particularly (ALLOYed with CARBON and other elements) in steel. It occurs in various ores, chief of which are haematite (*USA*: hematite), limonite and magnesite, which are refined in a blast furnace to produce pig IRON. Inorganic IRON compounds are used as pigments; the BLOOD PIGMENT HAEMOGLOBIN (*USA*: hemaglobin) is an organic IRON COMPOUND. At. no. 26; r.a.m. 55.847.

iron(II) (chemistry) An alternative term for FERROUS.

iron(II) sulphate (chemistry) $FeSO_4.7H_2O$. Green CRYSTALLINE COMPOUND, used in making inks, in printing and as a wood preservative. A white MONOHYDRATE is also known. Also termed: FERROUS SULPHATE (*USA*: ferrous sulfate). (*USA*: iron(II) sulfate)

iron(III) (chemistry) An alternative term for FERRIC.

iron(III) chloride (chemistry) $FeCl_3.6H_2O$ Brown CRYSTALLINE COMPOUND, used as a CATALYST, a mordant and for etching COPPER in the manufacture of printed circuits. Also termed: FERRIC CHLORIDE.

iron(III) oxide (chemistry) Fe_2O_3. Red INSOLUBLE COMPOUND, the principal constituent of haematite (*USA*: hematite). It is used as a PIGMENT, CATALYST and polishing COMPOUND. Also termed: FERRIC OXIDE.

irradiance (physics) The POWER of LIGHT falling on an AREA of a surface. It can be measured in watts per square METRE.

irradiation (1 physics; 2 radiology) 1 RADIANT ENERGY per UNIT of intercepting AREA. 2 TREATMENT by exposure to RADIATION of any kind, but usually refers to TREATMENT by ionising RADIATION. *See* RADIATION.

irrational number (mathematics) REAL NUMBER that cannot be expressed as a FRACTION, *i.e.* as the ratio of two integers; *e.g.* π, 2.

irreversible reaction (chemistry) CHEMICAL REACTION that takes place in one direction only, therefore proceeding to completion.

irrigation (medical) The washing-out of a cavity or WOUND by a stream of WATER or other LIQUID.

irritability (physiology) Ability to respond to a STIMULUS, evident in all living material.

irritants (toxicology) Any non-corrosive substance that, on immediate, prolonged or repeated contact with NORMAL living TISSUE produces a local inflammatory REACTION.

ISCB (society) An abbreviation of 'I'nternational 'S'ociety for 'C'ell 'B'iology.

ISCERG (society) An abbreviation of 'I'nternational 'S'ociety for 'C'linical 'E'lectro'R'etino'G'raphy.

ischaemia (medical) Inadequate BLOOD supply to a part of the body, caused by

spasm or disease of the BLOOD VESSELs or failure of the general circulation; if it is prolonged and severe, the TISSUE dies. (*USA*: ischemia).

ischiorectal abscess (medical) An ABSCESS occurring between the RECTUM and the ischium, part of the PELVIS.

ISCP (society) An abbreviation of 'I'nternational 'S'ociety of 'C'linical 'P'athology.

ISGE (society) An abbreviation of 'I'nternational 'S'ociety of 'G'astro-'E'nterology.

ISH (society) An abbreviation of 'I'nternational 'S'ociety of 'H'aematology.

ISHAM (society) An abbreviation of 'I'nternational 'S'ociety for 'H'uman and 'A'nimal 'M'ycology.

islets of langerhans (histology/ biochemistry) Clusters of specialized secretory CELLS in the PANCREAS. They control the LEVEL of GLUCOSE in the BLOOD by secreting the HORMONES INSULIN and GLUCAGON.

isobar (1, 2 physics) 1 Curve that relates to qualities measured at the same PRESSURE. 2 One of a SET of atomic nuclei having the same total of protons and neutrons (*i.e.* the same NUCLEON NUMBER or MASS NUMBER) but different numbers of protons and therefore different identities.

isochromosome (genetics) an ABNORMAL CHROMOSOME in which two identical arms have become joined at the CENTROMERE because the CENTROMERE divided transversely and not longitudinally during CELL DIVISION.

isochrony (physics) The property of having the same time interval.

isocyanide (chemistry) A COMPOUND of GENERAL FORMULA R-NC, rather than R-CN, where R is an organic or inorganic RADICAL. Also termed: ISONITRILE; CARBYLAMINE.

isoelectric point (pI) (biochemistry) The HYDROGEN ION CONCENTRATION (PH) at which a SPECIES (AMINO ACID, PROTEIN or COLLOID) is electrically NEUTRAL.

See also ISOELECTRIC FOCUSING.

isoelectric focusing (biochemistry) A method used to separate mixtures containing proteins of different pI. The migration of ampholytes (e.g. proteins) occurs through a PH GRADIENT under an applied ELECTRIC FIELD. Molecules possessing an ELECTRIC CHARGE migrate towards a region in which they are isoelectric.

See also ISOELECTRIC POINT.

isoenzymes (biochemistry) A SET of ENZYMES all carrying out the same CHEMICAL REACTION. Several ISOENZYMES may be present within the same organism, as they are coded for by genes at different loci. Also termed ISOZYMES. Compare ALLOZYME.

isogamy (biology) Sexual FISSION of gametes that are similar in structure and size. It occurs in some PROTOZOA, FUNGI and ALGAe.

See also ANISOGAMY.

isolation (1 medical; 2 microbiology) 1 The separation of an infective patient from others, so that the infecting organism is not spread. 2 The GROWTH and separation of MICRO-ORGANISMS.

isoleucine (biochemistry) CRYSTALLINE AMINO ACID; it is a constituent of proteins, and essential in the diet of human beings.

isomer (chemistry) Substance that exhibits chemical ISOMERISM.

isomerism (1 chemistry; 2 physics) 1 In chemistry, the existence of substances that have the same molecular composition (and therefore the same CHEMICAL FORMULA), but different structures. See also OPTICAL ISOMERISM. 2 In physics, the existence of atomic nuclei with the same ATOMIC NUMBERS and the same MASS NUMBERS, but different ENERGY states.

isoniazid (pharmacology) A powerful drug used in the TREATMENT of TUBERCULOSIS.

isonitrile (chemistry) An alternative term for ISOCYANIDE.

isopropanol (chemistry) $(CH_3)_2CHOH$ One of the two isomers of PROPANOL. Also termed: ISOPROPYL ALCOHOL.

isopropyl alcohol (chemistry) An alternative term for ISOPROPANOL.

isothermal process (physics) Process that occurs at a CONSTANT or uniform TEMPERATURE; e.g. the compression of a GAS under CONSTANT TEMPERATURE conditions.

See also ADIABATIC PROCESS.

isotonic (chemistry) Solutions which have the same OSMOTIC PRESSURE. Such solutions will not bring about DIFFUSION one into the other through an intervening MEMBRANE.

isotope (physics) A chemical ELEMENT which has the same ATOMIC NUMBER as another, but a different ATOMIC MASS. It has the same number of protons in the NUCLEUS, but a different number of neutrons. RADIOACTIVE ISOTOPEs change into another ELEMENT over the course of time, the change being accompanied by the emission of ELECTROMAGNETIC RADIATIONS.

isotopic number (chemistry) Difference between the number of neutrons in an ISOTOPE and the number of protons. Also termed: NEUTRON EXCESS.

isotopic weight (chemistry) ATOMIC WEIGHT of an ISOTOPE. Also termed: isotopic MASS.

isotropic (chemistry) Describing a substance whose physical properties are the same in all directions (*e.g.* most liquids).

Isozymes (biochemistry) *See* ISOENZYMES.

ISV (quality standards) An abbreviation of 'I'nternational 'S'cientific 'V'ocabulary.

ITP (biochemistry) An abbreviation of 'I'nosine 'T'ri'P'hosphate.

IU (measurement) An abbreviation of 'I'nternational 'U'nit(s)

IUAT (society) An abbreviation of 'I'nternational 'U'nion 'A'gainst 'T'uberculosis.

IUB (society) An abbreviation of 'I'nternational 'U'nion of 'B'iochemistry.

IUBS (society) An abbreviation of 'I'nternational 'U'nion of 'B'iological 'S'ciences.

IUCD (medical) An abbreviation of 'I'ntra-'U'terine 'C'ontraceptive 'D'evice.

IUCr (society) An abbreviation of 'I'nternational 'U'nion of 'Cr'ystallography.

IUD (medical) An abbreviation of 'I'ntra'U'terine 'D'evice.

IUPAB (society) An abbreviation of 'I'nternational 'U'nion of 'P'ure and 'A'pplied 'B'iophysics.

IUT (medical) An abbreviation of 'I'ntra 'U'terine 'T'ransfusion.

IV (medical) An abbreviation of 'I'ntra'V'enous.

J

J (measurement) An abbreviation of 'j'oule.

Jacksonian epilepsy (medical) Focal epilepsy usually the result of a localised AREA of disease *e.g.* TUMOUR (*USA:* tumor), or injury in the motor CORTEX of the BRAIN, the attack begins in a definite place and spreads from there in a definite PROGRESSION. Named after the English neurologist, J. H. Jackson (1835-1911).

jail fever (microbiology) *See* TYPHUS.

Jakob-Creutzfeldt disease (medical) *See* Creutzfeldt-Jakob disease.

jaundice (medical) A condition characterised by a yellow appearance of the whites of the eyes, the SKIN and MUCOUS MEMBRANES. This discolouration (*USA:* discoloration) is due to the presence of excess BILIRUBIN in the BLOOD. JAUNDICE is a common symptom of disorders of the GALL BLADDER or LIVER.

jaws (1, 2 anatomy) 1 In vertebrates, bony structure enclosing the mouth, often furnished with TEETH for grasping prey and/or chewing food, consisting of an upper MAXILLA and lower MANDIBLE. 2 In invertebrates, grasping structure surrounding the mouth.

J/deg. (measurement) An abbreviation of 'J'oule per 'deg'ree.

jejunectomy (medical) Excision of part of the JEJUNUM.

jejunitis (medical) INFLAMMATION of the JEJUNUM.

jejunum (anatomy) Part of the INTESTINE of mammals, located between the DUODENUM and the ILEUM, the main FUNCTION of which is ABSORPTION.

Jerne plaque assay (immunology) A method of quantitating ANTIBODY-producing CELLS.

J exon (immunology) *See* J GENE.

JG cells (histology) An abbreviation of 'J'uxta'G'lomerular CELLS.

J gene (immunology) A short sequence of DNA coding for part of the hyper-VARIABLE REGION of IMMUNOGLOBULIN LIGHT or heavy chains near to the site of joining to the CONSTANT region. Also termed J EXON.

jigger (parasitology) A flea *Tunga penetrans* which burrows into the SKIN of the feet, causing intense irritation and ulceration.

jnl (literary terminology) An abbreviation of 'j'our'n'a'l'. Also termed jl/ jour.

joint (anatomy) Point of articulation of limbs or bones. The bones are connected to each other by CONNECTIVE TISSUE ligaments, and are well lubricated. Common types of joints include ball-and-socket joints (*e.g.* the HIP JOINT), hinge joints (*e.g.* the elbow) and sliding joints (*e.g.* between vertebrae).

joint probability (statistics) The probability that two or more events will occur together.

Jonckheere test (statistics) A non-parametric planned comparison trend test of the HYPOTHESIS that the values of a VARIABLE of different samples are ordered in a specific sequence.

Jones methenamine silver stain (histology) A histological staining technique that may be used to make basement MEMBRANE and mesangium visible under the MICROSCOPE.

joule (J) (measurement) The SI UNIT of ENERGY, WORK and quantity of HEAT. Equal to the WORK done when one NEWTON of FORCE moves an OBJECT one METRE. Named after James Prescott Joule (1818-89).

joule's law (1, 2 physics) 1 INTERNAL ENERGY of a given MASS of GAS is dependent only on its TEMPERATURE and is independent of its PRESSURE and VOLUME. 2 If an ELECTRIC CURRENT I flows through a resistance R for a time t, the HEAT produced Q, in joules, is given by $Q = I^2Rt$.

Joule-Thompson effect (physics) When a GAS is allowed to undergo adiabatic expansion through a porous plug, the TEMPERATURE of the GAS usually drops. This results from the WORK done in breaking the INTERMOLECULAR FORCES in the GAS, and is a DEVIATION from JOULE'S LAW. The effect is important in the LIQUEFACTION OF GASES by cooling. Also termed: Joule-Kelvin effect. *See* ADIABATIC PROCESS.

jour. (literary terminology) An abbreviation of 'jour'nal.

journal (jour.) (literary terminology) A scientific/ medical etc. newspaper or periodical.

J region (immunology) An abbreviation of 'j'oining 'region'. The part of an IMMUNOGLOBULIN MOLECULE that lies between the CONSTANT and the VARIABLE REGIONS.

jugular vein (anatomy) One of a pair of veins draining the BRAIN and joining with the subclavian veins before discharging into the ANTERIOR VENA CAVA.

jumping genes (genetics) Genes that move within chromosomes. They influence the regulation of GENE activity, probably by physically removing a GENE from its PROMOTER. *See* OPERON.

junk DNA (genetics) Sequences of DNA in the GENOME that have no apparent genetic FUNCTION. Also known as 'SELFISH DNA'.

jurisprudence (medical) Medical jurisprudence, or forensic medicine, concerned with any aspect of medicine which relates to the LAW.

juv. (general terminology) An abbreviation of 'juv'enile.

juvenile (juv.) (general terminology) A minor; someone who has not reached the age of majority.

K

K (1 chemistry; 2 measurement; 3 biochemistry) 1 CHEMICAL SYMBOL for POTASSIUM, derived from Latin: Kalium. 2 An abbreviation of 'K'ilodalton/ 'K'elvin/ 'K'ilobyte/ 'K'ilogram. 3 A symbol for lysine.

K$_E$ (physiology/ biochemistry) A symbol for exchangeable body POTASSIUM.

Kahn test (bacteriology) A serological test formerly used in the diagnosis of syphilis, now superseded by the VENEREAL DISEASE Research Laboratories test (VDRL test). Named after the Lithuanuan-born American serologist, Reuben Leon Kahn (1887-1979).

Kala azar (microbiology) one of the forms of LEISHMANIASIS, caused by *Leishmania* organisms and spread to humans by the bite of sandflies. KALA AZAR occurs mainly in the Mediterranean AREA and in India, but is spreading westward into Europe. There is FEVER, ANAEMIA (*USA*: anemia), LYMPH NODE swelling, enlargement of the SPLEEN and LIVER, damage to the BONE MARROW, MALNUTRITION and loss of immune CAPACITY (IMMUNOSUPPRESSION). The condition can be diagnosed by the elisa test and is treated with drugs containing ANTIMONY. Also known as VISCERAL LEISHMANIASIS.

kallikreins (biochemistry) Proteases that release the peptides bradykinin and lysylbradykinin from the PRECURSOR proteins, high-molecular-WEIGHT kininogen and low-molecular-WEIGHT kininogen. There are two KALLIKREINS: PLASMA kallikrein, which circulates in an inactive form, and which with high-molecular-WEIGHT kininogen also catalyse the activation of FACTOR XII; and TISSUE kallikrein, which is located primarily on the apical membranes of CELLS concerned with transcellular ELECTROLYTE transport.

kanamycin (pharmacology) A broad SPECTRUM aminoglycoside ANTIBIOTIC derived from a soil actinomycete. KANAMYCIN is active against gram-negative organisms but is now largely replaced by gentamicin. The aminoglycosides can cause deafness, tinnitus and KIDNEY damage.

kaolin (chemistry) ALUMINIUM silicate, or china clay. It is used in the TREATMENT of mild DIARRHOEA (*USA*: diarrhea).

kaolinite (chemistry) HYDRATED ALUMINIUM silicate mineral.

Kaposi's sarcoma (medical) A MALIGNANT GROWTH formerly known to affect African children and Mediterranean men over the age of 50, who developed the TUMOUR (*USA*: tumor) on the legs. In the 1980s it became apparent that the TUMOUR was associated with the immunoDEFICIENCY DISEASE AIDS. Now about a quarter of those suffering with AIDS present with the TUMOUR (*USA*: tumor), which is thought to be due to a VIRUS INFECTION.

Kartagener's syndrome (medical) The COMBINATION of CONGENITAL malfunction of the brush borders of the respiratory HAIR CELLS (cilia) with bronchiectasis, sinusitis and reversal (TRANSPOSITION) of the internal organs of the body.

karyapsis (cytology) *See* KARYOGAMY.

karyo- (cytology) Combining form donoting a CELL NUCLEUS. From the Greek *karuon*, meaning 'a nut'.

karyogamy (cytology) the coming together and fusing of the nuclei of gametes.

karyogenesis (cytology) The formation of a CELL NUCLEUS.

karyokinesis (cytology) *See* MITOSIS.

karyolymph (cytology) The FLUID in the NUCLEUS of a CELL.

karyolysis (cytology) Destruction of a CELL NUCLEUS.

karyomegaly (cytology) An increase in the size of the nuclei of the CELLS of a TISSUE.

karyon (cytology) The CELL NUCLEUS.

karyoplasm (cytology) The PROTOPLASM of the CELL NUCLEUS.

karyorrhexis (cytology) Rupture of the CELL NUCLEUS in which the CHROMATIN disintegrates.

karyosome (cytology) A spherical MASS of aggregated CHROMATIN material in a resting (INTERPHASE) NUCLEUS.

karyotype (genetics) The chromosomal constitution of an individual as seen in the NUCLEUS of a SOMATIC CELL. It provides information about the SPECIES or strain, because a KARYOTYPE is CHARACTERISTIC to the CELL of a particular organism. The chromosomes are classified by their size and CENTROMERE position, and for convenience are usually shown in a specific ORDER in an IDIOGRAM.

Kastenbaum-Bowman test (statistics) A test of statistical significance used in calculation of MUTATION frequencies.

katal (measurement) A UNIT of ENZYME activity in the SI system. 1 international UNIT is equal to 16.6 nanokatal.

Katayama syndrome (medical /parasitology) A SET of allergic phenomena associated with the penetration of the SKIN and invasion of the body by the larval stage (cercariae) of SCHISTOSOMIASIS. The effects include local itching, URTICARIA, FEVER, headache, MUSCLE aches, abdominal pain, cough, patchy pneumonia and enlargement of the SPLEEN.

Kawasaki disease (medical) A world-wide disease of infants and young children that causes FEVER, swollen LYMPH NODES, a MEASLES-like rash, red eyes, inflamed TONGUE, dry cracking lips, peeling SKIN and, in just under half the cases, local widening (aneurysms) in the coronary arteries. These are usually transient but 10 per cent have long-term involvement of the coronaries. The disease is probably a RETROVIRUS INFECTION possibly spread by house-dust mites or cat fleas. ASPIRIN has been found useful in the TREATMENT and appears to reduce the INCIDENCE of HEART complications. Less than 1 per cent of affected children die from the disease and most make a complete recovery.

Kayser-Fleischer ring (toxicology) A golden-yellow coloured (*USA*: colored) ring seen near the edge of the corneas on examination with a slit-lamp MICROSCOPE in WILSON'S DISEASE. The ring is due to a deposition of COPPER.

k bar (measurement) An abbreviation of 'k'ilo'BAR'.

kc (measurement) An abbreviation of 'k'ilo'c'ycle.

Kcal (measurement) An abbreviation of 'K'ilo 'cal'orie. Also termed k.cal.

K cells (immunology) An abbreviation of 'K'iller CELLS.

K complex (physiology) An isolated slow WAVE occurring in the ELECTROEN-CEPHALOGRAM, usually during stage II sleep.

Kda (measurement) An abbreviation of 'K'ilo'da'lton.

Kell blood group system (haematology) A FAMILY of RED BLOOD CELL antigens designated as the allotypes KK, Kk, kk and K-k-. Antibodies to the K-ANTIGEN occur in about 10 per cent of people in England and can cause red CELL breakdown, haemolytic (*USA*: hemolytic), transfusion reactions. The GROUP system is next in importance to the ABO and rhesus systems and is named after a woman whose SERUM contained the antibodies.

keloid (histology) An overgrowth of scar TISSUE at the site of a cut or burn. The scar, instead of disappearing, spreads and sends out offshoots like claws which pucker the surrounding SKIN.

kelvin (K) (measurement) SI UNIT of thermodynamic TEMPERATURE with OK being ABSOLUTE ZERO [-273.15°C or -459.7°F]. One KELVIN DEGREE is equal to one Celsius DEGREE. The FREEZING POINT of WATER is 273.15K, 32°F, and 0°C. The BOILING POINT of WATER is 373.15K, 212°F, and 100°C. Named after the

British physicist Lord KELVIN (William Thomson) (1824-1907).

See also KELVIN TEMPERATURE.

Kelvin effect (physics) An alternative term for the Thomson effect.

Kelvin temperature (measurement) Scale of TEMPERATURE that originates at ABSOLUTE ZERO, with the triple point of WATER defined as 273.16K. The FREEZING POINT of WATER (on which the CELSIUS SCALE is based) is 273.15K. Also termed: KELVIN thermodynamic scale of TEMPERATURE.

Kendall's coefficient of concordance (*W*) (statistics) A measure of the extent to which two or more rank orderings agree with one another. Complete agreement between the rankings gives $W = 1$; lack of agreement gives $W = 0$ (or nearly 0).

Kendall's tau coefficient (statistics) A COEFFICIENT of rank correlation between two sets of scores based on the number of inversions of ranks in one ranking compared with the other.

kerat-, kerato- (histology) Combining form denoting CORNEA or horny keratosis. From the Greek 'keras', meaning horn.

keratin (biochemistry) A fibrous PROTEIN containing SULPHUR (*USA*: sulfur), the substance of which horn, HAIR, the outer layer of the SKIN, and the nails are composed. It is also part of the structure of the ENAMEL of the TEETH.

keratinization (histology) Replacement of the CYTOPLASM of CELLS in the EPIDERMIS by KERATIN, thus resulting in hardening of SKIN. Also termed: CORNIFICATION.

keratitis (medical) INFLAMMATION of the outer LENS of the EYE, the CORNEA. This implies a prior invasion of the CORNEA with BLOOD VESSELS (vascularization). KERATITIS commonly follows inadequately or incorrectly treated infections with cold sore (*HERPES simplex*) VIRUSES and is also a feature of TRACHOMA and CONGENITAL syphilis. There is pain, watering and ACUTE sensitivity to LIGHT. Vision is severely affected if the centre (*USA*: center) of the CORNEA is involved.

keratometer (measurement) An instrument for measuring the RADIUS OF CURVATURE of the CORNEA.

keratoscope (medical) An instrument for examining the CORNEA that makes it possible to detect irregularities of curvature.

kernicterus (biochemistry) The staining with BILIRUBIN of the basal ganglia of the BRAIN in infants suffering from haemolytic (*USA*: hemalytic) disease of the newborn. It may cause toxic degeneration of the NERVE CELLS with resulting disabilities including spasticity and mental DEFECT.

Kernig's sign (medical) An indication of irritation of the membranes surrounding the BRAIN and SPINAL CORD (the MENINGES) as in MENINGITIS. Inability to straighten the leg at the knee joint when the thigh is flexed at right angles to the trunk.

Kerr cell (physics) Chamber of LIQUID between two crossed polaroids that darkens or lightens in an ELECTRIC FIELD (applied between two electrodes). It can be used as a shutter or to modulate a LIGHT beam. It was named after the British physicist John Kerr (1824-1907).

ketene (chemistry) Unstable ORGANIC COMPOUND of GENERAL FORMULA R_2CCO, where R is an organic RADICAL. KETENES react with other UNSATURATED COMPOUNDS to form 4-membered rings.

ketoacidosis (biochemistry) ACIDOSIS resulting from the accumulation of KETONE bodies in the BLOOD.

ketoconazole (pharmacology) An IMIDAZOLE antifungal drug. Ketoconazole is absorbed into the BLOOD from the INTESTINE and can be used to treat internal (systemic) fungal infections as well as SKIN fungal infections. It can, however, damage the LIVER.

keto-enol tautomerism (chemistry) The existence of a chemical COMPOUND in two double-bonded structural forms, keto and ENOL, which are in EQUILIBRIUM. The keto changes to the ENOL by the migration of a HYDROGEN ATOM to form a HYDROXYL GROUP with the KETONE OXYGEN; the position of the DOUBLE BOND also changes.

ketogenesis (biochemistry) The formation of ACID KETONE bodies, as in uncontrolled DIABETES, starvation or as a result of a diet with a very high fat content.

ketogenic (biochemistry) (of an AMINO ACID) Giving rise to KETONE bodies.

ketonaemia (biochemistry) Raised KETONES in the BLOOD. Low levels are NORMAL. (*USA*: ketonemia).

ketone (chemistry) Member of a FAMILY of ORGANIC COMPOUNDS of GENERAL FORMULA RCOR', where R and R' are organic radicals and $=CO$ is a CARBONYL GROUP. KETONES may be made in various ways, such as the OXIDATION of a secondary ALCOHOL; *e.g.* OXIDATION of ISOPROPANOL gives ACETONE (propanone) $(CH_3)_2CO$.

Ketones are produced in the body by the imperfect breakdown of stored fats in severe DIABETES MELLITUS and starvation.

See also DIABETES MELLITUS.

ketosis (biochemistry) Poisoning caused by an accumulation of KETONES (acetoacetate, D-0-hydroxybutyrate, ACETONE) in the BLOOD.

ketotic (biochemistry) Pertaining to KETOSIS.

Kety method (physiology) Method for measuring cerebral BLOOD flow. The AVERAGE cerebral BLOOD flow in young adults is 54mL/ 100g/ min. The Kety method gives no information about regional differences in BLOOD flow.

keV (measurement) An abbreviation of 'k'ilo-'e'lectron 'V'olt, a UNIT of PARTICLE ENERGY equivalent to 10^3 ELECTRON volts.

keyboard (computing) COMPUTER INPUT DEVICE which a human OPERATOR uses to type in DATA as ALPHANUMERIC characters. It consists of a standard KEYBOARD, usually with additional FUNCTION keys.

Kf (physiology/ biochemistry) A symbol for glomerular ultrafiltration coefficient.

kg (measurement) An abbreviation of 'k'ilo'g'ram.

kg cal (measurement) An abbreviation of 'k'ilo'g'ram 'cal'oric.

kg cum (measurement) An abbreviation of 'k'ilo'g'rams per 'cu'bic 'm'etre.

kg m (measurement) An abbreviation of 'k'ilo'g'ram 'm'etre.

kg f (measurement) An abbreviation of 'k'ilo'g'ram 'f'orce.

kH (measurement) An abbreviation of 'k'ilo'H'ertz. Also termed kHz.

kidney (anatomy) One of a pair of excretory organs that FILTER waste products (particularly nitrogenous waste) from the BLOOD and concentrate them in URINE. Kidneys also have an important FUNCTION in the regulation of the BALANCE of WATER and salts in the body. The main processes of the KIDNEY occur in a large number of tubular structures called nephrons. WATER and waste products pass from the kidneys to the BLADDER via the ureters.

kidney cysts (histology) Small, FLUID-filled cavities in, the kidneys that are common and BENIGN and usually cause neither symptoms nor danger.

kidney failure (medical) The stage in KIDNEY disease in which neither ORGAN is capable of excreting body waste products fast enough to prevent their accumulation in the BLOOD.

kidney stones (biochemistry) CRYSTALLIZATION out of various substances dissolved in the URINE. Stones may occur in inherited disorders in which ABNORMAL amounts of substances such as CYSTINE and XANTHINE are excreted, but most KIDNEY STONES contain various combinations of CALCIUM, MAGNESIUM, PHOSPHORUS, and oxilate.

kidney transplant (medical) The INSERTION of a donated KIDNEY into the body and connection of its BLOOD VESSELS to the HOST vessels and its URETER to the HOST BLADDER.

killer cells (immunology) A subclass of large, granular LYMPHOCYTES. These are important elements in the IMMUNE SYSTEM and are the final effectors in the process by which damaged, infected or MALIGNANT CELLS are recognized and destroyed.

kilo- (measurement) Metric prefix meaning a thousand times (x 10^3) used with units of measurements.

kilobase (molecular biology) A UNIT of length of DNA or RNA of 1000 bases, used in describing genes or shorter sequences. When measuring double stranded DNA, it is actually BASE-PAIRS that are counted, so that the UNIT is comparable with counting bases in a single-stranded MOLECULE.

kilobyte (K) (computing) A COMPUTER term denoting 1,024 bytes of information or STORAGE space.

kilocalorie (Kcal) (measurement) 1,000 small calories [cal] or one large CALORIE [Cal]. This is a scientific UNIT of ENERGY required to burn off consumed food.

kilogram (kg) (measurement) SI UNIT of MASS, equal to 1,000 grams. 1 kg = 2.2046 lb.

kilohertz (kHz) (measurement) A UNIT of FREQUENCY equal to 1,000 hertz, or 1,000 cycles per second.

kilojoule (kj) (measurement) UNIT of ENERGY equal to 1,000 joules.

kilometre (km) (measurement) UNIT of length equal to 1,000 metres. 1 km = 0.62137 miles. (*USA:* kilometer).

kilowatt (kw) (measurement) A UNIT of electrical POWER equal to 1,000 watts.

kilowatt-hour (kwh or kwhr) (measurement) A UNIT of measure equal to 1,000 watts of POWER over the PERIOD of an hour. Also termed: UNIT.

kinaesthesis (physiology) Process by which sensory CELLS in muscles and organs relay information concerning the relative position of the limbs and the general orientation of an organism in space; a type of biological FEEDBACK.

kinase (chemistry) ENZYME that causes PHOSPHORYLATION by ATP.

kinematic viscosity (v) (physics) The COEFFICIENT of VISCOSITY of a FLUID divided by its DENSITY.

kinesis (biology) The simplest kind of orientation BEHAVIOUR (*USA:* behavior) that occurs in RESPONSE to a STIMULUS (*e.g.* the CONCENTRATION of a nutrient or an irritant). The speed of an ANIMAL's random motion increases until the STIMULUS reduces.

See also TAXIS.

kinetic energy (physics) The ENERGY possessed by an OBJECT because of its motion, equal to $1/2mv^2$, where m = MASS and v = velocity. The KINETIC ENERGY of the particles that make up any SAMPLE of MATTER determine its HEAT ENERGY and therefore its TEMPERATURE (except at ABSOLUTE ZERO, when both are equal to zero). *See* KINETIC THEORY.

kinetic theory (physics) Theory that accounts for the properties of substances in terms of the movement of their COMPONENT particles (atoms or molecules). The theory is most important in describing the BEHAVIOUR (*USA:* behavior) of gases (when it is referred to as the KINETIC THEORY of gases). An ideal GAS is assumed to be made of perfectly elastic particles that collide only occasionally with each other. Thus, *e.g.* the PRESSURE exerted by a GAS on its container is then the result of GAS particles colliding with the walls of the container.

See also KINETIC THEORY.

kinetics (chemistry) Study of the rates at which CHEMICAL REACTIONS take place.

kinetochore (cytology) The point of attachment of the spindle in a CELL.

kingdom (biology) Highest rank in the CLASSIFICATION of living organisms, which encompasses phyla (for animals) and divisions (for plants). Criteria determining members of a KINGDOM are broad, and consequently members are very diverse. Traditionally, there were two kingdoms: the plants and the animals. However, FUNGI, protists and prokaryotes are now often placed in kingdoms of their own.

kinins (biochemistry) VASODILATOR HORMONES. Two related VASODILATOR peptides called KININS are found in the body. One is the nanapeptide brabykinin and the other is the decapeptide lysylbradykinin, also known as kalidin.

kininase I (biochemistry) An ENZYME involved in the cardiovasular regulatory mechanism. A carboxypeptidase that metabolizes the KININS bradykinin and lysylbradykinin to inactive fragments by removing the C-terminal Arg.

kininase II (biochemistry) An ENZYME, like KININASE I, involved in the cardiovasular regulatory mechanism. It is a dipeptidyl-carboxypeptidase that inactivates bradykinin and lysylbradykinin by removing Phe-Arg from the C terminal. KININASE II is the same ENZYME as the angiotensin-converting ENZYME, which removes His-Leu from the C-terminal end of angiotensin I.

Kirchhoff's laws (1, 2 physics) Extensions of OHM'S LAW that are used in the ANALYSIS of complex electric circuits. 1 The sum of the currents flowing at any junction is zero. 2 Around any closed path, the sum of the EMFS equals the sum of the products of the currents and impedances.

kissing bug (parasitology) The reduviid BUG that transmits chagas' disease. It is so called because its nocturnal bite is barely felt.

kJ (measurement) An abbreviation of 'k'ilo'j'oule.

Klinefelter's syndrome (genetics) A disorder, limited to males, caused by having an extra X CHROMOSOME (YXY); the male characteristics tend to be diminished, and there is a predisposition to mental illness and mental retardation.

klino-taxis (biology) Movement of an ANIMAL in RESPONSE to LIGHT.

knowledge base (computing) The part of an expert system in which the expert knowledge is stored.

Koch's postulates (bacteriology) A SET of criteria to be obeyed before it is established that a particular organism causes a particular disease. The organism must be present in every case and must be isolated, cultured and identified; it must produce the disease when a pure culture is given to susceptible animals; and it must be recoverable from the diseased ANIMAL. Named after the German BACTERIOLOGIST, R. Koch (1843-1910).

Koplik's spots (virology) Tiny white spots, surrounded by a red BASE, occurring on the inside of the cheeks and the inner surface of the lower lip during the INCUBATION PERIOD of MEASLES. Named after the American paediatrician, H. Koplik (1858-1927).

Korsakoff's syndrome (medical) A condition that follows delirium and toxic states. Often due to alcoholism.

Kr (chemistry) The CHEMICAL SYMBOL for KRYPTON.

Krause end bulb (histology) An encapsulated SKIN RECEPTOR probably sensitive to cold.

Krebs cycle (biochemistry) A cyclical sequence of 10 bioCHEMICAL REACTIONS, brought-about by mitochondrial ENZYMES, that involves the OXIDATION of a MOLECULE of acetyl-CoA, to two molecules of CARBON DIOXIDE and WATER. It forms the second stage of AEROBIC RESPIRATION, in which PYRUVATE or LACTIC ACID produced by GLYCOLYSIS is oxidized to CARBON DIOXIDE and WATER, thus producing a large amount of ENERGY in the form of ATP molecules. It was named after the German-born British biochemist Hans Krebs (1900-82). Also termed: CITRIC ACID cycle; TRICARBOXYLIC ACID CYCLE.

Kruskal-Wallace test (statistics) A nonparametric rank test of the HYPOTHESIS that two or more independent samples have been drawn from the same population.

krypton Kr (chemistry) Gaseous non-metallic ELEMENT of GROUP 0 of the PERIODIC TABLE (the RARE GASes), which occurs in trace quantities in AIR (from which it is extracted). It is used in GAS-filled lamps and DISCHARGE tubes. At. no. 36; r.a.m. 83.80.

Kupffer cells (histology) The CELLS that line the fine BLOOD sinuses (capillaries) of the LIVER and act as scavengers to remove BACTERIA and other foreign material. Named after the German anatomist, K. W. von Kupffer (1829-1902).

kurchatovium (chemistry) An alternative term for the post-ACTINIDE ELEMENT RUTHERFORDIUM.

Kuru (medical) A disease of the BRAIN caused by a transmissible slow VIRUS, found in Papua New Guinea in 1957. It is fatal, and affects the CEREBELLUM and other parts of the BRAIN, resulting in progressive unsteadiness and inability to control movements. The disease was passed on by the practice of cannibalism and is thought to be caused by a prion.

kV (measurement) An abbreviation of 'k'ilo'V'olt.

kVA (measurement) An abbreviation of 'k'ilo'V'olt-'A'mpere.

Kveim test (medical) A test for SARCOIDOSIS involving the introduction of some TISSUE, prepared from a person suffering from the condition, into the SKIN. A typical TISSUE REACTION occurs after a few weeks. Named after the Norwegian physician, Morton Ansgar Kveim (1892-1966).

kw (measurement) An abbreviation of 'k'ilo'w'att.

kwashiorkor (biochemistry) A severe nutritional disorder of infants and young children which occurs when diet is extremely deficient of PROTEIN.

Kyasanur forest disease (virology) An arbovirus haemorrhagic FEVER (*USA*: hemorrhagic fever) that occurs in Mysore State, India, in the villages around the Kyasanur forest. The disease is caused by a VIRUS of the same GROUP as that causing Japanese B encephalitis and the INFECTION is transmitted by TICK bite.

L

L (biochemistry) A symbol for leucine.

l (measurement) An abbreviation of 'l'itre (*USA, liter*).

L- (biochemistry) A symbol for geometric isomer of D- form of chemical compound.

La (chemistry) The CHEMICAL SYMBOL for LANTHANUM.

lab. (general terminology) An abbreviation of 'lab'oratory.

label (chemistry) An ISOTOPE (RADIOACTIVE or STABLE) that replaces a STABLE ATOM in a COMPOUND. The course of a chemical or bioCHEMICAL REACTION or physical process can be followed by tracing the RADIO-ACTIVITY using a COUNTER or, in the case of STABLE isotopes, a MASS SPECTROMETER.

labiate (biology) Having lips or structures resembling lips.

labile (chemistry) Liable to change; usually applied with respect to particular conditions, *e.g.* HEAT-LABILE.

labium (anatomy) One of the folds of flesh at the entrance to the VAGINA.

laboratory (lab) (general terminology) A room for scientific experiments and demonstrations.

labour (physiology) PARTURITION, the process of giving birth. When PREGNANCY in the human has lasted for more or less 280 days the contractions of the UTERUS known as LABOUR (*USA:* LABOR) pains begin. LABOUR is divided into three stages: DILATION of the CERVIX, the neck of the womb; delivery of the child; and expulsion of the PLACENTA, the AFTER BIRTH. (*USA:* LABOR).

labyrinth (anatomy) Part of the INNER EAR of vertebrates, containing the COCHLEA and vestibular apparatus. Also known as the INNER EAR.

labyrinthitis (medical) INFLAMMATION of the INNER EAR, which causes vertigo, nausea and vomiting.

Lac operon (genetics) The GROUP of genes in *ESCHERICHIA COLI* that controls the METABOLISM of LACTOSE. It was the first OPERON to be discovered, and was found by Jacob and Monod in 1961.

lacrimal gland (anatomy) GLAND that produces tears. FLUID is continuously secreted to protect and moisten the CORNEA; it also contains the BACTERICIDAL ENZYME LYSOZYME. Also termed: lachrimal GLAND.

β-lactam (pharmacology) Member of a GROUP of antibiotics that include the PENICILLINS.

lactate (1 chemistry; 2 biology) 1 SALT or ESTER of LACTIC ACID (2-hydroxyPROPANOIC ACID). 2 To produce milk.

lactation (physiology/ biochemistry) The production of milk. May be physiological (after PREGNANCY) or pathological (galac-torrhoea).

lacteal (physiology) LYMPH VESSEL of the villi in the INTESTINE of vertebrates. Fat passes into the LACTEALS as an EMULSION of globules to be circulated in the LYMPHATIC SYSTEM.

lactic acid (biochemistry) $CH_3CH(OH)$-COOH Colourless (*USA*: colorless) LIQUID ORGANIC ACID. A MIXTURE of (+)-LACTIC ACID (DEXTROROTATORY) and (-)-LACTIC ACID (LAEVOROTATORY) is produced by BACTERIAL ACTION on the SUGAR LACTOSE in milk during souring. The (+)-form is produced in animals when ANAEROBIC RESPIRATION takes place in muscles because of an insufficient OXYGEN supply during vigorous activity. LACTIC ACID is used in the chemical and textile industries. Also termed: 2-hydroxyPROPANOIC ACID.

lactic dehydrogenase (LDH) (biochemistry) An ENZYME that catalyses the REDUCTION of PYRUVATE to LACTATE. The ENZYME is found in all CELLS capable of GLYCOLYSIS. LDH exists as several different ISOZYMES, and different tissues have either different ISOZYMES or different sets of ISOZYMES. Release of LDH into the BLOOD is a sign of TISSUE damage and can occur under many circumstances (*e.g.* MYOCARDIAL INFARCTION, HEPATOTOXICITY, nephrotoxicity, etc.). Identification of the particular isozyme can be used to identify the ORGAN involved. For example, the SERUM CONCENTRATION of LDH, is increased in LIVER injury, whereas LDH and LDH are increased in KIDNEY injury.

lactoflavin (biochemistry) An alternative term for RIBOFLAVIN.

lactose (chemistry) $C_{12}H_{22}O_{11}$ White CRYSTALLINE DISACCHARIDE SUGAR that occurs in milk, formed from the union of GLUCOSE and GALACTOSE. It is a REDUCING SUGAR. Also termed: milk-SUGAR.

laevorotatory (*l*-) (chemistry) Describing a COMPOUND with OPTICAL ACTIVITY that causes the plane of POLARIZED LIGHT to rotate in an anti-clockwise direction.

laevulose (chemistry) Fruit SUGAR, also called FRUCTOSE. A MONOSACCHARIDE CARBOHYDRATE.

lag phase (microbiology) PERIOD of slow microbial GROWTH, which occurs following INOCULATION of the culture medium.

Lamarckism (genetics) Discredited theory proposed by the French natuarlist Jean-Baptiste Lamarck (1744-1829) that evolutionary change could be achieved by the transmission of acquired characreristics from parents to offspring. The theory was superseded by Darwinism.

lambda (genetics) One of the most intensively studied of the bacteriophages. It attacks *ESCHERICHIA COLI*. The GENOME is double-stranded DNA, but with single-stranded, mutually complementary 'tails' that join up to make a circular DNA after entry into the HOST CELL.

lambda particle (physics) Type of ELEMENTARY PARTICLE with no ELECTRIC CHARGE.

lambda point (chemistry) TEMPERATURE at which LIQUID HELIUM (HELIUM I) becomes the superfluid known as HELIUM II.

Lambert's law (physics) Equal fractions of incident LIGHT RADIATION are absorbed by successive layers of equal thickness of the LIGHT-absorbing substance. It was named after the German mathematician and physicist Johann Heinrich Lambert (1728-77).

234

laminar flow (physics) Streamlined, or non-turbulent, flow in a GAS or LIQUID.

lanolin (chemistry) Yellowish sticky substance obtained from the grease that occurs naturally in wool. It is used in cosmetics, as an ointment and in treating leather. Also termed: lanoline; WOOL FAT.

lanthanide (chemistry) Member of the GROUP IIIB elements of ATOMIC NUMBER 57 to 71. The properties of these metals are very similar, and consequently they are difficult to separate. Also termed: lanthanoid; rare-EARTH ELEMENT.

lanthanum (La) (chemistry) SILVER-white metallic ELEMENT in GROUP IIB of the PERIODIC TABLE, the parent ELEMENT of the LANTHANIDE SERIES. It is used in making lighter flints. At. no. 57; r.a.m. 138.9055.

laparoscopy (medical) Inspection of intra-abdominal structures through a FIBRE-OPTIC (*USA*: fiberoptic) scope. Very widely used in GYNAECOLOGY (*USA*: gynecology).

LaPlace law (physics) An alternative term for AMPERE'S LAW.

large intestine (anatomy) *See* COLON; INTESTINE.

Larmor precession (physics) ORBITAL motion of an ELECTRON about the NUCLEUS of an ATOM when it is subjected to a small MAGNETIC FIELD. The ELECTRON processes about the direction of the MAGNETIC FIELD. It was named after the British physicist Joseph Larmor (1857-1942).

laryngitis (medical) INFLAMMATION of the LARYNX, usually caused by a VIRUS INFECTION such as in the common cold.

larynx (anatomy) Region of TRACHEA (windpipe) that usually houses the VOCAL CORDS (composed of MEMBRANE folds that vibrate to produce sounds).

laser (physics) An abbreviation of 'l'ight 'a'mplification by 's'timulated 'e'mission of 'r'adiation.

Lassa fever (virology) Lassa FEVER is a VIRUS INFECTION carried by the rat *Mastomys natalensis* found in sub-Saharan Africa. First seen in a town called Lassa in northern Nigeria in 1969, the INFECTION is thought to be spread to humans by contamination of food by rat's URINE, and from person to person by contact with BLOOD or other body fluids.

late genes (virology/ genetics) Genes that are expressed late in the process of a VIRUS infecting a BACTERIAL CELL. They usually code for the PROTEIN(s) that make up the VIRUS's coat.

latency period (biology) The PERIOD of time between the application of an agent to a living organism and a demonstrable effect of such application.

latent heat (physics) HEAT ENERGY that is needed to produce a change of state during the melting (SOLID-to-LIQUID change) or vaporisation (*USA*: vaporization) (LIQUID-to VAPOUR/ GAS change) of a substance; it causes no rise in TEMPERATURE. This HEAT ENERGY is released when the substance reverts to its former state (by FREEZING/ solidifying or condensing/ liquefying).

latent trait (genetics) Any trait that is not expressed in an organism's PHENOTYPE, but that can be passed on through its genes to descendants.

lateral (anatomy) Lying towards the side; away from the mid-line. *Contrast* MEDIAL.

lateral dorsal nucleus (cytology) A NUCLEUS that projects to the cingulate gyrus.

lateral horn (histology) GREY MATTER lying on either side of the SPINAL CORD between the DORSAL and VENTRAL horns, and forming part of the autonomic system.

latex (chemistry) Milky FLUID produced in some plants after damage, containing sugars, proteins and ALKALOIDs. It is used in manufacture, *e.g.* of rubber. A SUSPENSION of SYNTHETIC rubber is also called LATEX.

latin square design (statistics) An experimental design whose aim is to remove experimental error due to VARIATION arising from two sources. The design is identified with the rows and columns of a square. The number of conditions arising from each source and the number of treatments are the same, and each TREATMENT occurs once in each column and row.

LATS (physiology/ biochemistry) An abbreviation of 'L'ong-'A'cting 'T'hyroid 'S'timulator.

lattice energy (crystallography) Strength of an IONIC BOND; the ENERGY required for the separation of the ions in 1 mole of a crystal to an infinite distance from each other. Also termed: LATTICE ENTHALPY.

lattice (crystallography) Regular three-dimensional NETWORK of atoms, ions or molecules in a crystal. Also termed: CRYSTAL LATTICE.

laughing gas (chemistry) An alternative term for DINITROGEN OXIDE.

lauric acid (chemistry) $CH_3(CH_2)_{10}COOH$ White CRYSTALLINE CARBOXYLIC ACID, used in making soaps and detergents. Also termed: DODECANOIC ACID; dodecylic ACID.

lavage irrigation (medical/ toxicology) Usually used in referring to GASTRIC LAVAGE, the washing out of the STOMACH through a STOMACH tube for severe ALCOHOLic intoxication or poisoning.

law (science) A simple statement or mathematical expression for the generalisation (*USA*: generalization) of results relating to a particular phenomenon or known facts.

law of constant composition (physics/ chemistry) In any given chemical COMPOUND, the same elements are always combined in the same proportions by MASS.

law of equivalent proportions (chemistry) When two elements both form chemical compounds with a third ELEMENT, a COMPOUND of the first two contains them in the relative proportions they have in compounds with the third one *e.g.* CARBON combines with HYDROGEN to form methane, CH_4, in which the ratio of CARBON to HYDROGEN is 12:4; OXYGEN also combines with HYDROGEN to form WATER, H_2O, in which the ratio of OXYGEN to HYDROGEN is 16:2. CARBON and OXYGEN form the COMPOUND CARBON MONOXIDE, CO, in which (and in accordance with the LAW) the ratio of CARBON to OXYGEN is 12:16. Also termed: LAW of RECIPROCAL proportions.

law of mass action (chemistry) The driving FORCE of a HOMOGENEOUS CHEMICAL REACTION is proportional to the ACTIVE MASSes of the reacting substances.

law of octaves (chemistry) When the elements are arranged in ORDER of their RELATIVE ATOMIC MASSes, any one ELEMENT has properties similar to those of the ELEMENT eight places in front of it and eight places behind it in the list. It is a rejected idea of the relationship of elements. Also termed: Newland's LAW.

See also PERIODIC TABLE.

law of reciprocal proportions (chemistry) An alternative term for the LAW of equivalent proportions.

lawrencium (Lr) (chemistry) RADIOACTIVE ELEMENT in GROUP IIIB of the PERIODIC TABLE (the last of the ACTINIDES). At. no. 103; r.a.m. 257 (most STABLE ISOTOPE).

laws of reflection of light (1, 2 physics) 1 The ANGLE OF REFLECTION equals the ANGLE OF INCIDENCE. 2 The reflected RAY is in the same plane as the incident RAY and the NORMAL at the point of INCIDENCE.

laws of refraction of light (1, 2 optics) 1 For two particular media, the ratio of the sine of the ANGLE OF INCIDENCE to the sine of the ANGLE OF REFRACTION is CONSTANT (the REFRACTIVE INDEX). This is a statement of Snell's LAW. 2 The refracted RAY is in the same plane as the incident RAY and the NORMAL at the point of INCIDENCE.

LCAT (physiology/ biochemistry) 'L'eci-thin-'C'holesterol 'A'cyl'T'ransferase.

LCD (physics) An abbreviation of 'l'iquid-'c'rystal 'd'isplay.

LCM (mathematics) An abbreviation of 'l'owest 'c'ommon 'm'ultiple.

LCR (physiology) An abbreviation of 'L'ocus 'C'ontrol 'R'egion.

ld (toxicology) An abbreviation of 'l'ethal 'd'ose.

LD50 (toxicology) A term used to denote the dose of a substance that will kill 50 per cent of the organisms receiving it. LD50 tests are used on LABORATORY animals for testing the toxicity of drugs, toilet preparations, cosmetics, etc. designed for human use.

LDH (physiology/ biochemistry) An abbreviation of 'L'actate 'D'e'H'ydrogenase.

LDL (biochemistry) An abbreviation of 'L'ow-'D'ensity 'L'ipoPROTEIN.

Le Chatelier's principle (physics) If a change occurs in one of the factors (such as TEMPERATURE or PRESSURE) under which a system is in EQUILIBRIUM, the system will tend to adjust itself so as to counteract the effect of that change. It was named after the French physicist Henri Le Chatelier (1850-1936). Also termed: Le Chatelier-Braun principle.

leaching (chemistry) Washing out of a SOLUBLE material from a SOLID by a suitable LIQUID.

lead dioxide (chemistry) An alternative term for LEAD(IV) OXIDE.

lead equivalent (radiology) FACTOR that compares any form of shielding against RADIOACTIVITY to the thickness of LEAD that would provide the same measure of protection.

lead monoxide (chemistry) An alternative term for LEAD(II) OXIDE.

lead (Pb) (chemistry) SILVER-blue poisonous metallic ELEMENT in GROUP IVA of the PERIODIC TABLE, obtained mainly from its SULPHIDE (*USA*: sulfide) ore galena.

Various isotopes of LEAD are final elements in RADIOACTIVE DECAY SERIES. The METAL is used in building, as shielding against IONIZING RADIATION, as electrodes in ACCUMULATORs and in various ALLOYS (such as solder, metals for bearings and type METAL). Its INORGANIC COMPOUNDS are employed as pigments; tetraethyllead is used as an anti-knock agent in petrol. At. no. 82; r.a.m. 207.19.

lead tetraethyl(IV) (chemistry) An alternative term for tetraethyllead.

lead(II) (chemistry) An alternative term for PLUMBOUS.

lead(II) oxide (chemistry) PbO Yellow CRYSTALLINE substance, used in the manufacture of GLASS. Also termed: LEAD MONOXIDE; litharge.

lead(IV) (chemistry) An alternative term for PLUMBIC.

lead(IV) oxide (chemistry) PbO_2 Brown AMORPHOUS SOLID, a strong oxidising (*USA, oxidizing*) agent, used in lead-acid accumulators. Also termed: LEAD DIOXIDE; LEAD PEROXIDE.

leader sequence (molecular biology) The part of a MOLECULE of MESSENGER RNA between the 5' end and the start of the coding sequence. It contains sequences that are concerned with binding to the RIBOSOME.

leaders (histology) The popular name for tendons.

lecithin (biochemistry) Type of PHOS-PHOLIPID, a GLYCERIDE in which one ORGANIC ACID residue is replaced by a GROUP containing phosphoric ACID and the BASE CHOLINE. It is a major COMPONENT of a CELL MEMBRANE and found in large amounts in the BRAIN and NERVES as well as SEMEN and the YOLK of eggs. Also termed: PHOSPHATIDYL CHOLINE.

lectins (biochemistry) A general term for proteins or GLYCOPROTEINS of non-immune ORIGIN that have multiple highly specific CARBOHYDRATE-binding sites.

LED (physics) An abbreviation of 'L'ight-'E'mitting 'D'iode.

leeches (biology) The medicinal leech, *Hirudo medicinalis,* can sometimes help in the technique of SKIN grafting by reducing swelling in the grafted SKIN.

LEED (physics) An abbreviation of 'L'ow-'E'nergy 'E'lectron 'D'iffraction.

legionaires disease (medical/ bacteriology) Pneumonia caused by the BACTERIA *Legionella pneumophila.* The disease cannot be spread from person to person, but only in infected drops of WATER such as appears in some cooling towers and condensers in air-conditioning systems, which can give out AIR infected with the BACTERIA in fine drops of WATER.

leiomyoma (histology) a TUMOUR (*USA:* tumor) of the unstriped or INVOLUNTARY MUSCLE in an internal ORGAN.

leiomyosarcoma (histology) MALIGNANT TUMOUR (*USA:* maglignant tumor) of the UTERUS which may arise in fibroids.

Leishman stain (histology) A histological staining technique that may be used to make BLOOD CELLS and PARASITES visible under the MICROSCOPE.

Leishman-Donovan body (microbiology) Small, round INTRACELLULAR form (called amastigote or leishmanial stage) of *Leishmania* sp. and *Trypanosoma cruzi.*

Leishmaniasis (medical/ microbiology) INFECTION with a protozoon of the GENUS *Leishmania*, which is found in dogs and rodents and transmitted by sandflies. The INFECTION may be of the SKIN, where it produces indolent sores, or it may be in the internal organs. Named after the English BACTERIOLOGIST, Sir W. Leishman (1865-1926). *See* KALA AZAR.

lens (optics) Any TRANSPARENT substance with two opposite surfaces that refract LIGHT, most often used of a disc having a spherical curvature on one or both sides, which through REFRACTION can be used to form an IMAGE, to magnify an IMAGE, etc. By analogy also a CURRENT-carrying coil that focuses a beam of electrons (as in an ELECTRON MICROSCOPE). The mammalian EYE contains a single LENS with CONVEX faces, lying behind the CORNEA. By changing its convexity, it brings the IMAGE of objects at different distances into correct FOCUS on the RETINA. The refractive POWER of the human LENS is about 20 diopters. *See* ACCOMMODATION.

Lenz's law (physics) When a wire moves in a MAGNETIC FIELD, the ELECTRIC CURRENT induced in the wire generates a MAGNETIC FIELD that tends to oppose the motion. It was named after the Russian physicist Heinrich Lenz (1804-65).

LEPRA (society) An abbreviation of 'LEP'rosy 'R'elief 'A'ssociation.

leprosy (medical/ bacteriology) Also known as Hansen's disease, LEPROSY is caused by BACTERIA called *Mycobacterium leprae*. It now occurs in many tropical and subtropical countries, but has disappeared from Northern Europe. Named after the Norwegian physician, Gerhard Henrik Hansen (1841-1912).

leptokurtic (statistics) Of a FREQUENCY DISTRIBUTION, having a sharper peak than a reference distribution such as the NORMAL curve.

Leptospira (bacteriology) BACTERIA like very fine corkscrews which are in CONSTANT motion.

leptotene (genetics) One of the stages in MEIOSIS. One of the two processes of CELL DIVISION.

LES (physiology) An abbreviation of 'L'ower 'E'sophageal 'S'phincter.

Lesch-Nyhon syndrome (genetics) A human disease inherited as an X-linked RECESSIVE. It therefore affects boys who have inherited it from CARRIER mothers. The actual MUTATION is a failure to produce the ENZYME hypoxanthine phosphoribosyl transferase (HPRT), which is part of the process for metabolising purines; build-up of only partly metabolised purines leads to mental retardation and cerebral palsy. The condition is very rare. Female relatives of a sufferer, who may be carriers, can have a FOETUS (*USA*: fetus) prenatally diagnosed, as the lack of HPRT can be detected from conception.

lesion (medical) A region of damage to an ORGAN, whether produced deliberately or by PATHOLOGY.

lethal mutation (genetics) Any MUTATION that has such a severe effect on the organism as to cause early death. From the genetic point of view, a MUTATION is considered 'lethal' if the death occurs at any time before the individual reaches reproductive age. Common usage in relation to humans, however, includes only those MUTATIONS that cause death before birth or in early infancy. LETHAL

239

MUTATIONS can be DOMINANT, RECESSIVE or X-linked, and there are some known as 'semi-lethals'. LETHAL MUTATIONS are quite common in humans. Approximately 20 per cent of pregnancies end in spontaneous ABORTION (MISCARRIAGE), with either LETHAL MUTATIONS or CHROMOSOME abnormalities responsible for most cases.

Leu. (biochemistry) An abbreviation of 'Leu'cine.

leucine (Leu.) (biochemistry) $(CH_3)_2CH$-$CH_2CH(NH_2)COOH$ Colourless (*USA*: colorless) CRYSTALLINE AMINO ACID; a constituent of many proteins. Also termed: 2-amino-4-methylpentanoic acid.

leucine-amino peptidase stain (histology) An ENZYME histochemical staining technique.

leuco- (general terminology) Prefix denoting white; *e.g.* LEUCOCYTE. (The prefix is spelled *leuk in LEUKAEMIA*.)

leucocyte (haematology) Any kind of WHITE BLOOD CELL. They are classified as polymorphonuclear LEUCOCYTES or polymorphs, LYMPHOCYTES and monocytes. Granulocytes are further divided into neutrophils, basophils or eosinophils, according to their staining characteristics. In health they number approximately 4 to 11 x 10^9 per LITRE in the BLOOD, 60-70 per cent of which are neutrophils. Their number is raised (leucocytosis) in inflammatory conditions and abnormally low (leucopenia) in other conditions, such as poisoning of the BONE MARROW by drugs. (*USA*: leukocyte).

leucoderma (medical) A condition of the SKIN in which patches of white appear. It may be caused by diseases such as pityriasis versicolor or LEPROSY, or by vitiligo, an autoimmune condition which

is common. The only harm it causes is the social embarrassment of the patient; but the blemish may often be camouflaged by 'make-up'. It may affect coloured (*USA*: colored) people; about one in three patients are cured spontaneously.

leucoplakia (medical) A condition in which the patient develops thickened white patches on the TONGUE, cheeks or gums which cannot be scraped off. In many cases no cause is found, but leucoplakia is a precancerous condition and a number of cases develop MALIGNANT change.

leukaemia (haematology) A MALIGNANT disease involving overproduction of WHITE BLOOD CELLS. LEUKAEMIA (*USA*: leukemia) may be ACUTE or CHRONIC, and according to the type of CELL involved can be divided into myeloid or lymphatic. ACUTE LYMPHATIC LEUKAEMIA is mostly a disease of children, and ACUTE myeloid LEUKAEMIA a disease of those over 55; the CHRONIC leukaemias occur in people over 40. In ACUTE disease, there is failure of the NORMAL FUNCTION of the BONE MARROW, leading to a lack of RED BLOOD CELLS, platelets necessary for BLOOD clotting, and white CELLS necessary to fight disease, so that the patient becomes anaemic (*USA*: anemic), and liable to develop infections and haemorrhages (*USA*: hemorrhages). In addition the LIVER and SPLEEN are enlarged, as are the LYMPH GLANDS. In all leukaemias, the diagnosis is made by examination of the BLOOD. (*USA*: leukemia).

leucocytosis (haematology) Elevated WHITE BLOOD CELL count. (*USA*: leukocytosis).

leucopenia (haematology) Low WHITE BLOOD CELL count. (*USA*: leukopenia).

leucorrhoea (medical) An ABNORMAL white DISCHARGE from the VAGINA. (*USA*: leukorrhoea).

level (statistics) A sub-CLASSIFICATION of a FACTOR. The LEVEL of a FACTOR corresponds to the value of an independent or INTERVENING VARIABLE. A 'fixed LEVEL' is any one LEVEL of a FACTOR where all possible levels are investigated. A 'random LEVEL' is a LEVEL chosen to be representative of the FACTOR levels where only some levels are investigated.

levelling effect (statistics) The tendency after many trials for scores to cluster closely around the MEAN.

Lewis acid and base (chemistry) Concept of acids and bases in which an ACID is defined as a substance capable of accepting a pair of electrons, whereas a BASE is able to donate a pair of electrons to a BOND. It was named after the American chemist Gilbert Lewis (1875-1946).

LFO (physics) An abbreviation of 'L'ow 'F'requency 'O'scillator.

LH (biochemistry) An abbreviation of 'L'uteinising 'H'ormone.

LHRF (biochemistry) An abbreviation of 'L'uteinising 'H'ormone 'R'eleasing 'F'actor.

LHRH (physiology/ biochemistry) An abbreviation of 'L'uteinizing 'H'ormone-'R'eleasing 'H'ormone.

Li (chemistry) The CHEMICAL SYMBOL for LITHIUM.

libido (physiology) The sexual IMPULSE.

life cycle (biology) Progressive sequence of changes that an organism undergoes from FERTILIZATION to death. In the course of the CYCLE a new generation is usually produced. REPRODUCTION may be sexual or ASEXUAL, both MEIOSIS and MITOSIS may occur.

ligament (histology) The tough elastic CONNECTIVE TISSUE that hold the bones together and stabilise the joints.

ligand (1 chemistry; 2 biochemistry) 1 Any MOLECULE or ION that has at least one ELECTRON pair that donates its electrons to a METAL ION or other ELECTRON acceptor, often forming a CO-ORDINATE BOND. 2 Any MOLECULE that interacts with or binds to a RECEPTOR that has an AFFINITY for it.

ligase (biochemistry) ENZYME that repairs damage to the strands that make up DNA, widely used in RECOMBINATION techniques to seal the joins between DNA sequences.

ligation (molecular biology) The joining together of separate sequences of DNA by DNA LIGASE ENZYMES. It occurs during REPLICATION, DNA repair, and is also widely used in GENETIC ENGINEERING to stick DNA molecules together *IN VITRO*.

ligature (medical) A piece of material, *e.g.* thread or catgut, used to tie off BLOOD VESSELS or other structures.

light (physics) Visible part of the ELECTROMAGNETIC SPECTRUM, of wavelengths between about 400 and 760 nanometres.

light amplification by stimulated emission of radiation (LASER) (physics) A device that causes particles of a substance to amplify ELECTROMAGNETIC WAVES into the VISIBLE SPECTRUM. The powerful beam of

LIGHT ENERGY produced is increasingly used in surgery, and has proved particularly useful in OPHTHALMIC operations because the EYE is largely devoid of significant optical scatter, unlike other tissues, so that an optical beam can be focused on TISSUE deep inside the EYE; COAGULATION and cutting is then possible without the risk of INFECTION.

light intensity (physics) The RADIANT ENERGY emitted per UNIT time. The SI UNIT of measurement is the WATT. *Contrast* LUMINOUS INTENSITY.

light meter (physics) Instrument for measuring levels of illumination (*e.g.* in PHOTOGRAPHY), usually by means of a PHOTOCELL.

light-emitting diode (LED) (physics) Semi-conducting DIODE that gives off LIGHT, used to form letters and numbers on a DISPLAY panel.

lignocaine (pharmacology) A commonly used local ANAESTHETIC (*USA*: anesthetic).

likelihood ratio (statistics) The ratio of the likelihood of obtaining an observed SET of DATA under one HYPOTHESIS to the likelihood of obtaining the same DATA under another. It is widely used in significance tests.

lime (chemistry) General term for QUICKLIME (CALCIUM OXIDE, CaO), slaked LIME and HYDRATED LIME (both CALCIUM HYDROXIDE, $Ca(OH)_2$). They are obtained from limestone.

lime water (chemistry) A SOLUTION of CALCIUM HYDROXIDE ($Ca(OH)_2$) in WATER, used as a test for CARBON DIOXIDE (which turns LIME WATER milky when bubbled through it due to the PRECIPITATION of CALCIUM CARBONATE; after prolonged bubbling the SOLUTION goes clear again due to the formation of SOLUBLE CALCIUM HYDROGENCARBONATE).

limit (mathematics) Value to which a sequence or SERIES tends as more and more terms are included.

limiting friction (physics) Maximum value of a frictional FORCE.

limiting step (chemistry) An alternative term for RATE-DETERMINING STEP.

line breeding (genetics) The technique of breeding from animals as closely related as possible.

linea alba (histology) A whitish line running down the middle of the muscular wall of the ABDOMEN, formed by the junction of the flat tendons of the external oblique, internal oblique and transverse muscles after they have split to enclose the two longitudinal rectus muscles.

lineage (genetics) A sequence of SPECIES through evolutionary time, from the ancestral SPECIES to its present-day descendants.

linear (1 statistics; 2 mathematics) 1 Pertaining to a straight line or plane. 2 Describing an equation of the first ORDER. (*See* LINEAR EQUATION).

linear absorption coefficient (physics) Measure of a medium's ability to absorb a beam of RADIATION passing through it, but not to scatter or diffuse it.

linear accelerator (physics) Apparatus for accelerating charged particles.

linear attenuation coefficient (physics) Measure of a medium's ability to diffuse and absorb a beam of RADIATION passing through it.

linear energy transfer (LET) (physics) LINEAR rate of ENERGY DISPERSION of separate particles of RADIATION when they penetrate an absorbing medium.

linear equation (mathematics) Algebraic equation of the first ORDER. In co-ORDINATE geometry, the equation of a straight line, GENERAL FORMULA $y = mx + c$, where m is the GRADIENT (slope) of the line and c (a CONSTANT) is its intercept with the Y-AXIS.

linear function (1 statistics; 2 general terminology) 1 A sum of weighted variables; they can be graphically expressed as a line or plane. 2 Any FUNCTION describing the relationship of output to input in a LINEAR SYSTEM.

linear molecule (chemistry) MOLECULE whose atoms are arranged in a line.

linear regression (statistics) Fitting a straight line to the DATA points produced when one VARIABLE is plotted against another.

linear system (statistics) A system in which the output varies in direct proportion to the input, and in which if there is more than one input, the RESPONSE is proportional to the weighted sum of the inputs.

linear transformation (statistics) A TRANSFORMATION of scores (*e.g.* test scores) that changes their MEAN and STANDARD DEVIATION, but retains other aspects of the original distribution. *Compare* NORMALIZATION.

Lineweaver-Burk plot (statistics) One of several ways of linearising ENZYME- or RECEPTOR-binding DATA, based on derivations of the LAW of MASS ACTION.

linkage (genetics) Occurrence of two genes on the same CHROMOSOME. Genes that are close together are likely to be inherited together; genes that are further apart may become separated during CROSSING OVER.

linkage group (genetics) A GROUP of genes that can be observed to be linked together rather than to assort independently. In practice, a LINKAGE GROUP means a GROUP of genes all on the same CHROMOSOME.

Linnaean system (biology) System that classifies and names all organisms according to scientific principles. Each SPECIES has two names; the first indicates the organism's general type (GENUS), the second names the unique SPECIES. It was named after the Swedish botanist Carolus Linnaeus (1707-78). Also termed: BINOMIAL CLASSIFICATION.

lipaemia (biochemistry) Abnormally high LIPID LEVEL in the BLOOD. (*USA*, lipemia).

lipase (biochemistry) In vertebrates, an ENZYME in intestinal juice and pancreatic juice that catalyses the HYDROLYSIS of fats to GLYCEROL and FATTY ACIDS.

lipid (biochemistry) Member of a GROUP of naturally occurring fatty or oily compounds that share the property of being SOLUBLE in organic solvents, but sparingly SOLUBLE in WATER; they are an important part of the CELL MEMBRANE. Also, all LIPIDS yield MONOCARBOXYLIC ACIDS on HYDROLYSIS.

lipolyte (cytology) LIPID-containing CELL. Also termed: fat CELL.

lipoma (histology) A harmless TUMOUR (*USA*: tumor) composed of fat CELLS often occurring just below the SKIN.

lipoprotein (biochemistry) A molecule consisting of a protein complexed with a lipid. They exist in a wide range of forms. Some have a transport function within cells, and others have roles in the metabolism of cholesterol, particularly in the context of some forms of heart disease.

liposome (cytology) Droplet of fat in the CYTOPLASM of a CELL, particularly that of an EGG.

liq. (general terminology) An abbreviation of 'liq'uid.

liquefaction of gases (chemistry) All gases can be liquefied by a COMBINATION of cooling and compression. The greater the PRESSURE, the less the GAS needs to be cooled, but there is for each GAS a certain CRITICAL TEMPERATURE below which it must be cooled before it can be liquefied.

liquid (liq.) (physics) FLUID that, without changing its VOLUME, takes the shape of its container. According to the KINETIC THEORY, the molecules in a LIQUID are not bound together as rigidly as those in a SOLID but neither are they as free to move as those of a GAS. It is therefore a PHASE that is INTERMEDIATE between a SOLID and a GAS.

liquid crystal (chemistry) COMPOUND that is LIQUID at room TEMPERATURE and ATMOSPHERIC PRESSURE but shows charac-teristics normally expected only from SOLID CRYSTALLINE substances. Large groups of its molecules maintain their mobility but nevertheless also retain a form of structural relationship. Some LIQUID CRYSTALs change COLOUR (*USA*: color) according to the TEMPERATURE.

liquid-crystal display (LCD) (physics) A device displaying letters and numbers on objects such as control panels. These images are produced when an electrical FIELD causes a CAPSULE of TRANSPARENT LIQUID CRYSTAL to become OPAQUE.

See also LIGHT-EMITTING DIODE (LED).

liquid-liquid extraction (chemistry) An alternative term for SOLVENT EXTRACTION.

Listeria (bacteriology) A GENUS of BACTERIA associated with FOOD POISONING, *L. monocytogenes* being a member of this GENUS. The sources of the organism include tissues, URINE and milk of infected animals and the foods commonly associated with outbreaks include milk and milk products, eggs, meat and poultry.

liter (measurement) *See* LITRE.

litharge (chemistry) An alternative term for LEAD(II) OXIDE.

lithium (Li) (chemistry) SILVER-white metallic ELEMENT in GROUP IA of the PERIODIC TABLE (the ALKALI METALS), the SOLID with the least DENSITY. Its compounds are used in lubricants, ceramics, drugs and the plastics industry. LITHIUM, when given as a SALT partially replaces SODIUM in body tissues, thus affecting the PERMEABILITY of membranes. It is used to reduce mania, and on a long-term basis, to alleviate manic-depressive illness. At. no. 3; r.a.m. 6.941.

lithium aluminium hydride (chemistry) LiAlH$_4$ Powerful REDUCING AGENT, used in ORGANIC CHEMISTRY. Also termed: LITHIUM tetrahydridoaluminate(III).

litmus (chemistry) Dye made from certain lichens, used as an INDICATOR to distinguish acids from ALKALIS (*USA*: alkalies). NEUTRAL LITMUS SOLUTION or LITMUS paper is naturally violet-blue; acids turn it red, ALKALIS (*USA*: alkalies) turn it blue.

litre (l) (measurement) A BASIC UNIT of CAPACITY in the METRIC SYSTEM, determined by VOLUME of DISTILLED WATER at 4° Celsius. (*USA, liter*). 1 LITRE = 1.7598 pints.

liver (anatomy) In vertebrates, a large ORGAN in the ABDOMEN, the main FUNCTION of which is to regulate the chemical composition of the BLOOD by removing surplus carbohydrates and AMINO ACIDS, converting the former into GLYCOGEN for STORAGE and the latter into UREA for EXCRETION. Its glandular SECRETION is known as BILE, and it is secreted into the SMALL INTESTINE via the common BILE DUCT. In those SPECIES having a gallBLADDER, including humans, the common BILE DUCT originates at the point at which the HEPATIC duct, draining the intra-HEPATIC BILE passages, and comes together with the cystic duct that connects the gallBLADDER to the common duct. BILE salts FUNCTION in the DIGESTION of fats in the SMALL INTESTINE. The LIVER is supplied with BLOOD via the HEPATIC ARTERY and the HEPATIC PORTAL VEIN, and drains into the INFERIOR VENA CAVA via HEPATIC veins. The LIVER receives BLOOD, via the HEPATIC PORTAL VEIN, from the SMALL INTESTINE, thus receiving the products of DIGESTION and ABSORPTION of food. It forms GLYCOGEN from GLUCOSE, proteins from AMINO ACIDs and glycerides from FATTY ACIDS. It also carries out many reactions of intermediary METABOLISM. It is responsible for the EXCRETION of BILIRUBIN and biliverdin, products formed by DEGRADATION of haem (*USA*: heme).

liver enzymes, in blood (serum enzymes) (biochemistry) The measurement of HEPATIC ENZYMES released into the BLOOD as a consequence of injury has proven to be a sensitive INDICATOR of HEPATOTOX-ICITY. Since the ENZYMES may be of cytoplasmic or ORGANELLE ORIGIN, such measurements may also help define the subcellular site of damage. One or more of the following ENZYMES are measured: ALKALINE PHOSPHATASE; 5-nucleotidase; LEUCINE aminopeptidase; glutamyl transpeptidase; LACTIC DEHYDROGENASE ISOZYMES; isocitrate DEHYDROGENASE; ALCOHOL DEHYDROGENASE; FRUCTOSE mono- or diphosphate aldolase; arginase; QUININE OXIDASE; 0-hydroxybutyrate DEHYDRO-GENASE; glutamic-pyruvic transAMINASE; glutamic-oxaloacetic transAMINASE; SORBI-TOL DEHYDROGENASE. Some of these are measured only rarely; the ones utilized most commonly being the two transami-nases.

liver fluke (parasitology) *Clonorchis, Fasciola* and *Opisthorcis* are GENERA of FLUKES which infect the LIVER of humans. They live in the BILIARY tract, and their INTERMEDIATE HOSTS are snails. *Clonorchis and Opisthorcis* find a further secondary HOST in freshwater fish, and the INFECTION occurs where people eat raw fish, particularly in the Far East. FLUKES may infect fish-eating mammals other than man, such as cats and dogs. *Fasciola* is the sheep LIVER FLUKE, and the snail infects vegetation and WATER; in sheep and cattle raising countries the INFECTION spreads to humans through infected WATER. *See* FLUKES.

LL (general terminology) An abbreviation of 'L'ower 'L'imb.

LMA (physics) An abbreviation of 'L'ow 'M'oisture 'A'vidity.

LMRSH (education) An abbreviation of 'L'icentiate 'M'ember of the 'R'oyal 'S'ociety for the 'P'romotion of 'H'ealth.

loa loa (parasitology) A filarial worm of West Africa, which infests the SUB-CUTANEOUS TISSUES, causes transient swellings (Calabar swellings) and intense itching, and is sometimes seen crossing the EYE beneath the CONJUNCTIVA. It is spread by the mango fly, and treated with diethylcarbamazine citrate. *See* FILARIASIS.

lobe (anatomy) A well-defined part of an ORGAN, by virtue of their shape, by partitions of CONNECTIVE TISSUE, or by fissures in the ORGAN. The BRAIN, lungs, LIVER and THYROID GLAND are for example made up of lobes.

loc. cit. (literary terminology) An abbreviation of 'loc'o 'cit'ato. Latin, meaning 'in the place cited'. Used in papers and dissertations to cite a WORK previously referred to.

local anaesthesia (medical) Anaesthesia of a localised AREA of the body, as opposed to general anaesthesia, when the whole body is rendered insensitive to pain (*USA*: local anesthesia).

lochia (physiology) The NORMAL DISCHARGE from the womb after childbirth. It may last for one or two weeks.

lockjaw (bacteriology) *See* TETANUS.

locus (1 mathematics; 2 genetics) 1 Path traced by a moving point. *i.e.* a line that can be drawn through adjacent positions of a point, each position of that point satisfying a particular SET of conditions. 2 Position of a GENE on a CHROMOSOME. (pl. 'loci').

lodestone (chemistry) Fe_3O_4 Naturally occurring magnetic OXIDE of IRON. Also termed: loadstone; magnetite.

LOEL (toxicology) An abbreviation of 'L'owest 'O'bserved 'E'ffect 'L'evel.

log (mathematics) An abbreviation of 'log'arithm to base 10.

logarithm (mathematics) Number related to an ordinary number in such a way that addition or subtraction of logarithms corresponds to multiplication or DIVISION of ordinary numbers. Logarithms are given to a particular BASE. The LOGARITHM of a number to a given BASE is the POWER to which the BASE must be raised to give the number, *i.e.* if y is a number and x is the BASE, $y = x^n$ where n is the LOGARITHM of y to the BASE x; *e.g.* the LOGARITHM of 100 to the BASE 10 is 2, because 10^2 is 100.

See also CHARACTERISTIC; COMMON LOGARITHM; NATURAL LOGARITHM.

logarithmic phase (microbiology) PERIOD of maximal GROWTH rate of a MICRO-ORGANISM in a culture medium.

logarithmic scale (measurement) NON-LINEAR scale of measurement. For COMMON LOGARITHMS (to the BASE 10), an increase of one UNIT represents a tenfold increase in the quantity measured.

logic (1 mathematics; 2 computing) 1 The use of methods from mathematics and formal LOGIC to analyse the underlying principles on which mathematical systems are based. 2 In electronic DATA-processing systems, the principles that define the interactions of DATA in the form of physical entities.

lone pair of electrons (chemistry) Pair of unshared electrons of opposite spin (in the same ORBITAL) that under suitable conditions can form a CO-ORDINATE BOND *e.g.* the NITROGEN ATOM in AMMONIA has a lone pair of electrons; the OXYGEN in WATER has two lone pairs.

long sight (medical) An alternative term for HYPERMETROPIA.

longitudinal study (statistics) Any study of a GROUP of people over a long PERIOD of time, usually years. It avoids the problems that arise in retrospective studies and in cross-sectional studies, but cannot take into account the effects of repeated testing.

loop diuretics (pharmacology) DIURETICS such as ethacrnic acid which act on the ascending tubules of the loop of Henlé, inhibiting resorption of SODIUM, some POTASSIUM and water.

loptotene (genetics) Stage of PROPHASE in the first CELL DIVISION in MEIOSIS. At this stage, chromosomes can be seen to carry chromomeres.

louse (parasitology) A parasitic insect. There are many varieties of lice, but only two which breed on man, *Pediculus* and *Pthirus*. *Pediculus humanus capitis* lives on the HEAD, and is common in schools, where it is spread by direct contact and by combs and hairbrushes. *Pediculus humanus humanus* is the body LOUSE, bigger than the HEAD LOUSE and capable of spreading TYPHUS, relapsing FEVER and trench FEVER. It lives in the clothes rather than on the body. *Pthirus pubis* is the crab LOUSE, found in the pubic HAIR and usually spread by sexual intercourse.

low birthweight (physiology) Birthweight less than 2.5 kg. Babies either preterm (two thirds) or small-for-dates (one third).

lowest common denominator (mathematics) Number that is the LOWEST COMMON MULTIPLE of all the denominators of a SET of fractions, necessary in ORDER to add or subtract the fractions; *e.g.* the LOWEST COMMON DENOMINATOR of 1/2, 1/3 and 1/4 is 12 (because these fractions can be expressed as 6/12, 4/12 and 3/12, and thereby added).

lowest common multiple (LCM) (mathematics) Smallest number that all the members of a GROUP of numbers will divide into; *e.g.* the LOWEST COMMON MULTIPLE of 2, 3, 4 and 5 is 60.

low-pass filter (physics) A FILTER that transmits from a waveform only frequencies below a given FREQUENCY.

Lowry-Brönsted theory (chemistry) Concept of acids and bases in which an ACID is defined as a substance with a tendency to lose a PROTON and a BASE as a substance with a tendency to GAIN an ELECTRON. It was named after the British chemist Thomas Lowry (1874-1936) and the Danish chemist Johannes Brönsted (1879-1947), who proposed it independently. Also termed: Brönsted-Lowry theory.

See also LEWIS ACID AND BASE.

LOX (physics) An abbreviation of 'L'iquid 'OX'ygen.

Lp (general terminology) An abbreviation of 'L'im'p'.

lp (medical) An abbreviation of 'l'atent 'p'eriod.

Lr (chemistry) The CHEMICAL SYMBOL for LAWRENCIUM.

LRCVS (education) An abbreviation of 'L'icentiate of the 'R'oyal 'C'ollege of 'V'eterinary 'S'urgeons.

LRIC (education) An abbreviation of 'L'icentiate of the 'R'oyal 'I'nstitute of 'C'hemistry.

LRP (physiology/ biochemistry) An abbreviation of 'L'DL 'R'eceptor-related 'P'rotein.

LSD (pharmacology) An abbreviation of 'L'y'S'ergic ACID 'D'iethylamide.

LSHTM (education) An abbreviation of 'L'ondon 'S'chool of 'H'ygiene and 'T'ropical 'M'edicine.

LTD (medical) An abbreviation of 'L'ong-'T'erm 'D'epression.

LTH (1 biochemistry; 2 education) 1 An abbreviation for 'L'uteo'T'ropic 'H'ormone. 2 An abbreviation of 'L'icentiate in 'T'ropical 'M'edicine.

LTP (physiology) An abbreviation of 'L'ong-'T'erm 'P'otentiation.

Lu (chemistry) The CHEMICAL SYMBOL for LUTETIUM.

lubricant (physics) Any substance used to reduce friction between surfaces in contact; *e.g.* oil, graphite, molybdenum disulphide (*USA*: molybdenum bisulfide), silicone grease.

luciferase (biochemistry) ENZYME that initiates the OXIDATION of LUCIFERIN.

luciferin (biochemistry) Substance that occurs in the LIGHT-producing ORGAN of some animals, *e.g.* firefly. When oxidized (through the ACTION of LUCIFERASE) it produces BIOLUMINESCENCE.

Lugol's iodine (chemistry) A SOLUTION of IODINE 5 per cent and POTASSIUM IODIDE 10 per cent in WATER.

lum. (1 medical; 2 physics) 1 An abbreviation of 'lum'bago. 2 An abbreviation of 'lum'inous.

lumbar (anatomy) Pertaining to the lower back, a region that comes between the sacral and thoracic regions.

lumbar puncture (medical) The introduction of a hollow needle into the spinal canal in ORDER to draw off a specimen of CEREBROSPINAL FLUID for LABORATORY examination, or to introduce drugs, spinal ANAESTHETICS (*USA*: spinal anesthetics) or RADIO-OPAQUE substances for X-RAY investigations. The puncture is made between the third and fourth or fourth and fifth LUMBAR vertebrae, where the point of the needle cannot harm the SPINAL CORD, for it ends at the LEVEL of the second spinal VERTEBRA. The puncture is usually made under LOCAL ANAESTHESIA (*USA*: local anesthesia).

lumen (1 physics; 2 biology) 1 The SI UNIT of LUMINOUS FLUX, equal to the amount of LIGHT emitted by source of 1 candela through UNIT SOLID angle. 2 The space enclosed by a duct, VESSEL or tubular ORGAN.

luminance (L) (physics) The photometric INTENSITY of the LIGHT emitted or reflected by a surface per UNIT AREA. The standard UNIT is candela per square METRE.

luminescence (physics) Emission of LIGHT by a substance without any appreciable rise in TEMPERATURE. *See* BIOLUMINESCENCE; FLUORESCENCE; INCANDESCENCE; PHOSPHORESCENCE.

luminosity (physics) The apparent brightness of a surface or LIGHT source. It tends to be used to MEAN the apparent INTENSITY of a LIGHT as derived from the luminous efficiency FUNCTION.

luminosity curve (physics) A curve showing the relative RADIANT POWER needed by LIGHT of different wavelengths in ORDER for them to appear equally bright.

luminous efficiency function (physics) A FUNCTION that can be applied to LIGHT of any MIXTURE of wavelengths to yield its apparent brightness or LUMINOSITY. It weights the INTENSITY of each WAVELENGTH according to the sensitivity of a hypothetical standard observer to that WAVELENGTH *e.g.* yellow LIGHT receives a higher weighting than blue. Different functions are used for scotopic, mesopic, and photopic conditions. The photometric functions are only an approximation to those of real observers. *Compare* LUMINOSITY CURVE.

luminous flux (physics) The total amount of LIGHT per UNIT time emitted from a source, as measured by PHOTOMETRY; the standard UNIT of measurement is the LUMEN. *See* PHOTOMETRY.

luminous intensity (physics) The LUMINOUS FLUX emitted per UNIT SOLID angle (steradian) by a LIGHT source; the standard UNIT of measurement is the candela. *See* PHOTOMETRY.

lunar caustic (chemistry) SILVER NITRATE.

lung (anatomy) The paired or single RESPIRATORY ORGAN located in the THORAX. Its surface contains a large AREA of thinly folded, moist EPITHELIUM MEMBRANE so that it occupies little VOLUME. This MEMBRANE is richly supplied by BLOOD capillaries which allow for efficient and easy gaseous exchange. AIR enters and leaves lungs through the BRONCHUS, which branches into bronchioles ending in clusters of alveoli, where the main gaseous exchange takes place. The respiratory system consists of the lungs, AIR passages, the muscles that control BREATHING, and the PLEURAL cavities.

lupus (medical) LUPUS vulgaris is TUBERCULOSIS of the SKIN, now increasingly rare; it occurs mostly on the face and nose, taking the form of small nodules which leave scars behind. It responds to the anti-tubercular drugs.

luteal phase (physiology) The stage of the MENSTRUAL CYCLE that starts with OVULATION and ends, unless FERTILIZATION occurs, with the onset of MENSTRUATION; during this stage PROGESTERONE is secreted by the CORPUS LUTEUM.

luteinizing hormone (LH) (biochemistry) GLYCOPROTEIN HORMONE that is secreted by the PITUITARY under regulation by the HYPOTHALAMUS. In females, it stimulates the formation of the CORPUS LUTEUM and GRAAFIAN FOLLICLE, which in turn stimulates OESTROGEN (*USA*: estrogen) production. LH is also essential for OVULATION. In males, it stimulates INTERSTITIAL CELLS of the TESTIS to produce ANDROGENS.

luteotrophin (biochemistry) An alternative term for PROLACTIN.

lutetium (Lu) (chemistry) Metallic ELEMENT in GROUP IIIB of the PERIODIC TABLE (one of the LANTHANIDES). The irradiated METAL is a BETA-PARTICLE emitter, used in catalytic processes. At. no. 71; r.a.m. 174.97.

lux (measurement) SI UNIT of illumination, equal to one LUMEN per square METRE. Also termed: METRE-CANDLE.

See also PHOTOMETRY.

luxol fast blue/cresyl violet stain (histology) A histological staining technique that may be used to make myelin and nissl substance visible under the MICROSCOPE.

luxury gene (genetics) A term rarely used nowadays. A GENE that codes for a PRODUCT specific to one particular type of CELL, in contrast to HOUSEKEEPING GENES. An example of a LUXURY GENE would be the GENE for INSULIN, which is active only in certain CELLS in the PANCREAS, though present in all CELLS. LUXURY GENES are switched off in all CELLS except the ones where their FUNCTION is needed. While they are inactive, the DNA of LUXURY GENES is highly condensed as HET-EROCHROMATIN, and it shows up as a dark-staining band.

lv (physics) An abbreviation of 'l'ow 'v'oltage.

LVET (physiology) An abbreviation of 'L'eft 'V'entricular 'E'jection 'T'ime.

LVI (physics) An abbreviation of 'L'ow 'V'iscosity 'I'ndex.

LVS (education) An abbreviation of 'L'icentiate in 'V'eterinary 'S'cience.

lye (chemistry) SOLUTION of strong CAUSTIC ALKALI (*e.g.* POTASSIUM HYDROXIDE, SODIUM HYDROXIDE).

Lyman series (physics) SERIES of lines in SPECTRUM of HYDROGEN. It was named the physicist Theodore Lyman (1874-1954).

Lyme disease (microbiology) First described as the result of cases occurring in Lyme in the USA in 1977, the disease is caused by the MICRO-ORGANISM *Borrelia bergdorferi,* and spread by TICKS, mosquitoes and biting flies. The disease may continue, some months after the original INFECTION, to involve the joints, especially the knee; the HEART, with irregular PULSE, shortness of breath and pain in the chest; and the central and PERIPHERAL NERVOUS SYSTEM, with encephalitis and neuritis. Similar illnesses have occurred in Europe where the TICK *Ixodes ricinus* is found to carry the disease, possibly from dogs.

lymph (histology) The FLUID found in the LYMPH vessels; it is clear and slightly yellow, containing LYMPH CELLS and, if it derives from intestinal vessels, particles of fat. It is similar in SALT CONCENTRATION to PLASMA, but possesses a lower PROTEIN CONCENTRATION. It originates in the TISSUE spaces, being derived from the FLUID which filters through the walls of the CAPILLARY BLOOD VESSELs. It may contain particles as big as BACTERIA if it is draining from an infected AREA.

lymph node (histology) Flat, oval structure made of LYMPHOID TISSUE that lies in the lymphatic vessels and occurs in clusters in the neck, armpit or groin. Its main FUNCTION is the manufacture of antibodies and leueocytes. LYMPH NODES also act as a defence barrier against the spread of INFECTION by filtering out foreign bodies and BACTERIA, thus preventing their entry into the bloodstream. Also termed: LYMPH GLAND. Also known as LYMPH GLANDS.

lymphadenitis (histology) INFLAMMATION of LYMPH GLANDS, or nodes.

lymphadenopathy (medical) Disease of the LYMPH NODES.

lymphatic leukaemia (haematology) *See* LEUKAEMIA.

lymphatic system (histology) TISSUE FLUID, consisting mainly of FLUID forced out of the capillaries by the PRESSURE of circulating BLOOD, is known as LYMPH, and is in part recirculated by a system known as the LYMPHATIC SYSTEM. The LYMPHATIC SYSTEM arises as capillaries in the tissues that come together to form an interconnecting NETWORK of progressively larger vessels, similar to veins in structure. Flow is maintained largely by contraction of body muscles with valves preventing back flow; the system empties into the VENA CAVA via the thoracic duct. As LYMPH moves through the system it passes through LYMPH NODES (LYMPH GLANDS is not correct usage). LYMPH NODES contain T and B CELLS derived from the BONE MARROW STEM CELLS and remove foreign particles by PHAGOCYTOSIS. The SPLEEN and the THYMUS are both largely composed of LYMPHOID TISSUE.

See also B CELLS; SPLEEN; THYMUS.

lymphocytes (haematology) The primary nucleated CELLS of the LYMPHATIC SYSTEM. Resting LYMPHOCYTES are small, densely staining and have little CYTOPLASM. Activated LYMPHOCYTES enlarge and have increased CYTOPLASM. LYMPHOCYTES comprise 20-80 per cent of the nucleated BLOOD CELLS and more than 99 per cent of the CELLS in the LYMPHATIC SYSTEM. LYMPHOCYTES originate from STEM CELLS in the BONE MARROW and migrate to secondary lymphoid organs for further maturation. The two major classes of

LYMPHOCYTES, which are morphologically indistinguishable, are the B CELLS, the EFFECTOR CELLS of the humoral IMMUNE RESPONSE, and T CELLS, the EFFECTOR CELLS of the cellular IMMUNE RESPONSE. LYMPHOCYTES circulate through the BLOOD stream and lymphatic vessels, passing through the SPLEEN and LYMPH NODES, which have filtered and retained ANTIGEN for presentation to the B and T CELLS. They enter the LYMPH NODES from the bloodstream via high endothelial venules (HEV) in the NODE, percolate through the LYMPH NODE and exit via the EFFERENT lymphatics that drain into the venous system at the thoracic duct. The SPLEEN is primarily a BLOOD-filtering ORGAN, and LYMPHOCYTES enter and exit via the capillaries.

See also B CELLS; T CELLS.

lymphogranuloma (medical/ microbiology) Lymphogranuloma venercum is a SEXUALLY TRANSMITTED DISEASE caused by INFECTION with the organism *Chlamydia trachomatis*. The INFECTION is found in Africa, the Caribbean, South America and South-East Asia.

lymphoid tissue (histology) TISSUE found in dense aggregations in LYMPH NODES, tonsils, THYMUS and SPLEEN. It produces LYMPHOCYTES and macrophagocytic CELLS, which ingest BACTERIA and other foreign bodies. Also termed: lymphatic TISSUE.

lymphokines (biochemistry) Biologically active molecules produced by LYMPHOCYTES that have diverse effects on many differenT CELL types. They can be produced in RESPONSE to stimulation by ANTIGEN, CELL contact or other LYMPHOKINES. The majority of LYMPHOKINES have been defined only functionally, although the structures of a few, such as interleukin are known. Most LYMPHOKINES have actions on several different target CELLS.

lymphoma (medical) A number of conditions that involve swelling of the LYMPH NODES which is not caused by INFLAMMATION, METASTATIC MALIGNANT disease or HODGKIN'S DISEASE, have been called lymphomas. They are rare, and the diagnosis is made on microscopical examination of LYMPH NODES removed at BIOPSY. TREATMENT is by RADIOTHERAPY or CHEMOTHERAPY, according to the particular needs of each case.

Lyon hypothesis (genetics) The theory that, in female mammals (SEX CHROMOSOMES XX), one X in each CELL is inactivated so as to achieve dosage compensation, the individual then having the same amount of X-CHROMOSOME activity as the male (XY). The X CHROMOSOME to be inactivated is chosen at random, and this happens in different tissues at different times during the development of the EMBRYO (EMBRYOGENESIS). Once one X has been inactivated in one CELL, all CELLS derived from that CELL will have the same X inactivated. The female mammal is a naturally occurring MOSAIC. The inactivated X CHROMOSOME can be seen microscopically as the BARR BODY. The theory is called after the British geneticist Mary F. Lyon. Also termed: inactive-X hypothesis.

lyophilic (chemistry) Possessing an AFFINITY for liquids.

lyophilized (chemistry) Freeze dried.

lyophobic (chemistry) LIQUID-repellent, having no attraction for liquids.

Lys (biochemistry) An abbreviation of 'Lys'ine.

lysergic acid diethylamide (LSD) (pharmacology) A SYNTHETIC substance, similar to some FUNGUS ALKALOIDS, which provokes hallucinations and extreme mental disturbance if taken, even in extremely small quantities.

lysergide (pharmacology) *See* LSD.

lysine (chemistry) $H_2N(CH_2)_4CH(NH_2)$-COOH ESSENTIAL AMINO ACID that occurs in proteins and is responsible for their BASE-neutralizing powers because of its two -NH_2 groups. Also termed: diaminocaproic acid.

lysis (biology) The break-up of a CELL after the rupture of its CELL wall. This can be the result of attack by chemicals (*e.g.* detergents) or INFECTION (as happens when BACTERIA are invaded by bacteriophages), or the CELL may simply dissolve itself (AUTOLYSIS).

See also VIRUS.

lysogeny (genetics) The colonisation of a HOST CELL by a VIRUS, which gets itself replicated by the HOST's genetic machinery.

lysosome (cytology) MEMBRANE-bound ORGANELLE of eukaryotes that contains a range of digestive ENZYMES, such as proteases, phosphatases, lipases and nucleases. The functions of lysosomes include contributing ENZYMES to WHITE BLOOD CELLS during PHAGOCYTOSIS and the destruction of CELLS and TISSUE during NORMAL development. Lysosomes may be produced directly from the ENDOPLASMIC RETICULUM or by BUDDING of the GOLGI APPARATUS.

lysozyme (biochemistry) ENZYME in SALIVA, EGG white, tears and MUCUS. It catalyses the destruction of BACTERIAL

CELL walls by HYDROLYSIS of their mucopeptides, and thus has a BACTE-RICIDAL effect.

M

M (1 general terminolgy; 2 biochemistry) 1 An abbreviation of 'M'ale. 2 An abbreviation of 'M'ethionine.

m (measurement) An abbreviation of 'm'etre (*USA*: meter).

ma (general terminology) An abbreviation of 'm'enstrual 'a'ge.

MA (general terminology) An abbreviation for 'M'ental 'A'ge.

mA (physics) milliAMPERE.

mAb (immunology) An abbreviation of 'm'onoclonal 'A'nti'b'ody.

mabp (physiology) An abbreviation of 'm'ean 'a'rterial 'b'lood 'p'ressure.

Macchiavello stain (histology) A histological staining technique that may be used to make RICKETTSIAE, viral inclusions, visible under the MICROSCOPE.

MACD (education) An abbreviation of 'M'ember of the 'A'ustralasian 'C'ollege of 'D'ermatologists.

maceration (histology) The softening of a SOLID by FLUID. In medicine, the softening and damaging of the tissues by WATER, as in the case of a corpse many hours drowned.

Macheth illuminometer (physics) A device for measuring LUMINANCE; an observer views a surface through it and adjusts a LIGHT of known INTENSITY to appear the same brightness as the LIGHT from the surface.

machine code (computing) The BASIC SET of instructions for a COMPUTER, which are in BINARY CODE and can be directly implemented by the CENTRAL PROCESSOR. They are limited in both number and scope. These instructions are used to construct the more complex and versatile instructions of high-LEVEL languages, which must be translated back into MACHINE CODE when a higher-LEVEL PROGRAM is run.

machine language (computing) *See* MACHINE CODE.

macro (computing) A procedure or OPERATOR built from a sequence of other procedures or operators.

macro- Prefix meaning large or long in size or duration.

macrocephaly (medical) A CONGENITAL disorder in which the HEAD is swollen through excess CEREBROSPINAL FLUID and the person is mentally retarded.

macrocyclic (chemistry) Describing a chemical COMPOUND whose molecules have a large ring structure.

macrolides (pharmacology) *See* ANTIBIOTIC.

macromolecule (chemistry) Very large MOLECULE containing hundreds or thousands of atoms; *e.g.* natural polymers such as CELLULOSE, rubber and

STARCH, and SYNTHETIC ones, including plastics.

macronutrient (biology) Food substance needed in fairly large amounts by living organisms, which may be an inorganic ELEMENT (*e.g.* PHOSPHORUS or POTASSIUM in plants) or an ORGANIC COMPOUND (*e.g.* AMINO ACIDS and carbohydrates in animals).

See also VITAMINS; TRACE ELEMENT.

macrophages (cytology) Large CELLS present in CONNECTIVE TISSUE and in the walls of BLOOD VESSELS. They can be found in the PLEURAL and peritoneal cavities, the lungs (ALVEOLAR MACROPHAGES), the LIVER (KUPFFER CELLS), CONNECTIVE TISSUE (histiocytes), the LYMPH NODES and other tissues. MACROPHAGES are highly phagocytic and serve in the first line of defence against MICROORGANISMS. They form part of the reticulo-endothelial system.

MACS (education) An abbreviation of 'M'ember of the 'A'merican 'C'hemical 'S'ociety.

macula (anatomy) Any small blemish, used in anatomy to MEAN an AREA distinguishable from its surroundings by its COLOUR (*USA*: color) or other peculiarity *e.g.* the MACULA of the RETINA is a YELLOW SPOT at the back of the RETINA, which has in it a central depression called the FOVEA, where the RETINA is thinnest and the vision most ACUTE.

macule (histology) A flat discoloured (*USA*: discolored) spot in the SKIN, as distinct from a papule, which is a raised spot.

Madura foot (medical/ mycology) A disease of the tropics in which the foot swells and its tissues and bones become riddled with sinuses caused by INFECTION with a FUNGUS. It is one of a GROUP of CHRONIC infections called mycetomas, caused by FUNGI or ACTINOMYCETES. The disease may attack many areas of the body but the legs and feet are most commonly affected.

mag (physics) An abbreviation of 'mag'net/ 'mag'netic/ 'mag'netism.

magnesia (chemistry) MAGNESIUM OXIDE, MgO, particularly a form that has been processed and purified. It is used as an ANTACID.

magnesium (chemistry) A metallic ELEMENT used in medicine in the form of its salts: MAGNESIUM CARBONATE, HYDROXIDE and trisilicate are used as antacids in the TREATMENT of PEPTIC ULCERS and GASTRITIS. MAGNESIUM HYDROXIDE MIXTURE (milk of MAGNESIUM) has a slight laxative ACTION, and MAGNESIUM SULPHATE (*USA*: magnesium sulfate) (EPSOM SALTS) a more powerful one. The ELEMENT is a constituent of chlorophyll, and so an essential part of life; it is essential for human beings, playing a part in the functioning of NERVES and muscles, and in ENERGY METABOLISM. A NORMAL diet supplies the requirements.

magnesium carbonate (chemistry) $MgCO_3$ White CRYSTALLINE COMPOUND, SOLUBLE in acids and INSOLUBLE in WATER and ALCOHOL, which occurs naturally as magnesite and dolomite. It is used, often as the BASIC CARBONATE, as an ANTACID.

magnesium chloride (chemistry) $MgCl_2$ White CRYSTALLINE COMPOUND obtained from sea-WATER and the mineral carnallite, used as a source of MAG ESIUM.

magnesium hydroxide (pharmacology) $Mg(OH)_2$ White CRYSTALLINE COMPOUND, used as an ANTACID.

magnesium Mg (chemistry) Reactive SILVER-white metallic ELEMENT in GROUP IIA of the PERIODIC TABLE (the ALKALINE EARTHS). It burns in AIR with a brilliant WHITE LIGHT, and is used in flares and lightweight ALLOYS. It is the METAL ATOM in chlorophyll and an important TRACE ELEMENT in plants and animals. At. no. 12; r.a.m. 24.305.

magnesium oxide (chemistry) MgO White CRYSTALLINE COMPOUND INSOLUBLE in WATER and ALCOHOL, made by heating MAGNESIUM CARBONATE. It is used as a refractory and ANTACID. Also termed: MAGNESIA.

magnesium silicate (chemistry) *See* TALC.

magnesium sulphate (pharmacology) *See* EPSOM SALT.

magnet (physics) OBJECT possessing the property of MAGNETISM, either permanently (a permanent MAGNET, made of a ferromagnetic material) or temporarily under the influence of another MAGNET or the MAGNETIC FIELD associated with an ELECTRIC CURRENT (an ELECTROMAGNET).

See also PARAMAGNETISM.

magnetic amplifier (physics) TRANSDUCER so arranged that a small controlling DIRECT CURRENT input can produce large changes in coupled ALTERNATING CURRENT circuits.

magnetic circuit (physics) Completely closed path described by a given SET of lines of MAGNETIC FLUX.

magnetic core (computing) COMPUTER STORAGE DEVICE consisting of a ferromag-

netic ring wound with wires; a CURRENT flowing in the wires polarizes the CORE, which can therefore adopt one of two states (making it a bistable device).

magnetic disk (computing) Device for direct-access STORAGE and retrieval of DATA, used in computers and similar systems. It consists of a rotatable flexible or rigid plastic disc (*i.e.* a floppy or HARD DISK) coated on one or both surfaces with magnetic material, such as IRON OXIDE. DATA is stored or retrieved through one or more read/write heads. Also termed: magnetic disc.

magnetic domain (physics) GROUP of atoms with aligned magnetic moments that occur in a ferromagnetic material. There are many randomly oriented domains in a permanent MAGNET.

magnetic drum (computing) COMPUTER STORAGE DEVICE consisting of a rotatable drum coated with magnetic material, such as IRON OXIDE. DATA is stored or retrieved through one or more read/write heads.

magnetic field (physics) FIELD of FORCE in the space around the magnetic poles of a MAGNET.

magnetic field strength (physics) An alternative term for MAGNETIC INTENSITY.

magnetic flux (physics) Measure of the total size of a MAGNETIC FIELD, defined as the scalar PRODUCT of the flux DENSITY and the AREA. Its SI UNIT is the WEBER.

magnetic flux density (physics) PRODUCT of MAGNETIC INTENSITY and PERMEABILITY. Its SI UNIT is the tesla (formerly WEBER m^{-2}).

magnetic induction (physics) In a magnetic material, MAGNETIZATION induced in it, *e.g.* by placing it in the electromagnetic field of a CURRENT-carrying coil or by stroking it with a permanent MAGNET.

magnetic intensity (physics) Magnitude of a MAGNETIC FIELD. Its SI UNIT is the AMPERE m^{-2}. Also termed: MAGNETIC FIELD STRENGTH; magnetizing FORCE.

magnetic lens (microscopy) Arrangement of electromagnets used to FOCUS a beam of charged particles (*e.g.* electrons in an ELECTRON MICROSCOPE).

magnetic resonance imaging (MRI) (physics) *See* NUCLEAR MAGNETIC RESONANCE I(NMR) MAGING.

magnetism (physics) Presence of magnetic properties in materials. Diamagnetism is a weak effect common to all substances and results from the ORBITAL motion of electrons. In certain substances this is masked by a stronger effect, PARAMAGNETISM, due to ELECTRON spin. Some paramagnetic materials such as IRON also DISPLAY FERROMAGNETISM, and are permanently magnetic.

magnetization (physics) Difference between the ratio of the MAGNETIC INDUCTION to the pemicability and the MAGNETIC INTENSITY; its SI UNIT is the AMPERE m^{-1}. It represents departure from randomness of MAGNETIC DOMAINS.

magnetochemistry (chemistry) Study of the magnetic properties of chemicals.

magnetohydrodynamics (MHD) (physics) Branch of physics that deals with the BEHAVIOUR (*USA*: behavior) of a conducting FLUID under the influence of a MAGNETIC FLUX.

magnetometer (physics) Instrument for measuring the strength of a MAGNETIC FIELD, used, *e.g.* in prospecting for minerals.

magneton (measurement) UNIT for the magnetic moment of an ELECTRON. Also termed: Bohr-magneton.

magnification (optics) The ratio y'/y, where y is the height of an OBJECT perpendicular to the OPTICAL AXIS and y' is the corresponding height of its magnified IMAGE. For a single LENS this is equivalent to the ratio of the IMAGE distance to the OBJECT distance.

maintenance level (physiology) The LEVEL of GROWTH at which further physical development ceases.

major histocompatibility complex (genetics) The GROUP of genes that control the HLA (human LEUCOCYTE ANTIGEN) system.

See also IMMUNE SYSTEM.

mal (medical) Sickness, disease.

malaise (medical) A vague feeling of general discomfort.

malaria (parasitology) An INFECTIOUS DISEASE in which the RED BLOOD CELLS are attacked by the Protozoan PARASITE Plasmodium, which is transmitted from one infected person to another by *Anopheles* mosquitoes. MALARIA is common in tropical areas, and used also to be common around the Mediterranean until mosquito numbers were reduced, partly through loss of their habitat as marshes were drained and partly by insecticidal campaigns. In those areas still affected by MALARIA, prevention is better than cure, and SYNTHETIC QUININE-like drugs are effective in deterring the *Plasmodium* PARASITE. MALARIA, which causes high FEVER that often recurs for years after the original INFECTION, is a dangerous disease, so it is not surprising that in areas where it is (or was) ENDEMIC genes that confer protection against it have been selected for and are common in the population. Unfortunately, in most cases these genes 'buy' protection against MALARIA at the cost of giving people who are HOMOZYGOUS for the GENE another disease: the two best examples are sickle-CELL ANAEMIA (*USA*: sickle-cell anemia) and THALASSAEMIA (*USA*: thalassemia), and another is GLUCOSE-6-PHOSPHATE DEHYDROGENASE deficiency (but one ANTIGEN in the Duffy BLOOD GROUP SERIES seems to give protection without deleterious effects)

malic acid (chemistry) COOHCH$_2$CH(OH)-COOH Colourless (*USA*: colorless) CRYSTALLINE CARBOXYLIC ACID with an agreeable sour TASTE resembling that of apples, found in unripe fruit. It is used as a flavouring agent.

malignant (medical) When used of a TUMOUR (*USA*: tumor) it means cancerous; the term is also applied to dangerous conditions which progress rapidly such as MALIGNANT MALARIA or MALIGNANT HYPERTENSION.

malignant hyperthermia (medical) MALIGNANT HYPERTHERMIA ia a lethal complication related to anaesthesia (*USA*: anesthesia). This SYNDROME is a CHAIN REACTION of abnormalities triggered in susceptible individuals by commonly used general anaesthetics. The signs include greatly increased body METABOLISM, MUSCLE rigidity, and eventual hyperthermia that may exceed 44^{0}C. Death can result from CARDIAC arrest, BRAIN damage, internal hemorrhaging or failure of other body systems. Susceptibility is inherited, although the basis varies from a single defective GENE from

one parent to more complex genetic patterns. VOLATILE gaseous inhalation anaesthetics, as well as the MUSCLE relaxant succinylcholine, can trigger it, whereas injectable local anesthetics, barbiturates, opioids, other SEDATIVE-hypnotics, and NITROUS OXIDE, are safe for persons susceptible to this disorder.

malignant tertian malaria (microbiology) MALARIA caused by *Plasmodium falciparum*.

malleus (anatomy) A small hammer-shaped BONE in the MIDDLE EAR, one of the OSSICLES. It is SET in motion by the EAR DRUM and transmits sound vibrations to the INCUS.

Mallory cell (physics) An alternative term for MERCURY CELL.

malnutrition (biochemistry) A condition arising from deficiency in the diet or deficiency in the ABSORPTION or METABOLISM of food.

Malpighian body (anatomy) Part of the mammalian KIDNEY, BOWMAN'S CAPSULE and GLOMERULUS. Its FUNCTION is to FILTER BLOOD. It was named after the Italian biologist Marcello Malpighi (1628-1694).

Malta fever (bacteriology) *See* BRUCELLOSIS.

maltose (chemistry) C$_{12}$H$_{22}$O$_{11}$ Common DISACCHARIDE SUGAR, composed of two molecules of GLUCOSE. It is found in STARCH and GLYCOGEN, and used in the food and brewing industries.

mammalian cell mutation tests (toxicology) The mutagenicity of chemicals is tested in cultured mammalian CELLS, such as Chinese hamster OVARY CELLS or mouse LYMPHOMA CELLS.

mammary gland (histology) The GLAND in the female breast that secretes milk.

mammillary bodies (histology) Two protrusions at the bottom of the POSTERIOR HYPOTHALAMUS - the MEDIAL and LATERAL mammillary nuclei. They are implicated in emotion and the sexual drive.

mammogram (radiology) A radiological examination of the breast to identify or exclude tumours (*USA*: tumors). It is simple, and recommended as a three-yearly routine in women between the ages of 50 and 65.

man. (general terminology) An abbreviation of 'man'ual. A guidebook explaining the use of a PRODUCT or the operations of an organisation.

mandible (anatomy) The lower jawbone.

mandibular nerve (anatomy) Sensory nerve which supplies the TEETH, the temple, the floor of the mouth and the back part of the TONGUE.

manganese Mn (chemistry) An ELEMENT that is essential as a cofactor for many ENZYMES, including hexokinase, XANTHINE OXIDASE and SUPEROXIDE dismutase. Although the ELEMENT is essential for life, only MINUTE quantities are needed; no cases of MANGANESE deficiency have been recorded. It may be used in medicine in the form of POTASSIUM PERMANGANATE as an ANTISEPTIC. If MANGANESE fumes or dust are inhaled to excess, patients develop a condition very like Parkinson's disease.

manganese dioxide (chemistry) An alternative term for MANGANESE (IV) OXIDE.

manganese Mn (chemistry) Metallic ELEMENT in GROUP VIIA of the PERIODIC TABLE, used mainly for making special ALLOY steels and as a deOXIDIZING AGENT. It is also an essential TRACE ELEMENT for plants and animals. At. no. 25; r.a.m. 54.9380.

manganese(IV) oxide (chemistry) MnO_2 Black AMORPHOUS COMPOUND, used as OXIDIZING AGENT, CATALYST and depolarizing agent in dry batteries. Also termed: MANGANESE DIOXIDE.

manganic (chemistry) An alternative term for MANGANESE(III) in MANGANESE compounds.

manganous (chemistry) An alternative term for MANGANESE(II) in MANGANESE compounds.

Mann Whitney U Test (statistics) A nonparametric test of whether two independent samples come from the same population. It is equivalent to Wilcoxon's test. The test compares each value in one SAMPLE with each value in the other but does not require ranking, as in Wilcoxon's ALGORITHM. It is a nonparametric version of a T-TEST for independent samples. *Compare* KRUSKAL-WALLACE TEST.

mannitol (chemistry) $HO.CH_2(CHOH)_4$-CH_2OH SOLUBLE hexahydric ALCOHOL that occurs in many plants, and is used in medicine as a diuretic.

manometer (physics) A device for measuring FLUID PRESSURE.

manoptoscope (measurement) A device for measuring EYE dominance.

mantissa (mathematics) Fractional part of a LOGARITHM (the other part is the CHARACTERISTIC); *e.g.* in the LOGARITHM 2.3010, the .3010 part is the MANTISSA.

Mantoux test (bacteriology) A test for INFECTION with tuberculosis. An injection of a SOLUTION of purified PROTEIN DERIVATIVE of tuberculin (PPD) is made into the SKIN, and a POSITIVE REACTION of INFLAMMATION in the SKIN over 10 mm in size is likely to indicate an INFECTION. The Heaf test is a VARIATION of the MANTOUX TEST. Named after the French physician, Charles Mantoux (1877-1947).

MAO (biochemistry) An abbreviation for 'M'ono'A'mine 'O'xidase.

MAOI (biochemistry) An abbreviation for 'M'ono'A'mine 'O'xidase 'I'nhibitors.

map unit (genetics) A measure of the distance between two loci on the same CHROMOSOME. Loci are 1 MAP UNIT apart if cross-over occurs between them in 1 per cent of cases. A MAP UNIT has the formal name of centimorgan.

marasmus (medical) Progressive wasting away, particularly in infants.

Marburg disease (virology) A VIRUS INFECTION first described in 1967 when it affected LABORATORY workers in Marburg who had been in contact with a GROUP of vervet monkeys from Uganda. In 1976 there was an outbreak of severe haemorrhagic FEVER (*USA*: hemorrhagic fever) in the Sudan and Zaire which was found to be caused by a VIRUS identical with the Marburg VIRUS, but carrying a different ANTIGEN. This was called the Ebola VIRUS. Both infections are now referred to as African haemorrhagic FEVER, and a number of cases have occurred. Although the cases at Marburg were connected with monkeys, it has not been proved that monkeys are the carriers of the disease. INFECTION from monkey to man was by contact with

infected body fluids, and the same is true of INFECTION from man to man.

Marchi stain (histology) A histological stain that makes myelinated NERVE FIBRES (*USA*: nerve fibers) visible.

Marfan's Syndrome (medical/ genetics) An inherited SYNDROME characterised by long thin fingers, toes, arms and legs, increased height, deformity of the SPINE and BREASTBONE, and abnormality of the HEART and eyes. The aortic VALVE in the HEART is incompetent, and the LENS of the EYE is dislocated. These various effects are the result of a single DOMINANT GENE, though the biochemical mode of action is not known. The symptoms do not cause any ill health until middle age, when the HEART deformities often prove fatal; thus people with the SYNDROME have usually already had children by the time they are diagnosed, and the GENE has been passed on to the next generation. About one person in 25,000 has Marfan's SYNDROME. Named after the French physician, Bernard Jean Antonin Marfan (1858-1942).

marihuana (toxicology) An alternative spelling of MARIJUANA.

marijuana (toxicology) A NARCOTIC prepared from hemp. It has mildly hallucinogenic effects.

marrow (histology) The MARROW of the bones in an adult is red or yellow. Red MARROW is found in the SKULL, ribs, PELVIS, BREASTBONE, the bodies of the vertebrae and the ends of the long bones. It is actively engaged in making the CELLS of the BLOOD. Yellow MARROW is full of fat; in early life, it is active and red, but by the end of the PERIOD of GROWTH it has become inactive. In times of crisis it is still capable of regaining activity, and it then becomes red again.

Martinotti cells (cytology) Spindle-shaped cells with CELL bodies in the internal GRANULAR LAYER of the CORTEX, and with axons extending to the CELL bodies of the outer pyramidal layer.

MAS (education) An abbreviation of 'M'aster of 'A'pplied 'S'cience. Also termed MASc.

maser (physics) An abbreviation of 'm'icrowave 'a'mplification by 's'timulated 'e'mission of 'r'adiation. A precise ENERGY-emitting device that amplifies ELECTROMAGNETIC WAVES into the MICROWAVE SPECTRUM.

mass (physics) Quantity of MATTER in an OBJECT, and a measure of the extent to which it resists ACCELERATION if acted on by a FORCE (*i.e.* its INERTIA). The SI UNIT of MASS is the KILOGRAM.

See also WEIGHT.

mass decrement (chemistry) *See* MASS DEFECT.

mass defect (1, 2 chemistry) 1 Difference between the MASS of an atomic NUCLEUS and the masses of the particles that make it up, equivalent to the BINDING ENERGY of the NUCLEUS (expressed in MASS units). 2 MASS of an ISOTOPE minus its MASS NUMBER. Also termed: mass decrement; mass excess.

mass number (A) (chemistry) Total number of protons and neutrons in an atomic NUCLEUS. Also termed: NUCLEON NUMBER.

See also ISOTOPE.

mass spectrograph (physics) VACUUM system in which POSITIVE rays of charged atoms (ions) are passed through electric and MAGNETIC FIELDS so as to separate them in ORDER of their CHARGE/ MASS ratios on a photographic plate. It measures precisely the RELATIVE ATOMIC MASSes of isotopes.

mass spectrometer (physics) MASS SPECTROGRAPH that uses electrical methods rather than photographic ones to detect charged particles.

mass spectrum (physics) Indication of the distribution in MASS, or in mass/ charge ratio, of ionized atoms or molecules produced by a MASS SPEC- TROGRAPH.

massage (medical) A manipulative TREATMENT used in physiotherapy. The masseur or masseuse uses passive movements of the muscles, limbs and joints, and by stroking, pinching, pressing and kneading stimulates the tissues.

mass-energy equation (physics) A deduction from Einstein's special theory of RELATIVITY that ENERGY has MASS; $E = mc^2$, where E is the ENERGY, m is the amount of MASS, and c the speed of LIGHT.

Masson/Fontana stain (histology) A histological staining technique that may be used to make MELANIN visible under the MICROSCOPE.

massons trichome (histology) A histo- logical staining technique that may be used to make CONNECTIVE TISSUE visible under the MICROSCOPE.

mast cells (cytology) Large CELLS found in many places in the body, particularly in CONNECTIVE TISSUES and the mucosal surfaces. If they are damaged, or activated by an ANTIBODY-ANTIGEN REACTION, they release HISTAMINE and other substances which increase the passage of FLUID from the BLOOD VESSELS, lower the BLOOD PRESSURE, increase SECRETION from the MUCOUS MEMBRANES, and contract SMOOTH MUSCLEs. They also attract WHITE BLOOD CELLS. Massive activation of the MAST CELLS results in anaphylactic shock.

mastectomy (medical) The removal of the breast. Simple MASTECTOMY is the removal of the breast alone; RADICAL MASTECTOMY, which may be carried out for CANCER, involves removal of the breast together with the muscles on which it lies and the LYMPH NODEs in the armpit.

mastic (microscopy) A RESIN derived from the tree *Pisiacia lentiscus,* used in microscopy and dentistry.

masticatory nerve (histology) An alternative term for MANDIBULAR NERVE.

mastitis (medical) ACUTE MASTITIS is an INFLAMMATION of the breast which most commonly occurs in nursing mothers in association with cracked or depressed nipples. TREATMENT is by PENICILLIN; feeding from the NORMAL breast may not have to be stopped, although the milk should be expressed manually from the infected breast while it is inflamed. CHRONIC MASTITIS is not an INFECTION, but a name used for changes which produce BENIGN lumps in the breast, possibly in association with cysts; the changes are probably dependent on hormonal imbalance, for it is found that the condition is improved by the contraceptive pill.

mastoiditis (medical) INFLAMMATION of the AIR CELLS in the mastoid process of the temporal BONE, once not uncommon in association with middle EAR disease, but since the advent of antibiotics rarely seen.

mat. (medical) An abbreviation of 'mat'ernity.

matched groups (statistics) Groups assigned to different experimental conditions but not differing in other ways, *e.g.* in IQ or age, that might be relevant to the outcome of the experiment. The expression is sometimes used of the MATCHED PAIRS METHOD, which is a special case.

matched pairs method (statistics) Obtaining two MATCHED GROUPS by matching each member of one GROUP against a member of the other GROUP by reference to qualities other than those under investigation.

matched sample (1 statistics; 2 general terminology) A SAMPLE chosen in such a way that each member of it is the same on some CHARACTERISTIC or characteristics (other than those being investigated) as a member of another SAMPLE to be compared with it; *e.g.* the same subjects may each be run under two conditions. In this case a paired comparison test can be run on the differences in the effects of the two conditions. *Contrast* independent samples. 2 A SAMPLE chosen in such a way that its members are on AVERAGE the same on some category as those of another SAMPLE, but are not necessarily matched pair by pair.

maternal effect (genetics) The situation in which the PHENOTYPE of the offspring is determined not by its own GENOTYPE but by its mother's. There is some evidence to suggest that left-handedness in humans is inherited in this way.

See also MATERNAL INHERITANCE.

maternal inheritance (genetics) Any effect on the offspring that is not genetically transmitted but is passed on through the CYTOPLASM of the EGG, *i.e.* cytoplasmic INHERITANCE. MATERNAL INHERITANCE is the explanation of the situation in which a cross between a Strain A female and a Strain B male gives a different result from a cross between a Strain B female and a Strain A male (assuming that X-LINKAGE has been ruled out).

See also MATERNAL EFFECT.

mathematical probability (mathematics) Expression of the extent to which an event is likely to occur, given a value between 0 (an impossibility) and 1 (a certainty); *e.g.* the probability of getting a 6 on one roll of a dice is 1/6 or 0.16666...

mathematics (mathematics) Branch of science concerned with the study of numbers, quantities and space.

mating system (genetics) The system within a population by which mates are chosen. At one extreme are PARTHE-NOGENESIS and self-FERTILIZATION; at the other is random mating. There may be systematic INBREEDING or outbreeding, or assortative mating in respect of one or more traits. Some MATING SYSTEMS involve equal numbers of both sexes; in others, members of one sex have multiple mates. All MATING SYSTEMS have an effect on the genetic constitution of the succeeding generations: under random mating, it stays the same; INBREEDING and POSITIVE assortative mating increase

homozygosity; outbreeding and negative assortative mating increase heterozygosity.

matrix (1 biology; 2 mathematics) 1 EXTRACELLULAR substance that embeds and connects CELLS, *e.g.* CONNECTIVE TISSUE. 2 Square or rectangular ARRAY of elements, *e.g.* numbers.

matter (physics) Substance that occupies space and has the property of INERTIA. These two characteristics distinguish MATTER from ENERGY, the various forms of which make up the rest of the material universe.

See also MASS.

max. (measurement) An abbreviation of 'max'imum. The highest amount possible.

maxilla (anatomy) The BONE of the upper JAW, which also takes part in the formation of the orbit or EYE-socket, the nose and the hard palate. It contains the maxillary ANTRUM or SINUS, a hollow cavity which communicates with the nose and is liable to become inflamed in sinusitis.

maximum and minimum thermometer (physics) THERMOMETER that records the maximum and minimum temperatures attained during a given PERIOD of time.

maximum individual risk (MIR) (toxicology) Increased risk for an individual exposed to the highest measured or predicted CONCENTRATION of a TOXICANT.

maximum likelihood principle (statistics) The principle that we should estimate the value of a population parameter as the value which maximizes the likelihood of the obtained DATA.

maximum residue limit (MRL) (toxicology) The LIMIT on the amount of an 'additive' that may be present in food.

maxwell (measurement) C.g.s. UNIT of MAGNETIC FLUX, the SI UNIT being the WEBER. 1 maxwell = 10^{-8} WEBER. It was named after the British physicist James Clerk Maxwell (1831-79).

May Grunwald-Giemsa (histology) A histological stain for AIR dried cytology preparations.

MB (education) An abbreviation of '*M'edicinae 'B'accalaureus.* [Latin, meaning 'Bachelor of Medicine'.]

mb (measurement) An abbreviation of 'm'illi'b'ar.

MBAC (education) An abbreviation of 'M'ember of the 'B'ritish 'A'ssociation of 'C'hemists.

mbc (physiology) An abbreviation of 'm'aximum 'b'reathing 'c'apacity.

MBCO (education) An abbreviation of 'M'ember of the 'B'ritish 'C'ollege of 'O'phthalmic 'O'pticians/ 'O'ptometrists.

mbp (physiology) An abbreviation of 'm'ean 'b'lood 'p'ressure.

mbr (general terminology) An abbreviation of 'm'em'b'e'r'.

mc (1, 2 measurement) 1 An abbreviation of 'm'ega'c'ycle. 2 An abbreviation of 'm'illi'c'uries, a measurement for RADIUM.

M cells (histology) An abbreviation of 'M'icrofold 'CELLs'.

mcg (measurement) An abbreviation of 'm'i'c'ro'g'ram. (1/1,000,000 of a gram). Scientifically expressed as μg.

Mcnemar's test (statistics) A nonparametric test for the significance of the difference between two proportions in MATCHED SAMPLES, usually used when the same SET of subjects are tested at two different times.

MCPA (education) An abbreviation of 'M'ember of the 'C'ollege of 'P'athologists of 'A'ustralia.

MCRA (education) An abbreviation of 'M'ember of the 'C'ollege of 'R'adiologists of 'A'ustralia.

M-CSF (physiology) An abbreviation of 'M'acrophage 'C'olony-'S'timulating 'F'actor.

MD (1, 2 education; 3 medical) 1 An abbreviation of 'M'edical 'D'epartment. 2 An abbreviation of 'M'edicinae 'D'octor. [Latin, meaning, 'Doctor of Medicine'. The graduate DEGREE awarded to a student who has successfully completed a predetermined course of study in medicine.] 3 An abbreviation of 'M'uscular 'D'ystrophy.

Md (chemistry) The CHEMICAL SYMBOL for ELEMENT 101, MENDELEVIUM.

MDM (pharmacology) *See* MDMA.

MDMA (pharmacology) An abbreviation of 'M'ETHYLENE'D'ioxy-'M'eth'A'mphetamine. An antidepressant used in THERAPY. Commonly referred to as Ecstasy.

mdr (physiology) An abbreviation of 'm'inimum 'd'aily 'r'equirement.

MDSc (education) An abbreviation of 'M'aster of 'D'ental 'Sc'ience.

ME (1 forensics; 2 physiology) 1 An abbreviation of 'M'edical 'E'xaminer. 2 An abbreviation of 'M'etabolizable 'E'nergy.

mean (statistics) The arithmetical AVERAGE, *i.e.* the sum of all the values divided by the number of individuals.

See also MEDIAN; MODE; NORMAL DISTRIBUTION.

mean average (mathematics) *See* ARITHMETIC MEAN; GEOMETRIC MEAN.

mean corpuscular haemoglobin (haematology) A measure of the HAEMOGLOBIN (*USA*: hemaglobin) content of RED BLOOD CELLS. (*USA*: mean corpuscular hemaglobin).

mean corpuscular volume (haematology) A measure of the VOLUME of RED BLOOD CELLS.

mean deviation (statistics) Of a GROUP of numbers, the sum of all deviations from the ARITHMETIC MEAN divided by the quantity of numbers in the GROUP.

mean life (1 satistics; 2 physics) 1 AVERAGE time for which the unstable NUCLEUS of a radioisotope exists before decaying. 2 AVERAGE time of survival of an ELEMENTARY PARTICLE, ION, etc. in a given medium or of a CHARGE CARRIER in a semiconductor.
mean square (statistics) The ARITHMETIC MEAN of the squared deviations from the MEAN, *i.e.* the VARIANCE.

measles (virology) An ACUTE VIRUS INFECTION which appears in epidemics, often in the winter and spring. It commonly affects children between the ages of three and six; up to a year old, children are protected by the antibodies passed to them by their mother. The infecting organism is a paramyxovirus, which is spread in droplets by coughing or sneezing. One attack of MEASLES confers IMMUNITY for life.

meatus (anatomy) Duct or channel between body parts, *e.g.* external AUDITORY MEATUS, the opening to the EAR.

mechanoreceptor (physiology) A RECEPTOR sensitive to a mechanical FORCE, *e.g.* PRESSURE receptors, hair-cells, MUSCLE receptors.

Meckel's diverticulum (histology) A hollow blind appendage sometimes found growing from the SMALL INTESTINE about 50 cm from the ileo-caecal junction. It varies in size, the AVERAGE length being about 5 cm. It is the remains of a structure in the EMBRYO called the vitello-intestinal duct, which in the early stages of development connects the YOLK SAC to the midgut. It may be connected to the UMBILICUS by a fibrous cord. In later life it may be the seat of INFECTION, or ulceration, because in some cases it contains GASTRIC CELLS. It is possible for the GUT to become twisted round a persisting connection to the UMBILICUS, causing an obstruction. Named after the German anatomist, Johann Friedrich Meckel II (1781-1833).

meconium (physiology) A dark green semi-FLUID material consisting of BILE, MUCUS, desquamated CELLS, and debris discharged from the infant's BOWEL at birth or immediately afterwards.

MED (pharmacology) An abbreviation of 'M'inimal 'E'ffective 'D'ose.

med. (1 medical; 2 statistics) 1 An abbreviation of 'med'ical/ 'med'icine. 2 An abbreviation of 'med'ium/ 'med'ian.

medial (anatomy) Toward the mid-line of the body or of an ORGAN. *Contrast* LATERAL.

medial dorsal nucleus (cytology) An alternative term for dorsomedial NUCLEUS.

medial forebrain bundle (MFB) (histology) A tract of axons passing through the LATERAL HYPOTHALAMUS and running in both directions between the FOREBRAIN and brainstem. It has many connections with the limbic system and self-stimulation can readily be obtained from it.

medial geniculate nucleus (cytology) A NUCLEUS in the THALAMUS relaying AUDITORY information received from the INFERIOR colliculus to the CORTEX.

medial hypothalamic area (histology) A region of the HYPOTHALAMUS, stimulation of which tends to arouse the parasympathetic system.

medial lemniscus (histology) A NERVE tract which is part of the lemniscus and which conveys somaesthetic information from the MEDULLA to the THALAMUS.

medial plane (histology) The vertical plane that divides the body into two symmetrical halves.

medial rectus (histology) An extraocular MUSCLE that pulls the EYE inward towards the nose.

median (1 statistics; 2 anatomy) 1 The value in a distribution that comes halfway between the highest and the lowest. *See also* MEAN; MODE; NORMAL DISTRIBUTION. 2 An alternative term for MEDIAL.

median eminence (histology) A swelling at the BASE of the HYPOTHALAMUS that releases HORMONES into the portal circulation of the ANTERIOR PITUITARY.

median lethal dose (toxicology) *See* LD50.

median nerve (histology) One of the NERVES of the arm. It originates in the brachial PLEXUS of NERVES in the ROOT of the neck, runs down the upper arm, passes in front of the elbow, down the forearm and ends in the palm of the hand.

median test (statistics) A nonparametric test for the significance of the difference between two or more samples. The MEDIAN for all samples combined is calculated; in each SAMPLE the number of values above and below the combined MEDIAN is found and the results are evaluated by a chi square test.

mediastinum (anatomy) The space in the chest between the two lungs. It contains the HEART and great vessels, the OESOPHAGUS (*USA*: esophagus), the lower end of the TRACHEA, the thoracic duct, various NERVES, the THYMUS GLAND and LYMPH NODES.

Medical Examiner (ME) (medical) A forensics specialist, coroner, or other official authorized to perform autopsies.

Medical Research Council (MRC) (governing body) A government organization that supports MRC research institutes in the UK, as well as providing funds for research projects carried out at universities.

Medicines Act (legislation) UK legislation, passed in 1968, that restricts the supply and manufacture of all medicines to license-holders.

Mediterranean fever (bacteriology) *See* BRUCELLOSIS.

med. lab. (general terminology) An abbreviation of 'med'ical 'lab'oratory.

Med.RC (education) An abbreviation of 'Med'ical 'R'esearch 'C'ouncil. Also termed MRC.

Med Sc D (education) Doctor of Medical Science.

Med. Tech. (education) An abbreviation of 'Med'ical 'Tech'nology.

medulla (1, 2 histology) 1 The inner part of a structure or ORGAN or TISSUE (*e.g.* adrenal MEDULLA). *See also* CORTEX. 2 An alternative term for MEDULLA OBLONGATA.

medulla oblongata (anatomy) The lower of the two divisions of the hindbrain; it is immediately above the SPINAL CORD and below the pons. It contains many NERVE tracts, and also the autonomic nuclei implicated in the control of BREATHING, HEARTBEAT, and is concerned with the co-ordination of NERVE IMPULSES from hearing, touch and TASTE receptors.

medullary layer (histology) The innermost of the three layers of the cerebellar CORTEX.

medullary sheath (histology) An alternative term for myelin.

medullated nerve fibre (histology) *See* NERVE FIBRE.

mega- (measurement) Metric prefix meaning million times; x 10^6 (*e.g.* megahertz).

megabyte (computing) A COMPUTER term denoting a million bytes of STORAGE space.

megacolon (histology) ABNORMAL enlargement of the COLON, which may happen in consequence of prolonged use of certain laxatives such as senna and cascara. It may be CONGENITAL as in Hirschsprung's disease (aganglionic MEGACOLON) where there are no NERVE GANGLION CELLS in the wall of the RECTUM and the absence of NERVE CELLS may extend upwards into the COLON. The affected part of the GUT causes failure of PERISTALSIS and obstruction, above which the COLON becomes loaded with FAECES (*USA*: feces) and grossly distended. Named after the Danish physician, Harald Hirschsprung (1830-1916).

megahertz (MHz) (measurement) UNIT of FREQUENCY of one million hertz.

megloblastic anaemia (haematology) An ANAEMIA (*USA*: anemia) due to deficiency of VITAMIN B_{12} or FOLIC ACID. In this type of ANAEMIA the red CELLS are immature and larger than NORMAL. *See* PERNICIOUS ANAEMIA. (*USA*: megloblastic anemia)

megrim (medical) Another term for headache; migraine.

meibomian cyst (histology) A cyst on the inside of the eyelid caused by blockage of-the duct from one of the meibomian GLANDS which normally open at the edge of the eyelid. Named after the German anatomist, Heinrich Meibom (1638-1700).

meiosis (genetics) The central event in HEREDITY. Type of CELL DIVISION in which the number of chromosomes in the DAUGHTER CELLS is halved; thus they are in the HAPLOID state. Two successive divisions occur in the process, giving four DAUGHTER CELLS. The first DIVISION takes place in four stages: PROPHASE, META-PHASE, ANAPHASE and TELOPHASE. The second DIVISION has three stages: METAPHASE, ANAPHASE and TELOPHASE. In animals MEIOSIS occurs in the formation of gametes, *e.g.* eggs and SPERM. Also termed: REDUCTION DIVISION.

See also MITOSIS.

meiotic (genetics) Describing or referring to MEIOSIS.

meiotic drive (genetics) Any mechanism that causes unequal proportions of the possible gametes to be formed at MEIOSIS. One example is B chromosomes, which tend to be included preferentially in the OVUM during MEIOSIS in the female.

Meissner's corpuscle (physiology) A SKIN RECEPTOR thought to be sensitive to PRESSURE.

meknuria (histology) Dark-coloured (*USA*: dark-colored) URINE, or URINE which turns dark if left standing, found in cases of melanotic tumours (*USA*: melanotic tumors), and the rare conditions of alcaptonuria and porphyria.

melaena (haematology) Black motions, caused by altered BLOOD originating from HAEMORRHAGE (*USA*: hemorrhage) in the STOMACH or intestines, by IRON taken as a medicine, or by some red wines.

melanin (biochemistry) The black or dark brown PIGMENT that gives COLOUR (*USA*: color) to SKIN, HAIR and eyes in animals, including humans. MELANIN production in melanocytes is stimulated by ULTRAVIOLET RADIATION, either natural (*i.e.* from the sun) or artificial, and is catalysed by the ENZYME tyrosinase, lack of which causes ALBINISM.

melanism (biochemistry/ histology) Occurrence in populations of dark-coloured (*USA*: colored) individuals having an excess of MELANIN in their tissues.

melanocyte (histology) A pigmented CELL in the SKIN containing MELANIN.

melanocyte-stimulating hormone (MSH) (biochemistry) A PEPTIDE HORMONE produced by the INTERMEDIATE LOBE of the PITUITARY that increases production of MELANIN.

melanoma (histology) A TUMOUR (*USA*: tumor) of CELLS containing MELANIN. The TUMOUR is MALIGNANT, and produces secondary deposits. It occurs most often on the legs in women, and on the neck, HEAD and trunk in men. The darker the SKIN, the less likely it is to develop a MELANOMA; the INCIDENCE varies according to the amount of ULTRAVIOLET RADIATION to which the SKIN is exposed, but it is not more common in outdoor than indoor workers, being related more to sunbathing. ULTRAVIOLET RADIATION is not the only FACTOR concerned in the development of the TUMOUR, for it may develop in those who never expose the SKIN to the sun. MALIGNANT melanomas may arise in previously existing moles, and if one starts to grow, bleed or change in any way, medical advice is necessary.

melatonin (biochemistry) A substance found in the PINEAL GLAND that is implicated in CIRCADIAN RHYTHMS.

melting point (physics) TEMPERATURE at which a SOLID begins to liquefy, a fixed (and therefore CHARACTERISTIC) TEM-PERATURE for a pure substance.

melting profile (genetics) A GRAPH that shows how much DNA in a SAMPLE melts over time in an increasing TEMPERATURE. DNA melts in the range 60-80°C (140-175°F). DNA with a preponderance of A-T BASE-pairs melts at lower temperatures than DNA with more G-Cs, so the MELTING PROFILE gives a crude indication of the composition of the SAMPLE.

membrane (1 physics; 2 biology) 1 Any thin material, *e.g.* plastic FILM. 2 Structure that forms a dynamic INTERFACE, *e.g.* the outer MEMBRANE between a CELL and its surroundings. The structure may be selective in allowing the passage of certain molecules through (*e.g. a* -PERMEABLE MEMBRANE) or specific (*e.g.* in ACTIVE TRANSPORT). Membranes are widely distributed and very important in all organisms.

See also PLASMA MEMBRANE.

membrane potential (physics) The VOLTAGE difference between the inside and outside of a CELL's MEMBRANE, particularly of a NERVE MEMBRANE.

membranous labyrinth (anatomy) *See* EAR.

memo. (general terminology) An abbreviation of 'memo'randum.

memory (1 computing; 2 medical) 1 Part of a COMPUTER that stores DATA and instructions (programs), usually referring to the immediate access store. *See also* RANDOM ACCESS MEMORY (RAM); READ-ONLY MEMORY (ROM). 2 Defects in MEMORY may result from faulty perception during preoccupation with other matters and paying little attention to what is going on

or being said; but a deficient MEMORY may be an early sign of cerebral disease such as ALZHEIMER'S DISEASE.

See also AMNESIA, KORSAKOFF'S SYNDROME.

memory cells (immunology) MEMORY, or the ability to mount a quantitatively and qualitatively different RESPONSE upon secondary exposure to a specific ANTIGEN, is one of the hallmarks of the VERTEBRATE IMMUNE RESPONSE. In the humoral, or ANTIBODY, secondary RESPONSE, ANTIBODY is produced more quickly, in larger quantities, for a longer PERIOD of time, and of different classes and affinities than in a primary RESPONSE. The secondary RESPONSE in CELL-mediated IMMUNITY produces faster elimination of viral antigens, faster and more severe delayed-type HYPERSENSITIVITY reactions and decreased GRAFT rejection time. The ability to mount a secondary IMMUNE RESPONSE is due to the generation of ANTIGEN-specific MEMORY CELLS during the primary RESPONSE. MEMORY B CELLS and probably MEMORY T CELLS, as well as EFFECTOR B CELLS (PLASMA CELLS) and EFFECTOR T CELLS (CYTOTOXIC T CELLS) are produced from naive B and T CELLS during the primary RESPONSE to that ANTIGEN. The EFFECTOR CELLS are generally short-lived, but a CLONE of long-lived ANTIGEN-primed MEMORY CELLS is thought to survive and provide for the heightened secondary RESPONSE by bypassing the early stages of clonal expansion.

See also IMMUNE SYSTEM.

menarche (physiology) The first appearance of the menstrual PERIODS.

mendelevium Md (chemistry) RADIOACTIVE ELEMENT in GROUP IIIB of the PERIODIC TABLE (one of the ACTINIDES); it has several isotopes, with half-lives of up to 54 days. At. no. 101; r.a.m. 258 (most STABLE ISOTOPE).

Mendelism (genetics) Study of IN-HERITANCE, and therefore genetics. The principles of genetics put forward by the Austrian monk Gregor Mendel (1822-84), who postulated the existence of genes, both DOMINANT and RECESSIVE, and the rules governing their transmission. *See* MENDEL'S LAWS.

See also HEREDITY.

Mendel's laws (genetics) Conclusions drawn from WORK on INHERITANCE carried out by Gregor Mendel in breeding experiments. The first is the LAW of SEGREGATION: an inherited CHARACTERISTIC is controlled by a pair of factors (ALLELEs), which separate and become incorporated into different gametes. The second is the LAW of INDEPENDENT ASSORTMENT: the separated factors are independent of each other when gametes form.

Ménière's disease (medical) A disorder of the INNER EAR, causing recurrent ACUTE vertigo, deafness and tinnitus. As time goes by, the deafness becomes worse but the attacks of giddiness improve. The noises in the EAR are usually present all the time, but are worse during the attacks of giddiness, which are bad enough to make the patient vomit and collapse. Attacks last about a day, but are liable to come in groups, with intervals of a few weeks or months. Those affected are usually 40 or 50 years old. The cause is thought to be excessive FLUID in the INNER EAR. Named after the French physician, Prosper Ménière (1799-1862) *See* EAR.

meninges (histology) The three layers of protective TISSUE that enclose the BRAIN and SPINAL CORD, which are, from outside to inside, the dura mater, arachnoid layer, and pia mater.

meningioma (histology) A fibrous TUMOUR (*USA*: tumor) arising from the MENINGES; it is not MALIGNANT unless it penetrates the SKULL, when the portion that breaks through may give rise to secondary tumours, but removal may prove difficult and dangerous when the TUMOUR grows about the BASE of the BRAIN. It produces symptoms according to its position by direct pressure on the BRAIN, and it also competes with the BRAIN for the limited space within the skull, thus producing symptoms of increased INTRACRANIAL PRESSURE such as severe headache, deterioration of vision, and in extreme cases vomiting and disturbance of consciousness. The TREATMENT is surgical removal; the operation for removal of a MENINGIOMA on the upper surface of the BRAIN is one of the most satisfactory in neurosurgery.

meningitis (medical/ microbiology) INFLAM-MATION of the MENINGES, membranes that cover the BRAIN and SPINAL CORD. It is possible for the MENINGES to become infected as a result of injury to the SKULL, or INFECTION of the MIDDLE EAR, but in general MENINGITIS is caused by a VARIETY of BACTERIA, VIRUSES and sometimes FUNGI. The symptoms of MENINGITIS are in general headache, FEVER, nausea, vomiting, backache, and dislike of LIGHT (photophobia). There is stiffness of the neck, and in children possibly convul-sions, and there may be a history of respiratory INFECTION. Often the meningeal irritation is due to a VIRUS INFECTION, the commonest being mumps; MEASLES can be responsible, as can a VARIETY of other VIRUSES, including the HERPES VIRUS, but they do not usually cause accompanying INFECTION of the BRAIN (encephalitis) and recovery is the rule. INFECTION due to the poliomyelitis VIRUS is now rarely seen because of the success of the IMMU-NISATION programme, and it is hoped that mumps and MEASLES will for the same reason become increasingly rare. BACTERIAL MENINGITIS is usually caused by *Neisseria meningitidis, STREPTOCOCCUS pneumoniae or Haemophilus influenzae.* INFECTION is spread by droplets from the nose and is encouraged by crowded conditions. In meningococcal infections (spotted FEVER) patients, who are often under five years old, may develop a rash. The diagnosis is confirmed by LUMBAR PUNCTURE. Since the introduction of antibiotics the mortality of BACTERIAL MENINGITIS has decreased from about 75 per cent to less than 5 per cent. Tuberculous MENINGITIS has become rare in the West, but is still to be found in developing countries where it is a serious disease.

meniscus (1 anatomy; 2 physics) 1 A semicircular or crescentic CARTILAGE in a JOINT, usually used to refer to the semilunar cartilages in the knee. 2 Curved surface of a LIQUID where it is in contact with a SOLID. The effect is due to SURFACE TENSION.

menopause (physiology) Final cessation of MENSTRUATION. The CAPACITY for REPRODUCTION in women begins to decrease at about the age of 40 to 45, and the PERIODS cease at about 50, either abruptly or more frequently gradually, with increasing intervals between. There is a gradual change in the FUNCTION of the ovaries, and there is a decrease in the LEVEL of oestrogens (*USA:* estrogens) in the BLOOD. *See* MENSTRUAL CYCLE.

menorrhagia (medical) Excessive BLOOD loss at the monthly PERIOD. It may be due to a number of factors: nervous and emotional causes are not uncommon, or

there may be a DEFECT in the clotting mechanism of the BLOOD. Any bleeding which happens after the MENOPAUSE is also a sign that investigation is needed.

menorrhea (medical) The NORMAL DISCHARGE of the MENSES.

menses (medical) The monthly flow of BLOOD from the genital tract of a woman.

menstrual age (medical) The age of the fetus, starting from the beginning of the mother's last MENSTRUATION.

menstrual cycle (physiology) HORMONE-regulated CYCLE of female reproductive BEHAVIOUR (*USA:* behavior) during which OVULATION occurs; it occurs in some primates, including human beings. The end of the CYCLE is marked by a monthly shedding of the endometrium (lining of the womb) accompanied by a DISCHARGE of BLOOD from the VAGINA, known as MENSTRUATION. The CYCLE begins with the MENARCHE at the beginning of puberty and ends at the MENOPAUSE. Also termed: sexual CYCLE.

See also OESTROUS CYCLE.

menstruation (physiology) *See* MENSTRUAL CYCLE.

mensuration (measurement) Science of measurement.

mental age (MA) (medical) A measure of mental ability derived from tests. The score is expressed as the AVERAGE age at which children on AVERAGE perform as well as the person being tested.

menthol (chemistry) $C_{10}H_{19}OH$ White SOLID ALICYCLIC COMPOUND. It is an ALCOHOL with a minty SMELL and TASTE, used as a flavouring and in medicines.

mercaptan (chemistry) An alternative term for a thiol.

mercuric (chemistry) An alternative term for MERCURY(II).

mercurous (chemistry) An alternative term for MERCURY(I).

mercury Hg (chemistry) Dense LIQUID metallic ELEMENT in GROUP IIB of the PERIODIC TABLE (a TRANSITION ELEMENT), used in lamps, batteries, switches and scientific instruments. It ALLOYS with most metals to form AMALGAMS. Its compounds are used in drugs, explosives and pigments. Also termed: QUICKSILVER. At. no. 80; r.a.m. 200.59.

mercury arc (chemistry) Bright blue-green LIGHT obtained from an electric DISCHARGE through a VAPOUR of MERCURY.

mercury cell (1, 2 physics) 1 ELEC-TROLYTIC CELL that has a CATHODE made of MERCURY. *See* POLAROGRAPHY. 2 DRY CELL that has a MERCURY ELECTRODE. Also termed: Mallory cell.

mercury(II) oxide (chemistry) HgO Red or yellow COMPOUND, slightly SOLUBLE in WATER, which reduces to metallic MERCURY on heating. Also termed: MERCURIC OXIDE.

mercury(I) chloride (chemistry) HgCl White CRYSTALLINE COMPOUND, used as an INSECTICIDE and in a MERCURY CELL. Also termed: MERCUROUS CHLORIDE; CALOMEL.

mercury(II) chloride (chemistry) $HgC1_2$ Extremely poisonous white COMPOUND. Also termed: MERCURIC CHLORIDE; CORROSIVE SUBLIMATE.

mercury(II) sulphide (chemistry) HgS Red COMPOUND, which occurs naturally as cinnabar, used as a PIGMENT (vermilion) and source of MERCURY. (*USA*: mercury(II) sulfide).

mercury-vapour lamp (physics) Lamp that uses a MERCURY ARC in a QUARTZ tube; it produces ULTRAVIOLET RADIATION.

mescaline (pharmacology/ toxicology) Powerful drug derived, from the Mexican mescal cactus (peyote), which has a similar effect to LYSERGIC ACID DIETH-YLamide (LSD), and causes hallucinations and mental disturbance.

mesencephalon (anatomy) An alternative term for mid-BRAIN.

mesentery (histology) Vertical fold of TISSUE on the inner surface of the body wall of animals, which supports internal organs or associated structures.

meso- (biology) Prefix meaning middle.

mesoderm (histology) TISSUE in an ANIMAL EMBRYO that develops into tissues between the GUT and ECTODERM.

mesomerism (chemistry) Phenomenon in which a chemical COMPOUND can adopt two or more different structures by the alteration of (covalent) bonds, the atoms in the molecules remaining in the same relationship to each other. Also termed: RESONANCE.

See also TAUTOMERISM.

meson (physics) Member of a GROUP of unstable ELEMENTARY PARTICLES with masses INTERMEDIATE between those of electrons and nucleons, and with POSITIVE, negative or zero CHARGE. MESONS are emitted by nuclei that have been bombarded by high-ENERGY electrons.

messenger RNA (mRNA) (molecular biology) RIBONUCLEIC ACID that conveys instructions from DNA by copying the code of DNA in the CELL NUCLEUS and passing it out to the CYTOPLASM. It is translated into a POLYPEPTIDE chain formed from AMINO ACIDS which join in a sequence according to the instructions in the messenger RNA.

See also TRANSCRIPTION.

Met. (pharmacology) An abbreviation of 'Met'hionine.

metabolism (biochemistry) CHEMICAL REACTIONS that occur in CELLS and are a CHARACTERISTIC of all living organisms. Metabolic reactions are initiated by ENZYMES and liberate ENERGY in a usable form. ORGANIC COMPOUNDS may be broken down to simple constituents (CATABOLISM) and used for other processes. Simple compounds may be built up to more complex ones (ANABOLISM).

metabolite (biochemistry) A MOLECULE participating in METABOLISM, which may be synthesized in an organism or taken in as food. Autotrophic organisms need only to take in inorganic metabolises; heterotrophs also need organic metabolises.

metal (chemistry) Any of a GROUP of elements and their ALLOYs with general properties of strength, hardness and the ability to conduct HEAT and ELECTRICITY (because of the presence of FREE ELECTRONS). Most have high MELTING POINTS and can be polished to a shiny finish. Metallic elements (about 80 per cent of the total) tend to form cations.

See also METALLOID.

metallocene (chemistry) Member of a GROUP of chemicals formed between a METAL and an AROMATIC COMPOUND in which the OXIDATION state of the METAL is zero; *e.g.* FERROCENE.

metalloid (chemistry) An ELEMENT with physical properties resembling those of metals and chemical properties typical of NON-METALS (*e.g.* ARSENIC, GERMANIUM, SELENIUM). Many metalloids are used in semiconductors.

metallurgy (chemistry) Scientific study of metals.

metaphase (genetics) Second stage of MITOSIS and MEIOSIS, in which chromosomes are lined up along the equator of the nuclear spindle. Also termed: ASTER PHASE.

metaplasia (cytology) TRANSFORMATION of one NORMAL TISSUE type into another as a RESPONSE to a disease or ABNORMAL condition.

metastasis (histology) Process by which disease-bearing CELLS are transferred from one part of the body to another via the LYMPH and BLOOD VESSELs; the term is usually applied to the spread of cancers. The term also applies to the newly diseased AREA arising from the process.

metastatic (chemistry) Describing electrons that leave an ORBITAL shell, either entering another shell or being absorbed into the NUCLEUS.

metatarsal (anatomy) One of the ROD-shaped bones that forms the lower hind limb or part of the hind foot in tetrapods and the arch of the foot in human beings.

methanal (chemistry) HCHO An alternative term for FORMALDEHYDE.

methanoic acid (chemistry) HCOOH An alternative term for FORMIC ACID.

methanol (chemistry) CH_3OH Simplest PRIMARY ALCOHOL, a poisonous LIQUID used as a SOLVENT and added to ETHANOL to make METHYLATED SPIRITS. Also termed: METHYL ALCOHOL; WOOD SPIRIT.

methionine (chemistry) $CH_3S(CH_2)_2CH$-$(NH_2)COOH$ SULPHUR (*USA*: sulfur) containing AMINO ACID; a constituent of many proteins. Also termed: 2-amino-4-methylthiobutanoic ACID.

methyl alcohol (chemistry) An alternative term for METHANOL.

methyl chloroform (chemistry) An alternative term for 1,1,1-trichloroethane.

methyl cyanide (chemistry) An alternative term for acetonitrile.

methyl orange (chemistry) Orange dye used as a PH INDICATOR.

methyl red (chemistry) Red dye used as a PH INDICATOR.

methyl salicylate (chemistry) Methyl ESTER of SALICYLLIC ACID, used in medicine. Also termed: oil of wintergreen.

methylamine (chemistry) CH_3NH_2 Simplest primary AMINE, a GAS smelling like ammonia, used in making herbicides.

methylaniline (chemistry) An alternative term for TOLUIDINE.

methylated spirits (chemistry) General SOLVENT consisting of ABSOLUTE ALCOHOL.

methylation (chemistry) A CHEMICAL REACTION in which a methyl GROUP is added to a chemical COMPOUND.

methylbenzene (chemistry) An alternative term for TOLUENE.

methylbutadiene (chemistry) An alternative term for isoprene.

methylene blue (chemistry) Blue dye used as a PH INDICATOR.

methylphenol (chemistry) $CH_3C_6H_4OH$ DERIVATIVE of PHENOL in which one of the hydrogens of the BENZENE RING has been substituted by a methyl GROUP. There are three isomers (ortho-, meta- and para-), depending on the positions of the substituents in the ring. Also termed: cresol.

metre (m) (measurement) SI UNIT of length. 1 m = 39.37 inches. (*USA*: meter).

metre-candle (measurement) An alternative term for LUX. (*USA*: meter-candle).

metric system (measurement) Decimal-based system of units. *See* SI UNITS.

MGP (physiology/ biochemistry) An abbreviation of 'M'atrix 'G'la 'P'rotein.

MHC (1,2 physiology) 1 An abbreviation of 'M'ajor 'H'istocompatibility 'C'omplex; 2 An abbreviation of 'M'yosin 'H'eavy 'C'hain.

mho (measurement) UNIT of CONDUCTANCE. Also termed: RECIPROCAL OHM.

MHPG (biochemistry) An abbreviation of 3-'M'ethoxy-4-'H'ydroxy'P'heny'G'lycol.

micro- (measurement) Metric prefix meaning a millionth; x 10^{-6} (*e.g.* microfarad). It is sometimes represented by the Greek letter μ (*e.g.* μF).

274

microbalance (equipment) A BALANCE capable of weighing very small masses (*e.g.* down to 10^{-5} mg).

microbe (microbiology) Imprecise term for any MICRO-ORGANISM.

microbiology (microbiology) Biological study of MICRO-ORGANISMS.

micrometre (measurement) Small UNIT of length equal to 10^{-6} m, formerly called a micron. (*USA*: micrometer).

micron (μ) (measurement) Former name for the micrometre.

micronutrient (biochemistry) General term for any of the TRACE ELEMENTS or VITAMINS.

micro-organism (microbiology) Organism that may be seen only with the aid of a MICROSCOPE. MICRO-ORGANISMS include microscopic FUNGI and ALGAe, BACTERIA, VIRUSES and single-celled animals (*e.g.* protozoans).

microprocessor (computing) *See* COMPUTER.

microscope (microscopy) Instrument that produces magnified images of structures invisible to the naked EYE. There are two major optical types: the simple MICROSCOPE, consisting of one short focal-length CONVEX LENS giving a virtual IMAGE, and the COMPOUND MICROSCOPE, consisting of two short focal-length CONVEX lenses which combine to give high MAGNIFICATION. Highest magnifications are produced by an ELECTRON MICROSCOPE.

microtome (histology) Instrument for cutting thin slices (of the ORDER of a few micrometres) of biological materials for microscopic examination.

microtubule (histology) MINUTE cylindrical unbranched tubule composed of globular PROTEIN subunits found either singly or in groups in the CYTOPLASM of EUKARYOTIC CELLS, in which it has the skeletal FUNCTION of maintaining their shape. Microtubules are also associated with spindle formation, and hence are responsible for chromosomal movement during NUCLEAR DIVISION.

microwave (physics) ELECTROMAGNETIC RADIATION with a WAVELENGTH in the approximate range I mm to 0.3 m, *i.e.* between INFRA-RED RADIATION and radio waves.

microwave spectroscope (physics) Study of atomic and/or molecular resonances in the MICROWAVE region.

midazolam (pharmacology) A benzodiazepine drug that, administered by injection, can be used as an ANXIOLYTIC and sedative in preoperative medication.

mid-brain (anatomy) Part of BRAIN that connects the fore-BRAIN to the hind-BRAIN, concerned with processing visual information passed from the fore-BRAIN. Fishes, amphibians and birds have a well developed mid-BRAIN roof, the tectum, which forms the INTEGRATION centre (*USA*: center) of their BRAIN. Mammals have a less well developed mid-BRAIN. Also termed: mesencephalon.

middle ear (anatomy) AIR-filled part of the EAR that is inside the EAR DRUM and transmits sound waves from the OUTER EAR to the INNER EAR. Also termed: tympanic cavity.

mifepristone (pharmacology) A uterine stimulant that, administered orally or topically via vaginal pessaries, is used for termination of uterine PREGNANCY.

mil (1, 2 measurement) 1 A millilitre. 2 One-thousandth of an INCH, equivalent to 0.0254 mm.

mile (measurement) UNIT of length equal to 1,760 yards or 5,280 feet. 1 mile = 1.60934 kilometres. A nautical mile is 6,080 feet (= 1.85318 km).

milk sugar (chemistry) An alternative term for LACTOSE.

milk teeth (anatomy) First of two sets of TEETH possessed by most mammals. Human beings have 20 MILK TEETH. Also termed: deciduous TEETH.

milli- (measurement) Metric prefix meaning a thousandth; x 10^{-3} (*e.g.* milligram).

milligram (mg) (measurement) Thousandth of a gram.

millilitre (ml) (measurement) Thousandth of a LITRE, equivalent to a CUBIC centimetre (cc or cm^3).

millimetre (mm) (measurement) Thousandth of a METRE, equal to a tenth of a centimetre. 1 mm = 0.03937 inches. (*USA*: millimeter).

millimetre of mercury (mmHg) (measurement) UNIT of PRESSURE, equal to 1/760 atmospheres. (*USA*: millimeter of mercury).

milrinone (pharmacology) A phosphodiesterase inhibitor which can be administered by INTRAVENOUS injection or infusion to treat congestive HEART FAILURE and in acute HEART FAILURE.

min (measurement) An abbreviation of 'min'ute(s).

mineral acid (chemistry) INORGANIC ACID such as sulphuric (*USA*: sulfuric), hydrochloric or NITRIC ACID.

mineral oil (chemistry) HYDROCARBON oil obtained from mineral sources or petroleum (as opposed to an ANIMAL oil or vegetable oil).

mineral salts (chemistry) Dissolved salts that occur in soil, derived from weathered rock and decomposed plants. They contain essential nutrients for plant GROWTH, which are in turn utilized by herbivores (and carnivores that feed on them).

minute (1, 2 measurement) 1 UNIT of time equal to 1/60 of an hour. 2 UNIT of angular measure equal to 1/60 of a DEGREE. Both types of minutes are made up of 60 seconds.

MIS (physiology/ biochemistry) An abbreviation of 'M'üllerian 'I'nhibiting 'S'ubstance.

miscarriage (medical) An alternative term for a spontaneous ABORTION.

miscible (chemistry) Describing two or more liquids that will mutually dissolve (mix) to form a single PHASE. They can be separated by FRACTIONAL DISTILLATION.

MIT (biochemistry) An abbreviation of 'M'ono'I'odo'T'yrosine.

mitochondrion (cytology) CELL ORGANELLE in the CYTOPLASM of EUKARYOTIC CELLS, concerned with AEROBIC RESPIRATION and hence ENERGY production from the REDUCTION of ATP to ADP. Its shape varies from spherical to cylindrical. Large concentrations of mitochondria are observed in areas of high ENERGY consumption, such as MUSCLE TISSUE. Also termed: CHONDRIOSOME.

mitosis (genetics) The usual type of CELL DIVISION in which the parent NUCLEUS splits into two identical daughter nuclei, which contain the same number of chromosomes and identical genes to that of the parent NUCLEUS. Also termed: KARYOKINESIS.

See also MEIOSIS.

mixed number (mathematics) Sum of a whole number (INTEGER) and a FRACTION (*e.g.* 3 2/3, 12 15/16).

mixture (chemistry) COMBINATION of two or more substances that do not react chemically and can be separated by physical methods (*e.g.* a SOLUTION).

m.k.s. unit (measurement) METRE-KILOGRAM-second UNIT, a metric UNIT used in science in preference to c.g.s. units and now superseded by SI UNITS. Also termed: MKS UNIT; Giorgi UNIT (after the Italian physicist Giovanni Giorgi (1871-1950), who devised it).

M Med (education) Master of Medicine; -(Sc.) Master of Medical Science

mode (statistics) Of a GROUP of numbers, the number that occurs most often in the GROUP.

See also MEDIAN.

modem (computing) Acronym of 'mo'dulator/ 'dem'odulator, a device for transmitting COMPUTER DATA over long distances (*e.g.* by telephone line).

molality (m) (chemistry) CONCENTRATION of a SOLUTION given as the number of moles of SOLUTE in a KILOGRAM of SOLVENT.

molar (1 chemistry; 2 anatomy) 1 Describing a quantity of a substance that is proportional to its MOLECULAR WEIGHT (a mole). *See* MOLARITY. 2 Molar TOOTH.

molar concentration (chemistry) *See* MOLARITY.

molar conductivity (physics) Electrical CONDUCTIVITY of an ELECTROLYTE with a CONCENTRATION of 1 mole of SOLUTE per LITRE of SOLUTION. Expressed in siemens cm^2 mol^{-1}.

molar heat capacity (measurement) HEAT required to increase the TEMPERATURE of 1 mole of a substance by 1 KELVIN. Expressed in joules K^{-1} mol^{-1}.

molar solution (chemistry) SOLUTION that contains 1 mole of SOLUTE in 1 LITRE of SOLUTION.

molar tooth (anatomy) One of the rearmost TEETH of a mammal, used for crushing and grinding food. They are absent from the MILK TEETH.

molar volume (chemistry) VOLUME occupied by 1 mole of a substance under specified conditions.

molarity (M) (chemistry) CONCENTRATION of a SOLUTION given as the number of moles of SOLUTE in a LITRE of SOLUTION.

mole (mol) (chemistry) SI UNIT of amount of substance. In chemistry, it is the amount of a substance in grams that corresponds to its MOLECULAR WEIGHT, or the amount that contains particles equal in number to the AVOGADRO CONSTANT. Also termed: gram-MOLECULE.

molecular biology (molecular biology) Study of biological macromolecules (*e.g.* NUCLEIC ACIDS, proteins).

molecular formula (chemistry) Method of describing the composition of a MOLECULE of a chemical COMPOUND, using the CHEMICAL SYMBOLS of the constituent elements with numerical suffixes that indicate the number of atoms of each ELEMENT in the MOLECULE *e.g.* H_2O and Na_2SO_4 are the MOLECULAR FORMULAe of WATER and SODIUM SULPHATE (*USA*: sodium sulfate), respectively. The MOLECULAR FORMULA gives no indication how the COMPONENT atoms are arranged.

See also EMPIRICAL FORMULA; STRUCTURAL FORMULA.

molecular orbital (chemistry) Region in space occupied by a pair of ELECTRONS that form a COVALENT BOND in a MOLECULE, formed by the overlap of two ATOMIC ORBITALS.

molecular oxygen (chemistry) O_2 DIATOMIC molecular form of OXYGEN.

molecular sieve (chemistry) Method of separating substances by trapping (absorbing) the molecules of one within cavities of another, usually a natural or SYNTHETIC ZEOLITE. MOLECULAR SIEVES are used in ION EXCHANGE, desalination and as supports for catalysts.

molecular spectrum (physics) *See* SPECTRUM.

molecular weight (chemistry) *See* RELATIVE MOLECULAR MASS.

molecule (chemistry) GROUP of atoms held together in fixed proportions by CHEMICAL BONDs; the fundamental UNIT of a chemical COMPOUND. The simplest molecules are DIATOMIC molecules, consisting of two atoms (*e.g.* O_2, HCl); the most complex are biochemicals and macromolecules. The atoms may be joined by COVALENT BONDS, DATIVE BONDS or bonds.

monatomic (chemistry) Describing a MOLECULE that contains only one ATOM (*e.g.* the RARE GASES).

mongolism (medical) An alternative term for DOWN'S SYNDROME.

Mono- (general terminology) Prefix meaning one (*e.g.* monobasic).

monoamine-oxydase inhibitors (MAOIs) (Pharmacology/ biochemistry) Drugs sometimes used in cases of depression. They take about three weeks to become effective, and have the disadvantage that they interact with certain substances to stimulate the release of NORADRENALINE (*USA*: norepinephrine) at the NERVE endings; this results in a sudden dangerous elevation of the BLOOD PRESSURE. The main substance liable to produce this effect is tyramine, which is found in many foods, *e.g.* cheese, or meat or YEAST extracts. Substances used in proprietary cough medicines and cold cures may have the same effect. The principal MAOIs are phenelzine and isocarboxazid.

Monobasic acid (chemistry) ACID that on solvation produces 1 mole of HYDROXONIUM ION (H_3O^+) per mole of ACID; an ACID with one replaceable HYDROGEN ATOM in its MOLECULE (*e.g.* HYDROCHLORIC ACID, HCl, and NITRIC ACID, HNO_3). It cannot therefore form ACID salts.

monocarboxylic acid (chemistry) CARBOXYLIC ACID with only one carboxylic GROUP (*e.g.* acetic (ethanoic) ACID, CH_3COOH).

monochromatic light (physics) LIGHT of a single WAVELENGTH.

monochromator (physics) *See* SPECTROMETER.

monoclinic (crystallography) Crystal form in which all three axes are unequal, with one of them perpendicular to the other two, which intersect at an angle inclined at other than a right-angle.

monoclonal (immunology) Derived from a single parent CLONE.

monoclonal antibody (immunology) ANTIBODY produced by a single-CELL CLONE and hence consisting of a single AMINO ACID sequence. Such CELL clones are produced by the artificial FUSION of cancerous and ANTIBODY-forming CELLS from the mouse SPLEEN. The HYBRID CELLS are grown in vitro as clones of cells, with each producing only a single type of ANTIBODY MOLECULE.

monocyte (haematology) Largest phagocytic LEUCOCYTE, of order of about 10 to 12 micrometres. Monocytes have monogranulated CYTOPLASM with a large oval NUCLEUS.

monohydrate (chemistry) Chemical COMPOUND (a HYDRATE) that contains 1 mole of WATER OF CRYSTALLIZATION in each of its molecules *e.g.* IRON(II) SULPHATE (*USA*: iron(II) sulfate) forms a MONOHYDRATE, $FeSO_4.H_2O$.

monohydric (chemistry) Describing a chemical COMPOUND that has one HYDROXYL GROUP in each of its molecules (*e.g.* ETHANOL, C_2H_5OH, is a MONOHYDRIC ALCOHOL).

monomer (chemistry) Small MOLECULE that can polymerize to form a larger MOLECULE. *See* POLYMER.

monosaccharide (chemistry) $C_nH_{2n}O_n$ Member of the simplest GROUP of carbohydrates, which cannot be hydrolysed to any other smaller units; *e.g.* the sugars GLUCOSE, FRUCTOSE.

monosodium glutamate (MSG) (chemistry) White CRYSTALLINE SOLID, a SODIUM SALT of the AMINO ACID GLUTAMIC ACID, made from soya bean PROTEIN and used as a flavour enhancer. Eating it can cause an allergic REACTION in certain susceptible people.

monovalent (chemistry) Having a VALENCE of one. Also termed: UNIVALENT.

morphine (pharmacology) SEDATIVE, NARCOTIC ALKALOID drug isolated from OPIUM, used for pain relief. Also termed: morphia.

morpholine (chemistry) C_4H_9O HETEROCYCLIC secondary AMINE, used as a SOLVENT.

morphology (biology) Study of the ORIGIN, development and structures of organisms.

mosaic (genetics) Organism derived from a single EMBRYO that displays the characteristics of different genes in different parts of its body. *See* CHIMAERA.

Moseley's law (physics) The X-RAY SPECTRUM of an ELEMENT can be divided into several distinct line SERIES: K, L, M and N. The LAW states that for certain elements the SQUARE ROOT of the FREQUENCY *f* of the CHARACTERISTIC X-RAYS of one of these SERIES is directly proportional to the ELEMENT's ATOMIC NUMBER *Z*. It was named after the British physicist Henry Moseley (1887-1915).

motile (biology) Describing an organism or structure that can move.

motor neurone (cytology) NERVE CELL that transmits impulses from the SPINAL CORD or the BRAIN to a MUSCLE. Also termed: motor neuron; motor NERVE.

MPGF (physiology/ biochemistry) An abbreviation of 'M'ajor 'P'ro'G'lucagon 'F'ragment.

MPP⁺ (biochemistry) An abbreviation of 1-'M'ethyl-4-'P'henyl'P'yridinium.

MPR (physiology/ biochemistry) An abbreviation of 'M'annose-6-'P'hosphate 'R'eceptor.

m pt (physics) An abbreviation of 'm'elting 'p'oint.

MPTP (biochemistry) An abbreviation of 1-'M'ethyl-4-'P'henyl-1,2,5,6-'T'etra-hydro'P'yridine.

MRI (physics) An abbreviation of 'M'agnetic 'R'esonance 'I'maging.

mRNA (physiology/ biochemistry) An abbreviation of 'm'essenger 'RNA'.

M.Sc. (education) - (Med.) Master of Science in Medicine; -(Med.Sc.) Master of Science in Medical Science; -(N) Master of Science in Nursing; -(Nutr.) Master of Science in Nutrition; -(Pharm.) Master of Science in Pharmacy; -(V. of Sc.) Master of Veterinary Science.

MSH (physiology/ biochemistry) Abbreviation of 'M'elanocyte-'S'timulating 'H'ormone.

MT (biochemistry) An abbreviation of 3-'M'ethyoxy'T'yramine.

mucin (biochemistry) Any of a number of GLYCOPROTEINS that occur in MUCUS.

mucous membrane (histology) Moist, MUCUS-lined EPITHELIUM which itself lines VERTEBRATE internal cavities, including the alimentary, respiratory and reproductive tracts, which are continuous with the outer ENVIRONMENT.

mucus (cytology) Slimy substance secreted by the GOBLET CELLS of MUCOUS MEMBRANE. It lubricates and protects the epithelial layer on which it is secreted.

multicellular (biology) Describing plants and animals that have bodies consisting of many CELLS.

multi-CSF (physiology/ biochemistry) An abbreviation of 'multi'potential 'C'olony-'S'timulating 'F'actor.

multifactorial inheritance (genetics) Existence of more than two ALLELES for one GENE; *e.g.* as in A, B, O blood grouping.

multimeter (physics) Instrument that can be used as a galvanometer, AMMETER and VOLTMETER.

multiple bond (chemistry) CHEMICAL BOND that contains more electrons than a SINGLE BOND (which contains 2 electrons); *e.g.* a DOUBLE BOND (4 electrons) or a TRIPLE BOND (6 electrons).

muscle (histology) ANIMAL TISSUE that contracts (by means of MUSCLE fibres [*USA*: muscle fibers]) to produce movement, tension and mechanical ENERGY. *See* INVOLUNTARY MUSCLE; VOLUNTARY MUSCLE.

mutagen (toxicology) Chemical or physical agent that induces or increases the rate of MUTATION; *e.g.* ETHYL methane sulphonate (*USA*: ethyl methan-sulfonate), ultra-violet LIGHT, X-RAYS and gamma-rays.

mutant (molecular biology) Organism that arises by MUTATION.

mutarotation (chemistry) Change in the OPTICAL ACTIVITY of a SOLUTION containing photo-active substances, such as sugars.

mutation (molecular biology) Alteration in the sequence of bases encoded by DNA, resulting in a permanent inheritable change in the GENE and consequently the PROTEIN encoded. MUTATIONS may occur in different ways and may be induced by a MUTAGEN or occur spontaneously. A MUTATION can be detrimental, *e.g.* those thought to be involved in CARCINOGENESIS (formation of CANCER). However, some MUTATIONS can be advantageous, *e.g.* in EVOLUTION, where favourable characteristics may be endowed.

mutualism (biology) Relationship between two organisms from which each benefits (*e.g.* CELLULOSE-digesting MICRO-ORGANISMS and animals, such as ruminants, whose GUT they inhabit).

See also SYMBIOSIS.

MVV (physiology) An abbreviation of 'M'aximal 'V'oluntary 'V'entilation.

mycelium (mycology) MASS of hyphae that form the body of a FUNGUS.

mycology (mycology) Scientific study of FUNGI.

Mycota (taxonomy) Division (PHYLUM) that includes the FUNGI, usually included in the plant KINGDOM but sometimes accorded a KINGDOM of its own.

mycotoxin (toxicology/ mycology) TOXIN produced by a FUNGUS.

myelin sheath (cytology) Thin fatty layer of membranes, produced by SCHWANN CELLS, that covers the AXON of most VERTEBRATE neurones (NERVE CELLS).

myeloid tissue (histology) TISSUE usually present in BONE MARROW which produces RED BLOOD CELLS and other BLOOD constituents.

myocardial (anatomy) Relating to MYO-CARDIUM.

myocardium (histology) MUSCLE TISSUE of the VERTEBRATE HEART.

myoglobin (biochemistry) In VERTEBRATE MUSCLE FIBRE (*USA*: muscle fiber), a haem (*USA*: heme) PROTEIN capable of binding with one ATOM of OXYGEN per MOLECULE.

myology (histology) Study of muscles.

myopia (medical) Short-sightedness, a VISUAL DEFECT in which the eyeball is too long (front to back) so that rays of LIGHT entering the EYE from distant objects are brought to a FOCUS in front of the RETINA. It can be corrected with spectacles or contact lenses made from diverging (CONCAVE) lenses.

See also HYPERMETROPIA.

myosin (biochemistry) Fibrous PROTEIN which, with ACTIN, makes up MUSCLE. Movement of MYOSIN fibres (*USA*: myosin fibers) between ACTIN fibres (*USA*: actin fibers) causes MUSCLE contraction.

myxoedema (medical/ biochemistry) A disorder caused by lack of HORMONES from the THYROID GLAND; if present at birth it causes cretinism.

N

N (biochemistry) A symbol for asparagine.

Na (chemistry) The CHEMICAL SYMBOL for SODIUM. The symbol is derived from Latin *natrium*.

NA (1, 2 general terminology) 1 An abbreviation of 'N'ot 'A'pplicable. 2 An abbreviation of 'N'ot 'A'vailable.

Na$_E$ (physiology/ biochemistry) A symbol for exchangeable body SODIUM.

NAD (biochemistry) An abbreviation of 'N'ictinamide-'A'denine 'D'inucleotide. Co-ENZYME form of the VITAMIN NICOTINIC ACID, necessary in certain ENZYME-catalysed OXIDATION-REDUCTION REACTIONS in CELLS. Its reduced form is a PRECURSOR in the fixation of CARBON DIOXIDE in chloroplasts during PHOTOSYNTHESIS.

NADP (biochemistry) An abbreviation of 'N'icotinamide-'A'denine 'D'inucleotide 'P'hosphate.

nail (histology) Layer of KERATIN that grows on the upper surface of the fingers of human beings and other primates (except tree-shrews, which have claws).

nano- (measurement) Prefix meaning a thousand-millionth; x 10^{-9}; *e.g.* 1 NANOSECOND is 10^{-9} s.

nanometre (measurement) Thousand-millionth of a METRE (*USA*: meter).; 10^{-9} m. It is the usual UNIT for wavelengths of LIGHT. (*USA*: nanometer).

nanosecond (nS) (measurement) One billionth of a second. Also termed nsec.

naphthalene (chemistry) $C_{10}H_8$ SOLID aromatic HYDROCARBON that consists of two fused BENZENE RINGS, INSOLUBLE in WATER but SOLUBLE in hot ETHANOL. It is a starting material in the manufacture of dyes.

Napierian logarithm (mathematics) LOGARITHM to the BASE e ($e = 2.71828...$), named after the Scottish mathematician John Napier (1550-1617). Also termed: NATURAL LOGARITHM.

narc. (biochemistry) An abbreviation of 'narc'otic.

narcosis (medical) A state of unconsciousness or extreme drowsiness induced by a NARCOTIC drug.

narcotic (pharmacology) ANALGESIC drug that, in addition to killing pain, causes loss of sensation or consciousness (*e.g.* MORPHINE and other opiates).

narcotic antagonist (pharmacology) Any drug that reduces the effects of a NARCOTIC.

nares (anatomy) The external openings of the nose; the nostrils.

NAS (education) An abbreviation of 'N'ational 'A'cademy of 'S'cience.

nasal cavity (anatomy) Cavity located in the HEAD of tetrapods, containing the OLFACTORY SENSE ORGANS.

nasopharyngeal (anatomy) Pertaining to the part of the PHARYNX above the LEVEL of the SOFT PALATE.

National Science Foundation (NSF) (governing body) An American government agency supporting research and education programmes (*USA*: programs) to encourage interest in science.

natural abundance (chemistry) Relative proportion of the various isotopes in a naturally occurring SAMPLE of an ELEMENT.

natural cytotoxic cells (immunology) *See* KILLER CELLS.

natural logarithm (mathematics) An alternative term for NAPIERIAN LOGARITHM.

natural number (mathematics) One of the SET of ordinary counting numbers (*e.g.* 1, 2, 3, 4, etc.).

natural selection (genetics) One of the conclusions drawn by the British naturalist Charles Darwin (1809-82) from the theory of EVOLUTION: certain organisms with particular characteristics are more likely to survive and hence pass on their characteristics to their offspring, *i.e.* survival of the fittest. Thus the characteristics of a population are controlled by this process.

Naumenko/Feigin stain (histology) Histological staining technique for astrocytes.

Nauta stain (histology) Histological staining technique. A SILVER stain that is taken up by degenerating axons, and hence identifies dead or degenerating neurons.

Nb (chemistry) The CHEMICAL SYMBOL for NIOBIUM.

NB (general terminology) An abbreviation of *'N'ota 'B'ene,* Latin, meaning 'note well'.

near infra-red or ultraviolet (physics) Parts of the INFRA-RED or ULTRAVIOLET regions of the ELECTROMAGNETIC SPECTRUM that are close to the visible region.

nearsightedness (medical) An alternative term for MYOPIA.

NEFA (physiology/ biochemistry) An abbreviation of 'Non'E'sterified free 'F'atty 'A'cid.

negative feedback (cybermetics) *See* FEEDBACK.

negative number (mathematics) Number less than zero.

Nematoda (parasitology) PHYLUM of INVERTEBRATE animals that contains round, thread and eel WORMS. They have unsegmented bodies that taper at each end. Many nematodes are PARASITES (*e.g.* filaria).

nematode (parasitology) Worm of the PHYLUM NEMATODA.

neo- (general terminology) Prefix meaning new.

neodymium Nd (chemistry) Metallic ELEMENT in GROUP IIIB of the PERIODIC TABLE (one of the LANTHANIDES), used in special GLASS for lasers. At.no. 60; r.a.m. 144.24.

neo-Lamarckism (genetics) *See* LAMARCK-ISM.

neon Ne (chemistry) Gaseous nonmetallic ELEMENT in GROUP 0 of the PERIODIC TABLE (the RARE GASES) which occurs in trace quantities in AIR (from which it is extracted). It is used in DISCHARGE tubes (for advertising signs) and INDICATOR lamps. At. no. 10; r.a.m. 20.179.

neonatal (medical) Concerning the new-born.

neoplasm (histology) TUMOUR (*USA*: tumor) or GROUP of CELLS with uncontrolled GROWTH. It may be BENIGN and localized, or if CELLS move from their NORMAL position in the body and invade other organs the TUMOUR is MALIGNANT.

See also CANCER; METASTASIS.

NEP (biochemistry) An abbreviation of 'N'eutral 'E'ndo'P'eptidase.

nephritis (medical) INFLAMMATION of the KIDNEY.

nephroblastoma (medical) A MALIGNANT TUMOUR (*USA*: malignant tumor) of the KIDNEY arising from primative kidney-forming tissue. Also termed Wilm's tumour. (*USA*: Wilm's tumor).

nephron (histology) Functional filtering UNIT of the VERTEBRATE KIDNEY, consisting of BOWMAN'S CAPSULE and the GLOMERULUS.

neptunium Np (chemistry) RADIOACTIVE ELEMENT in GROUP IIIB of the PERIODIC TABLE (one of the ACTINIDEs); it has several isotopes. At. no. 93; r.a.m. 237 (most STABLE ISOTOPE).

nerve (anatomy) Structure that carries nervous impulses to and from the CENTRAL NERVOUS SYSTEM, consisting of a bundle of NERVE FIBRES (*USA*: nerve fibers).

See also NERVE FIBRE; NEURONE.

nerve cell (cytology) An alternative term for a NEURONE.

nerve cord (histology) Cord of nervous TISSUE in invertebrates that forms part of their CENTRAL NERVOUS SYSTEM.

nerve fibre (histology) Extension of a NERVE CELL. NERVE FIBRES (*USA*: nerve fibers) may be surrounded by a MYELIN SHEATH (except at the nodes of Ranvier), as in many vertebrates; or they may be unmyelinated and bound by a PLASMA MEMBRANE. (*USA*: nerve fiber).

nerve impulse (physiology) Electrical signal conveyed by a NERVE to carry information throughout the NERVOUS SYSTEM. External stimuli trigger NERVE IMPULSES in RECEPTOR CELLS, and travel along AFFERENTS towards the CENTRAL NERVOUS SYSTEM. Alternatively the impulses are generated within the CENTRAL NERVOUS SYSTEM and travel along efferents towards organs and tissues (*e.g.* along motor NERVES to muscles).

nervous system (anatomy) System that provides a rapid means of communication within an organism, enabling it to be aware of its surroundings and to react accordingly. In most animals it consists of a CENTRAL NERVOUS SYSTEM (CNS) that integrates the sensory input from PERIPHERAL NERVES which transmit stimuli from receptors (afrerents) to the CNS, allowing the appropriate RESPONSE from the electors.

net weight (nt wt) (measurement) Used on packaging and labelling to show the WEIGHT of the PRODUCT itself, not including the WEIGHT of the packaging the PRODUCT is stored in.

nettle rash (immunology) *See* URTICARIA.

network (physics/ computing) System of interconnected points and their connections; *e.g. a* grid of ELECTRICITY supply lines or a SET of interconnected terminals online to one or more computers.

neur. (medical) An abbreviation of 'neur'ological/ 'neur'ology. Also termed neurol.

neural (anatomy) Pertaining to NERVE CELLS or neurons, or pertaining to the NERVOUS SYSTEM.

neurinoma (histology) a BENIGN TUMOUR (*USA*: benign tumor) arising from the sheath of a NERVE. Also termed a neurofibroma.

neuro. (medical) An abbreviation of 'neuro'tic.

neuroanatomy (anatomy) The study of the structure of the NERVOUS SYSTEM, its constituents, and their connections.

neurochemistry (biochemistry) The study of the chemistry of neurons.

neuroglia (histology) CONNECTIVE TISSUE between NERVE CELLS (neurones) of the BRAIN and SPINAL CORD.

neurohumour (biochemistry) Any chemical substance specifically secreted by neurons, particularly substances involved in synaptic transmission such as NEUROTRANSMITTERS.

neurol. (medical) *See* neur.

neurology (medical) A medical speciality dealing with the diagnosis and TREATMENT of patients with damage to, or disorders of, the NERVOUS SYSTEM, and with the causation of the symptoms. It is not concerned with mental diseases that have no known pathological basis.

neuroma (histology) A TUMOUR (*USA*: tumor) composed of NERVE CELLS or NERVE FIBRES (*USA*: nerve fibers); a TUMOUR growing from a NERVE.

neuromuscular junction (anatomy) The INTERFACE between a motor NERVE FIBRE (*USA*: motor nerve fiber) and a skeletal MUSCLE.

neurone (cytology) BASIC CELL of the NERVOUS SYSTEM which transmits NERVE IMPULSES. Each CELL BODY typically possesses a NUCLEUS and fine processes: short dendrites and a long AXON. The AXON carries impulses to distant EFFECTOR CELLS and other neurones. Neurones also make functional contacts over the surface of shorter, thread-like projections from the CELL BODY (dendrites). Also termed: neuron; NERVE CELL.

neuropathology (medical) The branch of PATHOLOGY that is concerned with diseases of the NERVOUS SYSTEM.

neuropharmacology (pharmacology) The study of the effects of drugs on the NERVOUS SYSTEM.

neurosecretory cell (biochemistry) A neuron that secretes a HORMONE into the EXTRACELLULAR FLUID.

neurosurgery (medical) The medical speciality concerned with surgery on the NERVOUS SYSTEM, particularly on the BRAIN.

neurotoxicology (biochemistry) The branch of toxicology that deals with toxicants affecting the central and/or PERIPHERAL NERVOUS SYSTEM and with the nature and mechanisms of the process of toxic injury and recovery of these aspects of the NERVOUS SYSTEM.

neurotransmitter (biochemistry) Chemical released by NEURONE endings to either induce or inhibit transmission of NERVE IMPULSES across a SYNAPSE. NEURO-TRANSMITTERS are typically stored in small vesicles near the SYNAPSE and released in RESPONSE to arrival of an IMPULSE. There are more than 100 different types, *e.g.* acetylcholine, NORADRENALINE (*USA*: norepinephrine) and SEROTONIN. Also termed: transmitter.

neurotrophic (biology) Having a selective AFFINITY for NERVE tissue. RABIES for example, is caused by a NEUROTROPHIC VIRUS.

neutral (1 physics; 2 chemistry) 1 Having neither POSITIVE nor negative electrical CHARGE; *e.g.* a NEUTRON is a NEUTRAL SUBATOMIC PARTICLE. 2 Describing a SOLUTION with pH equal to 7 (*i.e.* neither acidic nor ALKALINE).

neutral oxide (chemistry) OXIDE that is neither an ACIDIC OXIDE nor a BASIC OXIDE (*e.g.* DINITROGEN OXIDE [N_2O], WATER [H_2O]).

neutralization (chemistry) CHEMICAL REACTION between an ACID and a BASE in which both are used up; the products of the REACTION are a SALT and WATER. The completion of the REACTION (end-point) can be detected by an INDICATOR.

neutron (chemistry) Uncharged PARTICLE that is a constituent of the atomic NUCLEUS, having a rest MASS of 1.67482 x 10^{-27} kg (similar to that of a PROTON). Free neutrons are unstable and disintegrate by BETA DECAY to a PROTON and an ELECTRON; outside the NUCLEUS

they have a MEAN LIFE of about 12 minutes.

neutron diffraction (chemistry) Technique for determining the crystal structure of solids by DIFFRACTION of a beam of neutrons. Similar in principle to ELECTRON DIFFRACTION, it can be used as a substitute for X-RAY CRYSTALLOGRAPHY.

neutron excess (chemistry) An alternative term for ISOTOPIC NUMBER.

neutron flux (chemistry) PRODUCT of the number of free neutrons per UNIT VOLUME and their MEAN speed. Also termed: NEUTRON FLUX DENSITY.

neutron number (chemistry) Number of neutrons in an atomic NUCLEUS, the difference between the NUCLEON NUMBER of an ELEMENT and its ATOMIC NUMBER.

neutropaenia (haematology) *See* AGRANU-LOCYTOSIS.

neutrophil (haematology) A granular leucocyte important in the IMMUNE SYSTEM because it ingests BACTERIA, whose PROTOPLASM can be stained by NEUTRAL dyes. Neutrophils have a NUCLEUS with 3 to 5 lobes connected.

newton (N) (measurement) SI UNIT of FORCE, defined as the FORCE that provides a MASS of 1 kg with an ACCELERATION of 1 m s^{-2}. It was named after the British mathematician and physicist Isaac NEWTON (1642-1727).

Newton per metre (N/m) (measurement/physics) A UNIT of SURFACE TENSION. (*USA*: Newton per meter).

Newton's formula (optics) For a LENS, the distances *p* and *q* between two conjugate points and their respective foci (f) are related by $pq = f^2$.

Newton's rings (optics) Circular INTERFERENCE fringes formed in a thin gap between two reflective media, *e.g.* between a LENS and a GLASS plate with which the LENS is in contact. There is a central dark spot around which there are concentric dark rings.

N gen (microbiology) An abbreviation of 'N'ew 'gen'us.

NGF (physiology/ biochemistry) An abbreviation of 'N'erve 'G'rowth 'F'actor.

niacin (biochemistry) VITAMIN B$_3$, the only one of the B VITAMINS that is synthesized by ANIMAL tissues. It is used by the body to manufacture the ENZYME nictinamide-adenine dinucleotide (NAD), and a deficiency causes the disease pellagra. Also termed: NICOTINIC ACID.

NIAID (education) An abbreviation of 'N'ational 'I'nstitute of' 'A'llergy and 'I'nfectious 'D'iseases.

NIC (chemistry) An abbreviation of 'NI'tro'C'ellulose.

niche (physiology) Status or way of life of an organism (or GROUP of organisms) within an ENVIRONMENT, which it cannot share indefinitely with another competing organism. Also termed: ECOLOGICAL NICHE.

nickel Ni (chemistry) SILVER-yellow metallic ELEMENT in GROUP VIII ofthe PERIODIC TABLE (a TRANSITION ELEMENT). It is used in VACUUM tubes, electroplating and as a CATALYST, and its ALLOYS (*e.g.* stainless steel, cupronickel, German SILVER, NICKEL SILVER) are used in making cutlery, hollow-ware and coinage. At. no. 28; r.a.m. 58.71.

nickel-iron accumulator (physics) Rechargable ELECTROLYTIC CELL (BATTERY) with a POSITIVE ELECTRODE of NICKEL OXIDE and a negative ELECTRODE of IRON, in a POTASSIUM HYDROXIDE ELECTROLYTE. Also termed: EDISON ACCUMULATOR; NIFE CELL.

Nicol prism (optics) Pair of calcite crystals glued together and cut in such a way that they polarize a beam of LIGHT passing through them. It was named after the British physicist William Nicol (1768-1851). *See* POLARIZED LIGHT.

nicotine (biochemistry) Poisonous ALKALOID, found in tobacco, which potentially binds to the RECEPTOR for the NEUROTRANSMITTER acetylcholine. It is used as an INSECTICIDE.

nicotinic acid (biochemistry) An alternative term for NIACIN.

NIDA (education) An abbreviation of 'N'ational 'I'nstitute of 'D'rug 'A'buse.

NIDDM (medical/ biochemistry) Abbreviation of 'N'on-'I'nsulin-'D'ependent 'D'iabetes 'M'ellitus.

NIDR (education) An abbreviation of 'N'ational 'I'nstitute of 'D'ental 'R'esearch.

NiFe cell (physics) An alternative term for NICKEL-IRON ACCUMULATOR.

NIH (institute) An abbreviation of 'N'ational 'I'nstitutes of 'H'ealth.

niobium Nb (chemistry) Metallic ELEMENT in GROUP VB of the PERIODIC TABLE (a TRANSITION ELEMENT). Its ALLOYS are used in high-TEMPERATURE applications and superconductors. At. no. 41; r.a.m. 92.9064.

nitrate (chemistry) SALT of NITRIC ACID, containing the NO_3^- ANION. NITRATES are employed as OXIDIZING AGENTS and commonly used as fertilizers, which may give rise to pollution of WATER supplies.

nitration (chemistry) CHEMICAL REACTION in which a nitro GROUP ($-NO_2$) is incorporated into a chemical structure, to make a NITRO COMPOUND. NITRATION of ORGANIC COMPOUNDS is usually achieved using a MIXTURE of concentrated nitric and SULPHURIC ACIDS (*USA*: sulfuric acid) (known as nitrating MIXTURE).

nitre (chemistry) Old term for POTASSIUM NITRATE, KNO_3, also commonly known as SALTPETRE.

nitric acid (chemistry) HNO_3 Strong extremely corrosive MINERAL ACID. It is manufactured commercially by the catalytic OXIDATION of AMMONIA to NITROGEN MONOXIDE (NITRIC OXIDE) and dissolving the latter in WATER. Its salts are NITRATES. The main use of the ACID is in making explosives and fertilizers.

nitric oxide (chemistry) An alternative term for NITROGEN MONOXIDE.

nitrification (chemistry) Conversion of AMMONIA and nitrites to NITRATES by the ACTION of nitrifying BACTERIA. It is one of the important parts of the NITROGEN CYCLE, because NITROGEN cannot be taken up directly by plants except as NITRATES.

nitrile (chemistry) Member of a GROUP of ORGANIC COMPOUNDS that contain the NITRITE GROUP (-CN). Also termed: CYANIDE.

nitrite (chemistry) SALT of NITROUS ACID, containing the NO_2^- ANION. Nitrites are used to preserve meat and meat products.

nitro compound (chemistry) ORGANIC COMPOUND in which a nitro GROUP ($-NO_2$) is present in the BASIC molecular structure. Usually made by NITRATION, some NITRO COMPOUNDS are commercial explosives.

nitrobenzene (chemistry) $C_6H_5NO_2$ An aromatic LIQUID ORGANIC COMPOUND in which one of the HYDROGEN atoms in BENZENE has been replaced by a nitro GROUP ($-NO_2$). It is used to make ANILINE and dyes.

nitrocellulose (chemistry) An alternative term for CELLULOSE trinitrate.

nitrogen N (chemistry) Gaseous non-metallic ELEMENT in GROUP VA of the PERIODIC TABLE. It makes up about 80 per cent of AIR by VOLUME, and occurs in various minerals (particularly NITRATES) and all living organisms. It is used as an INERT filler in electrical devices and cables, and is an essential plant nutrient. At. no. 7; r.a.m. 14.0067.

nitrogen cycle (biochemistry) Circulation of NITROGEN and its compounds in the ENVIRONMENT. The main reservoirs of NITROGEN are NITRATES in the soil and the GAS itself in the ATMOSPHERE (formed from NITRATES by DENITRIFICATION). NITRATES are also taken up by plants, which are eaten by animals, and after their death the NITROGEN-containing proteins in plants and animals form AMMONIA, which NITRIFICATION converts back into NITRATES. Some atmospheric NITROGEN undergoes fixation by lightning or BACTERIAL ACTION, again leading to the eventual formation of nitrogen dioxide NO_2.

nitrogen fixation (biology) *See* FIXATION OF NITROGEN.

nitrogen monoxide (chemistry) NO Colourless (*USA*: colorless) GAS made commercially by the catalytic OXIDATION of AMMONIA and used for making NITRIC ACID. It reacts with OXYGEN (*e.g.* in AIR) to form nitrogen dioxide. Also termed: NITRIC OXIDE.

nitrogen oxides (chemistry) Compounds containing NITROGEN and OXYGEN in various ratios, including N_2O, NO, N_2O_3, NO_2, N_2O_4, N_2O_3, N_2O_5, NO_3 and N_2O_6. The most important are DINITROGEN OXIDE, NITROGEN DIOXIDE and NITROGEN MONOXIDE.

nitro-reduction (biochemistry/ microbiology) The REDUCTION of aromatic amines by either BACTERIAL or mammalian nitro-reductase systems.

nitrous acid (chemistry) HNO_2 Weak, unstable MINERAL ACID, made by treating a SOLUTION of one of its salts (nitrites) with an ACID.

nitrous oxide (chemistry) An alternative term for DINITROGEN OXIDE.

nits (microbiology) The EGG containers of lice. *See* LOUSE.

NK (general terminology) An abbreviation of 'N'ot 'K'nown.

nm (measurement) An abbreviation for 'n'ano'm'etre.

NMDA (biochemistry) An abbreviation of 'N'-'M'ethyl-'D'-'A'spartate.

nmr (physics) Abbreviation of 'n'u-clear 'm'agnetic 'r'esonance.

No (chemistry) The CHEMICAL SYMBOL for NOBELIUM.

nobelium No (chemistry) RADIOACTIVE ELEMENT in GROUP IIIB of the PERIODIC TABLE (one of the ACTINIDES); it has various isotopes with half-lives of up to 3 min. At. no. 102; r.a.m. 255 (most STABLE ISOTOPE).

noble gas (chemistry) Any of the elements in GROUP 0 of the PERIODIC TABLE: HELIUM, NEON, ARGON, KRYPTON, XENON and RADON. They have a complete SET of outer electrons, which gives them great chemical stability (very few NOBLE GAS compounds are known); RADON is RADIOACTIVE. Also termed: INERT GAS; RARE GAS.

noble metal (chemistry) Highly unreactive METAL, *e.g.* GOLD and PLATINUM.

nocturia (medical) Excessive urination at night.

node (1 anatomy; 2 mathematics; 3 physics) 1 Thickening or junction of an anatomical structure, *e.g.* LYMPH NODE (GLAND), sinoatrial NODE, NODE OF RANVIER. 2 Meeting point of one or more arcs on a NETWORK. 3 Stationary point (*i.e.* point with zero AMPLITUDE) on a standing WAVE.

node of ranvier (histology) One of several regular constrictions along the MYELIN SHEATH of a NERVE FIBRE (*USA*: nerve fiber). It was named after the French histologist Louis-Antoine Ranvier (1835-1922).

non-homologous chromosomes (genetics) Any CHROMOSOMES that do not have an exactly matching pair. The main example is the SEX CHROMOSOMES, in which the X and Y are non-HOMOLOGOUS.

non-metal (chemistry) Substance that does not have the properties of a METAL. Nonmetallic elements are usually gases (*e.g.* NITROGEN, halogens, NOBLE GASes) or low-MELTING POINT solids, *e.g.* PHOSPHORUS, SULPHUR (*USA*: sulfur), IODINE; BROMINE is exceptional in being LIQUID at ordinary temperatures. They have poor electrical and THERMAL CONDUCTIVITY, form ACIDIC OXIDEs, do not react with acids and tend to form COVALENT BONDs. In ionic compounds they usually form anions.

non-Newtonian fluid (physics) FLUID that consists of two or more phases at the same time. The COEFFICIENT of VISCOSITY is not a CONSTANT but is a FUNCTION of the rate at which the FLUID is sheared as well as of the relative CONCENTRATION of the phases.

non-parametric (statistics) Describing significance tests that do not involve the assumptions of normality or HOMOGENEITY OF VARIANCE. In such tests, no assumptions are made about the distribution or parameters of the population from which the observations were sampled. The chi-square test is an example of a commonly employed NON-PARAMETRIC test. *Contrast* PARAMETRIC.

nonsense codon (genetics) One of the three codons that specify the end of a genetic message. These codons do not code for any AMINO ACID but signal the TERMINATION of the PROTEIN being synthesised. They are UAG ('amber'), UAA ('OCHRE') and UGA ('opal'). Also known as 'stop codon'. *See* GENETIC CODE; PROTEIN SYNTHESIS.

nonsense mutation (genetics) A MUTATION in which a codon that codes for an AMINO ACID is changed to a codon that codes for 'stop', resulting in a shortened PROTEIN. The DEGREE to which the PROTEIN is shortened depends on how far along the GENE the NONSENSE MUTATION occurs. *See*

GENETIC CODE; NONSENSE CODON; PROTEIN SYNTHESIS.

non-specific urethritis (medical/ microbiology) One of the most commonly encountered SEXUALLY TRANSMITTED DISEASES which produces FREQUENCY of micturition, some pain and a DISCHARGE. It is in many cases caused by the organism *Chlamydia trachomatis,* the organism of TRACHOMA, in others possibly by *Ureaplasma urealyticum;* the TREATMENT is by TETRACYCLINES or erythromycin.

nonsporulating (microbiology) Does not produce spores.

nonstoichiometric compound (chemistry) Chemical whose molecules do not contain small whole numbers of atoms.

See also STOICHIOMETRIC COMPOUND.

non-viable (microbiology) Not capable of independent life.

noradrenaline (biochemistry) HORMONE secreted by the MEDULLA of the ADRENAL GLANDS for the regulation of the CARDIAC MUSCLE, glandular TISSUE and SMOOTH MUSCLEs. It is also a NEUROTRANSMITTER in the SYMPATHETIC NERVOUS SYSTEM, where it acts as a powerful vasoconstrictor on the vascular SMOOTH MUSCLEs. In the BRAIN, levels of NORADRENALINE (*USA*: norepinephrine) are related to NORMAL mental FUNCTION, *e.g.* lowered levels LEAD to mental depression. (*USA*: norepinephrine).

norepinephrine (biochemistry) An alternative term for NORADRENALINE.

norm. (general terminology) An abbreviation of 'norm'al.

normal (1 mathematics; 2 chemistry) 1 A plane or line that is perpendicular to another.' At any point on a curve, the NORMAL is perpendicular to the tangent to the curve at that point. 2 Describing a SOLUTION that contains 1 gram-equivalent of SOLUTE in 1 LITRE of SOLUTION. It is denoted by the symbol N and its multiples (thus 3N is a CONCENTRATION of 3 times NORMAL; N/10 or decinormal is a CONCENTRATION of one-tenth NORMAL).

normal distribution (statistics) The statistical distribution in which the FREQUENCY of occurrences of values decreases with their distance from the MEAN. When plotted as a GRAPH, a NORMAL DISTRIBUTION looks symmetrically bell-shaped. The MEAN (the AVERAGE of all the individual values), the MODE (the value that occurs most often) and the MEDIAN (the half-way point between the highest and the lowest values) all coincide. The STANDARD DEVIATION is a measure of how steep-sided the 'bell' is. In biological DATA, many traits that show continuous VARIATION conform to a NORMAL DISTRIBUTION. Also termed Gaussian distribution.

normalization (statistics) Transforming DATA by mathematical operations to make them fit a preconceived pattern.

normoblast (haematology) Immature RED BLOOD CELL which still has a NUCLEUS. As the CELL matures and enters the bloodstream, the NUCLEUS breaks up, and the CELL containing the remains of the NUCLEUS is called reticulocyte. Finally, when it is mature, the RED BLOOD CELL has no NUCLEUS. Normoblasts are not seen in the circulation unless new red CELLS are being formed abnormally quickly.

Northern blotting (biochemistry) A similar procedure to SOUTHERN BLOTTING, except that the NUCLEIC ACID being transferred is RNA and not DNA. NUCLEIC ACIDS, previously resolved by agarose GEL ELECTROPHORESIS, are transferred to a NITROCELLULOSE FILTER by CAPILLARY ACTION. They are then bound to the sheet by heating and can be probed with RADIOACTIVE labelled (USA: labeled) NUCLEIC ACIDS followed by AUTORADIOGRAPHY. Whereas SOUTHERN BLOTTING was called after its inventor, NORTHERN BLOTTING got its name by analogy.

See also WESTERN BLOTTING.

nos. (general terminology) Numbers. The plural of no.

not applicable (NA) (general terminology) Term used in tables and charts to indicate that the information is not pertinent.

not available (NA) (general terminology) Term used in tables and charts to indicate that the information is not available.

notifiable diseases (microbiology) Certain communicable diseases that are by LAW notifiable to the appropriate authority.

Np (chemistry) The CHEMICAL SYMBOL for neptunium.

NPH insulin (physiology/ biochemistry) An abbreviation of 'N'eutral 'P'rolamine 'H'agedorn insulin.

NPN (physiology/ biochemistry) An abbreviation of 'N'on'P'rotein 'N'itrogen.

npt (physics) An abbreviation of 'n'ormal 'p'ressure and 't'emperature.

NREM sleep (physiology) An abbreviation of 'N'on'R'apid 'E'ye 'M'ovement sleep.

nS (measurement) An abbreviation of 'n'ano's'econd.

NSAID (pharmacology) An abbreviation of 'N'on-'S'teroidal 'A'nti-'I'nflammatory 'D'rugs.

NSF (governing body) An abbreviation of 'N'ational 'S'cience 'F'oundation.

NSILA (physiology/ biochemistry) An abbreviation of 'N'on'S'uppressible 'I'nsulin'L'ike 'A'ctivity.

NSILP (physiology/ biochemistry) An abbreviation of 'N'on'S'uppressible 'I'nsulin'L'ike 'P'rotein.

nsp (microbiology) An abbreviation of 'n'ew 'sp'ecies.

NSS (chemistry) An abbreviation of 'N'ormal 'S'aline 'S'olution.

nt (physics) An abbreviation of 'n'ormal 't'emperature.

N terminal (biochemistry) A term for the end of peptide or PROTEIN having a free - NH2 group.

NTP (physics) An abbreviation of 'N'ormal 'T'emperature and 'P'ressure.

See also STANDARD TEMPERATURE AND PRESSURE (STP).

NTS (physiology) An abbreviation of 'N'ucleus of the 'T'ractus 'S'olitarius.

nt wt (physics) An abbreviation of 'n'e't' 'w'eigh't'.

nuclear barrier (chemistry) Region of high POTENTIAL ENERGY that a charged PARTICLE must pass through in ORDER to enter or leave an atomic NUCLEUS.

nuclear division (genetics) *See* MEIOSIS; MITOSIS.

nuclear envelope (cytology) The double MEMBRANE that surrounds the NUCLEUS of EUKARYOTIC CELLS.

nuclear force (chemistry) Strong FORCE that operates during interactions between certain SUBATOMIC PARTICLES. It holds together the protons and neutrons in an atomic NUCLEUS.

nuclear isomerism (chemistry) Property exhibited by nuclei with the same MASS NUMBER and ATOMIC NUMBER but different RADIOACTIVE properties.

nuclear magnetic resonance (nmr) (physics) An effect observed when radio-frequency radiation is absorbed by matter. NUCLEAR MAGNETIC RESONANCE spectroscopy is used in chemistry for the study of molecular structure.

See also NUCLEAR MAGNETIC RESONANCE IMAGING.

nuclear magnetic resonance (nmr) imaging (medical/ physics) A technique of imaging by computer using a strong magnetic field and radio frequency signals to examine thin slices of the body. It has the advantage over computed tomography in that no X-rays are used, thus no biological harm is thought to be caused to the subject.

See also NUCLEAR MAGNETIC RESONANCE

nuclear medicine (medical/ radiology) The use of RADIOACTIVE substances in medicine. A common use of a RADIO-ACTIVE substance in the TREATMENT of disease is the use of RADIOACTIVE IODINE in THYROTOXICOSIS.

nuclear membrane (cytology) MEMBRANE that encloses the NUCLEUS of a CELL.

nuclease (biochemistry) Type of ENZYME that splits the 'chain' of the DNA MOLECULE. Nucleases that act at specific sites are called RESTRICTION ENZYMES.

nucleic acid (molecular biology) Complex ORGANIC ACID of high MOLECULAR WEIGHT consisting of chains of nucleotides. NUCLEIC ACIDS commonly occur, CONJUGATED with proteins, as nueleoproteins, and are found in CELL nuclei and PROTOPLASM. They are responsible for storing and transferring the GENETIC CODE. *See* DNA (DEOXYRIBONUCLEIC ACID); RNA (RIBONUCLEIC ACID).

nucleoid (cytology) In a PROKARYOTIC CELL, the DNA-containing region, similar to the NUCLEUS of a EUKARYOTIC CELL but not bounded by a MEMBRANE.

nucleolus (cytology) Spherical body that occurs within nearly all nuclei of EUKARYOTIC CELLS. It is associated with RIBOSOME SYNTHESIS and is thus abundant in CELLS that make large quantities of PROTEIN. It contains PROTEIN DNA and much of the nuclear RNA.

nucleon (chemistry) A comparatively massive PARTICLE in an atomic NUCLEUS; a PROTON or NEUTRON.

nucleon number (chemistry) Total number of neutrons and protons in an atomic NUCLEUS. *See* MASS NUMBER.

nucleophile (chemistry) ELECTRON-rich chemical REACTANT that is attracted by ELECTRON-DEFICIENT COMPOUNDS. Examples include an ANION such as CHLORIDE (Cl⁻) or a COMPOUND with a lone pair of electrons such as AMMONIA (NH_3).

See also ELECTROPHILE.

nucleophilic reagent (chemistry) Chemical REACTANT that contains ELECTRON-rich groups of atoms.

nucleophilic substitution (chemistry) SUBSTITUTION REACTION that involves a NUCLEOPHILE.

nucleoprotein (molecular biology) A COMPOUND that is a COMBINATION of a NUCLEIC ACID (DNA, RNA) and a PROTEIN. For example, in EUKARYOTIC CELLS DNA is associated with HISTONES and protamines; RNA in the CYTOPLASM is associated with PROTEIN in the form of the ribosomes.

nucleoside (molecular biology) COMPOUND formed by partial HYDROLYSIS of a NUCLEOTIDE. It consists of a BASE, such as PURINE or PYRIMIDINE, linked to a SUGAR, such as RIBOSE or DEOXYRIBOSE; *e.g.* ADENOSINE, cytidine and uridine.

nucleotide (molecular biology) COMPOUND that consists of a SUGAR (RIBOSE or DEOXYRIBOSE), BASE (PURINE, PYRIMIDINE or PYRIDINE) and phosphoric ACID. These are the BASIC units from which NUCLEIC ACIDS are formed.

nucleus (1 chemistry/ physics; 2 cytology) 1 The most massive, central part of the ATOM of an ELEMENT, having a POSITIVE CHARGE given by Ze, where Z is the ATOMIC NUMBER of the ELEMENT and e the CHARGE on an ELECTRON. It is composed of chiefly protons and (except for HYDROGEN) neutrons, and is surrounded by orbiting electrons. *See also* ISOTOPE. 2 The largest CELL ORGANELLE (about 20 micrometres in DIAMETER), found in nearly all EUKARYOTIC CELLS. It is spherical to oval, containing the genetic material DNA, and hence controlling all CELL activities. A NUCLEUS is absent from mature mammalian ERYTHROCYTES (RED BLOOD CELLS) and the mature sieve-tube elements of plants. It is surrounded by a double MEMBRANE that forms the NUCLEAR ENVELOPE.

nucleophilic addition (chemistry) A CHEMICAL REACTION in which a nucleophile adds onto an ELECTROPHILE.

null method (measurement) Any measuring system that establishes an unknown value from other known values, when a particular instrument registers zero, *e.g.* a POTENTIOMETER. Also termed: ZERO METHOD.

numeral (mathematics) A symbol that represents a number; *e.g.* Arabic NUMERALS 1, 2, 3, 4, 5, 6 etc. or ROMAN NUMERALS I, II, III, IV, V, VI etc.

numerator (mathematics) Top part of a FRACTION (the lower part being the DENOMINATOR).

NZAB (society) An abbreviation of 'N'ew 'Z'ealand 'A'ssociation of 'B'acteriologists.

NZASc (society) An abbreviation of 'N'ew 'Z'ealand 'A'ssociation of 'Sc'ientists.

O

object (optics) With a mirror, LENS or optical instrument, the source of LIGHT rays that form an IMAGE.

objective (microscopy) LENS of an optical system (*e.g.* MICROSCOPE) that is nearest the OBJECT.

obligate anaerobe (microbiology) MICRO-ORGANISM that grows only in complete or nearly complete absence of AIR or MOLECULAR OXYGEN.

OBP (physiology/ biochemistry) Abbreviation of 'O'dorant-'B'inding 'P'rotein.

obtuse (mathematics) Describing an angle that is more than 90 degrees but less than 180 degrees.

occlusion (1 biology; 2 chemistry) 1 Closure of an opening (*e.g.* the way an ANIMAL's TEETH meet when the mouth closes). 2 ABSORPTION of a GAS on a SOLID MASS or on the surface of SOLID particles by forming a SOLID SOLUTION, by the formation of a chemical COMPOUND, or by the CONDENSATION of the GAS on the surface of the SOLID.

ochre (chemistry) Mineral of clay and IRON(III) OXIDE (Fe_2O_3), used as a LIGHT yellow to brown PIGMENT.

OCR (computing) An abbreviation of 'o'ptical 'c'haracter 'r'ecognition.

octa-/ octo- (general terminology) Prefix meaning eight.

octadecanoic acid (chemistry) An alternative term for STEARIC ACID.

octahedral compound (chemistry) A chemical COMPOUND whose molecules have a central ATOM joined to six atoms or groups located at the vertices of an octahedron.

octahydrate (chemistry) A chemical containing eight molecules of WATER OF CRYSTALLIZATION. *See* HYDRATE.

octanoic acid (chemistry) $C_7H_{15}COOH$ Colourless (*USA*: colorless) oily CARBOX-YLIC ACID, used in the manufacture of dyes and perfumes. Also termed: CAPRYLIC ACID.

octet (chemistry) STABLE GROUP of eight electrons; the CONFIGURATION of the outer ELECTRON shell of most RARE GASes, and the arrangement achieved by the atoms of other elements as a result of most cases of CHEMICAL COMBINATION between them. Also termed: ELECTRON OCTET.

odd-even nucleus (chemistry) Atomic NUCLEUS with an odd number of protons and an even number of neutrons.

odd-odd nucleus (chemistry) Atomic NUCLEUS with an odd number of both protons and neutrons; it is usually unstable.

oedema (medical) A swelling due to the accumulation of excess tissue fluid. (*USA*: edema).

oesophagus (anatomy) Muscular tube between the PHARYNX and STOMACH (the gullet), through which food passes by PERISTALSIS. (*USA*: esophagus).

oestrogen (biochemistry) Female SEX HORMONE, a member of a GROUP of STEROID HORMONES that act on the sex organs. The most important is oestradiol, which is responsible for the GROWTH and activity of much of the female reproductive system. (*USA*: estrogen).

oestrous cycle (physiology) Reproductive CYCLE of female mammals during which there is a PERIOD of oestrus or 'HEAT', when OVULATION occurs and the female may be successfully impregnated by a male to achieve FERTILIZATION. The CYCLE is regulated by HORMONES. (*USA*: estrous cycle).

See also MENSTRUAL CYCLE.

OGF (physiology/ biochemistry) An abbreviation of 'O'varian 'G'rowth 'F'actor.

ohm Ω (measurement) The SI UNIT of ELECTRICAL RESISTANCE. It is the resistance of a CONDUCTOR in which the CURRENT is 1 AMPERE when a POTENTIAL DIFFERENCE of 1 VOLT is applied across it. It was named after the German physicist Georg OHM (1787-1854).

Ohm's law (physics) Relationship stating that the VOLTAGE across a CONDUCTOR is equal to the PRODUCT of the CURRENT flowing through it and its resistance. It is written $V = IR$, where V is VOLTAGE, I CURRENT and R resistance.

oil of vitriol (chemistry) Old name for SULPHURIC ACID (*USA*: sulfuric acid).

oil of wintergreen (chemistry) An alternative term for METHYL SALICYLATE.

-ol (chemistry) Chemical suffix that denotes an ALCOHOL or PHENOL.

oleate (chemistry) ESTER or SALT of OLEIC ACID.

olefin (chemistry) An alternative term for ALKENE.

oleic acid (chemistry) $C_{17}H_{33}COOH$ UNSATURATED FATTY ACID that occurs in many FATS AND OILS. It is a colourless (*USA*: colorless) LIQUID that turns yellow on exposure to AIR, and is used in varnishes.

oleum (chemistry) $H_2S_2O_7$ Oily SOLUTION of SULPHUR TRIOXIDE (*USA*: sulfur trioxide) (SO_3) in concentrated SULPHURIC ACID (*USA*: sulfuric acid). Also termed: DISULPHURIC ACID (*USA*: disulfuric acid); fuming SULPHURIC ACID (*USA*: fuming sulfuric acid).

olfaction (physiology) Process of smelling. In vertebrates, the incoming NERVE IMPULSES from the OLFACTORY SENSE ORGANS are processed in the OLFACTORY lobes of the BRAIN.

olfactory (physiology) Concerning the sense of SMELL.

oligo- (general terminology) Prefix that denotes small or few in number.

oligomer (chemistry) POLYMER formed from the COMBINATION of a few MONOMER molecules.

oncogenic (toxicology) CANCER-producing.

See also CARCINOGENIC.

oncology (histology) The study of MALIGNANT tumours (*USA*: maglignant tumors).

oncovirus (virology) An alternative term for RETROVIRUS.

on-line (computing) Describing part of a COMPUTER (*e.g.* an INPUT DEVICE) that is linked directly to and under the control of the CENTRAL PROCESSOR.

oocyte (biology) CELL at a stage of oogenesis before the complete development of an OVUM. A primary OOCYTE undergoes the first MEIOTIC DIVISION to give the secondary OOCYTE, which after the second MEIOTIC DIVISION produces an OVUM. *See* MEIOSIS.

opaque (physics) Not allowing a WAVE motion (*e.g.* LIGHT, sound, X-RAYS) to pass; not transmitting LIGHT, not TRANSPARENT.

operand (mathematics) An entity or quantity on which a mathematical OPERATOR acts.

operator (1 mathematics; 2 molecular biology) 1 Symbol or term that represents a mathematical operation to be carried out on a particular OPERAND. 2 Region of DNA to which a MOLECULE or repressor may bind to regulate the activity of a GROUP of closely linked structural genes.

operon (genetics) Groups of closely linked structural genes which are under control of an OPERATOR GENE. The OPERATOR may be switched off by a repressor, produced by a regulator GENE separate from the OPERON. Another substance, the EFFECTOR, may inactivate the repressor.

ophthalmic (medical) Pertaining to the EYE.

ophthalmology (medical) The branch of medicine dealing with the EYE and its diseases.

opium (pharmacology) Dried juice from a SPECIES of poppy; a bitter nauseous-tasting brown MASS with a heavy, CHARACTERISTIC SMELL. Its NARCOTIC ACTION, for which it is used both medicinally and as an abused drug, depends on the ALKALOIDs it contains.

See also MORPHINE.

optic (optics) Concerning the EYE and vision.

optic nerve (histology) CRANIAL NERVE of vertebrates that transmits stimuli from the EYE to the BRAIN.

optical activity (chemistry) Phenomenon exhibited by some chemical compounds which, when placed in the path of a beam of plane-POLARIZED LIGHT, are capable of rotating the plane of POLARIZATION to the left (LAEVOROTATORY) or right (DEXTROROTATORY). Also termed: OPTICAL ROTATION.

optical axis (optics) Line that passes through the OPTICAL CENTRE (*USA*: optical center) and the CENTRE OF CURVATURE (*USA*: center of curvature) of a spherical LENS or mirror. Also termed: principal AXIS.

optical centre (optics) Point at the centre of a LENS through which a RAY continues straight on and undeviated. (*USA*: optical center).

optical character reader (computing) COMPUTER INPUT DEVICE that 'reads' printed or written ALPHANUMERIC characters and feeds the information into a COMPUTER system.

optical character recognition (OCR) (computing) Technique that uses an OPTICAL CHARACTER READER.

optical fibre (optics) *See* FIBRE OPTICS.

optical glass (microscopy) Very pure GLASS free from streaks and bubbles, used for lenses, etc.

optical isomerism (chemistry) Property of chemical compounds with the same molecular structure, but different configurations. Because of their molecular asymmetry they exhibit OPTICAL ACTIVITY.

optically active (chemistry) Describing a substance that exhibits OPTICAL ACTIVITY.

optical rotation (chemistry) An alternative term for OPTICAL ACTIVITY.

optics (optics) Branch of physics concerned with the study of LIGHT.

oral (anatomy) Concerning the mouth and, in some contexts, speech.

orange oxide (chemistry) An alternative term for URANIUM(VI) OXIDE.

orbital (chemistry) Region around the NUCLEUS of an ATOM in which there is high probability of finding an ELECTRON. *See* ATOMIC ORBITAL; MOLECULAR ORBITAL.

orbital electron (chemistry) ELECTRON that orbits the NUCLEUS of an ATOM. Also termed: planetary ELECTRON. *See* ATOMIC ORBITAL; MOLECULAR ORBITAL.

order (taxonomy) In biological CLASSIFICATION, one of the groups into which a CLASS is divided, and which is itself divided into families; *e.g.* Lagomorpha (lagomorphs), Rodentia (rodents).

order of reaction (chemistry) CLASSIFICATION of CHEMICAL REACTIONS based on the POWER to which the CONCENTRATION of a COMPONENT of the REACTION is raised in the RATE LAW. The overall ORDER is the sum of the powers of the concentrations.

ordinal number (mathematics) Number that indicates the rank of a quantity; *e.g.* 1st, 2nd, 3rd, etc. (as opposed to ordinary counting or CARDINAL NUMBERS: 1, 2, 3, etc.).

ordinate (mathematics) In CO-ORDINATE geometry, the *y* CO-ORDINATE of a point (distance to the *x*-AXIS). The other (*x*) CO-ORDINATE is the ABSCISSA.

organ (anatomy) Specialized structural and functional UNIT made up of various tissues, in turn formed of many CELLS, found in animals and plants; *e.g.* HEART, KIDNEY, leaf.

organ culture (histology) Maintenance of an ORGAN in vitro (after removal from an organism) by the artificial creation of the bodily ENVIRONMENT.

organ of corti (anatomy) ORGAN concerned with hearing, located in the COCHLEA of the EAR. It was named after the Italian anatomist Alfonso Corti (1822-88).

organelle (histology) Discrete MEMBRANE-bound structure that performs a specific FUNCTION within a EUKARYOTIC CELL; *e.g.* NUCLEUS, MITOCHONDRION, chloroplast, ENDOPLASMIC RETICULUM.

organic acid (chemistry) An ORGANIC COMPOUND that can give up protons to a BASE; *e.g.* CARBOXYLIC ACIDS, PHENOL.

organic base (chemistry) An ORGANIC COMPOUND that can donate a pair of electrons to a BOND; *e.g.* amines.

organic chemistry (chemistry) Study of ORGANIC COMPOUNDS.

organic compound (chemistry) COMPOUND of CARBON, with the exception of its oxides and metallic carbonates and carbides. Other elements are involved in ORGANIC COMPOUNDS, principally HYDROGEN and OXYGEN but also NITROGEN, the halogens, and SULPHUR (*USA*: sulfur).

organic cyanide (chemistry) *See* NITRILE.

organometallic compound (chemistry) A chemical COMPOUND in which a METAL is directly bound to CARBON in an organic GROUP.

organosilicon compound (chemistry) A chemical COMPOUND in which SILICON is directly bound to CARBON in an organic GROUP.

origin (mathematics) In CO-ORDINATE geometry, the point where the x- and y-axes cross (and from which CARTESIAN CO-ORDINATES are measured).

ornithine (chemistry) $NH_2(CH2)_3CH(NH_2)$-COOH AMINO ACID, involved in the formation of UREA in animals. Also termed: 1,6-diaminovaleric ACID.

ornithosis (medical/ microbiology) A disease carried by birds and transmitted to man, caused by the organism *Chlamydia psitiaci*. The organisms can be carried by budgerigars, parrots, pigeons, poultry, sea-birds and other more exotic birds also carry it. The organism causes headache, FEVER and coughing, and the INFECTION may proceed to pneumonia, or enlargement of the LIVER and SPLEEN.

ortet (genetics) The original organism from which a CLONE is derived.

orth. (medical) An abbreviation of 'orth'opaedic (*USA*: orthopedic).

ortho- (chemistry) Prefix that denotes a BENZENE COMPOUND with substituents in the 1, 2 positions.

See also PARA-.

orthoarsenic acid (chemistry) *See* ARSENIC ACID.

orthopaedic (orth.) (medical) Relating to the medical science of treating injured bones and muscles (*USA*: orthopedic).

orthophosphoric acid (chemistry) An alternative term for PHOSPHORIC(V) ACID.

Os (chemistry) The CHEMICAL SYMBOL for OSMIUM.

oscillator (physics) Device or electronic CIRCUIT for producing an ALTERNATING CURRENT of a particular FREQUENCY, usually controlled by altering the value of a CAPACITOR in the OSCILLATOR CIRCUIT.

oscilloscope (physics) An instrument incorporating a cathode-ray tube, time-base generators, triggers etc. for displaying a wide range of waveforms by electron beam.

osm (measurement) An abbreviation of 'osm'ole(s).

osmium Os (chemistry) Metallic ELEMENT in GROUP VIII of the PERIODIC TABLE (a

TRANSITION ELEMENT). The densest ELEMENT, it is used in hard ALLOYS and as a CATALYST. At. no. 76; r.a.m. 190.2.

osmium(iv) oxide (chemistry) OsO_4 VOLATILE CRYSTALLINE SOLID with a CHARACTERISTIC penetrating odour (*USA*: odor) reminiscent of CHLORINE. It is used in the preparation of tissues for observation with an ELECTRON MICROSCOPE. Its AQUEOUS SOLUTIONS are used as a CATALYST in organic reactions. Also termed: OSMIUM tetroxide.

osmoregulation (physiology) Process that controls the amount of WATER and ELECTROLYTE (salts) CONCENTRATION in an ANIMAL's body. In a saltwater ANIMAL, there is a tendency for WATER to pass out of the body by OSMOSIS, which is prevented by OSMOREGULATION by the kidneys. In freshwater animals, OSMOREGULATION by the kidneys (or by CONTRACTILE VACUOLES in simple creatures) prevents WATER from passing into the ANIMAL by OSMOSIS.

osmosis (physics) Movement of a SOLVENT from a DILUTE to a more concentrated SOLUTION across a semi-PERMEABLE (or differentially PERMEABLE) MEMBRANE, thus tending to equal the CONCENTRATION of the SOLUTE on either side.

osmotic diuretics (pharmacology) Inert DIURETIC compounds such as MANNITOL which are secreted into the KIDNEY proximal tubules and not resorbed. They therefore carry water and salts with them into the URINE.

osmotic pressure (physics) The PRESSURE required to prevent OSMOSIS i.e. the flow of WATER through a SEMIPERMEABLE MEMBRANE to the side on which there is a greater CONCENTRATION of a SOLUTE.

ossicles (anatomy) Small bones; usually used to refer to the small bones of the MIDDLE EAR.

ossification (histology) Process by which BONE is formed, especially the TRANSFORMATION of CARTILAGE into BONE.

OST (governing body) An abbreviation of 'O'ffice of 'S'cience and 'T'echnology.

outer ear (anatomy) Part of the EAR that transmits sound waves from external AIR to the EAR DRUM.

output device (computing) Part of a COMPUTER that presents DATA in a form that can be used by a human OPERATOR; *e.g.* a PRINTER, visual DISPLAY UNIT (VDU), chart plotter, etc. A machine that writes DATA onto a portable magnetic medium (*e.g.* MAGNETIC DISK or tape) may also be considered to be an OUTPUT DEVICE.

oval window (histology) Membranous AREA at which the 'sole' of the stirrup (stapes) BONE of the INNER EAR makes contact with the COCHLEA. Also termed: fenestra ovalis.

ovarian follicle (histology) An alternative term for GRAAFIAN FOLLICLE.

ovary (anatomy) Female reproductive ORGAN. In vertebrates, there is a pair of ovaries, which produce the ova (eggs) and SEX HORMONES.

ovary ossicle (anatomy) An alternative term for an EAR OSSICLE.

oviduct (anatomy) Tube that conducts released ova (eggs) from the ovaries after OVULATION. Also termed: FALLOPIAN TUBE.

OVLT (physiology) An abbreviation of 'O'rganum 'V'asculosum of the 'L'amina 'T'erminalis.

ovulation (physiology) In vertebrates, DISCHARGE of an OVUM (EGG) from a mature GRAAFIAN FOLLICLE at the surface of an OVARY. In mature human females, OVULATION occurs from alternate ovaries at about every 28 days until the MENOPAUSE occurs.

ovum (cytology) Unfertilized non-MOTILE female GAMETE produced by the OVARY. Also termed: EGG CELL; EGG.

oxalate (chemistry) ESTER or SALT of OXALIC ACID.

oxalic acid (chemistry) $(COOH)_2.2H_2O$ White CRYSTALLINE poisonous DICARBOXYLIC ACID. It occurs in rhubarb, wood sorrel and other plants of the *Oxalis* GENUS. It is used in dyeing and VOLUMETRIC ANALYSIS. Also termed: ETHANEDIOIC ACID.

oxatyl (chemistry) An alternative term for CARBONYL GROUP.

oxidase (biochemistry) Collective name for a GROUP of ENZYMES that promote OXIDATION within plant and ANIMAL CELLS.

oxidation (chemistry) Process that involves the loss of electrons by a substance; the COMBINATION of a substance with OXYGEN. It may occur rapidly (as in COMBUSTION) or slowly (as in rusting and other forms of corrosion).

oxidation number (chemistry) Number of electrons that must be added to a CATION or removed from an ANION to produce a NEUTRAL ATOM. An OXIDATION NUMBER of zero is given to the elements themselves. In compounds, a POSITIVE OXIDATION NUMBER indicates that an ELEMENT is in an

oxidized state; the higher the OXIDATION NUMBER, the greater is the extent of OXIDATION. Conversely, a negative OXIDATION NUMBER shows that an ELEMENT is in a reduced state.

oxidation-reduction reaction (chemistry) An alternative term for a REDOX REACTION.

oxide (chemistry) COMPOUND of OXYGEN and another ELEMENT, usually made by direct COMBINATION or by heating a CARBONATE or HYDROXIDE.

See also ACIDIC OXIDE; BASIC OXIDE; NEUTRAL OXIDE.

oxidizing agent (chemistry) Substance that causes OXIDATION. Also termed: ELECTRON acceptor.

oxime (chemistry) COMPOUND containing the GROUP $-NH_2OH$, derived by the CONDENSATION of an ALDEHYDE or KETONE with hydroxylamine (NH_2OH).

2-oxopropanoic acid (chemistry) An alternative term for PYRUVIC ACID.

oxyacid (chemistry) ACID in which the acidic (*i.e.* replaceable) HYDROGEN ATOM is part of a HYDROXYL GROUP, *e.g.* organic CARBOXYLIC ACIDS and phenols, and inorganic acids such as PHOSPHORIC(V) ACID and SULPHURIC ACID (*USA*: sulfuric acid).

oxygen O (chemistry) Gaseous nonmetallic ELEMENT in GROUP VIA of the PERIODIC TABLE. A colourless (*USA*: colorless) odourless (*USA*: odorless) GAS, it makes up about 20 per cent of AIR by VOLUME, from which it is extracted, and is essential for life. It is the most abundant ELEMENT in the EARTH's crust, occurring in all WATER and most rocks. It has a triatomic ALLOTROPE, OZONE (O_3). At. no. 8; r.a.m. 15.9994.

oxygen debt (physiology) Physiological condition that induces ANAEROBIC RESPIRATION in an otherwise AEROBIC organism. It occurs during ANOXIA, caused *e.g.* by violent exercise.

oxyhaemoglobin (haematology) PRODUCT of RESPIRATION formed by the COMBINATION of OXYGEN and HAEMOGLOBIN (*USA*: hemaglobin). (*USA*: oxyhemoglobin).

ozone (chemistry) O_3 ALLOTROPE of OXYGEN that contains three atoms in its MOLECULE. It is formed from OXYGEN in the upper ATMOSPHERE by the ACTION of ULTRAVIOLET RADIATION, where it also acts as a shield that prevents excess ULTRAVIOLET RADIATION reaching the EARTH's surface. It is a powerful OXIDIZING AGENT, often used in ORGANIC CHEMISTRY.

P

P (biochemistry) An abbreviation of 'P'roline.

P450 (genetics) A GENE superfamily, consisting of large groups of genes that code for proteins (CYTOCHROMES) which metabolise drugs or other foreign chemicals. The P450 CYTOCHROMES are coded for by 20 different families of genes, ten of which are the same in all mammals. Any one mammalian SPECIES may have between 60 and 200 individual P450 genes, each making a unique CYTOCHROME. The drug or chemical acts in many cases as the INDUCER for the relevant P450 GENE. In humans, POLYMORPHISMS of P450 genes are responsible for many of the examples of patients' VARIABLE responses to clinical drugs.

P$_{50}$ (physiology/ biochemistry) An abbreviation of partial pressure of O_2 at which haemoglobin (*USA*: hemoglobin) is half-saturated with O_2.

p (1, 2 physics; 3 chemistry) 1 An abbreviation of 'p'article; 2 An abbreviation of 'p'roton; 3 An abbreviation of 'p'ara.

Pa (1 chemistry; 2 measurement) 1 The CHEMICAL SYMBOL for ELEMENT 91, PROTACTINIUM. 2 An abbreviation of 'Pa'scal (SI unit of pressure).

PABA (chemistry) An abbreviation of 'P'ara-'A'mino'B'enzoic 'A'cid. An ORGANIC ACID found in YEAST. It absorbs ULTRAVIOLET RADIATION and is used in suntan lotions.

pachymeningitis (histology) INFLAMMATION of the dura mater of the BRAIN. *See* MENINGITIS.

pachytene (genetics) A stage in PROPHASE or first DIVISION of MEIOSIS, in which the paired chromosomes shorten and thicken, appearing as two chromatids.

Pacinian corpuscle (histology) A small structure about 4 mm long found below the SKIN and in other parts of the body,which in SECTION is like an oval onion. It is attached to a sensory NERVE FIBRE (*USA*: nerve fiber), and is sensitive to PRESSURE. The structure is named after the Italian anatomist, F. Pacini (1812-83).

packing fraction (radiology) Difference between the actual MASS of an ISOTOPE and the nearest whole number divided by the MASS NUMBER.

paediatrics (medicine) The medical speciality concerned with childhood diseases and disorders. (*USA*: pediatrics).

PAF (physiology/ haematology) An abbreviation of 'P'latelet-'A'ctivating 'F'actor.

PAH (biochemistry) An abbreviation of 'P'ara-'A'mino'H'ippuric acid.

palladium Pd (chemistry) SILVER-white metallic ELEMENT in GROUP VIII of the PERIODIC TABLE (a TRANSITION ELEMENT), used as a CATALYST and in making jewellery. At. no. 46; r.a.m. 106.4.

palmitic acid (chemistry) $C_{15}H_{31}COOH$ Long-chain CARBOXYLIC ACID which occurs in oils and fats (*e.g.* palm oil) as its glyceryl ESTER, used in making SOAP.

PAM (physiology/ haematology) An abbreviation of 'P'ulmonary 'A'lveolar 'M'acrophage.

pancreas (anatomy) GLAND situated near the DUODENUM that has digestive and endocrine functions. The ENZYMES AMYLASE, trypsin and LIPASE are released from it during DIGESTION. Special groups of CELLS (the ISLETS OF LANGERHANS) produce the HORMONES INSULIN and glueagon for the control of BLOOD SUGAR levels.

pandemic (epidemiology) Describing a disease that affects people or animals throughout the world.

See also ENDEMIC; EPIDEMIC.

pantothenic acid (biochemistry) A constituent of COENZYME A, a CARRIER of ACYL GROUPS in biochemical processes. It is required as a B VITAMIN by many organisms, including vertebrates and YEAST.

papain (biochemistry) Proteolytic ENZYME, which digests proteins, found in various fruits and used as a meat tenderizer.

paper chromatography (chemistry) Type of CHROMATOGRAPHY in which the mobile PHASE is LIQUID and the stationary PHASE is porous paper. Compounds are separated on the paper, and can then be identified.

papovavirus (virology) Member of a GROUP of double-stranded DNA VIRUSES which infect the CELLS of higher vertebrates, in which they can cause tumours (*USA*: tumors).

para- (1, 2 chemistry) 1 Prefix that denotes the form of DIATOMIC MOLECULE in which both nuclei have opposite spin directions. 2 Relating to the 1, 4 positions in the BENZENE RING. Also termed *p-*.

See also meta-, ortho-.

paraffin wax (chemistry) MIXTURE of SOLID paraffins (ALKANES) which takes the form of a white TRANSLUCENT SOLID that melts below 80°C. It is used to make candles. Also termed: PETROLEUM WAX.

paraformaldehyde (chemistry) An alternative term for POLYMETHANAL.

paraldehyde (chemistry) $(CH_3CHO)_3$ A CYCLIC TRIMER formed by the polymerization of ACETALDEHYDE (ETHANAL), used as a sleep-inducing drug. Also termed: ETHANAL TRIMER.

parallel circuit (physics) Electrical circuit in which the voltage supply is connected to each side of all the components so that only a fraction of the total current flows through each of them.

See also SERIES CIRCUIT.

paramagnetism (physics) Property of substances that possess a small permanent magnetic moment because of the presence of odd (unpaired) electrons; the substance becomes magnetized in a MAGNETIC FIELD as the magnetic moments align.

parasite (parasitology) Organism that forms the beneficial partner in PARASITISM.

parasitism (parasitology) The intimate relationship between two organisms in which one (the PARASITE) derives benefit from the other (the HOST), usually to obtain food or physical support. PARASITISM can have minor or major effects on the survival of the HOST.

See also COMMENSALISM; SYMBIOSIS.

parasympathetic nervous system (anatomy) Branch of the AUTONOMIC NERVOUS SYSTEM used in involuntary activities, for which ACETYLCHOLINE is the transmitter substance. Effects of the PARASYMPATHETIC NERVOUS SYSTEM generally counteract those of the SYMPATHETIC NERVOUS SYSTEM.

parathyroid (anatomy) Four ENDOCRINE GLANDS embedded in the THYROID in the neck which release a HORMONE that controls the levels of CALCIUM in the BLOOD.

parietal cells (histology) Large CELLS in the lining of the STOMACH that secrete hydrochloric acid.

Parkinson's disease (medical) A disease of the nervous system first described by the British physician James Parkinson (1775-1824). PARKINSON'S disease is a result of a degenerative process in the substantia nigra, a pigmented NUCLEUS in the BRAIN stem, which employs the substance DOPAMINE as the transmitter of nerve impulses to the corpus striatum, one of the basal ganglia of the BRAIN, in which there is consequuently a deficiency of DOPAMINE.

parthenogenesis (biology) The development of an unfertilized egg into an adult organism. Virgin birth. This occurs naturally in bees and ants and in some animal species development of an ovum can be induced chemically or by pricking with a fine glass fibre (*USA*: glass fiber). The result is a clone of the mother cell identical in all respects. Only females can

be produced by PARTHENOGENESIS, as no Y chromosome is present.

partial derivative (mathematics) The DERIVATIVE of a FUNCTION with respect to one of its variables, all other variables in the FUNCTION being taken as CONSTANT. Also termed: partial differential.

partial fraction (mathematics) One of the COMPONENT fractions into which another FRACTION can be separated (so that the sum of the partial fractions equals the original FRACTION).

partial pressure (physics) *See* DALTON'S LAW OF PARTIAL PRESSURES.

particle (physics) MINUTE portion of MATTER, often taken to mean an ATOM, MOLECULE or ELEMENTARY PARTICLE or SUBATOMIC PARTICLE.

particle physics (physics) Branch of science concerned with the properties of ELEMENTARY PARTICLES.

partition coefficient (chemistry) Ratio of the concentrations of a single SOLUTE in two IMMISCIBLE solvents, at EQUILIBRIUM. It is independent of the actual concentrations.

parturition (physiology) Birth of a full-growth FOETUS (*USA*: fetus) at the completion of PREGNANCY (GESTATION).

PAS (histology) Abbreviation of 'P'eriodic 'A'cid – 'S'chiffs stain.

pascal (Pa) (measurement) SI UNIT of PRESSURE, equal to a FORCE of 1 NEWTON per square METRE (N m^{-2}). It was named after the French physicist and mathematician Blaise Pascal (1623-62).

pasteurization (microbiology) Process of heating food or other substances under controlled conditions. It was developed by the French chemist Louis Pasteur (1822-95) to destroy pathogens. It is widely used in industry, *e.g.* milk production.

patella (anatomy) BONE in front of the knee JOINT. Also termed: kneecap.

path. (general terminology) An abbreviation of 'path'ology.

pathetic nerve (histology) An alternative term for trochlear NERVE.

pathogen (microbiology) An organism, or other agent, capable of causing disease. Commonly used of MICRO-ORGANISMS such as BACTERIA and VIRUSES.

pathogenesis (microbiology) The ORIGIN and course of a disease.

pathogenic (microbiology) Producing disease.

pathognomonic (medical) Indicative of, or CHARACTERISTIC of, a particular illness.

pathognomy (1, 2 medical) 1 The study of how to recognize an illness from its symptoms. 2 Symptom or symptoms of an illness.

pathologic (medical) Due to or involving a morbid condition, as a PATHOLOGIC state.

pathology (path.) (medical) The study of morphological changes CHARACTERISTIC of ABNORMAL states, including both physiological (ENDOGENOUS) effects, effects caused by PATHOGENIC organisms and the adverse effects of EROGENOUS physical and chemical agents. It includes changes at the LEVEL of gross anatomy.

Paul-bunnell test (virology) A BLOOD test for infectious mononucleosis (GLANDULAR FEVER). Nameed after American physicians, J. Paul (1893-1971) and W.W. Bunnell (1902-1966).

Pb (chemistry) The CHEMICAL SYMBOL for ELEMENT 82, LEAD. The symbol is derived from Latin: plumbum.

PBI (biochemistry) An abbreviation of 'P'rotein-'B'ound 'I'odine.

p-block elements (chemistry) 30 nonmetallic elements that form Groups IIB, IVB, VB, VIB, VIIB and 0 of the PERIODIC TABLE (HELIUM is usually excluded), so called because their 1 to 6 outer electrons occupy p-orbitals.

P cells (1, 2 physiology) An abbreviation of 'P'rincipal CELLs in the renal tubules; 2 An abbreviation of 'P'acemaker CELLs of sinoatrial and atrioventricular nodes.

PCR (biochemistry) An abbreviation of 'P'olymerase 'C'hain 'R'eaction.

pd (physics) An abbreviation of 'p'otential 'd'ifference.

PDGF (physiology/ biochemistry) An abbreviation of 'P'latelet-'D'erived 'G'rowth 'F'actor.

PE (statistics) An abbreviation for 'P'robable 'E'rror.

PEC (physics) An abbreviation of 'P'hoto 'E'lectric 'C'ell.

peck (measurement) UNIT of dry CAPACITY equal to a quarter of a BUSHEL, or 2 gallons (= 9.092 LITRES).

pectin (chemistry) Complex POLYSAC-CHARIDE DERIVATIVE present in plant CELL walls, to which it gives rigidity. It can be converted to a GEL form in sugary ACID SOLUTION.

pectoral (medical) Relating to the chest.

pectoral (anatomy) Concerning the part of the front end of a VERTEBRATE's body which supports the shoulders and forelimbs.

pediat. (medical) An abbreviation of 'pediat'rics

pediatrics (medical) *See* PAEDIATRICS.

pediculosis (parasitology) INFESTATION with lice. *See* LOUSE.

pedigree (genetics) A diagram representing the genetic relationships between individuals. Usually drawn up with reference to one (or a few) specific traits, the PEDIGREE uses conventional symbols to show the sex of the individuals (usually squares for males, circles for females); a diagonal line through their symbol shows that the person is deceased. Whether or not the individual is affected with the trait in question is shown by having their symbol SOLID or open, perhaps with HETEROZYGOTES (proven or surmised) shaded.

peduncle (histology) Any bundle of NERVE FIBRES (*USA*: nerve fibers) in the BRAIN.

PEEP (physiology) An abbreviation of 'P'ositive 'E'nd-'E'xpiratory 'P'ressure breathing.

PEG (chemistry) An abbreviation of 'P'oly'E'thylene 'G'lycol.

PEL (toxicology) An abbreviation of 'P'ermissible 'E'xposure 'L'evel. *See* PERMISSIBLE DOSE.

pelvic (anatomy) Concerning the part of the rear end of a VERTEBRATE's body which supports the hindlimbs.

pelvis (1, 2 anatomy) 1 Part of the SKELETON (PELVIC girdle) to which a VERTEBRATE's hindlimbs are joined. 2 Cavity in the KIDNEY which receives URINE from the tubules and drains it into the URETER.

pemphigus (medical) A term used for SKIN diseases in which blisters develop.

penetrance (genetics) The FREQUENCY with which a DOMINANT ALLELE is expressed in the PHENOTYPE of the individual carrying it. A completely penetrant ALLELE is expressed in every case, and this is normally the position with DOMINANT ALLELEs having major effects. An ALLELE is said to have incomplete PENETRANCE if it is not always expressed (this will depend on the genetic background and on the ENVIRONMENT).

penicillin (pharmacology) Member of a CLASS of antibiotics produced by moulds (*USA*: molds) of the GENUS *Penicillium*. It inhibits GROWTH of some BACTERIA by interfering with CELL-wall BIOSYNTHESIS.

penicillinase (beta-lactamase I) (microbiology) ENZYME produced by some BACTERIAL SPECIES, which inactivates the antimicrobial activity of certain PENICILLINS (*e.g.* PENICILLIN G).

penis (anatomy) The male sex ORGAN through which SEMEN and URINE are discharged by way of the URETHRA. The shaft of the PENIS contains spongy TISSUE which fills with BLOOD during sexual excitement: the ensuing erection makes sexual intercourse possible.

pentahydrate (chemistry) A chemical containing five molecules of WATER OF CRYSTALLIZATION (*e.g.* $CUSO_4.5H_2O$).

pentane (chemistry) C_5H_{12} LIQUID ALKANE, extracted from petroleum and used as a SOLVENT and in organic SYNTHESIS. It has three isomers.

pentanoic acid (chemistry) $CH_3(CH_2)_3$ -COOH LIQUID CARBOXYLIC ACID with a pungent odour (*USA*: odor), used in perfumes. Also termed: valeric ACID.

pentavalent (chemistry) Having a VALENCE of five.

pentazocine (pharmacology) Mixed opioid AGONIST-ANTAGONIST used as an ANALGESIC. This is a NARCOTIC and, in the UK and US, a controlled substance.

pentose (chemistry) A MONOSACCHARIDE CARBOHYDRATE (SUGAR) that contains five CARBON atoms and has the GENERAL FORMULA $C_5H_{10}O_5$; *e.g.* RIBOSE and XYLOSE. Also termed: pentaglucose.

pentyl group (chemistry) An alternative term for AMYL GROUP.

pentylenetetrazole (pharmacology) Once believed to be a useful CNS stimulant as well as an ANALEPTIC agent. Because its effective dose is similar to doses that induce seizures, its only present utility is as a diagnostic aid in screening for latent epileptogenic foci, in characterizing the underlying cerebral disorders in individuals with documented cases of epilepsy and in BASIC research.

PEP (physiology) An abbreviation of 'P're'E'jection 'P'eriod.

pepsin (biochemistry) ENZYME produced in the STOMACH which, under ACID conditions, brings about the partial HYDROLYSIS of polypeptides which breaks down PROTEIN in the food.

peptic ulcer (medical) Ulcers in the STOMACH and DUODENUM are referred to as PEPTIC ULCERS. Duodenal ulcers are more common than those in the STOMACH, and more common in men than women, who are more liable to develop duodenal ulcers after the MENOPAUSE.

peptidase (biochemistry) ENZYME, often secreted in the body (*e.g.* by the INTESTINE), which degrades peptides into free AMINO ACIDS, thus completing the DIGESTION of proteins.

peptide (biochemistry) Compounds that consist of a relatively small number of AMINO ACIDS linked covalently through PEPTIDE BONDS (-NH-CO-). The PEPTIDE BOND is formed by the elimination of the atoms of WATER from the AMINO GROUP of one AMINO ACID and the CARBOXYL GROUP of another. Peptides polymerize to form proteins.

peptide bond (biochemistry) A BOND joining AMINO ACIDS to form peptides or proteins.

percentage (statistics) A FRACTION expressed in hundredths (with the DENOMINATOR omitted) *e.g.* one half = 1/2 = 50/100 = 50 per cent (often written 50%).

percentage composition (chemistry) Make-up of a chemical COMPOUND expressed in terms of the percentages (by MASS) of each of its COMPONENT elements *e.g.* ETHANE (C_2H_6), ETHENE (C_2H_4) both consist of CARBON and HYDROGEN but their respective approximate PERCENTAGE COMPOSITIONS are: ETHANE, 80 per cent CARBON + 20 percent HYDROGEN; ETHENE 85 per cent CARBON + 15 per cent HYDROGEN.

percentile (statistics) Hundredth part of a range of statistics (DATA) of equal FREQUENCY *e.g.* the 80th PERCENTILE is the value below which 80 per cent of all the values fall. The 50th PERCENTILE is the MEDIAN.

perdisulphuric(VI) acid (chemistry) H_2SO_5 White CRYSTALLINE COMPOUND, used as a powerful OXIDIZING AGENT. Also termed: CARO'S ACID; persulphuric acid (*USA*: perdisulfuric(VI) acid; peroxomonosulphuric acid (*USA*: peroxomonosulfuric acid).

perfect gas (chemistry) An alternative term for ideal GAS.

See also KINETIC THEORY.

perfect number (mathematics) Number that equals the sum of all its factors (except the number itself *e.g.* 28 (= 1 + 2 + 4 + 7 + 14) and 496 (= 1 + 2 + 4 + 8 + 16 + 31 + 62 + 124 + 248) are PERFECT NUMBERS.

periarteritis nodosa (histology) INFLAMMATION of the outer part of the wall of an ARTERY and the tissues immediately roundabout.

periarthritis (histology) INFLAMMATION of the tissues surrounding a JOINT.

pericarditis (medical) INFLAMMATION of the PERICARDIUM, the MEMBRANE surrounding the HEART. It may occur in association with coronary THROMBOSIS, VIRUS INFECTION, TUBERCULOSIS, rheumatic HEART disease or BACTERIAL INFECTION, or as the result of injury. There is pain in the chest, and if there is an EFFUSION of FLUID between the two layers of the PERI-CARDIUM the ACTION of the HEART may be affected. It may then be necessary to aspirate the FLUID.

pericardium (anatomy) The membranous sac which contains the HEART. It has two layers, between which is a CAPILLARY space containing a FILM of FLUID. This provides lubrication to assist the free movement of the HEART in relation to neighbouring structures. The outermost part of the PERICARDIUM is fibrous.

pericentric (genetics) *See* INVERSION.

perichondrium (histology) The thin MEMBRANE which covers CARTILAGE, except on free joint surfaces.

pericranium (histology) The periosteal MEMBRANE covering the SKULL.

perikaryon (cytology) An alternative term for CELL BODY.

perilymph (anatomy) The FLUID found in the INNER EAR separating the MEMBRANE of the LABYRINTH from the surrounding BONE. It does not communicate with the ENDOLYMPH, the FLUID inside the membranous LABYRINTH. *See* EAR.

perilymph (anatomy) FLUID that surrounds the COCHLEA of the EAR.

perimeter (medical) A device for measuring sensitivity of each part of the RETINA.

perimetry (medical) Measurement of the outer limits of the FIELD of vision of each EYE.

perinatal mortality rate (statistics) The number of stillbirths (babies born dead after 28 weeks) plus NEONATAL deaths (babies born alive but dying within aweek, regardless of gestational age at delivery) expressed as a proportion of 1000 total births.

perinatal period (physiology) The developmental PERIOD preceding birth; the last third of GESTATION.

perinephric (medical) Surrounding the KIDNEY.

perineum (anatomy) The fork, strictly the region between the genital organs in front and the ANUS behind.

period (1 chemistry; 2 physics) 1 One of the seven horizontal rows of elements in the PERIODIC TABLE. 2 Time taken to complete a regular CYCLE.

periodic acid - Schiff orange G (histology) A histological staining technique that may be used to make PITUITARY CELL types visible under the MICROSCOPE.

periodic acid - Schiff (PAS) (histology) A histological staining technique that may be used to make mucins and CARBO-HYDRATE groups, fungi etc. visible under the MICROSCOPE.

periodic disease (medical) Recurrent polyscrositis: a disease of unknown cause, inherited as a RECESSIVE trait, commonest among Arabs, Armenians, Jews and Turks, which usually starts before the age of 20; the patient suffers a VARIETY of symptoms.

periodic function (mathematics) FUNCTION that returns to the same value at regular intervals.

periodic law (chemistry) Properties of elements are a PERIODIC FUNCTION of their ATOMIC NUMBERS. Also termed: Mendeleev's LAW.

periodic table (chemistry) Arrangement of elements in ORDER of increasing ATOMIC NUMBER, with elements having similar properties, *i.e.* in the same FAMILY, in the same vertical column (GROUP). Horizontal rows of elements are termed PERIODS.

periodicity (chemistry) Regular increases and decreases of physical values for elements known to have similar chemical properties.

periods (physiology) *See* MENSTRUATION.

periorbita (medical) Periosteum of the bones of the orbit or EYE socket. (periorbital, adj.).

periosteum (histology) The thin MEMBRANE of CONNECTIVE TISSUE that surrounds the bones.

periostitis (medical) INFLAMMATION of the periosteum. It may follow injury, when the periosteum is stripped from the BONE and there is an extravasation of BLOOD, an open fracture, or BACTERIAL INFECTION in neighbouring tissues; it can be caused by TUBERCULOSIS and syphilis.

peripheral (1 computing, 2 medical) 1 Any device attached to COMPUTER but not forming part of the central processor or CORE store, *e.g.* a DISK, printer, visual DISPLAY UNIT. 2 A term applied to structures towards the outer parts or extremities, *e.g.* the PERIPHERAL as opposed to the CENTRAL NERVOUS SYSTEM.

peripheral nervous system (anatomy) That portion of the NERVOUS SYSTEM consisting of the NERVES and ganglia outside of the SPINAL CORD and BRAIN (CENTRAL NERVOUS SYSTEM, CNS).

peripheral neuropathy (medical) A disorder of the PERIPHERAL NERVOUS

SYSTEM. SOMATIC motor, sensory, and autonomic NEURONES may be equally or preferentially affected. Clinical manifestations reflect the distribution of the pathological changes among SOMATIC motor, sensory and autonomic NEURONES and include MUSCLE weakness, MUSCLE ATROPY, sensory disturbances and autonomic dysfunction. Neuropathies may be classified by AETIOLOGY (*USA*: etiology) as toxic, metabolic, hereditary, autoimmune, ischaemic, traumatic, neoplasmic, infectious or IDIOPATHIC.

peripheral unit (computing) Equipment that can be linked to a COMPUTER, including input, output and STORAGE DEVICES.

peristalsis (physiology) The process by which the contents are propelled along tubular organs, as in the intestines; contractions of the MUSCLE in the walls of the GUT pass in a WAVE-like motion along its length, being controlled by the nervous PLEXUS present there, *e.g.* in the OESOPHAGUS or INTESTINE to push food along.

peristriate cortex (histology) An alternative term for parastriate CORTEX.

peritoneal dialysis (medical) *See* DIALYSIS.

peritoneoscopy (laparoscopy) (medical) The examination of the peritoneal cavity and abdominal organs through an ENDOSCOPE passed through the abdominal wall.

peritoneum (histology) The MEMBRANE covering the inner walls of the abdominal cavity and the organs it contains. There are two layers, the MEMBRANE covering the wall of the cavity is the parietal layer, and that covering the abdominal organs the VISCERAL layer.

peritonitis (medical) INFLAMMATION of the PERITONEUM.

peritonsillar abscess (microbiology) (QUINSY) An ABSCESS round the TONSIL, usually occurring as the result of ACUTE INFECTION of the tonsils.

periventricular (medical) Near the ventricles of the BRAIN.

Perl's prussian blue ferric stain (histology) A histological staining technique that may be used to make FERRIC IRON visible under the MICROSCOPE.

permanent gas (chemistry) GAS that is incapable of being liquefied by PRESSURE alone; a GAS above its CRITICAL TEMPERATURE.

permanent magnet (physics) Ferromagnetic OBJECT that retains a permanent MAGNETIC FIELD and the magnetic moment associated with it after the magnetizing FIELD has been removed.

permanent teeth (anatomy) Second SET of TEETH used by most mammals in adult life (after they have displaced the first SET of milk or deciduous TEETH).

permanganate bleach (histology) A histological staining technique used for removing MELANIN.

permeability (1, 2 physics)1 Rate at which a substance diffuses through a porous material. 2 Extent to which a substance can pass through a MEMBRANE. Membranes may be semi-PERMEABLE, *e.g.* PLASMA MEMBRANE, which allows small molecules such as those of WATER to pass through. 3 MAGNETIZATION developed in a material placed in a MAGNETIC FIELD, equal to the flux DENSITY produced divided by the MAGNETIC FIELD STRENGTH. Also termed: magnetic PERMEABILITY.

permeable (physics) Porous; describing something (*e.g.* a MEMBRANE) that exhibits PERMEABILITY.

permissible dose (toxicology) That dose of a chemical that may be received by an individual without expectation of an adverse effect.

permutation (mathematics) Number of ways a SET of numbers can be arranged and ordered. For n numbers, there are $n!$ ways of arranging them n at a time, and $n!/(n - r)!$ ways of arranging them r at a time ($n!$ stands for FACTORIAL n).

pernicious anaemia (medical/ haematology) A condition resulting from the inability of the bone marrow to produce normal red blood cells because of the deprivation of a protein released by gastric glands, called the intrinsic factor, which is necessary for the absorption of vitamin B_{12} from food. An auto-immune mechanism may be responsible. (*USA*: pernicious anemia).

peroxide (1, 2 chemistry) 1 OXIDE of an ELEMENT containing more OXYGEN than does the NORMAL OXIDE of the ELEMENT. 2 OXIDE, containing the O_2^{2-} ION, that yields HYDROGEN PEROXIDE on TREATMENT with an ACID. Peroxides are powerful OXIDIZING AGENTS.

peroxomonosulphuric acid (chemistry) An alternative term for perdisulphuric (VI) ACID (*USA*: perdisulfuric acid). (*USA*: peroxomonosulfuric acid).

Perspex (chemistry) Trade name for the plastic polymethyl methacrylate.

persulphate (chemistry) SALT of PERDISULPHURIC(VI) ACID (*USA*: persulfuric(VI) acid), used as an OXIDIZING AGENT. (*USA*: persulfate).

persulphuric acid (chemistry) An alternative term for perdisulphuric(VI) acid (*USA*: perdisulfuric(VI) acid). (*USA*: persulfuric acid).

pertussis (medical/ bacteriology) An acute, highly infectious, disease of early childhood acquired by droplet infection and caused by the bacteria *Bordetella pertusis*. Also termed: whooping cough.

pesticide (toxicology) COMPOUND used in agriculture to destroy organisms that can damage crops or stored food, especially insects and rodents. Pesticides include FUNGICIDES, herbicides and insecticides. The effects of some of them, *e.g.* organic CHLORINE compounds such as dichloro-diphenyl-trichloroethane (DDT), can be detrimental to the ECOSYSTEM.

petri dish (laboratory equipment) Sterilizable circular GLASS plate with a fitted lid used in microbiology for holding media on which MICRO-ORGANISMS may be cultured. It was named after the German BACTERIOLOGIST Julius Petri (1852-1921).

petroleum wax (chemistry) An alternative term for parafin WAX.

P factor (physiology) An abbreviation of hypothetical 'P'ain producing substance produced in ischemic muscle.

PGO spikes (physiology) An abbreviation of 'P'onto-'G'eniculo-'O'ccipital spikes in rapid eye movement sleep.

PH (chemistry) Hydrogen ion concentration (grams of hydrogen ions per litre) expressed as its negative logarithm; a measure of acidity and alkalinity. *E.g.* a hydrogen ion concentration 10^{-4} grams per litre corresponds to a pH of 4, and is acidic. A pH of 7 is neutral while a pH of more than 7 is alkaline.

pH scale (chemistry) Scale that indicates the acidity or alkalinity of a SOLUTION. *See* PH.

phage (microbiology) *See* BACTERIOPHAGE.

phagocyte (cytology) CELL that exhibits PHAGOCYTOSIS.

phagocytosis (cytology) Engulfment of external SOLID material by a CELL, *e.g.* PHAGOCYTE. It is also the method by which some UNICELLULAR organisms (*e.g.* PROTOZOA) feed.

phalanges (anatomy) Bones in the digits of the hand or foot.

pharmacodynamics (pharmacology) The study of the effects of drugs upon the body.

pharmacokinetics (pharmacology) The study of how drugs are absorbed into, distributed and broken down in, and excreted from, the body.

pharmacology (pharmacology) The study of the action of drugs on living organisms; drug development, their use; their adverse effects and their beneficial effects.

pharmacy (general terminology) Preparation and dispensing of drugs, and the place where this is done.

pharynx (anatomy) AREA that links the BUCCAL CAVITY (mouth) to the OESOPHAGUS (gullet) and the nares (back of the nostrils) to the TRACHEA (windpipe). Food passes via the PHARYNX to the OESOPHAGUS when the EPIGLOTTIS closes the entrance of the TRACHEA.

phase (1 chemistry; 2 physics) 1 Any HOMOGENEOUS and physically distinct part of a chemical system that is separated from other parts of the system by definite boundaries, *e.g.* ICE mixed with WATER. 2 The part of a periodically varying waveform that has been completed at a particular moment, there being 360° or 2π RADIANS in a full CYCLE.

phase contrast microscope (microscopy) MICROSCOPE that uses the principle that LIGHT passing through materials of different refractive indices undergoes a change in PHASE, transmitting these changes as different intensities of LIGHT given out by different materials.

phase rule (physics) The number of degrees of freedom (F) of a HETEROGENEOUS system is related to the number of components (C) and of phases (P) present at EQUILIBRIUM by the equation $P + F = C + 2$.

Phe (biochemistry) An abbreviation of 'Phe'nylalanine.

phenanthrene (chemistry) $C_{14}H_{10}$ Tricyclic aromatic ORGANIC COMPOUND consisting of three BENZENE RINGS fused together, the BASIC SKELETON of steroids and many other biologically active compounds.

phenol (chemistry) C_6H_5OH Colourless (*USA*: colorless) CRYSTALLINE SOLID which turns pink on exposure to AIR and LIGHT. It has a CHARACTERISTIC, rather sweet odour (*USA*: odor). It is used as an ANTISEPTIC and disinfectant, and in the preparation of dyes, drugs, etc. Also termed: CARBOLIC ACID; HYDROXYBENZENE. Other compounds with one or more hydroxy groups bound directly to a BENZENE RING are also known as phenols. They give reactions typical of ALCOHOLS (*e.g.* they form esters and ethers), but they are more acidic and form salts by the ACTION of strong ALKALIS (*USA*: strong alkalies).

phenolphthalein (chemistry) An ORGANIC COMPOUND that is used as a laxative and as an INDICATOR in VOLUMETRIC ANALYSIS. It is red in ALKALIS (*USA*: alkalies) and colourless (*USA*: colorless) in acids.

phenotype (genetics) Outward appearance and characteristics of an organism, or the way genes express themselves in an organism. Organisms of the same PHENOTYPE may possess different genotypes; *e.g.* in a HETEROZYGOUS organism two ALLELES of a GENE may be present with the expression of only one.

phenyl group (chemistry) C_6H_5- MONOVALENT RADICAL derived from BENZENE.

phenyl methyl ketone (chemistry) An alternative term for ACETOPHENONE.

3-phenylpropenoic acid (chemistry) An alternative term for cinnamic ACID.

phenylalanine (chemistry) $C_6H_5CH_2CH-(NH_2)COOH$ ESSENTIAL AMINO ACID that possesses a BENZENE RING.

phenylamine (chemistry) An alternative term for ANILINE.

phenylethylene (chemistry) An alternative term for styrene.

phenylketonuria (biochemistry) An autosomal recessive inherited deficiency of the liver enzyme phenylalanine hydroxylase that converts the amino acid phenylalanine into tyrosine. Phenylalanine and its toxic derivatives accumulate in the body and can cause brain damage with mental retardation. In the UK babies are screened at birth by the Guthrie test and about 1 in 16,000 is found to have the condition.

pheromone (biochemistry) Chemical substance produced by an organism which may influence the BEHAVIOUR (*USA*: behavior) of another; *e.g.* in moths, pheromones act as sexual attractants; in social insects such as bees, pheromones have an important role in the development and BEHAVIOUR of the COLONY.

phon (acoustics) UNIT of loudness of sound (given as the number of decibels it appears to be above a reference tone of known FREQUENCY and INTENSITY).

phosgene (chemistry) $COCl_2$ Colourless (*USA*: colorless) GAS with penetrating and suffocating SMELL. It was formerly used as a war GAS, and is now used in organic SYNTHESIS. Also termed: CARBONYL CHLORIDE.

phosphate (chemistry) SALT of PHOSPHORIC(V) ACID, containing the ION PO_4^{3-}. Many phosphates occur naturally in minerals (*e.g.* APATITE, CALCIUM PHOSPHATE) and in biological systems, and some are of enormous commercial and practical importance, *e.g.* AMMONIUM PHOSPHATE fertilizers and ALKALI PHOSPHATE buffers. Also termed: orthophosphate. Because PHOSPHORIC(V) ACID is a tribasic ACID, it also forms hydrogenphosphates, HPO_4^{2-} and dihydrogenphosphates, $H_2PO_4^-$.

phosphatidyl choline (biochemistry) An alternative term for LECITHIN, a PHOSPHOLIPID constituent of PLASMA MEMBRANES.

phosphide (chemistry) A chemical COMPOUND of PHOSPHORUS and another ELEMENT.

phospholipid (chemistry) Member of a CLASS of complex LIPIDS that are major components of CELL MEMBRANES. They consist of molecules containing a PHOSPHORIC(V) ACID ESTER of GLYCEROL (*i.e.* phosphoglycerides), the remaining HYDROXYL GROUPS of the GLYCEROL being esterified by FATTY ACIDS. Also termed: phosphoglyceride; phosphatide; GLYCEROL phosphatide.

phosphonium ion (chemistry) ION PH_4^+.

phosphor (chemistry) Substance capable of LUMINESCENCE or PHOSPHORESCENCE, as used to coat the inside of a television screen or FLUORESCENT LAMP.

phosphorescence (chemistry) Emission of LIGHT, generally VISIBLE LIGHT, after ABSORPTION of LIGHT of another WAVELENGTH, usually ULTRAVIOLET RADIATION or near ULTRAVIOLET RADIATION or ELECTRONS. Phosphorescence continues after the stimulating source is removed.

See also FLUORESCENCE; LUMINESCENCE.

phosphoric(V) acid (chemistry) H_3PO_4 Tribasic ACID, a colourless (*USA*: colorless) CRYSTALLINE SOLID, made by dissolving PHOSPHORUS(V) OXIDE in WATER. It is used to form a corrosion-resistant layer on steel. Its salts, the phosphates, are of great biological and commercial importance. Also termed: phosphoric ACID; ORTHOPHOSPHORIC ACID.

phosphorus P (chemistry) Nonmetallic ELEMENT in GROUP VA of the PERIODIC TABLE. It exists as several ALLOTROPES, chief of which are red PHOSPHORUS and the poisonous and spontaneously inflammable white or yellow PHOSPHORUS. It occurs in many minerals (particularly phosphates) and all living organisms; it is an essential nutrient for plants.

PHOSPHORUS is made by heating CALCIUM PHOSPHATE (with CARBON and sand) in an electric furnace. It is used in matches and for making fertilizers. At. no. 15; r.a.m. 30.9738.

phosphorus(III) oxide (chemistry) P_2O_3 White waxy SOLID which readily reacts with OXYGEN to form PHOSPHORUS(V) OXIDE. Also termed: PHOSPHORUS trioxide.

phosphorus(III) bromide (chemistry) PBr_3 Colourless (*USA*: colorless) LIQUID, used in organic SYNTHESIS to replace a HYDROXYL GROUP with a BROMINE ATOM. Also termed: PHOSPHORUS tribromide.

phosphorus(III) chloride (chemistry) PCl_3 Colourless (*USA*: colorless) fuming LIQUID, used to make ORGANIC COMPOUNDS of PHOSPHORUS. Also termed: PHOSPHORUS trichloride.

phosphorus(V) bromide (chemistry) PBr_5 Yellow CRYSTALLINE SOLID, used as a brominating agent. Also termed: PHOSPHORUS pentabromide.

phosphorus(V) chloride (chemistry) PCl_5 Yellowish-white CRYSTALLINE SOLID, used as a chlorinating agent. Also termed: PHOSPHORUS pentachloride.

phosphorus(V) oxide (chemistry) P_2O_5 HYGROSCOPIC white powder which readily reacts with WATER to form PHOSPHORIC(V) ACID. It is used as a DESICCANT. Also termed: PHOSPHORUS pentoxide.

phosphorylation (chemistry) Process by which a PHOSPHATE GROUP is transferred to a MOLECULE of an ORGANIC COMPOUND. In some substances, *e.g.* atp, a high-ENERGY BOND may be formed by PHOSPHORYLATION, which is essential for ENERGY-transfer in living organisms. It is an important biochemical end-REACTION which modifies the CONFORMATION of molecules such as ENZYMES, receptors, etc.

photocell (physics) Device that converts LIGHT into an ELECTRIC CURRENT. It can be used for the detection and measurement of LIGHT. Also termed: PHOTOELECTRIC CELL; photoemissive CELL.

photochemical reaction (chemistry) A CHEMICAL REACTION that is initiated by the ABSORPTION of LIGHT. The most important phenomenon of this type is PHOTO-SYNTHESIS. It is also the basis of PHOTOGRAPHY.

photochemistry (chemistry) Branch of chemistry concerned with the ACTION of LIGHT in initiating CHEMICAL REACTIONS.

photoconductivity (physics) Change in electrical CONDUCTIVITY of a substance when it is exposed to LIGHT; *e.g.* SELENIUM, used in photoelectric LIGHT METERS.

photoelectric cell (physics) An alternative term for PHOTOCELL.

photoelectric effect (chemistry) A phenomenon that occurs with some semi-metallic materials. When photons strike them they are absorbed and the energized electrons produced flow in the material as an ELECTRIC CURRENT. It is the basis of photocells and instruments that employ them, such as photographers' LIGHT METERS and burglar alarms.

photoelectron (chemistry) An ELECTRON produced by the PHOTOELECTRIC EFFECT or by PHOTOIONISATION.

photoemission (chemistry) Emission of photoelectrons by the PHOTOELECTRIC EFFECT or by PHOTOIONISATION.

photographic fixing (PHOTOGRAPHY) The process for removing unexposed SILVER halides after development of a photographic EMULSION. It involves dissolving the SILVER salts by immersing the developed FILM in a fixing bath consisting of a SOLUTION of SODIUM or ammonium thiosulphate (*USA*: ammonium thiosulfate).

photography (photography) Process of taking photographs by the chemical ACTION of LIGHT or other RADIATION on a sensitive plate or FILM made of GLASS, celluloid or other TRANSPARENT material coated with a LIGHT-sensitive EMULSION. LIGHT causes changes in particles of SILVER salts in the EMULSION which, after development (in a REDUCING AGENT), form grains of dark metallic SILVER to produce a negative IMAGE. Unaffected SILVER salts are removed by fixing (in a SOLUTION of ammonium or SODIUM THIOSULPHATE [*USA*: sodium thiosulfate]).

photoionisation (chemistry) IONIZATION of atoms or molecules by LIGHT or other ELECTROMAGNETIC RADIATION.

photoluminescence (chemistry) LIGHT emission by a substance after it has itself been exposed to VISIBLE LIGHT or INFRA-RED or ULTRAVIOLET RADIATION.

photolysis (chemistry) PHOTOCHEMICAL REACTION that results in the DECOMPOSITION of a substance.

photometer (physics) Instrument for measuring the INTENSITY of LIGHT.

photometry (measurement) Measurement of the INTENSITY of LIGHT.

photomicrograph (microscopy/ photography) Photograph obtained through a MICROSCOPE.

photomultiplier (physics) PHOTOCELL of high sensitivity used for detecting very small quantities of LIGHT RADIATION. It consists of SERIES of electrodes in an evacuated ENVELOPE, which are used to amplify the emission CURRENT by ELECTRON multiplication. Also termed: ELECTRON MULTIPLIER.

photon (physics) QUANTUM of ENERGY in ELECTROMAGNETIC RADIATION, such as LIGHT or X-RAYS. The amount of ENERGY per PHOTON is hv, where h is PLANCK'S CONSTANT and v is the FREQUENCY of the RADIATION.

photoneutron (physics) NEUTRON resulting from the INTERACTION of a PHOTON with an atomic NUCLEUS.

photophosphorylation (biology) Process during PHOTOSYNTHESIS that results in the formation of ATP from ENERGY derived from sunlight via chlorophyll. The reactions also produce HYDROGEN, which is used in COMBINATION with CARBON DIOXIDE to make sugars. Also termed: photosynthetic PHOSPHORYLATION.

See also PHOSPHORYLATION-3 PHOTO-SYNTHESIS.

photoreceptor (physics) A RECEPTOR consisting of sensory CELLS that are stimulated by LIGHT, *e.g.* LIGHT-sensitive CELLS in the EYE.

photosynthesis (biology) Type of autotrophic nutrition employed by green plants which involves the synthesis of organic compounds (mainly sugars) from carbon dioxide and water. Sunlight is used as a source of energy, which is trapped by chlorophyll present in chloroplasts. The process consists of a light stage, in which energy is converted into ATP and water is split into hydrogen

and oxygen. Hydrogen is subsequently combined with carbon dioxide in the dark stage to form carbohydrates. Photosynthetic bacteria use different sources of hydrogen in the process.

photovoltaic cell (physics) An alternative term for a PHOTOCELL.

phthalic acid (chemistry) $C_6H_4(COOH)_2$ White CRYSTALLINE SOLID which on heating converts to its ANHYDRIDE. It is used in organic SYNTHESIS and to make polyester resins. Also termed: BENZENE-1,2-DICARBOXYLIC ACID.

phthalocyanine (chemistry) Member of an important CLASS of SYNTHETIC organic dyes and pigments. They are blue to green and used for colouring (*USA*: coloring) paints, printing inks, SYNTHETIC plastics and fibres (*USA*: fibers), rubber, etc.

phylogeny (taxonomy) Relationship between groups of organisms (*e.g.* members of a PHYLUM) based on the closeness of their evolutionary descent.

phylum (taxonomy) In biological CLASSIFICATION, one of the groups into which the ANIMAL KINGDOM is divided. The members of the GROUP, although often quite different in form and structure, share certain common features; *e.g.* the PHYLUM Arthropoda (arthropods) includes all animals with jointed legs and an exoskeleton. Phyla are subdivided into classes. The equivalent of a PHYLUM in the plant KINGDOM is a DIVISION.

physical change (chemistry) Reversible alteration in the properties of a substance that does not affect the composition of the substance itself (as opposed to a chemical change, which is difficult to reverse and in which composition is affected).

physical chemistry (chemistry) Branch of chemistry concerned with the physical properties of substances.

physical states of matter (chemistry) Three kinds of substances that make up MATTER: gases, liquids and solids.

physics (physics) Science concerned with the properties of MATTER, ENERGY and RADIATION, particularly in processes involving no change of chemical composition.

physiology (physiology) Branch of biology that is concerned with the functioning of living organisms (as opposed to anatomy, which deals with their structure).

Pi π (mathematics) Symbol for the ratio between the CIRCUMFERENCE of a circle and its DIAMETER. It is an IRRATIONAL NUMBER with the value 3.1415926536...

Pi (biochemistry) An abbreviation of 'P'hosphate- 'i'norganic.

picrate (chemistry) 1 SALT of PICRIC ACID 2 CHARGE-transfer complex of PICRIC ACID with aromatic HYDROCARBONS, amines and phenols; picrates are frequently used to identify these classes of compounds. *See* AROMATIC COMPOUND.

picric acid (chemistry) $C_6H_2(NO_3)_3OH$ Yellow CRYSTALLINE SOLID obtained by nitrating PHENOL SULPHONIC ACID (*USA*: phenol sulfonic acid). It has been used as an ANTISEPTIC, dye and explosive. Also termed: 2,4,6-TRINITROPHENOL.

pictogram (statistics) A method of graphically representing statistical DATA that uses symbols, each representing a given number of items of information; *e.g.* if a barrel is used to symbolize a million gallons of oil, a row of 7 barrels represents 7 million gallons. It is thus a sort of pictorial BAR CHART.

pie chart (statistics) A method of graphically representing statistical DATA that consists of a circular diagram divided into sectors whose size (determined by the angle they subtend at the centre [*USA*: center]) represents a number of items of information, calculated as a PERCENTAGE of the whole; *e.g.* an item allocated a quadrant (quarter of the PIE CHART) represents 25 per cent of the whole.

piezoelectric effect (physics) Production of a measurable ELECTRIC CURRENT by some crystals when they are subjected to mechanical compression.

piezoelectricity (physics) ELECTRICITY produced by the PIEZOELECTRIC EFFECT.

pigment (chemistry) INSOLUBLE colouring (*USA*: coloring) material, used for imparting various colours to paints, paper, polymers, etc. (SOLUBLE colouring materials are dyes). Some naturally occurring coloured substances are also known as pigments; *e.g.* green chlorophyll in plants and red HAEMOGLOBIN (*USA*: hemoglobin) in BLOOD.

PIH (physiology/ biochemistry) An abbreviation of 'P'rolactin-'I'nhibiting 'H'ormone.

pineal gland (anatomy) Club-shaped, elongated outgrowth from the roof of the VERTEBRATE FOREBRAIN. It may act as a third EYE in some lower bony fishes; in other vertebrates it serves as a HORMONE-producing ORGAN whose secretory FUNCTION is regulated by LIGHT entering the body via the eyes. In human beings its role is not clear. Also termed: pineal body; EPIPHYSIS.

pinna (anatomy) The part of the EAR that extends beyond the SKULL, consisting of a cartilaginous flap. It covers and protects the opening of the EAR.

pinocytosis (cytology) Uptake of particles and macromolecules by living CELLS. Also termed: endocytosis.

pint (measurement) UNIT of LIQUID measure equal to 20 FLUID ounces or one-eighth of a gallon. 1 pint = 0.56826 LITRES.

pipette (laboratory equipment) Device for transferring a known VOLUME of LIQUID. It consists of a GLASS tube, often with a swelling at its centre (*USA*: center), and may have a rubber bulb or GLASS 'cylinder' at one end. Pipettes are used in VOLUMETRIC ANALYSIS.

pituitary (anatomy) ENDOCRINE GLAND situated at the BASE of the BRAIN in vertebrates, responsible for the production of many HORMONES. The ANTERIOR (front) LOBE produces GROWTH HORMONE, LUTEINIZING HORMONE, FOLLICLE-stimulating HORMONE, thyrotrophic HORMONE, lactogenic HORMONE and ACTH. The POSTERIOR (rear) LOBE secretes oxytocin and VASOPRESSIN produced in the HYPOTHALAMUS. Also termed: PITUITARY GLAND; HYPOPHYSIS.

pk value (mathematics) Negative LOGARITHM of the EQUILIBRIUM CONSTANT for the DISSOCIATION of an ELECTROLYTE in AQUEOUS SOLUTION.

placenta (anatomy) Vascular ORGAN that attaches the FOETUS (*USA*: fetus) to the wall of the UTERUS (womb).

Planck's constant (*h*) (physics) Fundamental CONSTANT that relates the ENERGY of a QUANTUM of RADIATION to the FREQUENCY of the OSCILLATOR that emits it. The relationship is $E = hv$, where E is the ENERGY of the QUANTUM and v is its FREQUENCY. Its value is 6.62559 x 10^{-34} JOULE second. It was named after the German physicist Max Planck (1858-1947).

Planck's radiation law (physics) An OBJECT cannot emit or absorb ENERGY, in the form of RADIATION, in a continuous manner; the ENERGY can be taken up or given out only as INTEGRAL multiples of a definite amount, known as a QUANTUM. Also termed: Planck's LAW of RADIATION.

plasma (1 physics; 2 haematology) 1 STATE OF MATTER in which the atoms or molecules of a substance are broken into electrons and POSITIVE ions. All substances pass into this STATE OF MATTER when heated to a very high TEMPERATURE, *e.g.* in an electric ARC or in the interior of a star. 2 Colourless (*USA*: colorless) FLUID portion of BLOOD or LYMPH from which all CELLS have been removed.

plasma cell (cytology) Large EGG-shaped CELL with granular, basophilic CYTOPLASM except for a clear AREA around the small eccentrically placed NUCLEUS. Its FUNCTION is believed to be ANTIBODY SYNTHESIS. Also termed: plasmacyte.

plasma membrane (histology) Thin layer of TISSUE consisting of fat and PROTEIN that forms a boundary surrounding the CYTOPLASM of EUKARYOTIC CELLS and its organelles. It is a differentially PERMEABLE MEMBRANE that separates adjacent CELLS and cavities. Also termed: cytoplasmic MEMBRANE.

plasma protein (haematology/ biochemistry) PROTEIN in the PLASMA of BLOOD (*e.g.* antibodies and various HORMONES).

plasmasol (cytology) An alternative term for ENDOPLASM.

plaster of Paris (chemistry/ medical) $CaSO_4.1/2H_2O$ CALCIUM SULPHATE HEMIHYDRATE (*USA*: calcium sulfate hemihydrate), obtained by heating GYPSUM. When WATER is added, it sets hard, reforming GYPSUM. In doing so, it does not expand or contract much, and is therefore valuable as a moulding (*USA*: molding) material, particularly as a splint for broken bones and in the building industry.

platelet (haematology) Small non-nucleated oval or round fragment of CELLS from the red BONE MARROW found in mammalian BLOOD. There are about 250,000 to 400,000 per mm³ in human BLOOD, which are required to initiate BLOOD clotting by disintegrating and liberating thrombokinase. In some vertebrates platelets are represented by THROMBOCYTES, which are small spindle-shaped nucleated CELLS.

platinum Pt (chemistry) Valuable SILVER-white metallic ELEMENT in GROUP VIII of the PERIODIC TABLE (a TRANSITION ELEMENT). It is used for making jewellery, electrical contacts and in scientific apparatus. At. no. 78; r.a.m. 195.09.

Platyhelminthes (parasitology) PHYLUM of simple invertebrates; flatworms. Parasitic platyhelminths include FLUKES and tapeworms.

PLC (biochemistry) An abbreviation of 'P'hospho'L'ipase 'C'.

pleura (anatomy) Double MEMBRANE that covers the lungs and lines the chest cavity, with FLUID between the membranes. Also termed: PLEURAL membranes.

pleural (anatomy) To do with the lungs.

plexus (anatomy) NETWORK of interlacing NERVES.

plumbic (chemistry) An alternative term for LEAD(IV).

plumbous (chemistry) An alternative term for LEAD(II).

plutonium Pu (chemistry) RADIOACTIVE ELEMENT in GROUP IIIB of the PERIODIC TABLE (one of the ACTINIDES), produced from URANIUM-238 in a breeder REACTOR. It has several isotopes (with half-lives of up to 76 million years), some of which (*e.g.* Pu-239) undergo nuclear FISSION; all are very poisonous. At. no. 94; r.a.m. 244 (most STABLE ISOTOPE).

PMN (haematology) An abbreviation of 'P'oly'M'orphonuclear 'N'eutrophilic leukocyte.

pneumatic (physics) Operated by AIR PRESSURE.

PNMT (biochemistry) An abbreviation of 'P'henylethanolamine-'N'-'M'ethyl'T'ransferase.

poikilothermic (biology/ physiology) Describing an ANIMAL that is cold-blooded and relies on the HEAT of the ENVIRONMENT to warm its body; *e.g.* among vertebrates, fish, amphibians and reptiles.

See also HOMOIOTHERMIC.

poison (1 chemistry; 2 toxicology) 1 Substance that destroys the activity of a

CATALYST. 2 Substance that when introduced into a living organism in any way destroys life or causes injury to health; a TOXIN.

polar bond (chemistry) COVALENT BOND in which the bonding electrons are not shared equally between the two atoms.

polar crystal (crystallography) Crystal that has IONIC BONDS between its atoms. Also termed: IONIC CRYSTAL.

polar molecule (chemistry) MOLECULE that is polarized even in the absence of an ELECTRIC FIELD. *See* POLARIZATION.

polarimeter (physics) Instrument for measuring the OPTICAL ACTIVITY of a substance. Also termed: polariscope.

polarimetry (measurement) Measurement of OPTICAL ACTIVITY, used in chemical ANALYSIS.

polarity (physics) Designation that something is either positively or negatively charged (*e.g.* the CATHODE in an ELECTROLYTIC CELL has negative POLARITY).

polarization (1 chemistry; 2, 3 physics) 1 Separation of the POSITIVE and negative charges of a MOLECULE. 2 Lining up of the electric and MAGNETIC FIELDS of an ELECTROMAGNETIC WAVE, *e.g.* as in POLARIZED LIGHT. Only transverse waves can be polarized. 3 Formation of GAS bubbles or a FILM of deposit on an ELECTRODE of an ELECTROLYTIC CELL, which tends to impede the flow of ELECTRIC CURRENT.

polarized light (optics) LIGHT waves (which normally oscillate in all possible planes) with fixed orientation of the electric and MAGNETIC FIELDS. It may be created by passing the LIGHT through a polarizer consisting of a plate of tourmaline crystal cut in a special way, through a NICOL PRISM or by using a Polaroid sheet. Substances that are OPTICALLY ACTIVE have the property of rotating the plane of polarized LIGHT.

polarography (chemistry) Method of chemical ANALYSIS for substances in DILUTE SOLUTION in which CURRENT is measured as a FUNCTION of POTENTIAL between MERCURY electrodes in an ELECTROLYTIC CELL containing the SOLUTION.

polaroid (photography) Trade name for a thin TRANSPARENT FILM that produces plane POLARIZED LIGHT when LIGHT is passed through it.

pole (physics) ELECTRODE (particularly of a BATTERY).

pollen (biology) Dust-like microspore of a seed plant produced by microsporangium cones in gymnosperms and by anthers in angiosperms. Each grain contains male gametes. If these gametes are carried by an external agent such as wind, insects or WATER to the ovules of gymnosperms or to the stigma of angiosperms, they produce FERTILIZATION. In susceptible (*i.e.* sensitive) people, POLLEN can be a powerful ANTIGEN that results in a vigorous ALLERGIC RESPONSE. Also termed: FARINA. *See* ALLERGY.

polonium Po (chemistry) RADIOACTIVE metallic ELEMENT in GROUP VIA of the PERIODIC TABLE, used as a source of alpha-particles. It has 27 isotopes, more than any other ELEMENT, with half-lives of up to 100 years. At. no. 84; r.a.m. 209 (most STABLE ISOTOPE).

poly- (general terminology) A prefix meaning many (*e.g.* polychaete, polygon).

polyamide (chemistry) CONDENSATION POLYMER in which the units are linked by AMIDE groups (-CONH-); *e.g.* proteins, HAIR, wool fibres (*USA*: wool fibers), nylon.

polybasic (chemistry) Describing an ACID with two or more acidic (replaceable) HYDROGEN atoms in its MOLECULE; *e.g.* PHOSPHORUS(V) (orthophosphoric) ACID, H_3PO_4, with three replaceable hydrogens, is tribasic.

polycyclic (chemistry) Describing a substance that has more than one ring of atoms in its MOLECULE.

polyhydric alcohol (chemistry) ALCOHOL that contains three or more HYDROXYL GROUPS.

polyhydric (chemistry) Containing a number of HYDROXYL GROUPS.

polymer (chemistry) Long-chain MOLECULE built up of a number of smaller molecules called monomers, joined together by POLYMERIZATION. Natural polymers include STARCH, CELLULOSE and rubber. SYNTHETIC polymers include all kinds of plastics.

polymerization (chemistry) Process of joining together of small molecules, called monomers, to form larger molecules, polymers, often in the presence of a CATALYST. In CONDENSATION POLYMERIZATION, two types of MONOMER molecules condense to form long chains, with the elimination of a small MOLECULE, such as WATER. In addition POLYMERI- ZATION, long chains are formed by molecules of a single MONOMER joining together.

polymethanal (chemistry) POLYMER formed from METHANAL (FORMALDEHYDE). Also termed: PARAFORMALDEHYDE.

polymethyl methacrylate (chemistry/ optics) TRANSPARENT colourless (*USA*: colorless) thermoplastic. Its optical properties of high transmission of LIGHT and high internal REFLECTION, coupled with great strength, are responsible for its use in place of GLASS. Also termed: PERSPEX.

polymorphism (1 chemistry; 2 biology) 1 Occurrence of a substance in more than one CRYSTALLINE form. 2 Occurrence of an organism in more than one structural form during its LIFE CYCLE.

polynomial (mathematics) An ALGEBRAIC expression with only one VARIABLE.

polynucleotide (chemistry) POLYMER of many nucleotides.

polypeptide (chemistry) Chain of AMINO ACIDS which is a BASIC constituent of proteins. It may be broken down by ENZYME ACTION (DIGESTION) to form peptides. The functionally significant linking and folding of polypeptides makes up the three-dimensional structure of a PROTEIN.

polyploidy (genetics) Condition in which a CELL or organism has three to four times the NORMAL HAPLOID or gametic number. It is often made use of in plant breeding because it results in the production of larger and more vigorous crops. Because it disturbs the sex-determining mechanism, POLYPLOIDY is rare in animals, and would result in sterility.

polypus Pendulous but usually BENIGN TUMOUR (*USA*: benign tumor) that grows from MUCOUS MEMBRANE (*e.g.* in the nose or womb). Also termed: polyp.

polysaccharide (chemistry) High MOLECU-LAR WEIGHT CARBOHYDRATE, linked by

322

GLYCOSIDE bonds, that yields a large number of MONOSACCHARIDE molecules (*e.g.* simple sugars) on HYDROLYSIS or ENZYME ACTION. The most common POLYSACCHARIDES have the GENERAL FORMULA $(C_6H_{10}O_5)_n$; *e.g.* STARCH, CELLULOSE, etc.

polyvalent (1, 2 chemistry) 1 Having a VALENCE of more than one. 2 Having more than one VALENCY.

POMC (biochemistry) An abbreviation of 'P'ro-'O'pio'M'elano'C'ortin.

population genetics (genetics) Study of the theoretical and experimental consequence of Mendelian INHERITANCE on population levels, taking into account the genotypes, phenotypes, GENE frequencies and the MATING SYSTEMS.

population inversion (chemistry) A condition in which a higher ENERGY state in an atomic system is more populated with electrons than a lower ENERGY state.

porosity (physics) Property of substance that allows gases or liquids to pass through it.

porphyrin (chemistry) Member of an important CLASS of naturally occurring organic pigments derived from four PYRROLE rings. Many form complexes with METAL ions, as in *e.g.* chlorophyll, haem (*USA*: heme), CYTOCHROME, etc.

portal vein (anatomy) Any VEIN connecting two CAPILLARY networks, thus allowing for BLOOD regulation from one NETWORK by the others *e.g.* the HEPATIC PORTAL VEIN connects the INTESTINE with the LIVER.

positive (1 mathematics; 2 physics) 1 Describing a number or quantity greater than zero. 2 Describing an ELECTRIC CHARGE or ION that is attracted by a negative one.

positive feedback (general terminology) FEEDBACK in which the output adds to the input.

positron (physics) ELEMENTARY PARTICLE which has a MASS equal to that of an ELECTRON, and an electrical CHARGE equal in magnitude, but opposite in sign, to that of the ELECTRON.

posterior 1 In bilaterally symmetrical animals, the end of the body directed backwards during locomotion; the rear or hind end. In bipedal animals (*e.g.* human beings), it corresponds to the DORSAL side of quadrupeds.

post-matum (medical) Over-developed; used of an infant born after its time.

potash (chemistry) A substance that contains POTASSIUM, particularly POTASSIUM CARBONATE.

potassium K (chemistry) Highly reactive SILVER-white metallic ELEMENT in GROUP IA of the PERIODIC TABLE (the ALKALI METALS). Its compounds occur widely (particularly the CHLORIDE) and have many uses; POTASSIUM is an essential nutrient for plants. The METAL is used as a COOLANT in nuclear reactors. At. no. 19; r.a.m. 39.102.

potassium bicarbonate (chemistry) An alternative term for POTASSIUM hydrogen-carbonate.

potassium bromide (chemistry) KBr White CRYSTALLINE SALT, used in medicine and PHOTOGRAPHY.

potassium carbonate (chemistry) K_2CO_3 White granular SOLID, used in the manufacture of GLASS and SOAP. Also termed: POTASH.

potassium chloride (chemistry) KCl Colourless (*USA*: colorless) or white CRYSTALLINE SALT, used as a fertilizer and as a dietary SALT (SODIUM CHLORIDE) substitute when SODIUM intake must be limited.

potassium cyanide (chemistry) KCN White poisonous SOLID, used in metallurgy and electroplating.

potassium ferricyanide (chemistry) $K_3Fe-(CN)_6$ Red crystals, used as a chemical REAGENT and in the manufacture of pigments (*e.g.* Prussian blue). An alternative term: POTASSIUM hexacyanoferrate(III).

potassium ferrocyanide (chemistry) $K_4Fe-(CN)_6.3H_2O$ Yellow crystals. Also termed: POTASSIUM hexacyanoferrate(II).

potassium hydrogencarbonate (chemistry) $KHCO_3$ White granular SOLID, used in pharmaceuticals. Also termed: POTASSIUM BICARBONATE.

potassium hydrogentartrate (chemistry) $HOOC(CHOH)_2 COOK$ White CRYSTALLINE powder, used in baking powder. Also termed: CREAM OF TARTAR.

potassium hydroxide (chemistry) KOH Strongly HYGROSCOPIC white SOLID. A strong ALKALI, it is used in the manufacture of soft soaps. Also termed: CAUSTIC POTASH.

potassium iodide (chemistry) KI Colourless (*USA*: colorless) CRYSTALLINE SALT, used in chemical ANALYSIS and organic SYNTHESIS. Its SOLUTION dissolves IODINE.

potassium manganate(VII) (chemistry) An alternative term for POTASSIUM PERMANGANATE.

potassium nitrate (chemistry) KNO_3 Colourless (*USA*: colorless) CRYSTALLINE SALT, a powerful OXIDIZING AGENT. It is used in the manufacture of GLASS and explosives, and as a food preservative. Also termed: SALTPETRE; NITRE.

potassium permanganate (chemistry) $KMnO_4$ Purple crystals, a powerful OXIDIZING AGENT. It is used in the manufacture of chemicals, as a disinfectant and FUNGICIDE, and in VOLUMETRIC ANALYSIS. Also termed: permanganate of POTASH; POTASSIUM manganate(VII).

potassium-sparing diuretics (pharmacology) Weak DIURETICs such as amiloride which act on the distal tubule causing retention of POTASSIUM.

potassium thiocyanate (chemistry) KSCN Colourless (*USA*: colorless) HYGROSCOPIC SOLID, used in SOLUTION to test for IRON(III) (FERRIC) compounds, which give a BLOOD-red COLOUR (*USA*: color).

potency (pharmacology) The strength of a drug based on its effectiveness to cause change.

potential (physics) An alternative term for POTENTIAL DIFFERENCE or VOLTAGE.

potential difference (pd) (physics) Difference in electric POTENTIAL between two points in an ELECTRIC CURRENT-carrying CIRCUIT, usually expressed in volts (V). Also termed: VOLTAGE.

potentiometer (1, 2 physics) 1 Instrument for measuring POTENTIAL DIFFERENCE or ELECTROMOTIVE FORCE 2 VOLTAGE DIVIDER.

potentiometric titration (chemistry) Method of QUANTITATIVE ANALYSIS, using TITRATION, that involves the measurement of changes in ELECTRODE POTENTIAL of an ELECTRODE dipping into a SOLUTION.

pound (1 lb; 2 £) (1, 2 measurement) 1 UNIT of WEIGHT equal to 16 ounces; 14 lb 1 stone, 112 lb = 1 hundredweight (cwt). 1 lb = 0.4536 kg. 2 UNIT of currency equal to 100 pence.

power (1 physics; 2 optics; 3 mathematics) 1 Rate of doing WORK. The SI UNIT of POWER is the WATT (equal to 10^7 erg s^{-1} or 1/745.7 horsepower). 2 The extent to which a curved mirror, LENS or optical instrument can magnify an OBJECT. For a simple LENS, POWER is expressed in dioptres. 3 An EXPONENT or INDEX, written as a small superior NUMERAL; *e.g.* 3^2 is 3 to the POWER 2 (or 3 squared) = 9; 4^3 is 4 to the POWER 3 (or 4 cubed) = 256; x^5 is x to the POWER 5 (or x to the 5th).

poxvirus (virology) Member of a GROUP of large DNA-containing VIRUSES that are responsible for smallpox, cowpox and some ANIMAL tumours (*USA*: tumors).

PRA (physiology/ biochemistry) An abbreviation of 'P'lasma 'R'enin 'A'ctivity.

praseodymium Pr (chemistry) Metallic ELEMENT in GROUP IIIB of the PERIODIC TABLE (one of the LANTHANIDES). At. no. 59; r.a.m. 140.9077.

PRC (biochemistry) An abbreviation of 'P'lasma 'R'enin 'C'oncentration.

precipitate (chemistry) SOLID that forms in and settles out from a SOLUTION.

precipitation (chemistry) Process of PRECIPITATE formation. *See* DOUBLE DECOMPOSITION.

precursor (chemistry) INTERMEDIATE substance from which another is formed in a CHEMICAL REACTION.

pregnancy (physiology) Time that elapses between FERTILIZATION or IMPLANTATION of a fertilized OVUM and an ANIMAL's birth; the time that an ANIMAL spends as an EMBRYO or FOETUS (*USA*: fetus). Also termed: GESTATION. The time that an EMBRYO reptile or bird spends in an EGG between laying and hatching is usually termed incubation.

premolar (anatomy) Grinding and chewing TOOTH located behind the canine TEETH and in front of the MOLAR TEETH. An adult human being has eight premolars, two in each side of each JAW.

presbyopia (medical) Age-related loss of ACCOMMODATION of the human EYE. Loss of elasticity of the EYE LENS makes it difficult to FOCUS on near objects.

See also HYPERMETROPIA.

pressure (p) (physics) FORCE applied to, or distributed over, a surface. Measured as FORCE f per UNIT AREA a; $p = f/a$. At a depth d in a LIQUID, the PRESSURE is given by $p = gd$, where   is the LIQUID's DENSITY, d the depth and g is the ACCELERATION of free fall. The SI UNIT of PRESSURE is the PASCAL; other units include bars, millibars, atmospheres and millimetres of MERCURY.

See also ATMOSPHERIC PRESIURE.

pressure gauge (physics) Device for measuring FLUID PRESSURE (*e.g.* BAROMETER, MANOMETER).

primary alcohol /amine (chemistry) ALCOHOL or AMINE with only one ALKYL GROUP or ARYL GROUP.

primary cell (physics) ELECTROLYTIC CELL (BATTERY) in which the CHEMICAL REACTIONS that cause the CURRENT flow are not readily reversible and the CELL cannot easily be recharged, *e.g.* a DRY CELL.

See also SECONDARY CELL.

primary colour (1, 2 physics) 1 Red, green and violet, which give all other colours (*USA*: colors) when LIGHT producing them is combined in various proportions. All three mix to give white. 2 PIGMENT colours red, yellow and blue, which can also be combined to give pigments of all other colours. All three mix to give black. (*USA*: primary color).

prime number (mathematics) INTEGER (whole number) divisible only by itself and 1. All PRIME NUMBERS except 2 are odd.

principle of flotation (physics) A floating OBJECT displaces its own WEIGHT of FLUID (LIQUID or GAS). An OBJECT floats if its WEIGHT equals the upthrust on it.

See also ARCHIMEDES' PRINCIPLE.

printer (computing) COMPUTER OUTPUT DEVICE that produces HARD COPY as a printout. There are various kinds, including (in ORDER of speed) daisy-wheel, dot-MATRIX, line, barrel and LASER.

print-out (computing) Output (HARD COPY) from a COMPUTER PRINTER.

probability distribution of electrons (physics) Probability that an ELECTRON within an ATOM will be at a certain point in space at a given time. It predicts the shape of an ATOMIC ORBITAL.

proboscis (biology) Tube-like ORGAN of varying form and functions. In insects, a PROBOSCIS is a filamentous structure that projects outwards from the mouthparts, functioning as a piercing and sucking device for obtaining LIQUID food. In elephants, the PROBOSCIS is the trunk, and in some marine animals it is a tube-like PHARYNX that can be protruded.

product (1 mathematics; 2 chemistry) 1 The result of multiplying numbers together. 2 A substance formed as a result of a chemical change.

proenzyme (biochemistry) An alternative term for ZYMOGEN.

progesterone (biochemistry) $C_{21}H_{30}O_2$ STEROID SEX HORMONE secreted by the CORPUS LUTEUM of the mammalian OVARY, PLACENTA, TESTES and ADRENAL CORTEX. In females it prepares the UTERUS for the IMPLANTATION of a fertilized OVUM (EGG) and during PREGNANCY maintains nourishment for the EMBRYO by developing the PLACENTA, inhibiting OVULATION and MENSTRUATION, and stimulating the GROWTH of the MAMMARY GLANDS.

progestogen drugs (pharmacology) A group of drugs chemically and pharmacologically similar to the natural HORMONE progesterone. Administered orally they are used in oral contraceptives and to treat menstrual disorders.

program (computing) Sequence of instructions for a COMPUTER. Also termed: programme.

progression (mathematics) Mathematical SERIES of terms. *See* ARITHMETIC PROGRESSION; GEOMETRIC PROGRESSION.

prokaryote (biology) DNA-containing, single-celled organism with no proper NUCLEUS or ENDOPLASMIC RETICULUM; *e.g.* BACTERIA, BLUE-GREEN ALGAe (cyanophytes).

See also EUKARYOTE.

prokaryotic (biology) Describing or resembling a PROKARYOTE.

prolactin (biochemistry) PROTEIN HORMONE secreted by the ANTERIOR PITUITARY. In mammals it stimulates LACTATION and promotes functional activity of the CORPUS LUTEUM. Also termed: LUTEOTROPHIN; mammary stimulating HORMONE; mammogen HORMONE; mammotrophin.

proline (biochemistry) White CRYSTALLINE AMINO ACID that occurs in most proteins.

promethium Pm (chemistry) RADIOACTIVE metallic ELEMENT in GROUP IIIB of the PERIODIC TABLE (one of the LANTHANIDES). It has several isotopes (none of which occurs naturally), with half-lives of up to 20 years. At. no. 61; r.a.m. 145 (most STABLE ISOTOPE).

promoter (chemistry) Substance used to enhance the efficiency of a CATALYST. Also termed: activator.

proof (measurement) Measure of the ETHANOL (ETHYL ALCOHOL) content of a SOLUTION (gunpowder moistened with a 100 per cent PROOF SPIRIT will just ignite). A 100 per cent PROOF SOLUTION is 57. 1 per cent ETHANOL by VOLUME or 49.3 per cent ETHANOL by WEIGHT.

propanoic acid (chemistry) CH_3CH_2COOH LIQUID CARBOXYLIC ACID. Also termed: PROPIONIC ACID.

propanol (chemistry) ALCOHOL that occurs as two isomers. 1 n-PROPANOL C_3H_7OH is a colourless (*USA*: colorless) LIQUID, used as a SOLVENT and in making toilet preparations. Also termed: n-propyl ALCOHOL; propan-l-ol. 2 ISOPROPANOL $(CH_3)_2CHOH$ is also a colourless LIQUID, used for preparing esters, ACETONE (propanone), and as a SOLVENT. Also termed: ISOPROPYL ALCOHOL; propan-2-ol.

propranolol hydrochloride (pharmacology) A BETA-BLOCKER that can be administered orally or by injection and used as an ANTIHYPERTENSIVE, as an ANTI-ANGINA treatment, an ANTI-ARRHYTHMIC, and an ANTITHYROID, antimigraine and axiolytic treatment.

2-propanone (chemistry) An alternative term for ACETONE.

propellant (physics) GAS used in an AEROSOL to expel the contents through an atomizing jet.

2-propenal (chemistry) An alternative term for ACROLEIN.

propene (chemistry) $CH_3CH = CH_2$ Colourless (*USA*: colorless) gaseous ALKENE (OLEFIN), used in industry for the preparation of ISOPROPANOL, GLYCEROL, polypropene, etc. Also termed: propylene.

propenoic acid (chemistry) An alternative term for acrylic acid.

propenonitrile (chemistry) An alternative term for ACRYLONITRILE.

proper fraction (mathematics) FRACTION whose NUMERATOR is less than its DENOMINATOR (a FRACTION whose NUMERATOR is larger than its DENOMINATOR is an IMPROPER FRACTION).

prophase (genetics) First stage of CELL DIVISION in MEIOSIS and MITOSIS. During PROPHASE chromosomes can be seen to thicken and shorten and to be composed of chromatids. The spindle is assembled for DIVISION of chromosomes and the NUCLEAR MEMBRANE disintegrates. In MEIOSIS the first PROPHASE is extended into several stages.

propionaldehyde (chemistry) An alternative term for propanal.

propionic acid (chemistry) An alternative term for propanoic acid.

prostaglandin (biochemistry) Member of a GROUP of UNSATURATED FATTY ACIDS that contain 20 CARBON atoms. They are found in all human TISSUE, and particularly high concentrations occur in SEMEN. Their activities affect the NERVOUS SYSTEM, circulation, female reproductive organs and METABOLISM. Most prostaglandins are secreted locally and are rapidly metabolized by ENZYMES in the TISSUE.

prostate gland (anatomy) GLAND located at the BASE of the urinary BLADDER that forms part of the male reproductive system. The size of the GLAND and the quantity of its SECRETION are controlled by ANDROGENS. Its FUNCTION is SECRETION of a FLUID containing ENZYMES and antiglutinating FACTOR, which contributes to the production of SEMEN.

prosthetic group (biochemistry) Non-PROTEIN portion of a CONJUGATED PROTEIN, *e.g.* haem (*USA*: heme) GROUP in HAEMOGLOBIN (*USA*: hemoglobin).

Prot· (biochemistry) An abbreviation of 'Prot'ein anion.

protactinium Pa (chemistry) RADIOACTIVE ELEMENT in GROUP IIIB of the PERIODIC TABLE (one of the ACTINIDES). It has several isotopes, with half-lives of up to 20,000 years. At. no. 91; r.a.m. 231.0319.

protease (biochemistry) ENZYME that breaks down PROTEIN into its constituent peptides and AMINO ACIDS by breaking PEPTIDE linkages (*e.g.* PEPSIN, trypsin).

protein (biochemistry) Member of a CLASS of high MOLECULAR WEIGHT polymers composed of a VARIETY of AMINO ACIDS joined by PEPTIDE linkages. In CONJUGATED proteins, the AMINO ACIDS are joined to other groups. Proteins are extremely important in the physiological structure and functioning of all living organisms.

protein synthesis (biochemistry) Process by which proteins are made in CELLS. A MOLECULE of MESSENGER RNA decodes the sequence of copied DNA on ribosomes in the CYTOPLASM. A POLYPEPTIDE chain is generated by the linking of AMINO ACIDS in an ORDER instructed by the BASE sequence of MESSENGER RNA.

protist (biology) Member of the PROTISTA.

Protista (taxonomy) KINGDOM that contains simple organisms such as ALGAe, BACTERIA, FUNGI and PROTOZOA, although sometimes MULTICELLULAR organisms are excluded.

proton (physics) Fundamental ELEMENTARY PARTICLE with a POSITIVE CHARGE equal in magnitude to the negative ELECTRON CHARGE, and with a rest MASS of 1.67252×10^{-27} kg (about 1,850 times that of an ELECTRON). Protons are constituents of the NUCLEUS in every kind of ATOM.

proton number (chemistry) An alternative term for ATOMIC NUMBER.

protonic acid (chemistry) COMPOUND that releases solvated HYDROGEN IONS in a suitable polar SOLVENT (*e.g.* WATER).

proton pump (physiology/ biochemistry) The enzyme hydrogen-potassium ATP-ase which is involved in the final stage of acid production in the PARIETAL CELLS.

proton pump inhibitors (pharmacology) Drugs, *e.g.* omeprazole, that block the action of the proton pump in the PARIETAL CELLS of the STOMACH causing a reduction in acid secretion.

protoplasm (cytology) Material within a CELL, *i.e.* the CYTOPLASM and NUCLEUS.

Protozoa (taxonomy) Subkingdom or PHYLUM of microscopic UNICELLULAR organisms which range from plant-like forms to types which feed and behave like animals. They have no fundamental body shape but have specialized organelles. BASIC MODE of REPRODUCTION is by BINARY FISSION, although multiple FISSION and CONJUGATION occur in some SPECIES. Some protozoans are colonial and many are parasitic, inhabiting freshwater, marine and damp terrestrial environments.

5-PRPP (biochemistry) An abbreviation of '5'-'P'hospho'R'ibosyl 'P'yro'P'hosphate.

prussic acid (chemistry) An alternative term for HYDROCYANIC ACID.

P sac (anatomy) Pericardial cavity. The cavity within which the HEART lies.

pseudo- (general terminology) Prefix meaning false (*e.g.* PSEUDOPREGNANCY).

pseudopodium (biology) Part of an AMOEBA (*USA:* ameba) or similar protozoan that bulges out of its single CELL. Pseudopodia are used for locomotion and to engulf food particles (for DIGESTION).

pseudopregnancy (physiology) In some female mammals, physiological state resembling PREGNANCY without the formation of embryos. Also termed: FALSE PREGNANCY.

P Surg. (medical) An abbreviation of 'P'lastic 'Surg'ery.

psychiatry (medical) Study and TREATMENT of disorders of the mind (*i.e.* mental disorders).

psycho- (general terminology) Prefix meaning to do with the mind (*e.g.* psychiatry, psychology).

psychology (psychology) Scientific study of the mind.

PTA (haematology) An abbreviation of 'P'lasma 'T'hromboplastin 'A'ntecedent (clotting factor XI).

PTC (1, 2 physiology) 1 Abbreviation of 'P'lasma 'T'hromboplastin 'C'omponent (clotting factor IX); 2 An abbreviation of 'P'henyl'T'hio'C'arbamide.

p tgt (chemistry) An abbreviation of 'p'rimary 't'ar'g'e 't'.

PTH (physiology/ biochemistry) Abbreviation of 'P'ara'T'hyroid 'H'ormone.

PTHRP (physiology/ biochemistry) Abbreviation of 'P'ara'T'hyroid 'H'ormone-'R'elated 'P'rotein.

pulmonary artery (anatomy) In mammals, a paired ARTERY that carries deoxygenated BLOOD from the right VENTRICLE of the HEART to the lungs. It is the only ARTERY that carries deoxygenated BLOOD.

pulmonary (anatomy) Concerning the lungs and BREATHING.

pulmonary vein (anatomy) A paired VEIN that carries oxygenated BLOOD from the lungs to the right ATRIUM of the HEART. It is the only VEIN that carries oxygenated BLOOD.

pulse (1 physics; 2 physiology) 1 Brief disturbance propagated in a similar way as a WAVE, but not having the continuous periodic nature of a WAVE. 2 Regular expansion of the wall of an ARTERY caused by the BLOOD PRESSURE waves that accompany heartbeats.

pump (equipment) Mechanical device for transferring liquids or gases, or for compressing gases. A simple lift PUMP employs ATMOSPHERIC PRESSURE and cannot PUMP a LIQUID vertically more than about 10 m (32 feet); a FORCE PUMP does not have this restriction.

purine (chemistry) $C_5H_4N_4$ HETEROCYCLIC NITROGEN-containing BASE from which the bases CHARACTERISTIC of nucleotides and DNA are derived; *e.g.* ADENINE, GUANINE. Other PURINE derivatives include CAFFEINE and URIC ACID.

putrefaction (microbiology) ANAEROBIC DECOMPOSITION of organic MATTER by microscopic organisms (*e.g.* BACTERIA, FUNGI, etc.) which results in the formation of incompletely oxidized products.

pyranose (chemistry) Any of a GROUP of MONOSACCHARIDE sugars (hexoses) whose molecules have a six-membered HETEROCYCLIC ring of five CARBON atoms and one OXYGEN ATOM.

See also FURANOSE.

pyrazine (chemistry) $C_4H_4N_2$ HETEROCYCLIC AROMATIC COMPOUND whose ring contains four CARBON atoms and two NITROGEN atoms. Also termed: 1, 4-diazine.

pyrazole (chemistry) $C_3H_4N_2$ HETEROCYCLIC AROMATIC COMPOUND whose ring contains three CARBON atoms and two NITROGEN atoms. Also termed: 1, 2-diazole.

pyrene (chemistry) $C_{16}H_{10}$ AROMATIC COMPOUND consisting of four BENZENE RINGS fused together.

Pyrex (chemistry) Trade name for a HEAT-resistant BOROSILICATE GLASS, used for domestic and LABORATORY glassware.

pyridine (chemistry) C_5H_5N HETEROCYCLIC LIQUID ORGANIC BASE which occurs in the LIGHT oil FRACTION of coal-tar and in BONE oil. It forms salts with acids and is important in organic SYNTHESIS.

pyridoxine (chemistry) CRYSTALLINE substance from which the active COENZYME forms of VITAMIN B_6 are derived. It is also utilized as a potent GROWTH FACTOR for BACTERIA.

pyrimidine (chemistry) $C_4H_4N_2$ HETEROCYCLIC CRYSTALLINE ORGANIC BASE from which bases found in nuelcotides and DNA are derived; *e.g.* URACIL, THYMINE and CYTOSINE. Its derivatives also include BARBITURIC ACID and the BARBITURATE drugs.

pyro- (general terminology) Prefix that denotes strong HEAT, fire.

(pyro)Glu (biochemistry) An abbreviation of 'pyro''Glu'tamic acid.

pyroelectricity (chemistry) POLARIZATION of certain crystals by the application of HEAT.

pyrolysis (chemistry) DECOMPOSITION of a chemical COMPOUND by HEAT.

pyrometer (physics) Instrument for measuring high temperatures, above the range of LIQUID thermometers.

pyrometry (measurement) Measurement of high temperatures.

pyrrole (biochemistry) $(CH)_4NH$ HETEROCYCLIC LIQUID ORGANIC COMPOUND whose ring contains four CARBON atoms and one NITROGEN ATOM. An AROMATIC COMPOUND, its derivatives are important biologically; *e.g.* haem (*USA*: heme), chlorophyll.

pyruvate (chemistry) ESTER or SALT of PYRUVIC ACID.

pyruvic acid (biochemistry) $CH_3COCOOH$ Simplest keto-ACID, important in making ENERGY available from ingested food. It is the PRODUCT of the first stage of RESPIRATION (GLYCOLYSIS). If OXYGEN is available, the ACID is broken down in the KREBS CYCLE to yield ENERGY. Also termed: 2-OXOPROPANOIC ACID.

PYY (biochemistry) An abbreviation of 'P'olypeptide 'YY'.

PZI (biochemistry) An abbreviation of 'P'rotamine 'Z'inc 'I'nsulin.

Q

Q (biochemistry) A symbol for glutamine.

q (genetics) Symbol used to designate the long arm of a CHROMOSOME. Thus if a GENE's LOCUS is given as 22q, this means that it is on the long arm of CHROMOSOME 22. The short arm is called p.

Q&A (literature terminology) An abbreviation of 'Q'uestion 'and' 'A'nswer.

QC (quality standards) An abbreviation of 'Q'uality 'C'ontrol.

Q fever (microbiology) An ACUTE febrile illness caused by INFECTION with the MICRO-ORGANISM *Coxiella burnetii,* a SPECIES of *Rickettsia.* The organism normally infects sheep, cattle and goats, passing to them from wild animals via TICKS and lice, but humans acquire the INFECTION by inhaling dust from dried excreta or drinking infected milk.

QSAR (toxicology) An abbreviation of 'Q'UANTITATIVE 'S'TRUCTURE 'A'CTIVITY 'R'ELATIONSHIPS.

qty (general terminology) An abbreviation of 'q'uan't'it'y'.

quadrate (anatomy) One of a pair of bones in the upper JAW of amphibians, birds, fish and reptiles that has evolved into the INCUS (an EAR OSSICLE) in mammals.

quadratic equation (mathematics) Algebraic equation of the second ORDER (DEGREE) or square POWER, which has two possible solutions, known as the roots of the unknown. The roots may be real and different, real and the same (coincident) or imaginary. For the general QUADRATIC EQUATION $ax^2 + bx + c = 0$, the solutions are given by $x = [-b \pm (b^2 - 4ac)^{1/2}]/ 2a$.

quadriceps (anatomy) The large MUSCLE covering the front of the thigh. It is a COMBINATION of four muscles, the vastus medialis, vastus intermediug, vastus lateralis and rectus femoris.

quadriplegia (medical) Paralysis of all four limbs.

quadrivalent (chemistry) Having a VALENCE of four. Also termed: TETRA-VALENT.

quadruplets (genetics) Four babies born together. Human QUADRUPLETS may be identical or non-identical.

qual. (1, 2, 3 general terminology) 1 An abbreviation of 'qual'ification. 2 An abbreviation of 'qual'itative. 3 An abbreviation of 'qual'ity.

qualitative (chemistry) Dealing with the qualities or appearance of something only.

qualitative analysis (chemistry) Identification of the constituents of a substance or MIXTURE, irrespective of their amount.

quality assurance (quality standards) *See* QUALITY CONTROL.

quality control (QC) (quality standards) A term used to describe mechanisms and procedures planned as a part of experimental protocols that are designed to reduce the possibility of error, particularly human error. INTEGRAL parts of QUALITY CONTROL include the design of procedures in such a way as to minimise the possibility of human error, the collection of DATA not only on the results of the experiments, but also on the daily activities, personnel involved, etc.; and the proper training of all LABORATORY and ANIMAL room personnel. Activity and results forms must be designed in such a way that omissions are immediately apparent.

quanta (measurement) Plural of QUANTUM.

quantification (genetics) the application of measurement to experimental results.

quantitative (chemistry) Dealing with quantities of substances, *e.g.* MASS, VOLUME, etc., irrespective of their identity.

quantitative analysis (chemistry) Determination of the amounts of constituents present in a substance or MIXTURE, often by weighing or manipulating volumes of solutions.

See also GRAVIMETRIC ANALYSIS; VOLUMETRIC ANALYSIS.

quantitative structure-activity relationships (QSAR) (toxicology) The relationship between the physical and/or chemical properties of chemicals and their ability to cause a particular effect, enter into particular reactions, etc.

quantum (measurement) UNIT quantity (an indivisible 'packet') of ENERGY postulated in the QUANTUM THEORY. The PHOTON is the QUANTUM of ELECTRO-MAGNETIC RADIATION (such as LIGHT) and in certain contexts the MESON is the QUANTUM of the nuclear FIELD.

quantum electrodynamics (physics) Study of ELECTROMAGNETIC INTERACTIONS, in accordance with the QUANTUM THEORY.

quantum electronics (physics) Generation or amplification of MICROWAVE POWER, governed by QUANTUM MECHANICS.

quantum evolution (genetics) Evolutionary change in which new SPECIES are formed very rapidly. The circumstance in which this is likely to happen is the colonisation of new habitats by small populations, in which both founder effect and GENETIC DRIFT contribute to genetic change.

quantum mechanics (physics) Method of dealing with the BEHAVIOUR (*USA*: behavior) of small particles such as electrons and nuclei. It uses the idea of the PARTICLE WAVE duality of MATTER. Thus an ELECTRON has a dual nature, PARTICLE and WAVE, but it behaves as one or the other according to the nature of the experiment.

quantum number (physics) INTEGER or half-INTEGRAL number that specifies possible values of a quantitized physical quantity, *e.g.* ENERGY LEVEL, nuclear spin, angular momentum, etc.

quantum state (physics) State of an ATOM, ELECTRON, PARTICLE, etc; defined by a unique SET of QUANTUM NUMBERS.

quantum theory (physics) Theory of RADIATION. It states that RADIANT ENERGY is given out by a radiating body in separate units of ENERGY known as quanta; the same applies to the ABSORPTION of

333

RADIATION. The total amount of RADIANT ENERGY given out or absorbed is always a whole number of quanta.

quarantine (medical) The ISOLATION of people who are suspected of being infected with a particular INFECTIOUS DISEASE.

quart (measurement) UNIT of LIQUID measure equal to 2 pints. 1qt (imperial) = 1.13652 LITRES.

quartan malaria (microbiology) MALARIA caused by *Plasmodium malariae*.

quartile (statistics) Value below which one-quarter of a SET of DATA lies; the 25th PERCENTILE. The second QUARTILE equals the MEDIAN.

quartz (chemistry) SiO_2 Natural CRYSTALLINE silica (SILICON dioxide), one of the hardest of common minerals. Its crystals (which can generate piezoelectricity) are frequently colourless (*USA*: colorless) and TRANSPARENT. It is used as an abrasive and in mortar and cement.

quasi group (statistics) A collection of people, not yet a proper GROUP, but with the CAPACITY to become one.

quaternary ammonium compound (chemistry) Member of a GROUP of white CRYSTALLINE solids, SOLUBLE in WATER, and completely dissociated in SOLUTION. These compounds have the GENERAL FORMULA $R_4N^+X^-$, where R is a long-chain ALKYL GROUP. They have DETERGENT properties. Also termed: quaternary ammonium SALT.

quenching (chemistry) Rapid cooling.

Question and Answer (Q&A) (general terminolgy) Relating to speeches and lectures, the time when people in the audience can ask specific questions of the speaker or panel.

quicklime (chemistry) CaO Whitish powder prepared by roasting limestone, used in agriculture and in cements and mortar. Also termed: CALCIUM OXIDE; LIME.

quicksilver (chemistry) *See* MERCURY.

quinidine (pharmacology) A drug obtained from the cinchona tree and used to treat irregular HEART ACTION.

quinine (pharmacology) An ALKALOID made from the bark of the South American cinchona tree. It is used against chloroquine-resistant strains of *Plasmodium falciparum*, the organism of maglignant MALARIA.

quinine (pharmacology) Colourless (*USA*: colorless) CRYSTALLINE ALKALOID, obtained from the bark of the cinchona shrub, once much used in the TREATMENT and prevention of MALARIA.

quinoline (chemistry) C_9H_7N Colourless (*USA*: colorless) oily LIQUID HETEROCYCLIC BASE. It is an AROMATIC COMPOUND consisting of fused BENZENE and PYRIDINE rings.

quinolones (pharmacology) A GROUP of antibiotics comprising nalidixic ACID and cinoxacin, used in urinary infections, ciprofloxacin, used in Gram-negative and some Gram-POSITIVE infections that are resistant to other antibiotics, and enoxacin, which is used in SKIN infections, shigella infections, GONORRHOEA and urinary infections.

quinone (chemistry) Member of a GROUP of CYCLIC UNSATURATED diketones in which the DOUBLE BONDS and keto groups are CONJUGATED. Thus they are not AROMATIC

COMPOUNDS. Many quinones are used as dyes.

quinsy (medical) *See* PERITONSILLAR ABSCESS.

quotient (mathematics) Result of DIVISION.

qwerty (computing) Description of the standard ALPHANUMERIC KEYBOARD used on typewriters, typesetting machines, WORD PROCESSORS and computers (named after the first six letters on the top rank of letters).

R

R (radiology) An abbreviation of 'R'adiologist/ 'R'adiology.

Ra (chemistry) The CHEMICAL SYMBOL for ELEMENT 88, RADIUM.

rabies (medical) VIRUS disease, mainly affecting carnivores but which can affect any WARM-BLOODED SPECIES, that is usually transmitted by bites from infected animals, including foxes, wolves, jackals, mongooses, raccoons, skunks and bats. Also termed: HYDROPHOBIA.

race (biology) In CLASSIFICATION, an alternative term for SUBSPECIES.

racemic acid (chemistry) RACEMIC MIXTURE of TARTARIC ACID.

racemic mixture (chemistry) Optically inactive MIXTURE that contains equal amounts of DEXTROROTATORY and LAEVOROTATORY forms of an OPTICALLY ACTIVE COMPOUND.

racemization (chemistry) TRANSFORMATION of OPTICALLY ACTIVE compounds into RACEMIC MIXTUREs. It can be effected by the ACTION of HEAT or LIGHT, or by the use of chemical reagents.

rad (1 radiology; 2 measurement) 1 An abbreviation of 'r'adiation 'a'bsorbed 'd'ose. 2 UNIT of ABSORBED DOSE of IONIZING RADIATION, equivalent to 100 ergs per gram (0.01 J kg⁻¹) of absorbing material. The corresponding SI UNIT is the gray.

Rad. (radiology) An abbreviation of 'Rad'iologist; 'Rad'iology; 'Rad'io-therapist; 'Rad'iotherapy;

rada (radiology) An abbreviation of 'rad'io'a'ctive.

radial immunodiffusion (RID) (immunology) *See* IMMUNOASSAY.

radial symmetry (general terminology) SYMMETRY about any one of several lines or planes through the centre (*USA*: center) of an OBJECT or organism.

See also BILATERAL SYMMETRY.

radian (rad) (measurement) SI UNIT of plane angle; the angle at the centre (*USA*: center) of a circle subtended by an ARC whose length is equal to the RADIUS of the circle. 1 RADIAN = 57 degrees (approx.).

radiance (physics) (measurement) The RADIANT INTENSITY of a source in a given direction per unit transverse AREA. It is usually measured in WATTS METRE² per steradian.

radiant (physics) Describing something that emits electromagnetic RADIATION (*e.g.* LIGHT, HEAT rays).

radiant energy (physics) Electromagnetic ENERGY, which the part with wavelengths between about 380 and 750 nm is visible as LIGHT.

radiant flux (physics) The rate at which POWER is emitted or received by an OBJECT in the form of ELECTROMAGNETIC RADIATION.

radiant heat (physics) HEAT that is transmitted in the form of INFRA-RED RADIATION.

radiant intensity (physics) The INTENSITY of energy emitted by a source per UNIT SOLID angle, usually measured in WATT steradian.

radiation (physics) ENERGY that travels in the form of ELECTROMAGNETIC RADIATION, *e.g.* radio waves, INFRA-RED RADIATION, LIGHT, ULTRAVIOLET RADIATION, X-RAYS and GAMMA RAYS. The term is also applied to the rays of ALPHA PARTICLES and BETA PARTICLES emitted by RADIOACTIVE substances. PARTICLE rays and short-WAVELENGTH ELECTROMAGNETIC RADIATION may be harmful to tissues as they are IONIZING RADIATION. Radiation is one of the causes of raised MUTATION rates and of increased INCIDENCE of cancers.

radiation damage (physics) Alteration of properties of a material that results from exposure to IONIZING RADIATION.

radiation pressure (physics) MINUTE FORCE exerted on a surface by ELECTROMAGNETIC RADIATION that strikes it.

radiation sickness (medical/ radiology) Illness caused by exposure to excessive RADIATION. ALPHA PARTICLES cannot penetrate SKIN and are not dangerous internally. GAMMA RADIATION, X-RAYS and neutrons can penetrate the body and are thus the most harmful.

radiation unit (radiology) Activity of a RADIO-ISOTOPE expressed in units of disintegrations per second, called the BECQUEREL in SI UNITS. Formerly it was measured in curies.

radical (1 chemistry; 2 mathematics) 1 A GROUP of atoms within a MOLECULE that maintains its identity through chemical changes that affect the rest of the MOLECULE, but is usually incapable of independent existence; *e.g.* alkyl RADICAL. *See also* FREE RADICAL. 2 Relating to the ROOT of a number or quantity.

radiculitis (histology) INFLAMMATION of a ROOT, applied to INFLAMMATION of a NERVE ROOT.

radioactive (radiology) Possessing or exhibiting RADIOACTIVITY.

radioactive decay (radiology) Way in which a RADIO-ISOTOPE spontaneously changes into another ELEMENT or ISOTOPE by the emission of alpha or BETA PARTICLES or GAMMA RAYS. The rate at which it does so is represented by its HALF-LIFE.

radioactive equilibrium (radiology) A condition attained when a parent RADIOACTIVE ELEMENT produces a daughter RADIOACTIVE ELEMENT that decays at the same rate as it is being formed from the parent.

radioactive isotope (chemistry) A form of a chemical substance that emits RADIOACTIVITY.

radioactive series (radiology) One of three SERIES that describe the RADIOACTIVE DECAY of 40 or more naturally occurring RADIOACTIVE ISOTOPES of high ATOMIC NUMBER. They are known (after the ELEMENT at the beginning of each sequence) as the THORIUM SERIES, URANIUM SERIES and ACTINIUM SERIES.

radioactive standard (radiology) RADIO-ISOTOPE of known rate of RADIOACTIVE DECAY used for the CALIBRATION of RADIATION-measuring instruments.

radioactive tracers (radiology) RADIOACTIVE ISOTOPES whose passage and BEHAVIOUR (*USA*: behavior) through the body is monitored by recording their RADIATION, *e.g.* ^{14}C, ^{15}N.

radioactive waste (radiology) Hazardous RADIO-ISOTOPES (FISSION products) that accumulate as waste products in a nuclear REACTOR. They have to be periodically removed and stored safely or reprocessed. The term is also applied to the waste ('tailings') produced by the processing of URANIUM ores.

radioactivity (radiology) Spontaneous DISINTEGRATION of atomic nuclei, usually with the emission of ALPHA PARTICLES, BETA PARTICLES or GAMMA RAYS.

radiobiology (radiology) Study of IONIZING RADIATION in relation to living systems. It includes the effects of RADIATION on living organisms and the use of RADIO-ISOTOPES in biological and medical WORK.

See also RADIOTHERAPY.

radiochemistry (radiology) Chemistry of RADIOACTIVE elements and their compounds, and use of RADIO-ISOTOPES (*e.g.* for 'labelling' in chemical ANALYSIS).

radiodiagnosis (radiology) Branch of medical radiology that is concerned with the use of X-RAYS or RADIO-ISOTOPES in diagnosis.

radiograph (radiology) Photographic IMAGE that results from uneven ABSORPTION by an OBJECT being subjected to penetrating RADIATION. An X-RAY photograph is a common example.

radiography (radiology) PHOTOGRAPHY using X-RAYS or GAMMA RAYS, particularly in medical applications.

radio-isotope (radiology) ISOTOPE that emits RADIOACTIVITY (IONIZING RADIATION) during its spontaneous DECAY. RADIO-ISOTOPES are useful sources of RADIATION (*e.g.* in RADIOGRAPHY) and are used as tracers for radioactive tracing.

radiology (radiology) Study of X-RAYS, GAMMA RAYS and RADIOACTIVITY (including RADIO-ISOTOPES), especially as used in medical diagnosis and TREATMENT.

radioluminescence (radiology) FLUO-RESCENCE caused by RADIOACTIVITY.

radio-opaque (radiology) Resistant to the penetrating effects of RADIATION, especially X-RAYS, often used to describe substances injected into the body before a RADIOGRAPHY examination.

radiotherapy (radiology) TREATMENT of disorders (*e.g.* CANCER) by the use of IONIZING RADIATION such as X-RAYS or RADIATION from RADIO-ISOTOPES.

radium Ra (chemistry) SILVER-white RADIOACTIVE metallic ELEMENT in GROUP IIA of the PERIODIC TABLE (the ALKALINE EARTHS). It has several isotopes, with half-lives of up to 1,620 years. It is obtained from pitchblende (its principal ore), and used in RADIOTHERAPY and luminous paints. At. no. 88; r.a.m. 226.0254.

radius (1 mathematics; 2 anatomy) 1 Distance from the centre (*USA*: center) of a circle to the CIRCUMFERENCE, equal to half the DIAMETER or the CIRCUMFERENCE divided by 2π. 2 One of two bones in the forearm of a tetrapod VERTEBRATE (the other is the ULNA).

radius of curvature (mathematics) Of a point on a curve, the RADIUS of a circle that touches the inside of the curve at that point.

radon Rn (chemistry) A RADIOACTIVE gaseous ELEMENT in GROUP 0 of the PERIODIC TABLE (the RARE GASes), a RADIOACTIVE DECAY PRODUCT of RADIUM. It has several isotopes, with half-lives of up to 3.82 days. RADON coming out of the ground, particularly in hard-rock areas, is a source of BACKGROUND RADIATION that has been recognized as a health hazard. At. no. 86; r.a.m. 222 (most STABLE ISOTOPE).

raffinate (chemistry) LIQUID that remains after a substance has been obtained by SOLVENT EXTRACTION.

raffinose (chemistry) $C_{18}H_{32}O_{16}$ Colourless (USA: colorless) CRYSTALLINE TRISACCHARIDE CARBOHYDRATE that occurs in SUGAR beet, which hydrolyses to the sugars GALACTOSE, GLUCOSE and FRUCTOSE.

r.a.m. (chemistry) An abbreviation of 'r'elative 'a'tomic 'm'ass (formerly called ATOMIC WEIGHT).

RAM (computing) An abbreviation of 'r'andom 'a'ccess 'm'emory of a COMPUTER.

Raman effect (physics) Scattering of MONOCHROMATIC LIGHT, when it passes through a TRANSPARENT HOMOGENEOUS medium, into different CHARACTERISTIC wavelengths because of INTERACTION with the molecules of the medium. It was named after the Indian physicist Chandrasekhara Raman (1888-1970).

random access memory (RAM) (computing) Part of a COMPUTER's MEMORY that can be written to and read from.

See also ROM.

random sample (statistics) SAMPLE taken from a large GROUP in such a way that it is representative of the GROUP as a whole. Random sampling is an important method of carrying out QUALITY CONTROL for MASS-produced articles.

Rankine scale (measurement) A TEMPERATURE SCALE that expresses ABSOLUTE TEMPERATURES in degrees Fahrenheit (ABSOLUTE ZERO = 0°R). It was named after the British engineer and physicist William Rankine (1820-72).

rare earth (chemistry) Member of the SERIES of elements, in GROUP IIIB of the PERIODIC TABLE, known also as the LANTHANIDES. Also termed: RARE EARTH ELEMENT.

rare gas (chemistry) One of the uncommon, unreactive and highly STABLE gases in GROUP 0 of the PERIODIC TABLE. They are HELIUM, NEON, ARGON, KRYPTON, XENON and RADON. Also termed: INERT GAS; NOBLE GAS.

RAS (physiology) An abbreviation of 'R'eticular 'A'ctivating 'S'ystem.

raster (computing) DISPLAY of information in the form of a grid, usually referring to the IMAGE produced by the parallel scanning ACTION of a CATHODE-RAY TUBE.

rate constant (chemistry) CONSTANT of proportionality for the speed of a CHEMICAL REACTION at a particular TEMPERATURE. It can only be obtained experimentally. Also termed: velocity CONSTANT; specific RATE CONSTANT.

rate-determining step (chemistry) The slowest step of a CHEMICAL REACTION which determines the overall rate, provided the other steps are relatively rapid. Thus the KINETICS and ORDER OF REACTION are basically those of the rate determining step. Also termed: LIMITING STEP.

rate equation (chemistry) An alternative term for RATE LAW.

rate law (chemistry) Equation that relates the rate of a CHEMICAL REACTION to the CONCENTRATION of the individual reactants. It has the form rate $= k[X]^n$, where k is the RATE CONSTANT, X is the REACTANT and n is the ORDER OF REACTION. It can only be obtained experimentally. Also termed: RATE EQUATION.

rate of reaction (chemistry) Speed of a CHEMICAL REACTION, usually expressed as the change in CONCENTRATION of a REACTANT or PRODUCT per UNIT time. It can be affected by TEMPERATURE, PRESSURE and the presence of a CATALYST.

rational number (mathematics) Number that may be expressed as a ratio of two integers – *i.e.* in the form of a FRACTION.

See also IRRATIONAL NUMBER.

ray (physics) Beam of any type of RADIATION, *e.g.* LIGHT.

rbc (haematology) An abbreviation of 'r'ed 'b'lood 'c'ell(s).

RCBF (physiology) An abbreviation of 'R'egional 'C'erebral 'B'lood 'F'low.

RCMRO (physiology) An abbreviation of 'R'egional 'C'erebral 'M'etabolic 'R'ate for 'O'xygen.

R&D (education) An abbreviation of 'R'esearch 'and' 'D'evelopment.

RDS (medical) An abbreviation of 'R'espiratory 'D'istress 'S'yndrome.

Re. (measurement) An abbreviation of 'Re'ynolds' number.

reactant (chemistry) Substance that reacts with another in a CHEMICAL REACTION to form new substances.

reaction (chemistry) An alternative term for CHEMICAL REACTION.

reactive dye (chemistry) Dye that forms a COVALENT BOND with the FIBRE MOLECULE (*USA*: fiber molecule) of the textile being dyed. This provides excellent fastness. Such dyes are used to dye CELLULOSE fibres (*USA*: cellulose fibers) (*e.g.* rayon).

reactor (chemistry) VESSEL in which a CHEMICAL REACTION is carried out.

read-only memory (ROM) (computing) Part of a COMPUTER'S MEMORY that can only be read (and not written to).

See also RANDOM ACCESS MEMORY.

reagent (1, 2 chemistry) 1 Substance that takes part in a CHEMICAL REACTION; a REACTANT. 2 Common LABORATORY chemical used in chemical ANALYSIS and for experiments.

real gas (chemistry) GAS that never fully achieves 'ideal' BEHAVIOUR (*USA*: behavior).

See also KINETIC THEORY.

real image (optics) IMAGE brought to a FOCUS by a LENS, mirror or optical system that can be displayed on a screen (as opposed to a virtual IMAGE, which can not).

real number (mathematics) Any number, POSITIVE or negative, from among all RATIONAL NUMBERS and IRRATIONAL NUMBERS (as opposed to an imaginary number).

realgar (chemistry) As_2S_2 Natural red ARSENIC disulphide (*USA*: arsenic disulfide), used as a PIGMENT and in pyrotechnics.

receptors (1 chemistry/ physics; 2 pharmacology) 1 Sensory CELLS, which may be part of a GROUP that form a SENSE ORGAN capable of detecting stimuli. When a RECEPTOR is stimulated (*e.g.* by TEMPERATURE or LIGHT), it produces electrical or biochemical changes that are relayed to the NERVOUS SYSTEM for processing. 2 PROTEINs through which many drugs and natural mediators act to exert their effects.

recessive (genetics) Describing a GENE that is expressed in the PHENOTYPE when it is HOMOZYGOUS in a CELL (*i.e.* there have to be two RECESSIVE genes for their effect to be apparent). The presence of a DOMINANT ALLELE masks the effect of a RECESSIVE GENE (*i.e.* in a COMBINATION of a DOMINANT GENE and a RECESSIVE GENE, the DOMINANT GENE manifests itself.

recipient (biology) Organism that receives material from another, *e.g.* as in the taking up of DNA by one bacterium from another.

reciprocal (mathematics) The quantity obtained by dividing a number into 1; *i.e.* the RECIPROCAL of x is the number $1/x$. Zero has no RECIPROCAL.

reciprocal wavelength (physics) An alternative term for WAVE NUMBER.

recombinant DNA (molecular biology) Type of DNA that has genes from different sources, genetically engineered using RECOMBINATION.

recombination (molecular biology) The process by which new combinations of characteristics not possessed by the parents are formed in the offspring. It results from CROSSING OVER during MEIOSIS to form gametes that unite during FERTILIZATION to form a new individual. Genetic engineers have developed techniques for artificially recombining strands of DNA (to make RECOMBINANT DNA).

record (computing) A number of elements of DATA that together form one UNIT of stored information.

recrystallization (1, 2 chemistry) 1 Change from one crystal structure to another; it occurs on heating or cooling through a CRITICAL TEMPERATURE. 2 Purification of a substance by repeated CRYSTALLIZATION from SOLUTION.

rectification (1 chemistry; 2 physics) 1 Purification of a LIQUID using DISTILLATION. 2 Conversion of ALTERNATING CURRENT (ac) into DIRECT CURRENT (dc) using a RECTIFIER.

rectified spirit (chemistry) SOLUTION of ETHANOL (ETHYL ALCOHOL) that contains about 5 to 7 per cent WATER. It is a CONSTANT-boiling MIXTURE and the WATER cannot be removed by DISTILLATION.

rectifier (physics) Electrical device for converting an ALTERNATING CURRENT (ac) into a DIRECT CURRENT (dc). It may take the form of a plate RECTIFIER, a DIODE VALVE or a semiconductor DIODE.

rectilinear (mathematics) In or forming a straight line.

rectum (anatomy) Final part of the INTESTINE, through which FAECES (*USA*: feces) are passed after reABSORPTION of WATER.

recurring decimal (mathematics) Decimal that contains a number or block of numbers that repeat to INFINITY; *e.g.* the decimal for 2/3 = 0.666666...

See also TERMINAL DECIMAL.

red blood cell (haematology) An alternative term for an ERYTHROCYTE, also known as a red cell or red corpuscle.

red lead (chemistry) Pb_3O_4 Bright red powdery OXIDE of LEAD. An OXIDIZING AGENT, it is used in anti-rust and priming paints. Also termed: minium; dilead(II); LEAD(IV) OXIDE; LEAD tetraoxide; triplumbic tetroxide.

red tide (biology) Phenomenon that occurs on seas and estuaries when SPECIES of red ALGAE multiply abnormally, sometimes producing a floating crust several centimetres thick. The ALGAE produce toxins that POISON shellfish and which can be passed along food chains.

redox reaction (chemistry) CHEMICAL REACTION in which OXIDATION is necessarily accompanied by REDUCTION, and vice versa; an OXIDATION-REDUCTION REACTION.

reduced equation of state (physics) An equation of state of a gas in which the temperature, pressure and volume are replaced by their reduced values. *See* REDUCED TEMPERATURE, PRESSURE AND VOLUME.

reduced pressure distillation (chemistry) An alternative term for VACUUM DISTILLATION.

reduced temperature, pressure and volume (physics) The ratios of the TEMPERATURE, PRESSURE and VOLUME to the CRITICAL TEMPERATURE, CRITICAL PRESSURE and CRITICAL VOLUME respectively in the REDUCED EQUATION OF STATE.

reducing agent (chemistry) Substance that causes chemical REDUCTION, often by adding HYDROGEN or removing OXYGEN; *e.g.* CARBON, CARBON MONOXIDE, HYDROGEN. Also termed: ELECTRON DONOR; reluctant.

reducing sugar (chemistry) Any SUGAR that can act as a REDUCING AGENT.

See also BENEDICT'S TEST; FEHLING'S TEST.

reductase (biochemistry) ENZYME that causes the REDUCTION of an ORGANIC COMPOUND.

reduction (chemistry) CHEMICAL REACTION that involves the GAIN of electrons by a substance; the addition of HYDROGEN or removal of OXYGEN from a substance.

REF (physiology/ biochemistry) An abbreviation of 'R'enal 'E'rythropoietic 'F'actor.

reflectance (measurement) Ratio of the INTENSITY of reflected RADIATION to the INTENSITY of the incident RADIATION.

reflection (physics) Change in direction of an ELECTROMAGNETIC WAVE (*e.g.* LIGHT) or sound WAVE after it strikes a (smooth) surface (*e.g.* a mirror). *See* LAWS OF REFLECTION.

reflector (optics) OBJECT or surface that reflects electromagnetic RADIATION (*e.g.*

LIGHT, radio waves), particularly one around or inside a lamp to concentrate a LIGHT beam.

reflex (1 biology; 2 mathematics) 1 Sequence of NERVE IMPULSEs that produce a fast involuntary RESPONSE to an external STIMULUS. 2 Describing an angle that exceeds 180 degrees (but is less than 360 degrees).

reflux (chemistry) Boiling of a LIQUID for long periods of time. Loss by EVAPORATION is prevented by using a REFLUX CONDENSER.

reflux condenser (chemistry) Vertical CONDENSER used in the process of refluxing. It is attached to a VESSEL that contains the LIQUID to be refluxed and condenses the VAPOUR produced on boiling, which then runs back into the VESSEL.

reflux reduction division (genetics) An alternative term for MEIOSIS.

reforming (chemistry) Production of branched-chain ALKANES from straight-chain ones or the production of AROMATIC COMPOUNDS (*e.g.* BENZENE) from ALKENES, using cracking or a CATALYST.

refraction (physics) Change in direction of an ENERGY WAVE (*e.g.* LIGHT, sound) when it passes from one medium into another in which its speed is different.

refraction of light (optics) Change in direction of a LIGHT RAY as it passes obliquely from one TRANSPARENT medium to another of different REFRACTIVE INDEX.

refractive constant (physics) An alternative term for REFRACTIVE INDEX.

refractive index (*n***)** (physics) Ratio of the speed of electromagnetic RADIATION (such as LIGHT) in AIR or VACUUM to its speed in another medium. The speed depends on the WAVELENGTH of the RADIATION as well as on the DENSITY of the medium. For a refracted RAY of LIGHT, it is equal to the ratio of the sine of the ANGLE OF INCIDENCE i to the sine of the ANGLE OF REFRACTION r; *i.e.* $n = \sin i / \sin r$. Also termed: REFRACTIVE CONSTANT.

refractometer (physics) Instrument for measuring the REFRACTIVE INDEX of a substance.

refrigerant (chemistry) Substance used as the WORKING FLUID in a refrigerator (*e.g.* AMMONIA, fluon, CFCS).

refrigeration (physics) A method of maintaining a cool TEMPERATURE in a room or container by transferring HEAT from it to the exterior using a HEAT PUMP. Cooling is caused by the EVAPORATION of a VOLATILE LIQUID (REFRIGERANT) into a VAPOUR, which is compressed by a PUMP (compressor) to turn it back to a LIQUID.

regeneration (physiology) Regrowth of TISSUE to replace that which has been damaged or lost, *e.g.* WOUND healing.

relative atomic mass (r.a.m.) (physics) MASS of an ATOM relative to the MASS of the ISOTOPE CARBON-12 (which is taken to be exactly 12). Former name: ATOMIC WEIGHT.

relative density (physics) Ratio of the DENSITY of a given substance to the DENSITY of some reference substance. For liquids, relative densities are usually expressed with reference to the DENSITY of WATER at 4°C. Former name: SPECIFIC GRAVITY.

relative humidity (physics) Ratio of the PRESSURE of WATER VAPOUR present in AIR to the PRESSURE the WATER VAPOUR would have if the AIR were saturated at the same TEMPERATURE (*i.e.* to the saturated-WATER VAPOUR PRESSURE). It is expressed as a PERCENTAGE.

relative molecular mass (chemistry) Sum of the RELATIVE ATOMIC MASSes of all the atoms in a MOLECULE of a substance. Also termed: MOLECULAR WEIGHT.

relative permittivity (physics) The ratio of the capacitance of a capacitor with a specified medium between the plates, to the capacitance of the same capacitor with free space between the plates. Also termed: dielectric constant.

relativity (physics) Einstein's theory; scientific principle expressing in mathematical and physical terms the implications of the fact that observations depend as much on the viewpoint as on what is being observed.

rem (radiology) An abbreviation of 'r'öntgen 'e'quivalent 'm'an, the quantity of IONIZING RADIATION such.that the ENERGY imparted to a biological system per gram of living material has the same effect as one röntgen.

REM sleep (physiology) An abbreviation of 'R'apid 'E'ye 'M'ovement (paradoxical) sleep.

renin (biochemistry) ENZYME produced by the KIDNEY that constricts arteries and thus raises BLOOD PRESSURE.

rennin (biochemistry) ENZYME found in GASTRIC JUICE that curdles milk. It is the active ingredient of rennet.

replicase (biochemistry) ENZYME that promotes the SYNTHESIS of DNA and RNA within living CELLS.

replication (molecular biology) The process by which a new complete molecule of DNA is made, by one strand being used as a template for the assembly of another strand.

reproduction (biology) Procreation of an organism. SEXUAL REPRODUCTION involves the FUSION of SEX CELLS or gametes and the exchange of genetic material, thus bringing new vigour to a SPECIES. ASEXUAL REPRODUCTION does not involve gametes, but usually the vegetative proliferation of an organism.

resin (chemistry) ORGANIC COMPOUND that is generally a viscous LIQUID or semi-LIQUID which gradually hardens when exposed to AIR, becoming an AMORPHOUS, brittle SOLID. Natural resins, found in plants, are yellowish in COLOUR (*USA*: color) and INSOLUBLE in WATER, but are quite SOLUBLE in organic solvents. SYNTHETIC resins (types of plastics) also possess many of these properties.

resistor (physics) Device that provides resistance in electrical circuits.

resonance (1 chemistry; 2 physics) 1 Movement of electrons from one ATOM of a MOLECULE or ION to another ATOM of that MOLECULE or ION to form a STABLE RESONANCE HYBRID structure (*e.g.* as in an AROMATIC COMPOUND). 2 Phenomenon in which a system is made to vibrate at its natural FREQUENCY as a result of vibrations received from another source of the same FREQUENCY.

resorcinol (chemistry) $C_6H_4(OH)_2$ CRYSTALLINE dihydric PHENOL, used in the SYNTHESIS of drugs, dyes and plastics. Also termed: m-dihydroxybenzene; 1,3-benzenediol.

respiration (1, 2 physiology) 1 Release of ENERGY by living organisms from the breakdown of ORGANIC COMPOUNDS. In AEROBIC RESPIRATION, which occurs in most CELLS, OXYGEN is required and CARBON DIOXIDE and WATER are produced. ENERGY production is coupled to a SERIES of oxidation-reduction reactions, catalysed by ENZYMES. In ANAEROBIC RESPIRATION (*e.g.* FERMENTATION), food substances are only partly broken down, and thus less ENERGY is released and OXYGEN is not required. 2 An alternative term for BREATHING.

respiratory movement (physiology) Movement by an organism to allow the exchange of respiratory gases, *i.e.* the taking up of OXYGEN and release of CARBON DIOXIDE. In mammals such as human beings this entails BREATHING, involving movements of the chest and DIAPHRAGM. In fishes, WATER is passed over the gills for gaseous exchange.

respiratory organ (anatomy) ORGAN in which RESPIRATION (BREATHING) takes place. In mammals (*e.g.* human beings), the process is carried out in the LUNG; in fish, the gills. There gaseous exchange takes place (usually of OXYGEN and CARBON DIOXIDE).

respiratory pigment (biochemistry) Substance that can take up and carry OXYGEN in areas of high OXYGEN CONCENTRATION, releasing it in parts of the organism with low OXYGEN concentrations where it is consumed, *i.e.* by RESPIRATION in CELLS. In vertebrates the RESPIRATORY PIGMENT is HAEMOGLOBIN (*USA*: hemoglobin); in some invertebrates it is HAEMOCYANIN (*USA*: hemocyanin).

respiratory quotient (RQ) (measurement) Ratio of CARBON DIOXIDE produced by an organism to the OXYGEN consumed in a given time. It gives information about the type of food being oxidized; *e.g.* CARBOHYDRATE has an RQ of approximately 1, but if the RQ becomes high (*i.e.* little OXYGEN is available), ANAEROBIC RESPIRATION may occur.

response (physiology) Physical, chemical or behavioural (*USA*: behavioral) change in an organism initiated by a STIMULUS.

resting potential (physiology) POTENTIAL DIFFERENCE between the inner and outer surfaces of a resting NERVE, which is about -60 to -80 mV. It occurs when the NERVE is not conducting any IMPULSE, and is in contrast to the ACTION POTENTIAL, which occurs during the application of a STIMULUS and brings about a rise in the POTENTIAL DIFFERENCE to a POSITIVE value.

restriction enzyme (biochemistry) ENZYME (a NUCLEASE) produced by some BACTERIA that is capable of breaking down foreign DNA. It cleaves double-stranded DNA at a specific sequence of bases, and the DNA of the BACTERIA is modified for protection against DEGRADATION. RESTRICTION ENZYMES are used widely as tools in GENETIC ENGINEERING for cutting DNA. Also termed: restriction endonuclease.

retina (histology) LIGHT-sensitive TISSUE at the back of the VERTEBRATE EYE, made up of a NETWORK of interconnected NERVES. The first CELLS in the NETWORK are photoreceptors consisting of cones (which are sensitive to COLOUR [*USA*: color]) or rods (which are sensitive to LIGHT). They contain visual pigments (*e.g.* RHODOPSIN) which ultimately cause impulses to be transmitted to the visual centre (*USA*: center) of the BRAIN via the OPTIC NERVE.

retinol (biochemistry) Fat-SOLUBLE VITAMIN found in plants, in which it is formed from CAROTENE. Also termed: VITAMIN A.

retort (chemistry) Heated VESSEL used for the DISTILLATION of substances, as in the separation of some metals.

retrovirus (virology) Member of a GROUP of VIRUSES that contain RNA as their genetic material. They use an RNA-dependent DNA polymerase or reverse transcriptase ENZYME to carry out TRANSCRIPTION. Many RNA VIRUSES are CARCINOGENIC in their hosts, which include mammals. Also termed: ONCOVIRUS.

reversible process (chemistry) Process that can theoretically be reversed by an appropriate small change in any of the thermodynamic variables (*e.g.* PRESSURE, TEMPERATURE). Real natural processes are irreversible.

reversible reaction (chemistry) CHEMICAL REACTION that can go either forwards or backwards depending on the conditions.

RFLP (physiology/ biochemistry) An abbreviation of 'R'estriction 'F'ragment 'L'ength 'P'olymorphism.

rhabdovirus (virology) Member of a GROUP of VIRUSES that can infect multi-cellular animals and plants. One type causes RABIES.

rhenium Re (chemistry) Rare metallic ELEMENT of GROUP VIIB of the PERIODIC TABLE (a TRANSITION ELEMENT), used in making thermocouples. At no 75; r.a.m. 186.20.

rheology (physics) Study of flow within objects under STRESS.

rheostat (physics) VARIABLE electrical RESISTOR, generally used to control ELECTRIC CURRENT flow.

Rh factor (haematology) An abbreviation of 'Rh'esus factor.

rhesus factor (Rh) (haematology/ immunology) ANTIGEN present in the RED BLOOD CELLS of a majority of human beings, who are thus rhesus POSITIVE (Rh+). Unlike the ABO BLOOD GROUP system, a person with rhesus-negative (Rh-) BLOOD does not possess the rhesus ANTIBODY unless he or she receives rhesus-POSITIVE BLOOD (through transfusion or via the PLACENTA). This can be fatal to a rhesus-POSITIVE FOETUS (*USA*: fetus) in a rhesus-negative mother.

rhinovirus (virology) Member of a GROUP of VIRUSES that infect the respiratory tract of vertebrates and which are one of the main causative agents of the common cold.

rhodium Rh (chemistry) SILVER-white metallic ELEMENT in GROUP VIII of the PERIODIC TABLE (a TRANSITION ELEMENT), used as a CATALYST and in making thermocouples. At. no. 45; r.a.m. 102.9055.

rhodopsin (biochemistry) PROTEIN (derived from VITAMIN A) in the rods of the RETINA of the EYE which acts as a LIGHT-sensitive PIGMENT; the ACTION of LIGHT brings about a chemical change that results in the production of a NERVE IMPULSE. Also termed: VISUAL PURPLE.

riboflavin (biochemistry) Orange WATER-SOLUBLE CRYSTALLINE SOLID, member of the VITAMIN B complex. It plays an important role in GROWTH. Also termed: riboflavine; LACTOFLAVIN; VITAMIN B_2.

ribonucleic acid (molecular biology) *See* RNA.

ribose (chemistry) $C_5H_{10}O_5$ OPTICALLY ACTIVE PENTOSE SUGAR, a COMPONENT of the aucleotides of RNA (RIBONUCLEIC ACID).

ribosome (cytology) PARTICLE present in the CYTOPLASM of CELLS, often attached to the ENDOPLASMIC RETICULUM, that is essential in the BIOSYNTHESIS of proteins. Ribosomes are composed of PROTEIN and RNA, and are the site of attachment for MESSENGER RNA during PROTEIN SYNTHESIS. They may be associated in chains called polyribosomes.

rickets (medical) Disorder that results from a deficiency of VITAMIN D. It mainly affects children and can cause deformed limbs.

rickettsiae (microbiology) GROUP of MICRO-ORGANISMS, often classified as being part way between BACTERIA and VIRUSES, that are parasitic on the CELLS of arthropods (lice, mites and TICKS) and vertebrates. Some can cause serious disorders (*e.g.* TYPHUS in human beings).

ringer's fluid (chemistry) Physiological SALINE SOLUTION used for keeping tissues and organs alive outside the body (in vitro). It is similar in composition to the FLUID that naturally bathes CELLS and tissues, maintaining a CONSTANT internal ENVIRONMENT. It contains chlorides of SODIUM, POTASSIUM and CALCIUM. It was named after the British physiologist Sydney Ringer (1835-1910).

ringworm (mycology) *See* TINEA.

RMV (physiology) An abbreviation of 'Respiratory 'M'inute 'V'olume.

RNA (molecular biology) An abbreviation of 'R'ibo'N'ucleic 'A'cid, one of the NUCLEIC ACIDS present in CELLS, the other being DNA. It is composed of nucleotides that contain RIBOSE as the SUGAR. RNA contains the bases ADENINE, GUANINE, CYTOSINE and URACIL. MESSENGER RNA takes part in TRANSCRIPTION or copying of the GENETIC CODE from a DNA template. TRANSFER RNA and ribosomal RNA take part in TRANSLATION or PROTEIN SYNTHESIS, all of which occur in prokaryotes and eukaryotes.

RNA virus (virology) VIRUS that has RNA as its genetic material (instead of DNA).

rock salt (chemistry) Naturally occurring CRYSTALLINE SODIUM CHLORIDE, an important raw material in the chemical industry.

rod (cytology) Type of sensory CELL present in the RETINA of the VERTEBRATE EYE. It is stimulated by LIGHT and is concerned with vision in low illumination. The ABSORPTION of LIGHT ENERGY (photons) by the visual PIGMENT RHODOPSIN present in the ROD causes a nervous IMPULSE, which travels along the OPTIC NERVE to the BRAIN.

See also CONE.

roentgen (R) (measurement) UNIT of RADIATION; the amount of X-RAYS or GAMMA RAYS that produce a CHARGE of 2.58×10^{-4} coulomb of ELECTRICITY in 1 cm^3 of dry AIR. It was named after the German physicist Wilhelm Röntgen (1845-1923). Also termed: röntgen.

Roentgen rays (radiology) An alternative term for X-RAYS.

ROM (computing) An abbreviation of 'r'ead-'o'nly 'm'emory of a COMPUTER.

Roman numerals (mathematics) A number system, originally used by the Romans, based on letters: I = 1; V = 5; X = 10; L = 50; C = 100; D = 500;

M = 1,000. Other numbers are written using combinations of these; there is no zero.

röntgen (chemistry) An alternative term for roentgen.

root (1, 2 mathematics) 1 Number or quantity that when multiplied by itself some specified times gives the number again; *e.g.* the square ROOT of a number is that when multiplied by itself gives the number. 2 SOLUTION of an ALGEBRAIC equation.

root-mean-square (rms) (mathematics) AVERAGE equal to the SQUARE ROOT of the sum of the squares of a number of values divided by the total number of values.

rotatory (chemistry/ optics) OPTICALLY ACTIVE; capable of rotating the plane of POLARIZED LIGHT.

rotoscope (physics) An alternative term for STROBOSCOPE.

round window (histology) Lower of two membranous areas on the COCHLEA of the INNER EAR (the other is the OVAL WINDOW). Also termed: fenestra rotunda.

RPF (physiology) An abbreviation of 'R'enal 'P'lasma 'F'low.

R plasmid (genetics) Any plasmid carying a GENE for ANTIBIOTIC resistance.

RQ (physiology) An abbreviation of 'R'espiratory 'Q'uotient.

R technique (statistics) A FACTOR ANALYSIS based on the correlations between tests that attempts to derive a limited number of factors underlying the correlations.

rubella (medical) An acute infectious viral disease spread by droplet infection. Complications are rare, except when contracted in the early months of pregnancy, when it may produce foetal (*USA*: fetal) deformities. Also termed: German measles.

rubidium Rb (chemistry) Reactive SILVER-white METAL in GROUP IA of the PERIODIC TABLE (the ALKALI METALS), with a naturally occurring RADIOACTIVE ISOTOPE (Rb-87). At. no. 37; r.a.m. 85.4678.

rule of acceleration (genetics) The rule that in an organism's development the structures that are formed first are the ones most important to the organism's overall FUNCTION.

R unit (measurement) 1 An abbreviation of 'R'esistance unit in the cardiovascular system, mmHg divided by ml/s. 2 An abbreviation of 'R'oentgen unit.

ruthenium Ru (chemistry) SILVER-white metallic ELEMENT in GROUP VIII of the PERIODIC TABLE (a TRANSITION ELEMENT), used to add hardness to PLATINUM ALLOYS. At. no. 44; r.a.m. 101.07.

rutherfordium Rf (chemistry) ELEMENT no. 104. A RADIOACTIVE METAL with at least three very short-lived isotopes (half-lives up to 70 seconds) made by bombarding an ACTINIDE with CARBON, OXYGEN or NEON atoms. Also termed: KURCHATOVIUM.

S

S (1 chemistry; 2 biochemistry) 1 The CHEMICAL SYMBOL for SULPHUR (*USA*: sulfur). 2 An abbreviation of 'S'erine.

SA (physiology) An abbreviation of 'S'pecific 'A'ctivity.

SAB (1 governing body; 2 society) 1 An abbreviation of 'S'cience/ 'S'cientific 'A'dvisory 'B'oard. 2 An abbreviation of 'S'ociety of 'A'merican 'B'acteriologists.

saccharide (chemistry) Simplest type of CARBOHYDRATE, with the GENERAL FORMULA ($C_6H_{12}O_6$), common to many sugars. Also termed: SACCHAROSE.

See also DISACCHARIDE; MONOSACCHARIDE.

saccharimetry (measurement) Measurement of the CONCENTRATION of SUGAR in a SOLUTION from its OPTICAL ACTIVITY, by using a polarimeter.

saccharin (chemistry) $C_6H_4SO_2CONH$ White CRYSTALLINE ORGANIC COMPOUND that is about 550 times sweeter than SUGAR; an artificial sweetener. It is almost INSOLUBLE in WATER and hence it is used in the form of its SOLUBLE SODIUM SALT. Also termed: 2-sulphobenzimide (*USA*: 2-sulfobenzimide); saccharine.

Saccharomyces cerevisiae (toxicology/ genetics) A common SPECIES of YEAST which is frequently used in *in vitro* tests for mutagenic POTENTIAL of chemicals, genetic research, commercial GENE CLONING.

saccharose (chemistry) An alternative term for SACCHARIDE.

SADR (biochemistry) An abbreviation of 'S'uspected 'A'dverse 'D'rug 'R'eaction.

safranine O/ fast green stain (histology) A histological staining technique that may be used to make CARTILAGE visible under the MICROSCOPE.

sagittal fissure (histology) The FISSURE separating the CEREBRAL HEMISPHERES.

SAIMR (institution) An abbreviation of 'S'outh 'A'frican 'I'nstitute of 'M'edical 'R'esearch.

sal ammoniac (chemistry) Old name for AMMONIUM CHLORIDE.

salicylate (chemistry) ESTER or SALT of SALICYLLIC ACID.

salicyllic acid (chemistry) $C_6H_4(OH)COOH$ White CRYSTALLINE ORGANIC COMPOUND, a CARBOXYLIC ACID. It is used as an ANTISEPTIC, in medicine, and in the preparation of AZO DYES. Its acetyl ESTER is ASPIRIN. Also termed: 2-HYDROXYBENZOIC ACID.

saline (chemistry) Salty; describing a SOLUTION of SODIUM CHLORIDE (COMMON SALT).

saliva (biochemistry) NEUTRAL or slightly ALKALINE FLUID secreted by the salivary GLANDS in the mouth. It lubricates food during chewing and aids DIGESTION. It consists of a MIXTURE of MUCUS and the

ENZYME AMYLASE (ptyalin), which breaks down STARCH to MALTOSE.

salpingostomy (medical) An operation to open the FALLOPIAN TUBES.

salt (1, 2 chemistry) 1 PRODUCT obtained when a HYDROGEN ATOM in an ACID is replaced by a METAL or its equivalent (*e.g.* the AMMONIUM ION NH_4^+). It results from the REACTION between an ACID and a BASE.

See also ACID SALT; BASIC SALT. 2 COMMON SALT, SODIUM CHLORIDE.

saltcake (chemistry) An alternative term for crude SODIUM SULPHATE (*USA*: sodium sulfate).

salting out (chemistry) PRECIPITATION of a COLLOID (*e.g.* gelatine) by the addition of large amounts of a SALT.

saltpetre (chemistry) An alternative term for POTASSIUM NITRATE.

salvation (chemistry) The attachment between SOLVENT and SOLUTE molecules. The greater the POLARITY of the SOLVENT, the greater is the attraction between SOLUTE and SOLVENT molecules.

sal volatile (chemistry) Old name for AMMONIUM CARBONATE.

samarium Sm (chemistry) Metallic ELEMENT in GROUP IIIB of the PERIODIC TABLE (one of the LANTHANIDES). It is slightly RADIOACTIVE and arises from FISSION fragments in a nuclear REACTOR, where it acts as a 'POISON'. At. no. 62; r.a.m. 150.35.

sample (statistics) Part of a population, usually randomly selected to be representative of the whole population.

sample bias (statistics) Any way in which a SAMPLE is not representative of the population from which it was drawn.

sampling error (statistics) The difference between any value of a statistic obtained from a SAMPLE of a population.

sampling population (statistics) The population from which a SAMPLE is drawn.

sampling theory (statistics) The principles that govern the selection of representative samples.

sampling validity (statistics) The extent to which a test appears to SAMPLE those traits under test, and only those traits.

sampling with replacement (statistics) Sampling from a finite population while replacing each item sampled.

sampling without replacement (statistics) Sampling from a finite population without replacing the items sampled.

sanatorium (medical) A hospital that specialised in the TREATMENT of TUBERCULOSIS. Since the introduction of CHEMOTHERAPY for the disease, such hospitals are no longer necessary.

sandwich compound (chemistry) ORGANO-METALLIC COMPOUND whose molecules consist of two parallel planar rings with a METAL ATOM centred (*USA*: centered) between them (*e.g.* FERROCENE).

SA node (histology) An abbreviation of 'S'ino'A'trial node.

SANTA (society) An abbreviation of 'S'outh 'A'frican 'N'ational 'T'uberculosis 'A'ssociation.

saponification (chemistry) HYDROLYSIS of an ESTER, using an ALKALI, to produce a free ALCOHOL and a SALT of ORGANIC ACID.

saponification value (chemistry) Number of milligrams of POTASSIUM HYDROXIDE required for the complete SAPONIFICATION of 1 g of the substance being tested. Also termed: saponification number.

saprophyte (microbiology) Organism that feeds on dead or decaying organic MATTER (*e.g.* many BACTERIA and FUNGI). Saprophytic activity is the first step in the DECOMPOSITION of dead animals and plants, and consequently is important in the recycling of elements. Also termed: saprotroph.

saprotroph (microbiology) An alternative term for SAPROPHYTE.

sarcoidosis (medical) A disease of unknown cause featuring GRANULOMAs in many parts of the body, especially in the LYMPH NODES, LIVER, LUNGS, skin and EYES.

See also KVEIM TEST.

sarcoptes (microbiology) A GENUS of acarids, which includes *SARCOPTES scabiti,* the itch mite which causes scabies.

satellite chromosome (genetics) A part of a CHROMOSOME that is joined to the end of the main CHROMOSOME by a very fine thread of non-condensed CHROMATIN.

satellite DNA (molecular biology) A FRACTION of DNA with significantly different DENSITY and thus BASE composition from most of the DNA in an organism.

saturated compound (chemistry) ORGANIC COMPOUND that contains only SINGLE BONDS; all the atoms in the COMPOUND exert their maximum combining POWER (VALENCY) with other atoms, so that a chemical change can be effected only by a SUBSTITUTION REACTION and not in an ADDITION REACTION.

saturated solution (chemistry) SOLUTION that cannot take up any more SOLUTE at a given TEMPERATURE.

See also SUPERSATURATED SOLUTION.

saturated vapour pressure (physics) The PRESSURE exerted by a SATURATED VAPOUR. It is TEMPERATURE dependent.

saturated vapour (physics) VAPOUR that can exist in EQUILIBRIUM with its parent SOLID or LIQUID at a given TEMPERATURE.

saturation (chemistry) Point at which no more of a material can be dissolved, absorbed or retained by another.

SB (education) An abbreviation of 'S'cientiae 'B'accalaureus. Latin, meaning 'Bachelor of Science'.

s-block elements (chemistry) Metallic elements that form Groups IA and IIA of the PERIODIC TABLE, which include the ALKALI METALS, ALKALINE EARTHS and the LANTHANIDES and ACTINIDES (together also known as the RARE EARTHS); HYDROGEN is usually included as well. They are so called because their 1 or 2 outer electrons occupy s-orbitals.

Sc (chemistry) CHEMICAL SYMBOL for SCANDIUM.

scandium Sc (chemistry) Silvery-white metallic ELEMENT in GROUP IIIB of the PERIODIC TABLE (a RARE EARTH ELEMENT); its OXIDE, Sc_2O_3, is used as a catalyst. At. no. 21; r.a.m. 44.9559.

scanner (computing) An alternative term for OPTICAL CHARACTER READER.

scanning electron microscope (microscopy) ELECTRON MICROSCOPE that scans the SAMPLE to be examined with a beam of electrons.

scapula (anatomy) An alternative term for the SHOULDER BLADE.

scattering of light (physics) Irregular REFLECTION or DIFFRACTION of LIGHT rays that occurs when a beam of LIGHT passes through a material medium.

SCE (genetics) An abbreviation of 'S'ister 'C'hromatid 'E'xchange.

Schiff's base (chemistry) ORGANIC COMPOUND formed when an ALDEHYDE or KETONE condenses with a primary aromatic AMINE with the elimination of WATER. Also termed: aldimine; AZOMETHINE. It was named after the German chemist Hugo Schiff (1834-1915).

Schiff's reagent (chemistry) REAGENT for testing for the presence of aliphatic ALDEHYDEs, which quickly restore its magenta COLOUR (*USA*: color). It is prepared by dissolving rosaniline hydrochloride in WATER and passing SULPHUR DIOXIDE (*USA*: sulfur dioxide) through it until the magenta COLOUR is discharged.

schistosomiasis (parasitology) An alternative term for BILHARZIA.

schizogony (biology) Form of ASEXUAL REPRODUCTION employed by some single celled animals, in which a parent CELL divides into more than two independent CELLS.

See also BINARY FISSION.

schizont (microbiology) A stage in the development of the MALARIA PARASITE. *See* MALARIA.

Schmorl stain (histology) A histological staining technique that may be used to make lipofuscin visible under the MICROSCOPE.

Schwann cell (cytology) CELL that produces the myclin sheath that surrounds a NERVE CELL (NEURONE). SCHWANN CELLs are in close contact with the AXON of the NEURONE and are separated by gaps called NODES OF RANVIER. It was named after the German physiologist Theodor Schwann (1810-82).

scintillation counter (physics) Device that counts the INCIDENCE of photons upon a material by the visible or near-VISIBLE LIGHT which is emitted.

scintillation spectrometer (physics) SCINTILLATION COUNTER capable of measuring the ENERGY and the INTENSITY of GAMMA RADIATION emitted from a material.

scleroprotein (biochemistry) Member of a GROUP of fibrous proteins that provide organisms with structural materials (*e.g.* COLLAGEN, KERATIN).

sclerotic (histology) Outermost of the three layers that form the eyeball (outside the CHOROID and RETINA).

SCN (histology) An abbreviation of 'S'upra'C'hiasmatic 'N'ucleus.

scombroid poisoning (toxicology) A seafood poisoning named for the fish FAMILY Scombroidae, which contains some of the fish SPECIES frequently causing the toxicosis. The poisoning results most frequently from fish such as tuna, skipjacks, bonitos and mahi-mahi. The poisoning occurs about 2 to 16 hours following ingestion of fish which have typically not been kept sufficiently chilled before cooking, and is the result of the presence of HISTAMINE and other toxic factors. It is usually not fatal.

scrofula (medical/ microbiology) TUBERCULOSIS of the LYMPH NODES in the neck, in which the disease may slowly progress to the formation of fistulous openings.

scrotum (anatomy) Sac present in males of some mammals that contains the TESTES. Positioned outside the body cavity so that their TEMPERATURE is cool enough for SPERM production.

SD (statistics) Abbreviation of 'S'tandard 'D'eviation.

SDA (physiology) An abbreviation of 'S'pecific 'D'ynamic 'A'ction.

SDS (computing) An abbreviation of 'S'cientific 'D'ata 'S'ystems.

SDS-PAGE (chemistry) An abbreviation of 'S'odium 'D'odecyl 'S'ulphate – 'P'oly 'A'crylamide 'G'el 'E'lectrophoresis.

sebaceous gland (anatomy) Small GLAND found in large numbers in the SKIN of mammals, usually alongside a HAIR FOLLICLE, that secretes the protective SKIN oil SEBUM.

sebum (biochemistry) Waxy material secreted by SEBACEOUS GLANDs, which helps to keep SKIN waterproof.

sec (measurement) An abbreviation of 'sec'ond. A UNIT of time equal to 1/60 of a MINUTE.

second (measurement) 1 SI UNIT of time, defined as the duration of 9,192,631,770 PERIODS of the RADIATION between the two hyperfine levels of the GROUND STATE of the CAESIUM-133 (USA: cesium-133) ATOM. Abbreviated to sec or s. 2 Angle equal to 1/60 of a MINUTE or 1/360 of a DEGREE.

secondary cell (physics) ELECTROLYTIC CELL that must be supplied with ELECTRIC CHARGE before use by passing a DIRECT CURRENT through it, but it can be recharged over and over again. Also termed: ACCUMULATOR; STORAGE CELL.

See also PRIMARY CELL.

secondary colour (optics) COLOUR (USA: color) obtained by mixing PRIMARY COLOURS. (USA: secondary color).

secondary sexual characteristics (physiology) Features that develop in some animals after the onset of puberty, distinguishing males from females but not required for sexual FUNCTION. They result from the actions of SEX HORMONES, principally TESTOSTERONE and OESTROGEN (USA: estrogen).

secretion (biochemistry) Release of a substance by a CELL or GLAND with a specialized FUNCTION, *e.g.* SECRETION of digestive ENZYMES by CELLS of the SMALL INTESTINE, or SECRETION of HORMONES by the PITUITARY.

section (histology) A slice of TISSUE cut for examination under a MICROSCOPE.

sedative (pharmacology) Drug that calms without (in NORMAL doses) causing loss of awareness or consciousness. In larger doses, some sedatives become sleep-inducing drugs.

See also TRANQUILLIZER.

sedimentation (physics) Removal of SOLID particles from a SUSPENSION by gravitational force or in a CENTRIFUGE.

segregation (genetics) Separation of a pair of ALLELES in a DIPLOID organism during MEIOSIS in the formation of gametes. A GAMETE receives one of the two ALLELES in a DIPLOID organism because it receives only one of a pair of HOMOLOGOUS CHROMOSOMES.

selection pressure (genetics) The INTENSITY with which NATURAL SELECTION is acting upon a population to change the GENE frequencies from one generation to the next.

selective advantage (genetics) The increase in fitness of one GENOTYPE compared to others in the same population.

selectively permeable membrane (physics) An alternative term for SEMIPERMEABLE MEMBRANE.

selenium Se (chemistry) Nonmetallic ELEMENT in GROUP VIA of the PERIODIC TABLE, obtained from flue dust in refineries that use SULPHIDE (*USA*: sulfide) ores. One of its ALLOTROPES conducts ELECTRICITY in the presence of LIGHT, and is used in photocells and rectifiers. At. no. 34; r.a.m. 78.96.

self-absorption (radiology) Decrease in RADIATION from a large RADIOACTIVE source due to ABSORPTION by the material itself of some of the RADIATION produced. Also termed: self-shielding.

self-induced electromotive force (physics) Production of an ELECTROMOTIVE FORCE (e.m.f.) in an electric CIRCUIT when the CURRENT is varied.

self-induction (physics) Resistance to a change in ELECTRIC CURRENT in a CIRCUIT by the creation of a back ELECTROMOTIVE FORCE.

selfish DNA (molecular biology) Those parts of a DNA sequence in a SPECIES that serve no apparent useful FUNCTION, and which are thought to have survived EVOLUTION only because they do not actually harm the organism in any way.

SEM (statistics) An abbreviation of 'S'tandard 'E'rror of the 'M'ean.

semen (biochemistry) FLUID produced in male reproductive organs of many animals. It contains SPERM, and in mammals secretions from the accessory sex GLANDS.

semicarbazone (chemistry) CRYSTALLINE ORGANIC COMPOUND formed when an ALDEHYDE or a KETONE reacts with semicarbazide ($NH_2NHCONH_2$) with the elimination of WATER. Semicarbazones are used to identify the original ALDEHYDE or KETONE.

semicircular canal (anatomy) Part of the EAR that is involved in maintaining BALANCE.

semiferous tubule (anatomy) One of many tubes within the TESTES in which SPERM are made.

seminal vesicle (anatomy) ORGAN in the TESTES that is used for storing SPERM.

semipermeable membrane (physics) A porous MEMBRANE that permits the passage of some substances but not others; *e.g.* PLASMA MEMBRANE, which permits entry of small molecules such as WATER but not large molecules, allowing OSMOSIS to occur. Such membranes are extremely important in biological systems and are used in DIALYSIS. Also termed: SELECTIVELY PERMEABLE MEMBRANE.

sense organ (histology) A GROUP of RECEPTOR CELLS specialized to react to (detect) a certain STIMULUS (*e.g.* the EYE to LIGHT, the EAR to sound, and chemoreceptors in the TONGUE and nose to tastes and smells).

senses (physiology) The five primary SENSES, common to most vertebrates but sometimes lacking in less highly evolved animals, are sight, hearing, TASTE, SMELL and touch, to which may be added the sense of BALANCE. They are effected by various SENSE ORGANS.

septicaemia (medical) Disorder that results from the presence of BACTERIA, or their toxins, in the bloodstream. Also termed: BLOOD POISONING. (*USA:* septicemia).

septivalent (chemistry) Having a VALENCY of seven. Also termed: HEPTAVALENT.

septum (anatomy) Dividing wall found in biological systems, *e.g.* between the nostrils or between the two halves of the HEART.

sequela (medical) Any abnormality caused by an illness that has ended.

SER (histology) An abbreviation of 'S'mooth 'E'ndoplasmic 'R'eticulum.

Ser. (biochemistry) An abbreviation of 'Ser'ine.

series (1 chemistry; 2 physics) 1 Systematically arranged succession of chemical compounds (*e.g.* HOMOLOGOUS SERIES) or of numbers or ALGEBRAic terms (*e.g.* ARITHMETIC SERIES, EXPONENTIAL SERIES, GEOMETRIC SERIES). 2 Describing the arrangement of components in a SERIES CIRCUIT.

series circuit (physics) Electrical CIRCUIT in which the components are arranged one after the other so that the same ELECTRIC CURRENT flows through each of them. For a SERIES of resistors, the total resistance R is equal to the sum of the individual resistors; *i.e.* $R = R_1 + R_2 + R_3 + ...$ For a SERIES of capacitors, the RECIPROCAL of the total CAPACITANCE C is equal to the sum of the reciprocals of the individual capacitances; *i.e.* $1/C = 1/C_1 + 1/C_2 + 1/C_3 + ...$

See also PARALLEL CIRCUIT.

serine (chemistry) $CH_2OHCHNH_2COOH$ White CRYSTALLINE AMINO ACID, present in many proteins. Also termed: 2-amino-3-hydroxypropanoic acid.

seroconversion (immunology) The point at which an individual exposed to a VIRUS or other agent becomes serologically POSITIVE.

serology (immunology) Branch of immunology concerned with reactions between antibodies of one organism with antigens of the SERUM of another.

serotonin (physiology/ pharmacology) Substance derived from TRYPTOPHAN and found in BLOOD SERUM, used as a NEUROTRANSMITTER and vasoconstrictor. It mediates chemical messages on its release to excite or inhibit other nerves, and also interacts with a variety of RECEPTORS. A number of important drug classes have been developed that act by mimicking, modifying, or antagonising serotonin's actions. Also termed: 5H; 5 -hydroxytryptamine.

serous cyst adenocarcinoma (medical/ histology) The most common MALIGNANT ovarian TUMOUR (*USA*: maglignant ovarian tumor).

serum (haematology) Constituent of PLASMA of BLOOD, which contains all the substances in PLASMA except for FIBRINOGEN.

set (mathematics) A GROUP of things (elements) that have at least one property in common; *e.g.* the SET of all even numbers or the SET of all people with red HAIR.

sex cell (cytology) An alternative term for GAMETE.

sex chromosome (genetics) CHROMOSOME that carries the genes determining sex. In mammals the female possesses two identical SEX CHROMOSOMEs or X-chromosomes, whereas in the male the two SEX CHROMOSOMEs differ, one being an X- and the other a Y-CHROMOSOME.

See also HETEROGAMETIC; HOMOGAMETIC; SEX DETERMINATION.

sex determination (genetics) INHERITANCE of particular COMBINATION of SEX CHROMOSOMES, which is the deciding FACTOR in whether an organism is male or female. INHERITANCE of a HOMOLOGOUS pair of SEX CHROMOSOMEs predisposes the organism to one sex (*e.g.* in mammals, the female). INHERITANCE of a pair of dissimilar SEX CHROMOSOMEs determines the other sex (in mammals, the male).

See also HETEROGAMETIC; HOMOGAMETIC.

sexual dimorphism (biology) The existence of physical differences between the two sexes, other than the differences in the reproductive organs.

sex hormone (biochemistry) HORMONE that determines SECONDARY SEXUAL CHARACTERISTICS and regulates the reproductive BEHAVIOUR (*USA*: behavior) of an organism. In mammals, the sexual CYCLE of the female is controlled by such HORMONES. In males the GONADS are regulated. *See* OESTROUS CYCLE.

sex linkage (genetics) Distribution of genes according to the sex of an organism because they are carried on the SEX CHROMOSOMES. In human males a RECESSIVE GENE carried on the X-CHROMOSOME will be expressed because no corresponding ALLELE is present on the Y-CHROMOSOME to mask it. In the female the corresponding ALLELE will be present on the other X-CHROMOSOME, and for this reason human males have a predisposition to RECESSIVE sex-linked disorders *e.g.* HAEMOPHILIA (*USA*: hemophilia), COLOUR BLINDNESS (*USA*: color blindness).

sex ratio (measurement) Ratio of the number of males to the number of females in a population. It may be expressed as the number of males to every 100 females.

sexagesimal (mathematics) Describing a number system with the BASE 60.

sexual reproduction (physiology) REPRODUCTION of an organism that involves the FUSION of specialized SEX CELLS or gametes (which are HAPLOID) to form DIPLOID progeny. It is important in bringing new vigour to a SPECIES by the mixing of genetic material from the parents to give a genetically different organism.

See also ASEXUAL REPRODUCTION; EGG; FERTILIZATION; SPERM.

sexually transmitted disease (medical) Previously called venereal disease. The currently generally preferred term is genitourinary medicine.

SFO (anatomy) An abbreviation of 'Sub'F'ornical 'O'rgan.

sg (physics) An abbreviation of 's'pecific 'g'ravity.

SGLT 1 (physiology/ biochemistry) An abbreviation of 'S'ODIUM-dependent 'GL'ucose 'T'ransporter.

SGOT (biochemistry) An abbreviation of 'S'erum 'G'lutamic-'O'xaloacetic 'T'rans-aminase.

SH (biochemistry) An abbreviation of 'S'ulp'H'ydryl (*USA*: sulfhydryl).

shingles (medical) *See* HERPES VARICELLA ZOSTER VIRUS (HVZ).

shortsightedness (medical) An alternative term for MYOPIA.

shoulder blade (anatomy) An alternative term for SCAPULA.

shunt (1 physics; 2 medical) 1 Device that directs an ELECTRIC CURRENT in a known way. 2 A surgically implanted tube or VESSEL that diverts the flow of FLUID (*e.g.* to by-pass an obstruction).

SIADH (physiology/ biochemistry) An abbreviation of 'S'yndrome of 'I'nappropriate hypersecretion of 'A'nti'D'iuretic 'H'ormone (vasopressin).

sibling (medical) A brother or sister.

sibship (medical) All the brothers and sisters in a FAMILY.

side reaction (chemistry) A CHEMICAL REACTION that takes place at the same time as the main REACTION.

SIDS (medical) An abbreviation of 'S'udden 'I'nfant 'D'eath 'S'yndrome.

siemens (S) (measurement) SI UNIT of electric CONDUCTANCE, formerly expressed in RECIPROCAL ohms (mhos). It was named after the German physicist Ernst Werner von Siemens (1816-92).

sievert (Sv) (measurement) SI UNIT of RADIATION dose equivalent.

SIF cells (histology) An abbreviation of 'S'mall, 'I'ntensely 'F'luorescent CELLs in sympathetic ganglia.

significant figure (mathematics) DIGIT that gives information about a number containing it, and not a zero used simply to indicate a vacant place at the beginning or end of the number; a DIGIT that makes an actual contribution to the number. Also termed: significant DIGIT.

silica gel (chemistry) Porous AMORPHOUS VARIETY of silica (SiO_2) which is capable of absorbing large quantities of WATER and other solvents. It is used as a DESICCANT and ADSORBENT.

silicon Si (chemistry) Nonmetallic ELEMENT in GROUP IVA of the PERIODIC TABLE, which exists as AMORPHOUS and CRYSTALLINE ALLOTROPEs. It is the second most abundant ELEMENT, occurring as silicates in clays and rocks. Sand and QUARTZ consist of silica (SILICON dioxide, SiO_2). It is used in making refractory materials and TEMPERATURE-resistant GLASS. At. no. 14; r.a.m. 28.086.

silver Ag (chemistry) SILVER-white metallic ELEMENT in GROUP IB of the PERIODIC TABLE (a TRANSITION ELEMENT). It occurs as the free ELEMENT (native) and in various SULPHIDE (*USA*: sulfide) ores. It is used in jewellery, electrical contacts, batteries and mirrors. SILVER halides are used in photographic emulsions. At. no. 47; r.a.m. 107.868.

silver bromide (chemistry) AgBr Pale yellow INSOLUBLE CRYSTALLINE SALT, used for making LIGHT-sensitive photographic emulsions.

silver chloride (chemistry) AgCl White INSOLUBLE CRYSTALLINE SALT, used in the manufacture of pure SILVER and in photographic emulsions.

silver iodide (chemistry) AgI Pale yellow INSOLUBLE CRYSTALLINE SALT, used in photographic emulsions.

silver nitrate (chemistry) $AgNO_3$ Colourless (*USA*: colorless) CRYSTALLINE SALT, used in VOLUMETRIC ANALYSIS and SILVER plating, and as a CAUSTIC in medicine (*e.g.* for removing WARTS).

silver oxide (chemistry) Ag_2O Brown AMORPHOUS SOLID, only slightly SOLUBLE in WATER but SOLUBLE in AMMONIA SOLUTION. Also termed: silver(I) oxide.

simultaneous equations (mathematics) SET of algebraic equations that are all true for the same particular values of their variables.

sine wave (physics) Waveform that represents the periodic oscillations of CONSTANT AMPLITUDE as given by the sine of a LINEAR FUNCTION. Also termed: sinusoidal WAVE; sine curve.

single bond (chemistry) COVALENT BOND formed by the sharing of one pair of electrons between two atoms.

sinus (anatomy) Irregular cavity or depression that forms part of an ANIMAL's anatomy; *e.g.* sinuses in the bones of the face in mammals.

siphon (physics) Device consisting of an inverted U-shaped tube that moves a LIQUID from one place to another place at a lower LEVEL. The tube has to be initially filled with LIQUID in ORDER to FUNCTION.

SI units (measurement) An abbreviation for 'S'ystème 'I'nternational d'Unités, an international system of scientific units. It has seven BASIC units: METRE (m), KILOGRAM (kg), second (s), KELVIN (K), AMPERE (A), mole (mol) and candela (cd), and two supplementary units RADIAN (rad) and steradian (sr). There are also 18 derived units.

skeleton (anatomy) Structure that supports the tissues and organs of an ANIMAL and is attached to muscles to allow locomotion. An endoskeleton is internal, made of BONE or CARTILAGE, and possessed by vertebrates. Exoskeletons lie outside the muscles, *e.g.* in arthropods. Some invertebrates possess a hydrostatic SKELETON which consists of FLUID under PRESSURE.

skin (anatomy) ORGAN that protects the body from invasion by pathogens. In WARM-BLOODED animals the SKIN also takes part in TEMPERATURE regulation, *e.g.* through sweating and the constriction and DILATION of its BLOOD VESSELs. It consists of epithelial TISSUE and CONNECTIVE TISSUE arranged in two major layers, the thin outer EPIDERMIS and the thicker underlying DERMIS.

skull (anatomy) Bones that form the HEAD and face, including the CRANIUM and JAWS.

small intestine (anatomy) Part of the digestive tract in mammals which is composed of the DUODENUM and ILEUM, and is the main site of DIGESTION and ABSORPTION in the GUT. BILE, pancreatic juice and intestinal juice are liberated in it, to supply many digestive ENZYMES.

See also INTESTINE.

smell (physiology) One of the primary SENSES that enables animals to detect odours (*USA*: odors), using chemoreceptors usually located (in mammals) in OLFACTORY bulbs in the NASAL CAVITY.

smg (biochemistry) An abbreviation of 'sm'all 'g'TP-binding PROTEIN.

smooth muscle (histology) Type of MUSCLE in internal organs and tissues, not under voluntary control. Also termed: INVOLUNTARY MUSCLE.

SMS (medical) An abbreviation of 'S'tiff-'M'an 'S'yndrome.

soap (chemistry) SODIUM or POTASSIUM SALT of a FATTY ACID of high MOLECULAR WEIGHT (*e.g.* PALMITIC ACID, STEARIC ACID). Soaps are made by the HYDROLYSIS or SAPONIFICATION of fats with hot SODIUM HYDROXIDE or POTASSIUM HYDROXIDE, giving GLYCEROL as a BY-PRODUCT. They emulsify grease and act as wetting agents.

See also DETERGENT.

SOD (biochemistry) An abbreviation of 'S'uper'O'xide 'D'ismutase.

soda (chemistry) Imprecise term for a COMPOUND of SODIUM, usually referring to SODIUM CARBONATE.

See also CAUSTIC SODA; SODA ASH; SODA LIME.

soda ash (chemistry) Common name for ANHYDROUS SODIUM CARBONATE. LIME SOLID MIXTURE of SODIUM HYDROXIDE and CALCIUM OXIDE.

sodium Na (chemistry) Soft, silvery-white metallic ELEMENT in GROUP IA of the PERIODIC TABLE (the ALKALI METALS). It occurs widely, principally as its CHLORIDE (COMMON SALT, NACl) in seawater and as underground deposits, from which it is extracted by ELECTROLYSIS. The METALS many compounds are important in the chemical industry, particularly, in addition to the CHLORIDE, SODIUM HYDROXIDE (CAUSTIC SODA, NAOH) and SODIUM CARBONATE (SODA, Na_2CO_3). At. no. 11; r.a.m. 22.9898.

sodium acetate (chemistry) CH_3COONa White CRYSTALLINE SOLID, used in PHOTOGRAPHY and in the manufacture of ETHYL ETHANOATE (acetate) and various pigments. Also termed: SODIUM ETHANOATE.

sodium azide (chemistry) NaN_3 White poisonous CRYSTALLINE SOLID, used in the manufacture of detonators.

sodium bicarbonate (chemistry) An alternative term for SODIUM HYDROGENCARBONATE.

sodium bisulphate (chemistry) An alternative term for SODIUM HYDROGENSULPHATE (*USA*: sodium hydrogensulfate). (*USA*: sodium bisulfate).

sodium bisulphite (chemistry) An alternative term for SODIUM HYDROGENSULPHITE (*USA*: sodium hydrogensulfite). (*USA*: sodium bisulfite).

sodium borate (chemistry) An alternative term for BORAX.

sodium bromide (chemistry) NaBr White CRYSTALLINE SOLID, used in medicine.

sodium carbonate (chemistry) Na_2CO_3.-$10H_2O$ White CRYSTALLINE SOLID which exhibits EFFLORESCENCE and forms an ALKALINE SOLUTION in WATER. It is used in GLASS making, as a WATER softener, and for the preparation of SODIUM chemicals. Also termed: WASHING SODA; SODA; SODA ASH.

sodium chlorate (chemistry) $NaClO_3$ White SOLUBLE CRYSTALLINE SOLID. It is a powerful OXIDIZING AGENT, used as a weed-killer and in the textile industry. Also termed: SODIUM CHLORATE(V).

sodium chloride (chemistry) NaCl White SOLUBLE CRYSTALLINE SALT, .extracted from seawater or underground deposits. It is used for seasoning and preserving food. Industrially, it is used in the manufacture of a wide VARIETY of chemicals, including CHLORINE, SODIUM CARBONATE, SODIUM HYDROXIDE and HYDROCHLORIC ACID. Also termed: COMMON SALT; SALT; sea SALT; table SALT.

sodium dihydrogenphosphate(V) (chemistry) NaH_2PO_4 White SOLID, used in detergents and certain baking powders. Also termed: SODIUM dihydrogen orthophosphate.

sodium ethanoate (chemistry) An alternative term for SODIUM ACETATE.

sodium hydrogencarbonate (chemistry) $NaHCO_3$ White SOLUBLE powder, used in making baking powder, powder-based fire extinguishers and antacids. Also termed: SODIUM BICARBONATE; BAKING SODA.

sodium hydrogensulphate (chemistry) $NaHSO_4.H_2O$ White SOLID, used in the dyeing industry and in the manufacture of SULPHURIC ACID (*USA*: sulfuric acid). Also termed: SODIUM BISULPHATE (*USA*: sodium bisulfate). (*USA*: sodium hydrogensulfate).

sodium hydrogensulphite (chemistry) $NaHSO_3$ White powder, used in medicine as an ANTISEPTIC, and as a preservative. Also termed: SODIUM BISULPHITE (*USA*: sodium bisulfite). (*USA*: sodium hydrogensulfite).

sodium hydroxide (chemistry) NaOH White DELIQUESCENT SOLID; a STRONG BASE. It is made by the ELECTROLYSIS of BRINE (SODIUM CHLORIDE SOLUTION). It is used in the manufacture of soaps, rayon and paper and many other SODIUM compounds. Also termed: CAUSTIC SODA; SODA.

sodium nitrate (chemistry) $NaNO_3$ White CRYSTALLINE SALT, used as a food preservative and in the manufacture of explosives and fireworks. Also termed: CHILE SALTPETRE; SODA NITRE.

sodium peroxide (chemistry) Na_2O_2 Pale yellow powdery SOLID that reacts readily with WATER to give SODIUM HYDROXIDE and OXYGEN. It is an OXIDIZING AGENT, used as a BLEACH.

sodium pump (physiology) Process by which POTASSIUM and SODIUM ions are transported across membranes that surround ANIMAL CELLS.

sodium silicate (chemistry) $Na_2SiO_3.5H_2O$ Colourless (USA: colorless) CRYSTALLINE SOLID, used in various types of detergents and cleaning compounds, and as a bonding agent in many ceramic cements and in various refractory applications. Also termed: SODIUM metasilicate.

sodium silicate solution (chemistry) A concentrated SOLUTION of SODIUM silicate in WATER, used to prepare SILICA GEL and precipitated silica. Also termed: WATER GLASS.

sodium sulphate (chemistry) $NaSO_4.-10H_2O$ White CRYSTALLINE SALT, used in the manufacture of paper, GLASS, dyes and detergents. Also termed: Glauber's SALT; SALTCAKE. (USA: sodium sulfate).

sodium sulphide (chemistry) NaS_2 A reddish-yellow DELIQUESCENT AMORPHOUS SOLID, used in the manufacture of dyes. (USA: sodium sulfide).

sodium sulphite (chemistry) Na_2SO_3 White SOLUBLE CRYSTALLINE SOLID, used in bleaching and PHOTOGRAPHY. (USA: sodium sulfite).

sodium thiosulphate (chemistry) $Na_2S_2O_3$ White SOLUBLE CRYSTALLINE SOLID. It is a strong REDUCING AGENT, used as a photographic fixing agent (when it reacts with unexposed SILVER halides) and in dyeing and VOLUMETRIC ANALYSIS. Also termed: hypo. (USA: sodium thiosulfate).

soft palate (anatomy) Rear part of the roof of the mouth, consisting of MUSCLE TISSUE covered by MUCOUS MEMBRANE. The uvula hangs from the back of the SOFT PALATE.

soft radiation (radiology) RADIATION of relatively long WAVELENGTH whose penetrating POWER is very limited.

soft water (chemistry) WATER that lathers immediately with SOAP. WATER from which most of the CALCIUM and MAGNESIUM compounds have been removed.

See also HARDNESS OF WATER.

softening of water (chemistry) *See* ION EXCHANGE.

software (computing) PROGRAM that can be used on a COMPUTER; *e.g.* executive programs, operating systems and utility programs.

See also HARDWARE.

sol (chemistry) Type of COLLOID consisting of a SOLID dispersed in a LIQUID. It is usually LIQUID (unlike a GEL, which is a jelly-like SOLID).

solar cell (physics) PHOTOCELL that converts solar ENERGY directly into ELECTRICITY.

solenoid (physics) Cylindrical coil of wire, carrying an ELECTRIC CURRENT, used to produce a MAGNETIC FIELD. It may have an IRON CORE that moves, often to WORK a switch.

See also RELAY, ELECTRICAL.

solid (1 chemistry; 2 mathematics) 1 An alternative name for a substance in the solid state. 2 Having or relating to three dimensions.

solidifying point (physics) An alternative term for FREEZING POINT.

solubility (chemistry) Amount of a substance (SOLUTE) that will dissolve in a LIQUID (SOLVENT) at a given TEMPERATURE, usually expressed as a WEIGHT per UNIT

VOLUME (*e.g.* gm per LITRE) or a PER-CENTAGE.

See also CONCENTRATION.

solubility product (chemistry) The PRODUCT of the concentrations of the ions of a dissolved ELECTROLYTE when in EQUILIBRIUM with undissolved substance.

soluble (chemistry) Describing a substance (SOLUTE) that will dissolve in a LIQUID (SOLVENT).

solute (chemistry) A substance that dissolves in a SOLVENT to form a SOLUTION.

solution (1 chemistry; 2 general terminology) 1 HOMOGENEOUS MIXTURE of SOLUTE and SOLVENT. 2 Result of solving a problem (*e.g.* finding the unknown quantity in a mathematical equation).

solvent extraction (chemistry) Removal of a substance from a (usually AQUEOUS) SOLUTION by dissolving it in a (usually organic) SOLVENT. The resulting LIQUID containing the substance is called a RAFFINATE. Also termed: LIQUID-LIQUID EXTRACTION.

solvent (chemistry) Substance in which a SOLUTE dissolves; the COMPONENT of a SOLUTION which is in excess.

solvolysis (chemistry) CHEMICAL REACTION between SOLVENT and SOLUTE molecules.

See also HYDROLYSIS.

somatic cell (histology) Any CELL in the body other than its gametes, the SPERM in its TESTES or the eggs in its OVARY.

somatic (histology) Of the body. SOMATIC CELLS include all CELLS of an organism except for the gametes or sex-CELLS.

somatotrophin (biochemistry) An alternative term for GROWTH HORMONE.

sorbitol (chemistry) ALCOHOL formed by the REDUCTION of GLUCOSE, used as a sweetening agent.

Soret effect (physics) *See* THERMAL DIFFUSION.

SOT (society) An abbreviation of 'S'ociety 'O'f 'T'oxicology.

Southern blotting (molecular biology) DNA blotting. Named after Edwin Mellor Southern (1938-). *See* WESTERN BLOTTING; NORTHERN BLOTTING.

Southgates mucicarmine stain (histology) A histological staining technique that may be used for MUCIN.

sp (microbiology) An abbreviation of 'sp'ecies.

species (sp) (taxonomy) Smallest GROUP commonly used in biological CLASSIFICATION and into which a GENUS is divided. SPECIES are sometimes further divided into SUBSPECIES (races). Generally, no more than one type of organism is present in one SPECIES. Members of a SPECIES may breed with one another, but cannot generally breed with members of another SPECIES. Rarely, very closely related SPECIES interbreed to produce a HYBRID.

See also BINOMIAL NOMENCLATURE; VARIETY.

specific activity (physics) Number of disintegrations of a RADIO-ISOTOPE per UNIT time per UNIT MASS.

specific charge (physics) Ratio of ELECTRIC CHARGE to UNIT MASS of an ELEMENTARY PARTICLE.

specific gravity (physics) Former name for RELATIVE DENSITY.

specific latent heat (physics) Amount of LATENT HEAT per UNIT MASS of a substance.

specific rate constant (chemistry) *See* RATE CONSTANT.

SPECT (physics) An abbreviation of 'S'ingle 'P'hoton 'E'mission 'C'omputed 'T'omography.

spectral line (physics) Particular WAVELENGTH of LIGHT in a line.

spectral series (physics) Sequence of lines in a line SPECTRUM.

spectrochemistry (chemistry) Branch of chemistry concerned with the study of spectra of substances.

spectrometer (physics) SPECTROSCOPE that has some form of photographic or electrical detection device.

spectrometry (measurement) Measurement of the INTENSITY of SPECTRAL LINES or SPECTRAL SERIES as a FUNCTION of WAVELENGTH.

spectrophotometer (physics) Instrument that measures the INTENSITY of ELECTROMAGNETIC RADIATION absorbed or transmitted by a substance as a FUNCTION of WAVELENGTH, usually in the visible, INFRA-RED and ULTRAVIOLET regions of the ELECTROMAGNETIC SPECTRUM.

spectroscope (physics) Instrument for splitting various wavelengths of ELECTROMAGNETIC RADIATION into a SPECTRUM, using an OPTICAL PRISM or DIFFRACTION GRATING.

spectroscopy (physics) Study of the properties of LIGHT, using a SPECTROSCOPE; the production and ANALYSIS of spectra.

spectrum (1, 2 physics) 1 Band, continuous range, or lines of ELECTROMAGNETIC RADIATION emitted or absorbed by a substance under certain circumstances. 2 Coloured (*USA*: colored) band of LIGHT or bands of colours produced by splitting various wavelengths of ELECTROMAGNETIC RADIATION, using an OPTICAL PRISM or DIFFRACTION GRATING.

spectrum colours (physics) Visible colours that are observed in the SPECTRUM of WHITE LIGHT (*e.g.* in a rainbow). (*USA*: spectrum colors).

sperm (cytology) An abbreviation of 'SPERM'atozoan, the GAMETE (sex-CELL) produced by the male in many SPECIES of animals (in mammals, in the TESTES). It consists of a HEAD containing genetic material in the NUCLEUS (which is HAPLOID) and usually possesses cilia or flagelia for movement.

spermatocyte (cytology) CELL from which SPERM (spermatozoa) are derived through SPERMATOGENESIS. Primary spermatocytes are DIPLOID; after MEIOSIS, secondary spermatocytes which are HAPLOID are formed. These further divide to produce spermatids, which differentiate to form SPERM.

spermatogenesis (physiology) Formation of SPERM in the TESTIS. It commences with the repeated MITOSIS of primordial GERM CELLS to form spermatogonia, which grow to form a primary SPERMATOCYTE. This ultimately forms HAPLOID spermatozoa after MEIOSIS.

spermatozoon (cytology) *See* SPERM.

spherical aberration (optics) Type of ABERRATION in a LENS or mirror.

sphincter (histology) Circular MUSCLE that controls the flow of a LIQUID or semi-solid through an orifice (*e.g.* the anal SPHINCTER, round the ANUS).

sphygmomanometer (physics) Instrument for measuring BLOOD PRESSURE.

spinal column (anatomy) *See* SPINE.

spinal cord (anatomy) Part of the CENTRAL NERVOUS SYSTEM (CNS) in vertebrates that is enclosed within the SPINE. It consists of a hollow NERVE tube containing many interconnecting neurones and connected to the SPINAL NERVES.

spinal nerve (histology) Any of several PERIPHERAL NERVEs arising from the SPINAL CORD which are connected to receptors and effectors in other parts of the body.

spine (anatomy) BACKBONE; dorsally situated bony column composed of vertebrae, which enclose the SPINAL CORD. Also termed: SPINAL COLUMN.

spirit (1, 2 chemistry) 1 A VOLATILE LIQUID obtained by DISTILLATION; a VOLATILE DISTILLATE (*e.g.* aviation SPIRIT). 2 A SOLUTION that consists of a VOLATILE substance dissolved in ETHANOL (ETHYL ALCOHOL).

See also METHYLATED SPIRITS.

spirochaete (bacteriology) Member of a GROUP of BACTERIA characterized by a spiral shape, some of which are parasitic and cause disorders (*e.g.* syphilis, YAWS, infectious JAUNDICE).

splanchnology (biology) Branch of biology and medicine concerned with the organs within the central body cavity of vertebrates.

spleen (anatomy) ORGAN present in the ABDOMEN of some vertebrates that aids in defence against invading organisms. It produces LYMPHOCYTES and also stores and removes RED BLOOD CELLS (ERYTH-ROCYTES) from the BLOOD system.

spontaneous generation (philosophy) A theory (now disproved) that living MATTER can arise from non-living MATTER. Also termed: ABIOGENESIS.

See also BIOGENESIS.

spore (biology) Resting form of an organism that is highly resistant to adverse conditions, *e.g.* in BACTERIA.

sq cm (measurement) An abbreviation of 'sq'uare 'c'enti'm'eter(s) (*USA*: centi-meter[s]).

squamous (histology) Scaly or plate-like; a type of CELL.

squamous cell carcinoma (histology) A MALIGNANT NEOPLASM derived from SQUAMOUS EPITHELIUM.

square root (mathematics) Of a number, another number that when multiplied by itself gives the original number. It is indicated by the symbol or the INDEX (POWER) $\frac{1}{2}$; *e.g.* 16 (or $16^{1/2}$) = 4.

See also ROOT.

SR (society) An abbreviation of 'S'ociety of 'R'adiographers.

SRIF (physiology/ biochemistry) Abbreviation of 'S'omatotrophin 'R'elease-'I'nhibiting 'F'actor. (USA: somatotropin release-inhibiting factor).

SRNA (biochemistry) An abbreviation of 'S'oluble 'R'ibo'N'ucleic 'A'cid.

SRY (genetics) An abbreviation of product of 'S'ex-determining 'R'egion of 'Y' chromosome.

SS (society) An abbreviation of Royal 'S'tatistical 'S'ociety.

SS 14 (biochemistry) An abbreviation of 'S'omato'S'tatin 14.

SS 28 (biochemistry) An abbreviation of 'S'omato'S'tatin 28.

SSRI (pharmacology) An abbreviation of 'S'elective 'S'erotonin 'R'euptake 'I'nhibitors.

ssp. (microbiology) An abbreviation of 's'ub 'sp'ecies.

stable (1 chemistry; 2, 3 physics) 1 Relatively INERT (*e.g.* describing a RARE GAS) or hard to decompose (*e.g.* describing an OXIDE such as silica). 2 In atomic physics, describing an ISOTOPE or NUCLEUS that shows no tendency to decompose (*e.g.* by emitting RADIOAC-TIVITY). 3 Describing a type of EQUILIBRIUM that does not have a tendency to shift (as opposed to unstable EQUILIBRIUM).

standard deviation (statistics) Measure of the spread of a SET of numbers about their ARITHMETIC MEAN. It is the SQUARE ROOT of the MEAN (AVERAGE) of the squares of all the deviations from the MEAN value of the SET (ROOT-MEAN-SQUARE value). It is a measure of the compact-ness of a SET of numbers. Also termed: STANDARD ERROR.

standard electrode potential (physics) ELECTRODE POTENTIAL specified by compari-son with a standard ELECTRODE.

standard error (statistics) An alternative term for STANDARD DEVIATION.

standard solution (chemistry) SOLUTION of definite CONCENTRATION, *i.e.* having a known WEIGHT of SOLUTE in a definite VOLUME of SOLUTION.

standard state (chemistry) ELEMENT in its most STABLE physical form at a specified TEMPERATURE and a PRESSURE of 101,325 pascals (760 mm Hg).

standard temperature and pressure (s.t.p. or STP) (physics) SET of standard conditions of TEMPERATURE and PRESSURE. By convention, the standard TEMPERATURE is 273.15 K (0ºC) and the standard PRESSURE is 101,325 pascals (760 mm Hg).

stannic chloride (chemistry) An alternative term for TIN(IV) CHLORIDE.

stannous (chemistry) Also termed: TIN(IV).

stannous chloride (chemistry) An alternative term for TIN(II) CHLORIDE.

staphylococcus (bacteriology) Type of gram-POSITIVE BACTERIUM characterized by its shape, which takes the form of irregular clusters (resembling a miniature bunch of grapes). Staphylococci cause various inflammatory disorders (*e.g.* BOILS, IMPETIGO, osteomyelitis).

starch (chemistry) $(C_6H_{10}O_5)_n$ Complex POLYSACCHARIDE CARBOHYDRATE, a POLYMER of GLUCOSE, that occurs in all green plants, where it serves as a reserve ENERGY material. It forms GLUCOSE on complete HYDROLYSIS. Also termed: AMYLUM.

stat (general terminology) (Do) immediately.

state of matter (physics) An alternative term for physical STATE OF MATTER.

statistical analysis (statistics) Evaluation of DATA by the use of statistics.

statistics (statistics) Branch of science concerned with the collection and CLASSIFICATION of numerical DATA and facts, and their interpretation in mathematical terms, especially the determination of probabilities.

STD (medical) An abbreviation of 'S'exually 'T'ransmitted 'D'isease.

steam point (physics) NORMAL BOILING POINT of WATER; it is taken to be a TEMPERATURE of 100°C (at NORMAL PRESSURE).

stearate (chemistry) ESTER or SALT of STEARIC ACID.

See also SOAP.

stearic acid (chemistry) $CH_3(CH_2)_{16}COOH$ Long-chain FATTY ACID (a CARBOXYLIC ACID) that occurs in most FATS AND OILS. Its SODIUM and POTASSIUM salts are constituents of soaps. Also termed: OCTADECANOIC ACID.

stem cell (cytology) A cell that gives rise to a particular type of cell, as occurs in haematopoiesis (*USA*: hematopoiesis).

stereochemistry (chemistry) Branch of chemistry concerned with the study of the spatial arrangement of the atoms within a MOLECULE and the way that these affect the properties of the MOLECULE.

stereoisomer (chemistry) One of two or more isomers with the same MOLECULAR FORMULA, but different configurations (arrangements of atoms).

stereoisomerism (chemistry) ISOMERISM of compounds of the same MOLECULAR FORMULA that results when the spatial arrangement of the atoms within the molecules are different.

See also GEOMETRIC ISOMERISM; OPTICAL ISOMERISM.

stereoregular (chemistry) Describing a COMPOUND that has a regular spatial arrangement of atoms within its MOLECULE.

stereoscope (physics) Optical instrument that gives a three-dimensional illusion of depth, normally from a pair of flat photographs.

stereoscopic (physics) Describing an instrument or system of vision that allows objects to be viewed in three dimensions.

stereospecific (chemistry) Describing a CHEMICAL REACTION in which a different PRODUCT is formed from each geometric ISOMER of the REACTANT.

steric effect (chemistry) Phenomenon in which the shape of a MOLECULE affects its CHEMICAL REACTIONS.

sterilization (1 microbiology; 2 medical) 1 TREATMENT of an apparatus or substance (*e.g.* food) so that it contains no MICROORGANISMS that could cause disease or spoilage, usually by means of high temperatures, GAMMA RADIATION, etc. 2 Surgical TREATMENT of an ANIMAL so that it cannot have offspring (*e.g.* in mammals by cutting or tying the FALLOPIAN TUBES of the female or vasa deferentia of the male; removing the ovaries or TESTES is a more drastic way of achieving the same effect).

sternum (anatomy) BONE in tetrapod vertebrates on the VENTRAL side of the THORAX, parallel to the SPINE, to which most of the ribs are attached. Also termed: BREASTBONE.

steroid (biochemistry) Any of a GROUP of naturally occurring tetracyclic organic compounds, widely found in ANIMAL tissues. Most have very important physiological activities (*e.g.* adrenal HORMONES, BILE acids, SEX HORMONES, sterols). Some can be made synthetically (*e.g.* for use as contraceptive pills).

sterol (biochemistry) Subgroup of steroids or STEROID ALCOHOLS. They include CHOLESTEROL, abundant in ANIMAL tissues, which is the PRECURSOR of many other steroids.

stethoscope (medical) An instrument through which the physician listens to sounds made by internal organs (*e.g.* HEART, lungs).

STH (physiology/ biochemistry) An abbreviation of 'S'omato'T'rophin, growth 'H'ormone (*USA*: somatotropin growth hormone).

still (chemistry) Apparatus for the DISTILLATION of liquids.

stimulated emission (physics) Process by which a PHOTON causes an ELECTRON in an ATOM to drop to a lower ENERGY LEVEL and emit another PHOTON. It is the principle of the LASER.

stimulus (physics) Environmental FACTOR that is detected by a RECEPTOR and induces a RESPONSE from an EFFECTOR.

stoichiometric compound (chemistry) A chemical whose molecules have the COMPONENT elements present in exact proportions as demanded by a simple MOLECULAR FORMULA.

stoichiometric mixture (chemistry) A MIXTURE of reactants that in a CHEMICAL REACTION yield a STOICHIOMETRIC COMPOUND with no excess REACTANT.

stoichiometry (chemistry) Branch of chemistry that deals with the relative quantities of atoms or molecules taking place in a REACTION.

stomach (anatomy) Muscular sac present in vertebrates in which food is partly digested and stored after passage through OESOPHAGUS (gullet). HYDRO-CHLORIC ACID is secreted in the STOMACH, as is the ENZYME PEPSIN, which begins the DIGESTION of proteins.

storage (computing) COMPUTER MEMORY CAPACITY.

storage cell (physics) An alternative term for SECONDARY CELL.

storage device (computing) An alternative term for a COMPUTER MEMORY or store.

See also RANDOM ACCESS MEMORY (RAM); READ-ONLY MEMORY (ROM).

STP or s.t.p. (physics) An abbreviation of 's'tandard 't'emperature and 'p'ressure.

STPD (physics) An abbreviation of 'S'tandard 'T'emperature and 'P'ressure (0°C, 760mm Hg), 'D'ry.

str. (microbiology) An abbreviation of 'str'eptococcus.

stratum (histology) Layer of CELLS or TISSUE.

strep. (microbiology) An abbreviation of 'strep'tococcus.

streptococcus (bacteriology) Type of GRAM-POSITIVE BACTERIUM characterized by its shape, which takes the form of a chain. Streptococci cause various disorders (*e.g.* erysipelas, scarlet fever).

streptomycin (pharmacology) ANTIBIOTIC that works by inhibiting PROTEIN SYNTHESIS in BACTERIAL CELLS.

stress (biology) Any environmental FACTOR, or COMBINATION of factors, that has adverse effects on the structure or BEHAVIOUR (*USA*: behavior) of an organism.

striated muscle (histology) MUSCLE that contains well-aligned threads of PROTEIN, which enable it to contract strongly in a particular direction. Also termed: VOLUNTARY MUSCLE.

stroboscope (physics) An instrument consisting of a rapidly flashing lamp, employed for measuring speeds of rotation. It can also be used, by controlling the rate of flashing, to view objects that are moving rapidly with periodic motion and to see them as if they were at rest. Also termed: rotoscope.

stroke (medical) Sudden damage to the VASCULAR SYSTEM in the BRAIN, caused by the rupture or blockage of a BLOOD-VESSEL and usually resulting in impairment or loss of some functions.

stroma (histology) The TISSUE that forms the supporting framework of an ORGAN, as distinct from the parenchyma, the functioning TISSUE.

strong acid (chemistry) ACID that is completely dissociated into its COMPONENT ions (*e.g.* HYDROCHLORIC ACID).

strong base (chemistry) BASE that is completely dissociated into its COMPONENT ions (*e.g.* SODIUM HYDROXIDE).

strontium Sr (chemistry) Silvery-white metallic ELEMENT in GROUP IIA of the PERIODIC TABLE (one of the RARE EARTH elements). STRONTIUM compounds impart a bright red COLOUR (*USA*: color) to a flame, and are used in flares and fireworks. At. no. 38; r.a.m. 87.62.

strontium unit (measurement) Measure of the CONCENTRATION of the RADIO-ISOTOPE STRONTIUM-90 in substances such as BONE, milk or soil relative to their CALCIUM content.

See also STRONTIUM.

structural formulae (chemistry) Shorthand description of a chemical compound that indicates the arrangement of the atoms in its molecules as well as its composition *e.g.* H_2O.

See also EMPIRICAL FORMULA; MOLECULAR FORMULA.

structural isomerism (chemistry) The ISOMERISM of chemical compounds that have the same MOLECULAR FORMULA but different structural formulae. Structural isomers have different physical and chemical properties.

strychnine (chemistry) White CRYSTALLINE INSOLUBLE ALKALOID with a bitter TASTE, one of the most powerful poisons known. Also termed: VAUQUELINE.

STX (toxicology) An abbreviation of 'S'axi'T'o'X'in.

subatomic particle (physics) PARTICLE that is smaller than an ATOM or forms part of an ATOM (*e.g.* ELECTRON, NEUTRON, NUCLEUS, PROTON). Sometimes also called an ELEMENTARY PARTICLE.

subclinical infections (medical/ microbiology) Infections with minimal or no apparent symptoms.

subcutaneous (medical) Beneath the surface of the SKIN, but not necessarily beneath all the layers of SKIN, usually applied to injections.

subcutaneous tissue (histology) Layer of TISSUE below the DERMIS of the SKIN. It often contains deposits of fat.

sublimate (chemistry) SOLID formed by the process of SUBLIMATION.

sublimation (chemistry) Direct conversion of a SOLID substance to its VAPOUR state on heating without melting taking place (*e.g.* SOLID CARBON DIOXIDE (DRY ICE). The VAPOUR condenses to give a SUBLIMATE. The process is used to purify various substances.

sub-shell (physics) Subdivision of an ELECTRON shell.

subspecies (taxonomy) A GROUP of organisms within a SPECIES that have certain characteristics not possessed by other members of the SPECIES. Breeding may occur between members of different subspecies. Also termed: RACE.

substituent (chemistry) ATOM or GROUP that replaces another ATOM or GROUP in a MOLECULE of a COMPOUND.

substitution product (chemistry) PRODUCT formed from substitution.

substitution reaction (chemistry) A CHEMICAL REACTION that involves the direct replacement of an ATOM or GROUP in a MOLECULE of a COMPOUND (usually an ORGANIC COMPOUND) by some other ATOM or GROUP; *e.g.* the REACTION in which an ATOM of CHLORINE replaces an ATOM of HYDROGEN in a MOLECULE of BENZENE (C_6H_6) to form a MOLECULE of chlorobenzene (C_6H_5Cl). Also termed: DISPLACEMENT REACTION.

substrate (1 biochemistry; 2 biology) 1 The MOLECULE or COMPOUND upon which an ENZYME acts. Each SUBSTRATE is specific to its own ENZYME, and vice versa. 2 Substance upon which an organism grows or is attached to.

succinic acid (chemistry) $(CH_2COOH)_2$ White CRYSTALLINE DICARBOXYLIC ACID, used in the manufacture of dyes and in organic SYNTHESIS. It is an INTERMEDIATE in the KREBS CYCLE (CITRIC ACID or TRI-CARBOXYLIC ACID CYCLE). Also termed: BUTANEDIOIC ACID; ethylenedicarboxylic ACID.

sucrase (biochemistry) ENZYME that breaks down SUCROSE into simpler sugars. Also termed: invertase.

sucrose (chemistry) $C_{12}H_{22}O_{11}$ White OPTICALLY ACTIVE SOLUBLE CRYSTALLINE DISACCHARIDE which is obtained from SUGAR cane and SUGAR-beet; ordinary SUGAR, used to sweeten food. It is hydrolysed to FRUCTOSE and GLUCOSE. Also termed: CANE-SUGAR; beet-SUGAR; SUGAR.

sudden infant death syndrome (SIDS) (medical) A term applied to babies who die unexpectedly and of undetermined cause, usually during sleep. Also called cot (*USA*: crib) death.

sugar (1, 2 chemistry) 1 CRYSTALLINE SOLUBLE CARBOHYDRATE with a sweet TASTE; usually a MONOSACCHARIDE or DISACCHARIDE. 2 Common name for SUCROSE.

sulphate (chemistry) ESTER or SALT of SULPHURIC ACID (*USA*: sulfuric acid). (*USA*: sulfate).

sulphation (chemistry) Conversion of a substance into a SULPHATE (*USA*: sulfate). (*USA*: sulfation).

sulphide (chemistry) BINARY COMPOUND containing SULPHUR (*USA*: sulfur); a SALT of HYDROGEN SULPHIDE (*USA*: hydrogen sulfide). Organic sulphides (*USA*: sulfides) are called THIOETHERS. (*USA*: sulfide).

sulphite (chemistry) ESTER or SALT of SULPHUROUS ACID (*USA*: sulfurous acid). (*USA*: sulfite).

2-sulphobenzimide (chemistry) An alternative term for SACCHARIN. (*USA*: sulfobenzimide).

sulphonamide (pharmacology) Member of a CLASS of SYNTHETIC anti-BACTERIAL drugs which act by ENZYME INHIBITION. They are amides derived from SULPHONIC ACIDS (*USA*: sulfonic acids). (*USA*: sulfonamide).

sulphonate (chemistry) ESTER or SALT of a SULPHONIC ACID (*USA*: sulfonic acid). (*USA*: sulfonate).

sulphonation (chemistry) A SUBSTITUTION REACTION that involves the replacement of a HYDROGEN ATOM by the SULPHONIC ACID GROUP (*USA*: sulfonic acid group). (*USA*: sulfonation).

sulphonic acid (chemistry) ACID that contains the GROUP -SO_3H. Organic SULPHONIC ACIDS (*USA*: sulfonic acids) are used in the manufacture of dyes, detergents and drugs. (*USA*: sulfonic acid).

sulphonium compound (chemistry) A COMPOUND of the EMPIRICAL FORMULA R_3SX, where R is an organic RADICAL and X is an electronegative ELEMENT or RADICAL. (*USA*: sulfonium compound).

sulphoxide (chemistry) COMPOUND of EMPIRICAL FORMULA RSOR', where R and R' are organic radicals. (*USA*: sulfoxide).

sulphur S (chemistry) Yellow nonmetallic SOLID ELEMENT in GROUP VIB of the PERIODIC TABLE, which forms several ALLOTROPES including alpha- (rhombic) SULPHUR (*USA*: sulfur) and beta- (MONOCLINIC) SULPHUR. It occurs as the free ELEMENT in volcanic regions and as underground deposits and as sulphates and sulphides, which include important minerals (*e.g.* galena, PbS, and pyrites, FeS_2). Chemically it behaves like OXYGEN, and can replace it in ORGANIC COMPOUNDS (*e.g.* THIOETHERS and thiols). SULPHUR is used to make SULPHURIC ACID, matches, gunpowder, drugs, FUNGICIDES and dyes, and in the vulcanization of rubber. At. no. 16; r.a.m. 32.06. (*USA*: sulfur).

sulphur dichloride oxide (chemistry) An alternative term for thionyl CHLORIDE. (*USA*: sulfur dichloride oxide).

sulphur dioxide (chemistry) SO_2 Colourless (*USA*: colorless) poisonous

GAS with a strong pungent odour (*USA*: odor), made by burning SULPHUR (*USA*: sulfur), roasting SULPHIDE (*USA*: sulfide) ores or by the ACTION of acids on sulphites (*USA*: sulfites). It is also produced when SULPHUR containing compounds, such as fossil fuels, are burned, and from this source is a major atmospheric pollutant. It is used to make SULPHURIC ACID (*USA*: sulfuric acid) and, in AQUEOUS SOLUTION, as a BLEACH. It is also termed: SULPHUR(IV) OXIDE (*USA*: sulfur(IV) oxide). (*USA*: sulfur dioxide).

sulphur dye (chemistry) Dye made by heating certain ORGANIC COMPOUNDS with SULPHUR (*USA*: sulfur) or ALKALI polysulphides (*USA*: polysulfides), used for dyeing industrial fabrics. (*USA*: sulfur dye).

sulphur(IV) oxide (chemistry) An alternative term for SULPHUR DIOXIDE (*USA*: sulfur dioxide). (*USA*: sulfur(IV) oxide).

sulphur(V1) oxide (chemistry) An alternative term for SULPHUR TRIOXIDE (*USA*: sulfur trioxide). (*USA*: sulfur(VI) oxide).

sulphur trioxide (chemistry) SO_3 VOLATILE white SOLID made by the catalytic OXIDATION of SULPHUR DIOXIDE (*USA*: sulfur dioxide), usually stored in sealed tubes. It reacts with WATER to form SULPHURIC ACID (*USA*: sulfuric acid). Also termed: SULPHUR (VI) OXIDE (*USA*: sulfur(VI) oxide). (*USA*: sulfur trioxide).

sulphuric acid (chemistry) H_2SO_4 A corrosive, colourless (*USA*: colorless), oily LIQUID ACID, made mainly from SULPHUR DIOXIDE (*USA*: sulfur dioxide) by the contact process. It is a DESICCANT, and when hot a powerful OXIDIZING AGENT. It is produced in large quantities and used in the manufacture of other acids,

fertilizers, explosives, ACCUMULATORS, petrochemicals, etc. Its salts are sulphates (*USA*: sulfates). Also termed: VITRIOL; oil of VITRIOL; HYDROGEN SULPHATE (*USA*: hydrogen sulfate). (*USA*: sulfuric acid).

sulphurous acid (chemistry) H_2SO_3 Colourless (*USA*: colorless) AQUEOUS SOLUTION of SULPHUR DIOXIDE (*USA*: sulfur dioxide), used as a BLEACH and a REDUCING AGENT. Its salts are sulphites (*USA*: sulfites). (*USA*: sulfurous acid).

superconductivity (physics) A large increase in electrical CONDUCTIVITY exhibited by certain metals and ALLOYS at a TEMPERATURE a few degrees above ABSOLUTE ZERO. Also termed: supraconductivity.

superconductor (physics) METAL that exhibits SUPERCONDUCTIVITY.

supercooling (chemistry) Metastable state of a LIQUID in which its TEMPERATURE has been brought below the NORMAL FREEZING POINT without any solidification or CRYSTALLIZATION occurring.

superheated steam (chemistry) Steam (under PRESSURE) at a TEMPERATURE above the BOILING POINT of WATER (100°C). *See* SUPERHEATING.

superheating (chemistry) Metastable state of a LIQUID or GAS that has been heated above its BOILING POINT in the LIQUID state, by increasing the PRESSURE above that of the ATMOSPHERE. Also termed: overheating.

supernatant liquid (chemistry) Clear LIQUID that lies above a sediment or PRECIPITATE.

superoxide (chemistry) 1 COMPOUND that yields the FREE RADICAL O_2^-, which is highly toxic to living CELLS. 2 OXIDE that yields both HYDROGEN PEROXIDE and OXYGEN on TREATMENT with an ACID.

See also PEROXIDE.

supersaturated solution (chemistry) An unstable SOLUTION that contains more SOLUTE than a SATURATED SOLUTION would contain at the same TEMPERATURE. It easily changes to a SATURATED SOLUTION when the excess SOLUTE is made to crystallize.

surface active agent (chemistry) An alternative term for SURFACTANT.

surface tension (physics) FORCE per UNIT length acting along the surface of a LIQUID at right-angles to any line drawn in the surface. It has the effect of making a LIQUID behave as if it has a surface SKIN (which can support *e.g.* small aquatic insects), and is responsible for CAPILLARITY and other phenomena. It is measured in newtons per METRE (N m^{-1}).

surfactant (chemistry) Substance that reduces the SURFACE TENSION of a LIQUID, used in detergents, wetting agents and foaming agents. Also termed: SURFACE ACTIVE AGENT.

suspension (chemistry) MIXTURE of INSOLUBLE small SOLID particles and a FLUID in which the INSOLUBLE substance stays evenly distributed throughout the FLUID (because of molecular collisions and the FLUID'S VISCOSITY, which prevent PRECIPITATION). Also termed: suspensoid.

suspensory ligament (anatomy) One of the structures that hold the LENS of the EYE in position.

sweat (physiology) A watery FLUID containing salts secreted from GLANDS in the SKIN. EVAPORATION of SWEAT aids in cooling the body. Also termed: perspiration.

symbiosis (biology) Association between two organisms of different SPECIES in which both partners benefit.

See also COMMENSALISM; PARASITISM; SAPROPHYTE.

symmetry (mathematics) The property of being symmetrical, *i.e.* having the same shapes on each side of or around a point, AXIS or plane.

sympathetic nervous system (anatomy) Branch of the AUTONOMIC NERVOUS SYSTEM that is structurally different to the PARASYMPATHETIC NERVOUS SYSTEM. NORADRENALINE (*USA:* norepinephrine) is produced at the end of sympathetic nerve fibres (*USA:* sympathetic nerve fibers), unlike the parasympathetic system. Effects produced by each system are generally antagonistic.

synapse (histology) Point of connection between neurones (NERVE CELLS). It consists of a gap between the membranes of two CELLS, across which impulses are transmitted by a transmitter substance (*e.g.* acetylcholine). Specialized synapses occur at NERVE-MUSCLE junctions.

See also NEUROTRANSMITTER.

syndrome (medical) SET of symptoms occurring together all thought to be produced by the same illness. (*e.g.* nephrotic SYNDROME).

synergy (biology) Collective ACTION of two or more things (*e.g.* drugs, muscles) that is more effective than it would be if they acted on their own. Also termed: synergism.

synovial fluid (anatomy) LIQUID secreted by a SYNOVIAL MEMBRANE.

synovial membrane (anatomy) Lining of the CAPSULE that encloses a JOINT between bones. It secretes SYNOVIAL FLUID, which acts as a LUBRICANT to prevent friction in the JOINT during movement.

synthesis (chemistry) Formation of a chemical COMPOUND by combining elements or simpler compounds; the building of compounds through a planned SERIES of steps.

synthetic (chemistry) Formed by artificial means; describing a chemical COMPOUND that has been produced by SYNTHESIS.

systole (physiology) The contraction phase of the cardiac cycle, as opposed to the DIASTOLE.

T

T (biochemistry) A symbol for THREONINE.

T4 (1 genetics; 2 biochemistry) 1 One of the most intensively studied of the bacteriophages. It only attacks *ESCHERICHIA COLI*. The GENOME is double-stranded DNA, LINEAR, but with matching ends that can join up to make a circular DNA MOLECULE after entry into the HOST CELL. 2 THYROXINE. *See* THYROID.

t (general terminology) An abbreviation of 't'ime.

TAB (immunology) An abbreviation of 't'yphoid, paratyphoid 'A' and paratyphoid 'B' (VACCINE).

tabes dorsalis (medical/ microbiology) Degeneration of neurons in the SPINAL CORD, caused by syphilis.

tachycardia (medical) Rapid HEARTBEAT, above 100 beats per MINUTE.

taenia (microbiology) A GENUS of tapeworms. A parasitic worm which is long and flat, like a piece of tape; it is divided into segments. *TAENIA saginata and TAENIA solium* are those important in medicine, for man is the only natural HOST.

tail (statistics) The extreme part of a distribution, which when represented graphically looks like a tail.

talc (chemistry) $3MgO.4SiO_2.H_2O$ Finely powdered HYDROUS MAGNESIUM SILICATE. Soft white or grey-green mineral. Its purified form is a white powder, used in talcum powder, in medicine and in ceramic materials. Also termed: French CHALK; MAGNESIUM SILICATE MONOHYDRATE.

talus (anatomy) The ankle BONE.

tandum duplication (genetics) A form of duplication in which part of a CHROMOSOME duplicates itself, the second copy being inserted in line with the first.

tanin (chemistry) Yellow substance that is a member of a CLASS of ORGANIC COMPOUNDS, of vegetable ORIGIN (*e.g.* in tree bark, oak galls and tea), that are derivatives of POLYHYDRIC BENZOIC ACIDS. They are used in tanning hides to make leather.

See also TANNIC ACID.

tannic acid (chemistry) White AMORPHOUS SOLID ORGANIC ACID, a member of the CLASS of compounds called tannins. It is used in tanning and for making inks and dyes. Also termed: tannin.

tantalum Ta (chemistry) Hard blue-grey metallic ELEMENT in GROUP VA of the PERIODIC TABLE (a TRANSITION ELEMENT), used in electronic and chemical equipment, and for making surgical instruments. At. no. 73; r.a.m. 180.9479.

tapeworm (parasitology) *See* TAENIA.

target dose (biochemistry) The amount or CONCENTRATION of a chemical that gets to the site of ACTION, causing a measurable effect.

tarone test (statistics) A statistical test used in carcinogenicity studies to evaluate the significance of the time of observation of TUMOUR rather than death as an endpoint. This test is only appropriate under certain defined conditions such as when the number of animals dying early with a lethal TUMOUR (*USA*: tumor) is large and control survival has been large.

tarsal (anatomy) BONE that occurs in the feet of tetrapods. Human beings have seven tarsals in each foot, one of them modified to form the heel BONE (calcaneum).

tartar emetic (chemistry) POTASSIUM antimonyl TARTRATE, $K.SbO.C_4H_4O_6.-1/2H_2O$, a poisonous COMPOUND used as an INSECTICIDE and as mordant in dyeing.

tartaric acid (chemistry) HOOC.CH(OH)-CH(OH).COOH A white CRYSTALLINE hydroxycarboxylic acid that occurs in grapes and other fruits. It is used in dyeing and printing. Its salts, the tartrates, are used as buffers and in medicine. Also termed: 2,3-dihydroxy-butanedioic acid; DIHYDROXYSUCCINIC ACID.

tartrate (chemistry) ESTER or SALT of TARTARIC ACID.

tartrazine (toxicology) A food colour (*USA*: food color) that is often used in dairy products, juices, jams and marmalades, ketchup (*USA*: catsup), pickles, etc.; as well as in pharmaceuticals. The major METABOLITE is sultannilic acid, with lesser amounts of p-acetoamidobenzenesulphonic acid (*USA*: p-acetoamidobenzenesulfonic acid). A small, but significant number (about 1 to 5 per cent) of individuals with ASPIRIN sensitivity also have cross-reactivity to TARTRAZINE, and other benzoates, and individuals sensitive to TARTRAZINE are frequently sensitive to ASPIRIN. Allergic reactions include asthma, rhinitis, URTICARIA and angioedema, and these may be life-threatening. Pharmaceuticals containing this COLOUR (*USA*: color) are therefore labelled.

taste bud (physiology) Small SENSE ORGAN containing chemoreceptors for the sense of TASTE, located in the mouth (particularly on the upper surface of the TONGUE).

taste (physiology) Sense that enables animals to detect flavours, which in mammals involves TASTE BUDS.

TATA box (genetics) A sequence found in EUKARYOTE genes. Part of the PROMOTER region, it occurs about 35 BASE-pairs UPSTREAM from the point at which RNA TRANSCRIPTION is to start. PROKARYOTES have a 'Pribnow box'.

tautomerism (chemistry) EQUILIBRIUM between two organic isomers. It usually involves a shift in the point of attachment of a mobile HYDROGEN ATOM and a shift in the position of a DOUBLE BOND in a MOLECULE. Also termed: DYNAMIC ISOMERISM.

taxis (biology) Orientation of an organism, involving movement, with respect to a STIMULUS from a specific direction.

See also CHEMOTAXIS.

taxon (genetics) Any GROUP of living things, from the viewpoint of CLASSIFICATION. The key TAXON is the SPECIES; the higher taxa are for animals: GENUS, FAMILY, ORDER, CLASS, PHYLUM, KINGDOM. (pl. taxa).

taxonomy (genetics) Study of the CLASSIFICATION of living organisms. The arrangement of taxa into a system of CLASSIFICATION. A MODEM technique is numerical TAXONOMY, in which all attributes of the PHENOTYPE metric, biochemical or whatever, are given equal weighting, and groupings are worked out by COMPUTER.

TB (bacteriology) An abbreviation of 'T'u'B'erculosis.

Tb (chemistry) The CHEMICAL SYMBOL for TERBIUM.

TBG (physiology/ biochemistry) An abbreviation of 'T'hyroxine-'B'inding 'G'lobulin.

TBPA (physiology/ biochemistry) An abbreviation of 'T'hyroxine-'B'inding 'P're'A'lbumin.

TBW (physiology) An abbreviation of 'T'otal 'B'ody 'W'ater.

Tc (chemistry) The CHEMICAL SYMBOL for ELEMENT 43, TECHNETIUM.

TCA (chemistry) An abbreviation of 'T'ri'C'hloroacetic 'A'cid.

T cell (immunology) An abbreviation of 'T'hymus-derived CELL.

T8 cells (immunology) A subset of T CELLS that may kill VIRUS infected CELLS and suppress immune FUNCTION when the INFECTION is over.

TCP (pharmacology) Trichloro-phenyl-iodo-methyl-salicyl.

TDN (biochemistry) An abbreviation of 'T'otal 'D'igestible 'N'utrients.

Te (chemistry) The CHEMICAL SYMBOL for ELEMENT 52, TELLURIUM.

TEA (biochemistry) An abbreviation of 'T'etra'E'thyl'A'mmonium.

tech. (general terminology) Technical.

technetium Tc (chemistry) Artificial RADIOACTIVE metallic ELEMENT in GROUP VIIA of the PERIODIC TABLE (a TRANSITION ELEMENT), which occurs among the FISSION products of URANIUM. It has several isotopes, with half-lives of up to 2.12×10^5 years. At. no. 43; r.a.m. 99 (most STABLE ISOTOPE).

teeth (anatomy) *See* TOOTH.

teflon (chemistry) Trade name for polytetrafluoroethene (PTFE).

telangiectasis (histology) A red spot on the SKIN formed by dilated CAPILLARY or terminal arterial BLOOD VESSELS.

telluride (chemistry) BINARY COMPOUND that contains TELLURIUM.

tellurium Te (chemistry) Silvery-white semi-metallic ELEMENT in GROUP VIB of the PERIODIC TABLE, obtained as a BY-PRODUCT of the extraction of GOLD, SILVER and COPPER. It is used as a CATALYST and to add hardness to ALLOYS of LEAD or steel. At. no. 52; r.a.m. 127.60.

telodendria (histology) The very fine terminal branches of an AXON.

telophase (cytology) Final PHASE of CELL DIVISION that occurs in MITOSIS and MEIOSIS. During TELOPHASE chromatids, on reaching the poles of the CELL, become densely packed and the CELL divides. In ANIMAL CELLS, the PLASMA MEMBRANE constricts. In plants, a wall divides the CELL in two.

temp. (measurement) An abbreviation of 'temp'erature.

temperature (measurement) The DEGREE of hotness or coldness, a measure of the AVERAGE KINETIC ENERGY of its atoms or molecules. The AVERAGE body TEMPERATURE in health is 37°C (98.6°F). It is a little lower in the morning and higher in the evening.

temperature coefficient (physics) Change in a physical quantity with change in TEMPERATURE, usually given as per DEGREE rise of TEMPERATURE.

See also TEMPERATURE SCALE.

temperature gradient (physics) DEGREE or measured rate of the TEMPERATURE change between two points of reference in a substance or in an AREA.

temperature scale (physics) Method of expressing TEMPERATURE. There are various scales, based on different FIXED POINTS. The Fahrenheit scale has largely been replaced by the CELSIUS SCALE (formerly centigrade), all of which express temperatures in degrees (°F and °C). In science, temperatures are frequently expressed in KELVIN (K), the thermodynamic UNIT of TEMPERATURE in SI UNITS.

tendon (histology) Strong CONNECTIVE TISSUE that attaches muscles to bones. It consists of COLLAGEN fibres (*USA*: collagen fibers).

See also LIGAMENT.

tenesmus (medical) Straining painfully but ineffectively to pass a motion or pass URINE.

tenosynovitis (histology) INFLAMMATION of the sheath of a TENDON.

tenoxicam (pharmacology) A non-steroidal ANTI-INFLAMMATORY drug (NSAID) which, administered orally or by injection, is used as a non-narcotic ANALGESIC and ANTIRHEUMATIC to treat pain and inflammation in rheumatic disease and other musculoskeletal conditions.

teratogen (toxicology) Any substance, natural or artificial, that causes ABNORMAL development of an EMBRYO.

teratology (medical) Study of birth defects. The study of ABNORMAL development between conception and birth.

teratoma (histology) A TUMOUR (*USA*: tumor) composed of embryonic tissues including all three layers of developing CELLS, endoderm, MESODERM and ECTODERM. A SOLID TERATOMA may contain pieces of BONE, NERVE or INTESTINE, and is usually MALIGNANT; it may develop in the TESTIS, or in other places, and must be removed. Cystic teratomas may contain various rudimentary tissues such as SKIN, HAIR and TEETH, and are not MALIGNANT; they may contain ECTODERM to the exclusion of other tissues, and are then called dermoid cysts.

terbium Tb (chemistry) Silvery-grey metallic ELEMENT in GROUP IIIA of the PERIODIC TABLE (one of the LANTHANIDES), used in making semiconductors and phosphors. At. no. 65; r.a.m. 158.9254.

term (medical) A definite PERIOD of time, in medicine usually applied to the duration of a PREGNANCY; full term is 282 days from the first day of the last menstrual PERIOD.

terminal decimal (mathematics) Decimal quantity that has a finite number of digits after the decimal point.

See also RECURRING DECIMAL.

terminal fronsferase (genetics) An ENZYME that synthesises a 'tail' on to a DNA MOLECULE. It is used in GENETIC ENGINEERING to add a poly-A tail (one that consists only of repeated As) to the end of one DNA MOLECULE and a poly-T tail (one that consists only of repeated Ts) to the end of another so that they join up.

terminal (computing) An INPUT DEVICE or OUTPUT DEVICE that can handle DATA.

termination (medical) Commonly used to MEAN TERMINATION of PREGNANCY, or ABORTION.

tesla (measurement) SI UNIT of MAGNETIC FLUX DENSITY, named after the Croatian-born American physicist Nikola Tesla (1857-1943).

testes (anatomy) Plural OF TESTIS.

testis (anatomy) The male GONAD whose primary structures are the seminiferous tubules in which SPERMATOGENESIS occurs and the INTERSTITIAL CELLS (Leydig CELLS) which secrete ANDROGENS.

testosterone (biochemistry) SEX HORMONE. The most active ANDROGEN HORMONE. It is produced by the TESTES in the male, in small quantities by the ovaries in the female, and by the ADRENAL CORTEX in both sexes. It stimulates the development of the male reproductive organs and of male secondary sex characteris-

tics like body HAIR and strong muscles. It also raises the sexual drive in males, and increases aggression in some SPECIES, probably including man.

tetanic (medical) Pertaining to the frequently repeated stimulation of a neuron or GROUP of neurons.

tetanospasmin (toxicology/ bacteriology) *See* TETANUS TOXIN.

tetanus (lockjaw) (medical/ bacteriology) A disease caused by the MICRO-ORGANISM *Clostridium tetani*. The spores of this organism are found in the bowels of many animals, including man, and are very common in the soil. The bacilli are Gram-POSITIVE and ANAEROBIC, that is, they will only grow in the absence of OXYGEN. INFECTION occurs through a WOUND or ABRASION in the SKIN; it need only be a very minor WOUND, and in some cases no entry WOUND can be found. The organism produces a TOXIN called tetanospasmin, which spreads to the SPINAL CORD and the BRAIN, both through the BLOOD and along the NERVES.

tetanus toxin (toxicology/ bacteriology) A 150,000 dalton neurotoxic PROTEIN composed of one heavy and one LIGHT PEPTIDE chain linked by a disulphide (*USA*: disulfide) BOND. It is HEAT-LABILE and easily oxidized. Also termed: tetanospasmin.

tetany (medical) Not to be confused with TETANUS, TETANY is a condition in which there is ABNORMAL excitability of the NERVES and muscles. The condition is caused by lack of CALCIUM ions in the BLOOD, and may be due to deficiency of the PARATHYROID GLANDS, lack of VITAMIN D or deficient ABSORPTION of CALCIUM; it may also be due to ALKALOSIS of the BLOOD from taking excess of ALKALIS (*USA*: alkalies), as may happen in the overenthusiastic TREATMENT of a PEPTIC ULCER or a bout of hysterical over-BREATHING. *See* CALCIUM.

tetrabenazine (pharmacology) A drug that administered orally reduces the amount of DOPAMINE in the nerves in the BRAIN. It is used to lessen the extent of involuntary movements in cases of HUNTINGDON'S CHOREA and related disorders.

tetrachloroethene (chemistry) $CCl_2 = CCl_2$ LIQUID HALOGENOALKENE, used as a SOLVENT (especially as a de-greasing agent). Also termed: ETHYLENE TETRACHLORIDE; TETRACHLOROETHYLENE.

tetrachloroethylene (chemistry) An alternative term for TETRACHLOROETHENE.

tetrachloromethane (chemistry) CCl_4 Colourless (*USA*: colorless) LIQUID HALOGENOALKANE, used as a SOLVENT, cleaning agent and in fire extinguishers. Also termed: CARBON TETRACHLORIDE.

tetracycline (pharmacology) Member of a CLASS of antibiotics which act by inhibiting PROTEIN SYNTHESIS in BACTERIA. They have a broad SPECTRUM of activity, but many organisms have developed resistance to them and they are not as widely used as they once were.

tetrad (1, 2 genetics) 1 Four CELLS formed after the second DIVISION in MEIOSIS is complete. 2 Four spores formed by MEIOSIS in a SPORE mother CELL, often seen in FUNGI. *See* TETRAD ANALYSIS.

tetrahedral compound (chemistry) A COMPOUND that has a central ATOM joined to other atoms or groups at the four corners of a tetrahedron. It is the CONFIGURATION of CARBON in many SATURATED COMPOUNDS.

tetrahydrate (chemistry) A chemical containing four molecules of WATER OF CRYSTALLIZATION.

tetraploid (genetics) Describing an organism that has four sets of HOMOLOGOUS CHROMOSOMES.

See also DIPLOID; HAPLOID.

tetravalent (chemistry) Having a VALENCE of four. Also termed: QUADRIVALENT.

tetrodotoxin (TTX) (toxicology) A TOXIN contained in the OVARY and LIVER of puffer fish, in the eggs of the California newt and in some other animals. It is used as a chemical tool for the study of ION channels. The LD50 in mice is 10 mg/kg. It is a TOXICANT of NERVE and MUSCLE by blocking SODIUM channels, this ACTION causing NERVE and MUSCLE paralysis. Symptoms include weakening of VOLUNTARY MUSCLES, respiratory failure from paralysis of the DIAPHRAGM and HYPOTENSION. There is no ANTIDOTE. THERAPY involves artificial RESPIRATION.

TF/P (physiology/ biochemistry) An abbreviation of concentration of a substance in renal 'T'ubular 'F'luid divided by its concentration in 'P'lasma.

TGFA (physiology) An abbreviation of 'T'ransforming 'G'rowth 'F'actor 'A'lpha.

Th (chemistry) The CHEMICAL SYMBOL for THORIUM.

thalamus (anatomy) Part of the FOREBRAIN of vertebrates that is concerned with the routing of nervous impulses to and from the SPINAL CORD.

thalassaemia (haematology) An inherited DEFECT in the formation of HAEMOGLOBIN (*USA*: hemaglobin) common in Mediterranean countries and Africa; there are a number of types, of which the most important is beta-THALASSAEMIA (*USA*: beta-thalassemia). This produces profound ANAEMIA (*USA*: anemia) in children, which if not treated by transfusions is often fatal. (*USA*: thalassemia).

thalidomide (toxicology/ pharmacology) Formerly used therapeutically as a SEDATIVE hypnotic; currently used to treat LEPROSY. THALIDOMIDE is a TERATOGEN; major morphological abnormalities result from exposure during the first trimester of PREGNANCY. Its mode of action involves the formation of a toxic arene OXIDE METABOLITE.

thallium Tl (chemistry) A silver-grey metallic ELEMENT in GROUP IIIB of the PERIODIC TABLE, used in electronic equipment and to make pesticides. At. no. 81; r.a.m. 204.39.

THC (toxicology) An abbreviation of 'T'etra'H'ydro'C'annabinol.

T helper cells (immunology) A subset of T CELLS that carry the T4 marker and are essential for turning on ANTIBODY production, activating CYTOTOXIC T CELLS and initiating many other IMMUNE RESPONSEs.

theophylline (pharmacology) A xanthine that is used as a bronchodilator drug. Administered orally or by injection it is mainly used as an ANTI-ASTHMATIC and for the treatment of bronchitis.

theorem (philosophy) General conclusion in science or mathematics which makes certain assumptions in ORDER to explain observations.

See also HYPOTHESIS; LAW.

therap. (general terminology) An abbreviation of 'therap'eutic.

therapeutic index (T1) (pharmacology) A numerical estimate of the relationship between the toxic dose of a drug and its therapeutic dose.

therapeutic window (pharmacology) The range of PLASMA levels of a drug within which optimal therapeutic effects are obtained; below the range the drug has too little beneficial effect, while too high concentrations may either produce serious side effects or reduce the therapeutic effect.

therapeutics (pharmacology) The study of the science of treating disease.

therapy (pharmacology) The TREATMENT of disease.

thermal conduction (physics) Transmission of HEAT by materials.

thermal conductivity (physics) Thermal conducting POWER of a material.

thermal diffusion (physics) Process of forming a concentration gradient in a fluid mixture by the application of a temperature gradient. Also termed: Soret effect.

thermistor (physics) TEMPERATURE-sensitive semiconductor device whose resistance decreases with an increase in TEMPERATURE, used in electronic thermometers and switches.

thermobarograph (physics) Instrument for measuring and recording the TEMPERATURE and PRESSURE of the ATMOSPHERE. It consists of a thermograph and a BAROGRAPH.

thermochemistry (chemistry) Branch of chemistry that deals with the study of HEAT changes in relation to CHEMICAL REACTIONS. The measurement of heats of REACTION, specific HEAT capacities and BOND energies falls within its scope.

thermocouple (physics) A device for measuring TEMPERATURE which relies on the Seebeck effect: a heated junction between two dissimilar metals produces a measurable ELECTROMOTIVE FORCE (e.m.f.) which depends on the TEMPERATURE of the junction.

thermodynamic temperature (physics) An alternative term for ABSOLUTE TEMPERATURE.

thermodynamics (physics) Branch of physics concerned with the study of the effects of ENERGY changes in physical systems and the relationship between various forms of ENERGY, principally HEAT and mechanical ENERGY.

thermoelectricity (physics) ELECTRICITY produced from HEAT ENERGY, as in a THERMOCOUPLE.

thermograph (physics) THERMOMETER that records variations in TEMPERATURE over a PERIOD in time on a GRAPH; a self-registering THERMOMETER.

thermography (physics) Variations of TEMPERATURE over the surface of a body can be recorded by using photographic FILM sensitive to INFRA-RED RADIATION. The technique is called thermography, and the RECORD a thermogram. Because the surface TEMPERATURE of the body is determined by the state of the local circulation, and variations in the BLOOD supply to a part can be produced by underlying disease processes, thermog-

raphy may help in the diagnosis of diseases such as CANCER of the breast.

thermolabile (biology) Adversely affected by HEAT (as opposed to thermostable, not affected by HEAT).

thermometer (measurement) An instrument for measuring TEMPERATURE. The common LIQUID in-GLASS THERMOMETER relies on the expansion of the LIQUID (e.g. MERCURY or dyed ALCOHOL) in a calibrated sealed GLASS CAPILLARY tube.

thermopile (physics) A TEMPERATURE-measuring device consisting of several thermocouples connected in SERIES, with one SET of junctions blackened so as to absorb thermal RADIATION.

thermoreceptors (measurement) Sensory receptors sensitive to TEMPERATURE.

thermoregulation (physiology) The control of the body's TEMPERATURE: the main regulating centre (*USA*: center) is in the HYPOTHALAMUS, which contains THERMORECEPTORS and can control VASODILATION, sweating, etc.

THI (physics) An abbreviation of 'T'emperature 'H'umidity 'I'ndex.

thiamine (chemistry) White WATER-SOLUBLE CRYSTALLINE B VITAMIN, found in cereals and YEAST. Deficiency of THIAMINE causes the disorder beri-beri in human beings. Also termed: thiamin; ANEURIN; VITAMIN B_1.

thiazide and thiazide-like diuretics (pharmacology) Commonly used DIURETICS such as chlorothiazide which act by inhibiting SODIUM reabsorption at the distal tubule of the KIDNEY. Their action may cause POTASSIUM loss from the blood. They are used in the TREATMENT of HIGH BLOOD PRESSURE and HEART failure.

thiazine (chemistry) Member of a GROUP of HETEROCYCLIC compounds that contain SULPHUR (*USA*: sulfur) and NITROGEN (in addition to CARBON) in the ring.

thin-layer chromatography (TLC) (biochemistry) A chromatographic separation technique using a LIQUID mobile PHASE that moves by CAPILLARY ACTION through a thin layer of sorbent coated on an INERT, ridgid backing material or plate. Once separated, they can be identified.

thio- (chemistry) Prefix denoting the presence of SULPHUR (*USA*: sulfur) in a COMPOUND.

thiocarbamide (chemistry) An alternative term for THIOUREA.

thioether (chemistry) Member of a class of organic compounds, ANALOGOUS to ethers, in which SULPHUR (*USA*: sulfur) takes the place of OXYGEN. Also termed: alkyl or aryl SULPHIDE (*USA*: aryl sulfide).

thiopentone sodium (pharmacology) A barbiturate drug which, administered by injection, is used as a general anaesthetic for induction and maintenance of anaesthesia during operations of short duration.

thiourea (chemistry) NH_2CSNH_2 Colourless (*USA*: colorless) CRYSTALLINE ORGANIC COMPOUND, the SULPHUR (*USA*: sulfur) analogue of UREA. Its conversion to its ISOMER ammonium thiocyanate on heating was the first demonstration of an ORGANIC COMPOUND being changed directly into an inorganic one. It is used in medicine and as a photographic sensitizer. Also termed: THIOCARBAMIDE.

thoracoscopy (medical) The inspection of the interior of the thoracic cavity through an ENDOSCOPE.

thoracotomy (medical) The operation of opening the wall of the chest.

thorax (anatomy) Region of the body that contains the HEART and lungs; the chest. It is separated from the ABDOMEN by the DIAPHRAGM.

thoria (chemistry) An alternative term for THORIUM DIOXIDE.

thorium dioxide (chemistry) ThO_2 White INSOLUBLE powder, used as a refractory and in non-silica OPTICAL GLASS. Also termed: THORIA.

thorium Th (chemistry) Silvery-white RADIOACTIVE ELEMENT in GROUP IIIA of the PERIODIC TABLE (one of the ACTINIDES). It has several isotopes, with half lives of up to 1.39×10^{10} years. THORIUM-232 captures slow, or thermal, neutrons and is used to 'breed' the fissile URANIUM-233. Its refractory OXIDE (THORIA, ThO_2) is used in GAS mantles. At.no. 90; r.a.m. 232.0381.

Thr (biochemistry) An abbreviation of 'Thr'eonine.

threadworm (parasitology) PARASITES called *Oxyuris vermicularis*. Also termed: pinworm. *See* WORMS.

threonine (biochemistry) AMINO ACID that is essential in the diet of animals. Also termed: 2-amino-3-hydroxybutanoic ACID.

threshold (physics) The value of a physical STIMULUS at which it becomes detectable, 'absolute threshold', or the minimum difference in the values of two stimuli lying on the same DIMENSION at which they can be discriminated, 'difference threshold'. Within limits the value assigned to a THRESHOLD is arbitrary: it is usually taken to be that at which the STIMULUS (or the difference between two stimuli) is detected on 50 per cent of presentations.

throat (medical) A common site of INFECTION involving the tonsils alone or more usually the whole of the THROAT, when it is called pharyngitis. The INFECTION is most often due to a VIRUS; this may be complicated by secondary INFECTION with haemolytic streptococci, *Haemophilus influenzae* or *STREPTO-COCCUS pneumoniae.*

thrombin (biochemistry) An ENZYME concerned with the conversion of FIBRINOGEN into FIBRIN in the clotting of BLOOD following injury. *See* COAGULATION of the BLOOD.

thrombocytes (platelets) (haematology) The smallest of the formed elements in the BLOOD. They are fragments of megakaryocytes, giant PRECURSOR CELLS. Platelets adhere to COLLAGEN fibres (*USA*: collagen fibers) exposed at points of BLOOD VESSEL injury. Additional platelets aggregate at this point to form a PLATELET plug, which is the first step in HAEMO-STASIS (*USA*: hemostasis). They release factors to promote COAGULATION. A typical PLATELET count is 250,000 per CUBIC millimetre (*USA*: CUBIC millimeter). ASPIRIN interferes with PLATELET aggregation and may be useful in preventing clot formation.

See also THROMBOCYTOPENIA.

thrombocytopenia (haematology) A condition of low PLATELET concentrations, resulting in excessive bruising and bleeding from WOUNDS. This can result

from an autoimmune REACTION following the COMBINATION of such agents as ASPIRIN, digoxin, antihistamines or sulphonamides (*USA*: sulfonamides) with PLATELET proteins to form antigens.

thrombophlebitis (haematology) INFLAM-MATION of a VEIN with consequent THROMBOSIS, the formation of a clot. It is quite common in varicose veins, which become red and tender and sometimes painful enough to make walking difficult.

thrombosis (haematology) The formation of a clot or THROMBUS in a BLOOD VESSEL. It may occur in arteries, particularly when the wall has been roughened by atherosclerosis, or in the veins, especially when the BLOOD flow is stagnant or sluggish.

thrombus (medical) A SOLID MASS formed from the constituents of BLOOD within the BLOOD VESSELs or the HEART. Thrombi that form within the rapidly moving arterial circulation are composed largely of FIBRIN and platelets with only a few trapped red and white CELLS. (pl. thrombi).

thrush (mycology) A disease character-ised by the formation of whitish spots in the mouth. It is caused by the FUNGUS *Candida albicans.*

thulium Tm (chemistry) Silvery-white metallic ELEMENT in GROUP IIA of the PERIODIC TABLE (one of the LANTHANIDES). Its RADIOACTIVE ISOTOPES emit GAMMA RAYS and X-RAYS and are used in portable RADIOGRAPHY equipment. At. no. 69; r.a.m. 168.9342.

thymine (chemistry) $C_5H_6N_2O_2$ Colourless (*USA*: colorless) CRYSTALLINE HETEROCYCLIC COMPOUND, one of the pyrimidines. It is found in the nucleotides of DNA (along with CYTOSINE, ADENINE and GUANINE). In

RNA the corresponding BASE is URACIL. Also termed: 5-methyluracil; 5-methyl-2,4-dioxopyrimidine.

thymol (chemistry) $C_{10}H_{14}O$ Colourless (*USA*: colorless) CRYSTALLINE ORGANIC COMPOUND found in the oils of thyme and mint. It is used in ANTISEPTIC mouth washes. Alternative names: 2-hydroxy-p-cymene, 2-hydroxy-1-isopropyl-4-methyl-benzene.

thymus (anatomy) Twin-lobed ENDOCRINE GLAND, situated in the chest near the HEART, that plays an important role in the IMMUNE RESPONSE. After birth it produces many LYMPHOCYTES and induces them to develop into ANTIBODY-producing CELLS. It declines after puberty and atrophies in older adults.

See also LYMPHATIC SYSTEM; T CELLS.

thymus-derived cell (T-CELL) (haematology) A LYMPH CELL of the body that fights against INFECTION and foreign particles.

thyroid (biochemistry) An ENDOCRINE GLAND, located in the neck region, that produces three HORMONES: THYROXINE (tetraiodothyronine, T4); triiodothyronine (T3); thyrocalcitonin (CALCITONIN). The former two are the classic 'THYROID HORMONES'. THYROXINE is the CLEAVAGE PRODUCT of thyroglobulin found in the THYROID GLAND COLLOID. THYROXINE represents the predominant circulating form. The L-form is the THYROID HORMONE, whereas the D-form has an anticholesteremic ACTION. THYROXINE is metabolized within target CELLS to T3, which is five times more active than T4. T3 binds to nuclear receptors where it activates genes. Its primary actions are to increase METABOLISM, to increase PROTEIN SYNTHESIS, stimulate BASAL METABOLIC RATE and increase HEAT production. THYROID

HORMONE SYNTHESIS and SECRETION are under the control of THYROID-STIMULATING HORMONE from the ADENOHYPOPHYSIS. HYPOTHYROIDISM in the infant causes cretinism and in the adult myxedema. HYPERTHYROIDISM leads to Graves' disease. The third HORMONE from the THYROID GLAND, CALCITONIN, decreases BLOOD CALCIUM levels and acts antagonistically to PARATHYROID HORMONE in CALCIUM HOMEOSTASIS. CALCITONIN SECRETION is controlled by BLOOD CALCIUM levels and not by THYROID-stimulating HORMONE. In human beings, undersecretion (HYPOTHYROIDISM) causes cretinism in children and MYXOEDEMA in adults; overproduction (HYPERTHYROIDISM) may cause THYROTOXICOSIS, resulting in goitre. IODINE is needed in the diet for efficient functioning of the THYROID; deficiency of IODINE may cause the GLAND to swell and form a goitre.

thyroid-stimulating hormone (TSH) (biochemistry) Alternative name for THYROTROPHIN.

thyrotoxicosis (medical) Graves' disease is the commonest cause of this overaction of the THYROID GLAND. It is five times more common in women than men, and is thought to be an AUTOIMMUNE DISEASE; it runs in families. The THYROID GLAND is enlarged. Investigation shows high levels in the BLOOD of the THYROID HORMONES T3 and T4 and a low value of the PITUITARY HORMONE TSH. Named after the Dublin physician, R. Graves (1796-1853).

thyrotrophin TSH (biochemistry) A tropic HORMONE from the ADENOHYPOPHYSIS that causes the THYROID GLAND to proliferate, absorb more IODINE and synthesise and secrete the THYROID HORMONES THYROXINE and triiodothyronine, but not thyrocalcitonin. TSH SECRETION is under the control of THYROTROPHIN-releasing FACTOR (TRF) (USA: thyrotropin-releasing factor) from the HYPOTHALAMUS. Thyrotrophin is a GLYCOPROTEIN, consisting of two large PEPTIDE units (one of which is similar to LH and FSH). (*USA*: thyrotropin). Also termed: THYROID-STIMULATING HORMONE.

thyroxin (biochemistry) White CRYSTALLINE ORGANIC COMPOUND, an IODINE-containing AMINO ACID derived from TYROSINE. It is a HORMONE secreted by the THYROID, which promotes GROWTH in immature organisms and increases metabolic rate in PERIODS of increased activity.

thyroxine (T4) (biochemistry) *See* THYROID.

Ti (chemistry) The CHEMICAL SYMBOL for TITANIUM.

TI (pharmacology) An abbreviation of 'T'herapeutic 'I'ndex.

tiaprofenic (pharmacology) A non-steroidal ANTI-INFLAMMATORY drug (NSAID) which, administered orally, is used to treat pain and inflammation in rheumatic disease and other musculoskeletal conditions.

tibia (anatomy) One of the two bones below the knee in a tetrapod VERTEBRATE (the other is the FIBULA); the shinbone.

tibolone (pharmacology) A drug that, administered orally, has both OESTROGEN and PROGESTOGEN activity. It can be used to treat menopausal problems in HORMONE REPLACEMENT THERAPY (HRT).

tick (parasitology) A BLOOD-sucking insect. They may be separated into hard, *Ixodidae*, and soft, *Argasidae*, TICKS. TICKS carry several diseases, among them encephalitis, relapsing FEVER, LYME DISEASE, TYPHUS, spotted lever, Q FEVER, and babesiosis which is a protozoan parasitic disease common in wild and domestic animals in tropical and subtropical countries, passed on to man by hard TICKS.

tidal volume (physiology) The VOLUME of GAS inspired or expired during each respiratory CYCLE. It is an INDICATOR of the depth of BREATHING.

time series (statistics) DATA tabulated by the time which successive observations are made.

time-lapse photography (photography) Technique for producing a speeded-up FILM, achieved by introducing a delay between each frame exposed during filming. It is used to FILM very slow-moving or slow-developing processes.

tin Sn (chemistry) Soft silvery-white metallic ELEMENT in GROUP IVB of the PERIODIC TABLE, which forms three ALLOTROPES. It occurs mainly as TIN(IV) OXIDE, SnO_2, in ores such as cassiterite (tinstone). It is used mainly as a protective coating for steel (TIN plate) and in making ALLOYS with LEAD (solder, type METAL, pewter). Its compounds are used as catalysts, FUNGICIDES and mordants. Metallic TIN and inorganic TIN compounds are not toxic to humans. Some organo-TIN compounds are toxic. At. no. 50; r.a.m. 118.69.

tin(II) (chemistry) An alternative term for stannous.

tin(IV) (chemistry) An alternative term for stannic.

tin(II) chloride (chemistry) $SnCl_2$ White SOLUBLE SOLID. A REDUCING AGENT, it is used as a CATALYST in organic reactions and as an anti-sludge agent for oils. Also termed: stannous chloride; tin salt.

tin dioxide (chemistry) An alternative term for TIN(IV) OXIDE.

tin disulphide (chemistry) An alternative term for TIN(IV) SULPHIDE (*USA*: tin(IV) sulfide). (*USA*: tin disulfide).

tin(IV) hydride (chemistry) SnH_4 Unstable GAS, used as a REDUCING AGENT in ORGANIC CHEMISTRY. Also termed: stannane.

tin(IV) oxide (chemistry) SnO_2 White CRYSTALLINE SOLID, used as a PIGMENT and as a refractory material. Also termed: TIN DIOXIDE.

tin(IV) sulphide (chemistry) SnS_2 Yellow INSOLUBLE SOLID, used as a PIGMENT. Also termed: TIN DISULPHIDE (*USA*: tin disulfide). (*USA*: tin(IV) sulfide).

tin salt (chemistry) An alternative term for TIN(II) CHLORIDE.

tincal (chemistry) Naturally occurring crude BORAX.

tinea (mycology) A superficial FUNGUS INFECTION of the SKIN. TINEA pedis is athlete's foot, caused by the organisms *Trichophyton rubrum* and *T. interdigitale,* which produce moist itching lesions commonest between the toes, and sometimes blisters on the soles of the feet. *T. rubrum* may cause scaly patches on the toes and feet, and attack the nails. Infections of the groin are caused by *T. rubrum* or *Epidermophyton floccosum,* and are more common in males.

tinea (medical/ mycology) RINGWORM, a SKIN disorder characterized by raised, roughly circular and discoloured (*USA*:

discolored) patches, that results from an INFECTION by a FUNGUS.

tinnitis (medical) An abnormality of hearing in which an apparent persistent ringing sound is heard when in fact no such sound is present.

tis. (general terminology) An abbreviation of 'tis'sue.

tissue (histology) The tissues are the substance of the body; particular tissues such as connective or fatty TISSUE are collections of CELLS of the same type specialised in the same way to carry out a particular FUNCTION. In higher organisms tissues may combine to form a highly specialized ORGAN.

tissue culture (biology) Process by which CELLS or tissues are maintained outside the body (in vitro) in a suitable medium. The material is kept at a suitable TEMPERATURE, pH and OSMOTIC PRESSURE. The composition of the medium depends on the type of TISSUE CULTUREd. Depending on the type of CELL, a culture may be able to go on indefinitely, with CELLS dividing from time to time. CANCER CELLS (or NORMAL CELLS that have undergone TRANSFORMATION in culture) will go on dividing infinitely often, but most differentiated CELLS seem to lose the ability to divide after 30-40 divisions; this is known as the Hayflick phenomenon.

tissue fluid (biology) An alternative term for LYMPH.

tissue typing (histology) The identification of histocompatibility antigens in DONOR and RECIPIENT prior to transplant surgery.

titania (chemistry) An alternative term for TITANIUM(IV) OXIDE.

titanic chloride (chemistry) An alternative term for TITANIUM(IV) CHLORIDE.

titanium Ti (chemistry) A silvery-white metallic ELEMENT in GROUP IVA of the PERIODIC TABLE (a TRANSITION ELEMENT). Its corrosion-resistant lightweight ALLOYS are employed in the aerospace industry. Naturally occurring CRYSTALLINE forms of TITANIUM(IV) OXIDE (titania, TiO_2) are the semi-precious gemstone rutile. The powdered OXIDE is used as a white PIGMENT and a DIELECTRIC in capacitors. At. no. 22; r.a.m. 47.90.

titanium tetrachloride (chemistry) An alternative term for TITANIUM(IV) CHLORIDE.

titrant (chemistry) Chemical SOLUTION of known CONCENTRATION, *i.e.* a STANDARD SOLUTION, which is added during the course of a TITRATION.

titration (chemistry) A technique in VOLUMETRIC ANALYSIS in which one chemical SOLUTION of known CONCENTRATION is added (using a BURETTE) to a known VOLUME of another chemical SOLUTION of unknown CONCENTRATION (measured by a PIPETTE), and the CHEMICAL REACTION followed by observing changes in COLOUR (*USA*: color), pH, etc. An INDICATOR may be added to indicate the end-point of the REACTION, which allows the unknown CONCENTRATION to be determined.

titre (measurement) RECIPROCAL value of the highest possible DILUTION that illicits a RESPONSE or REACTION. (*USA*: titer).

Tk locus (thymidine KINASE LOCUS) (biochemistry) The TK LOCUS allows cultured mammalian CELLS to incorporate pyrimidines from the medium so that these pyrimidines may be converted into NUCLEIC ACIDS. A MUTATION at this LOCUS prevents uptake of pyrimidines, both NORMAL and toxic, such as bromodeoxy-uridine or trifluorothymidine; with toxic pyrimidines, such a MUTATION allows GROWTH of the cultured CELLS since they can produce pyrimidines by de novo SYNTHESIS. This concept is utilised in some mutagenicity tests in which cultured mammalian CELLS are exposed to toxic pyrimidines in addition to possible mutagens; GROWTH of these CELLS indicates that a MUTATION in the TK LOCUS has occurred.

Tl (chemistry) The CHEMICAL SYMBOL for ELEMENT 81, THALLIUM.

TLC (biochemistry) An abbreviation of 'T'hin-'L'ayer 'C'hromatography.

TLV (toxicology) An abbreviation of 'T'hreshold 'L'imit 'V'alue.

T lymphocytes (immunology) A GROUP of WHITE BLOOD CELLS involved in the IMMUNE SYSTEM. They have on their surfaces receptors that recognize histocompatibility antigens on the surfaces of CELLS, so that they bind on to these antigens on any foreign CELL that enters the body. They are therefore the main part of the body's RESPONSE to transplants. T LYMPHOCYTES (so called because they originate in the THYMUS) recognize the antigens by sequence (unlike B LYMPHOCYTES). T LYMPHOCYTES also release factors that induce proliferation of T LYMPHOCYTES and B LYMPHOCYTES.

Tm (1 chemistry; 2 physiology) 1 The CHEMICAL SYMBOL for ELEMENT 69, THULIUM. 2 An abbreviation of renal 'T'ubular 'm'aximum.

Tn (chemistry) The CHEMICAL SYMBOL for thoron.

TNF (histology/ biochemistry) An abbreviation of 'T'umour 'N'ecrosis 'F'actor (USA: tumor necrosis factor).

tocopherol (biochemistry) A VITAMIN isolated from plants that increases fertility in rats. Deficiency of it causes wasting of muscles in animals. It has been found to have ANTIOXIDANT activity, and it is important in maintaining membranes. Also termed: VITAMIN E.

tolbutamide (pharmacology) A sulphonyl-urea drug used as an orally administered treatment in non-insulin-dependent DIABETES MELLITUS.

tolerance (1 pharmacology; 2 immunology) 1 An ADAPTATIONal state when, after repeated exposure, a given dose of an agent produces a decreased effect or, conversely, when increasingly larger doses are necessary to obtain the effects observed with the original dose. Two mechanisms of acquired pharmacological TOLERANCE are generally recognized: (a) dispositional; (b) pharmacodynamic. Dispositional TOLERANCE results from alterations in the pharmacokinetic properties of the agent. Pharmacody-namic TOLERANCE results from adaptive changes within affected systems, such that the RESPONSE is reduced in the presence of the same CONCENTRATION of the agent. TOLERANCE may not develop uniformly to all the actions of an agent. The toxicological manifestation of TOLERANCE development is typically expressed as a progressive increase in the LD50 for a given agent, although it should be recognized that TOLERANCE development is not absolute. 2 A state of nonresponsiveness to a particular ANTIGEN or GROUP of antigens.

Tollens' reagent (chemistry) Ammoniacal SOLUTION of SILVER OXIDE used as a test for ALDEHYDES, which reduce it to deposit a mirror of SILVER. It was named after the German chemist Bernhard Tollens (1841-1918).

toluene (chemistry) $C_6H_5CH_3$ Colourless (USA: colorless) aromatic organic LIQUID that occurs in coal-tar, used as an industrial SOLVENT and starting point for making explosives. Also termed: METHYLBENZENE.

toluidine (chemistry) $CH_3C_6H_4NH_2$ One of three isomeric aromatic amines, used in the manufacture of dyes and drugs. The ortho- and meta- forms are colourless (USA: colorless) liquids; the para- ISOMER is a colourless CRYSTALLINE SOLID. Also termed: AMINOTOLUENE; METHYLANILINE.

toluidine blue in sorensons PH 6.8 buffer (histology) A histological staining technique that may be used to make helicobacter pylori visible under the MICROSCOPE.

toluidine blue stain (histology) A histological staining technique that may be used to make amyloid visible under the MICROSCOPE.

tomogram (radiology) An X-RAY taken to show structures lying in a selected plane in the body.

tomography (medical) Any non-invasive technique that yields information about the different spatial parts of the BRAIN, particularly about successive slices through it.

ton (measurement) UNIT of MASS equal to 20 cwt or 2,240 lb (an imperial, or long, ton); a short ton equals 2,000 lb.

See also TONNE.

tongue (anatomy) Muscular ORGAN located in the BUCCAL CAVITY (mouth) of some animals, used for manipulating food (and in human beings involved in speech).

tonne (measurement) UNIT of MASS equal to 1,000 kilograms. 1 tonne = 23204.62 lb, slightly less than the imperial ton (2,240 lb). Also termed: metric ton.

tonsil (anatomy) One of a pair of LYMPHOID TISSUE regions at the back of the mouth which help to prevent INFECTION by producing LYMPHOCYTES.

tooth (anatomy) A hard structure embedded in the JAW BONE and adapted for cutting and grinding food. TEETH are composed of a cavity containing capillaries and NERVE endings, a layer of DENTINE and a tough outer layer of ENAMEL.

See also CANINE TOOTH; INCISOR; MOLAR TOOTH; PREMOLAR.

torasemide (pharmacology) A powerful DIURETIC drug of the LOOP DIURETIC type which can be administered orally, by injection or infusion. It is used to treat OEDEMA (*USA*: edema), oliguria, and as a ANTIHYPERTENSIVE.

torr (measurement) UNIT of PRESSURE equivalent to that produced by a 1 mm column of MERCURY. It is equal to 133.3 newtons m^{-2}.

toxaemia (bacteriology) The presence of BACTERIAL toxins in the BLOOD. TOXAEMIA of PREGNANCY is a different condition, and is now called eclampsia. (*USA*: toxemia).

toxic shock syndrome (TSS) (medical/ bacteriology) A life-threatening but rare condition caused by the damaging effect of toxins of *STAPHYLOCOCCUS aureus* SPECIES on the lining of BLOOD VESSELs. The condition has been linked to sanitary tampon use.

toxicant (toxicology) Any chemical, of natural or SYNTHETIC ORIGIN, capable of causing a deleterious effect on a living organism. The term TOXIN should never be used as an alternative term for TOXICANT, being properly reserved for only those toxicants synthesised metabolically by a living organism.

toxicara (parasitology) An INFESTATION with *TOXICARA canis,* a worm that lives in the intestines of dogs and foxes. The eggs are passed in the excreta, and if humans eat contaminated food the larvae travel through the lungs and LIVER but normally do no harm and die in about a year. Occasionally however they reach the EYE, where they can SET up a granulomatous INFLAMMATION and affect the RETINA, causing a squint and loss of vision.

toxicol. (toxicology) An abbreviation of 'toxicol'ogical; 'toxicol'ogist; 'toxicol'ogy.

toxicology (toxicology) The science that deals with poisons (toxicants) and their effects. A POISON is defined as any substance that causes a harmful effect, either by accident or design, when administered to a living organism.

toxicosis (toxicology) The state of having been poisoned.

toxin (1, 2 toxicology) 1 A POISON; usually applied to those produced by a living organism. 2 Any harmful substance.

toxoid (toxicology) A BACTERIAL TOXIN so modified that it has lost its poisonous properties, but can still act as an ANTIGEN to provoke the formation of antibodies; TETANUS TOXOID is, for example, used by injection to induce IMMUNITY to TETANUS, but it does not produce symptoms of the disease.

toxoplasmosis (parasitology) INFECTION with the protozoan PARASITE *Toxoplama gondii*. Human beings may become infected from cats or by eating meat containing TISSUE cysts which has been badly cooked; the disease is common in sheep. In the vast majority of cases the INFECTION does no harm and passes unrecognized, but in some there may be enlargement of the LYMPH NODEs and rarely a rash, with general MALAISE which may last weeks; the disease resembles infectious mononucleosis. It usually resolves without trouble, but it may infect those suffering from IMMUNO-SUPPRESSIVE disorders such as AIDS or those who are taking IMMUNOSUPPRESSIVE drugs, when the disease may affect the BRAIN and produce encephalitis. Most importantly, however, mothers who become infected during PREGNANCY may pass the INFECTION on to the child. This may result in MISCARRIAGE, or the child may be born with abnormalities of the CENTRAL NERVOUS SYSTEM which are apparent at birth or become apparent later, perhaps after several years.

TPA (physiology/ biochemistry) An abbreviation of 'T'issue 'P'lasminogen 'A'ctivator.

TPN (biochemistry) An abbreviation of 'T'ri'P'hosphopyridine 'N'ucleotide.

TPNH (biochemistry) An abbreviation of reduced 'T'ri'P'hosphopyridine 'N'ucleo-tide.

Tr (chemistry) CHEMICAL SYMBOL for TERBIUM.

trace element (biochemistry) ELEMENT essential to METABOLISM, but necessary only in very small quantities (*e.g.* COPPER and COBALT in animals, molybdenum in ants). Such elements are usually poisonous if large quantities are ingested.

trachea (anatomy) Tube through which AIR is drawn into the lungs; windpipe.

tracheotomy (medical) The operation of cutting an opening into the TRACHEA.

trachoma (medical/ microbiology) An INFECTION of the EYE, caused by the MICROORGANISM *Chlamydia trachomatis*. Commonest in tropical Africa and India, it is worldwide the largest single cause of human sight loss.

tranexamic acid (pharmacology) An antifibrinolytic drug which administered orally or by injection, acts by inhibiting plasminogen, which is one of the blood's natural ANTICOAGULANT factors. It is used to stem bleeding in circumstances such as excessive period bleeding (MENOR-RHAGIA).

tranquillizer (pharmacology) Drug that acts on the CENTRAL NERVOUS SYSTEM (CNS), used for calming people and animals without affecting consciousness.

See also SEDATIVE.

trans configuration (genetics) One of the two possible arrangements for the ALLELEs in an individual that is HET-

EROZYGOUS for MUTATIONS at two linked loci. *Trans* (from the Latin meaning 'across') means that one of the MUTANT ALLELES is on one CHROMOSOME and the other is on the HOMOLOGOUS CHROMOSOME, *i.e.* the two chromosomes are a + and + b. The opposite is *cis*. Also termed: repulsion.

transamination (chemistry) Removal and transference of an AMINO GROUP from one COMPOUND (usually an AMINO ACID) to another.

transcendental (1, 2 mathematics) 1 IRRATIONAL NUMBER that is not the ROOT of a POLYNOMIAL equation. 2 FUNCTION that is not a finite POLYNOMIAL equation (*e.g.* logarithmic).

transcription (molecular biology) The process by which one strand of DNA is copied into a single strand of RNA; the first step in PROTEIN SYNTHESIS. The RNA MOLECULE is synthesized by RNA polymerase, copying the DNA message by following the base-pairing rules. The polymerase first recognizes the PROMOTER region, and actual TRANSCRIPTION begins at the start codon a few bases further downstream (going from the 5' towards the 3' end of the DNA strand). *See* GENETIC CODE.

transducer (physiology) A device that receives a signal in one physical form and outputs it in another; *e.g.* sensory receptors signal the STIMULUS received by a change in their MEMBRANE POTENTIAL.

transduction (genetics) The transfer of genetic information from one BACTERIUM to another when it is carried by a BACTERIOPHAGE.

transfer RNA (molecular biology) Small MOLECULE of RNA that acts as a CARRIER of specific amino acids in the SYNTHESIS of proteins. AMINO ACIDS are placed in a specific ORDER by the transfer RNA molecules according to instructions in the MESSENGER RNA, to form a POLYPEPTIDE chain.

transferases (biochemistry) *See* ENZYMES.

transference number (physics) An alternative term for TRANSPORT NUMBER.

transformation (genetics) This has two meanings in genetics. (1) A permanent change in the genetic characteristics of one BACTERIUM by exposure to DNA of a different ORIGIN. It was the phenomenon of TRANSFORMATION that led Avery to the discovery that DNA was the MOLECULE responsible for carrying genetic information. (2) A change in an ANIMAL CELL in TISSUE CULTURE so that it grows and divides in the same way as a CANCER CELL, possibly due to activation of a viral GENE. The relationship of this phenomenon to CANCER is not understood.

transformation constant (radiology) An alternative term for DISINTEGRATION CONSTANT.

transition (molecular biology) A MUTATION in which a PURINE BASE (ADENINE, GUANINE) is replaced with another PURINE, or a PYRIMIDINE (CYTOSINE, THYMINE) with another PYRIMIDINE.

See also TRANSVERSION.

transition element (chemistry) Member of a large GROUP of elements that have partly filled inner ELECTRON shells, which gives them their distinctive physical and chemical properties (particularly VARIABLE VALENCY and the tendency to form coloured [*USA*: colored] compounds). They occupy Groups IIIA, IVA, VA, VIA,

VIIA, VIII, IB and IIB of the PERIODIC TABLE. Many of these elements and their compounds are used as catalysts.

transition point (1, 2 chemistry) 1 TEMPERATURE at which the TRANSFORMATION of one form of a substance into another form can occur (usually one CRYSTALLINE modification into another). 2 TEMPERATURE at which two SOLID phases exist at EQUILIBRIUM. 3 TEMPERATURE at which a change to SUPERCONDUCTIVITY happens in a substance.

transition temperature (chemistry) The TEMPERATURE above and below which different ALLOTROPES are STABLE.

translation (biochemistry) Process by which PROTEIN is synthesized in CELLS. It occurs the ACTION of MESSENGER RNA, which attaches to a RIBOSOME in the CYTOPLASM. TRANSFER RNA molecules which are attached to a specific AMINO ACID then line up according to the sequence of AMINO ACIDS encoded in the MESSENGER RNA to form a POLYPEPTIDE chain. Also termed: PROTEIN SYNTHESIS.

translocation (genetics) A MUTATION consisting of the transfer of part of a CHROMOSOME to another part of the same CHROMOSOME or of a different CHROMOSOME.

translucent (chemistry) Describing a substance that transmits and diffuses LIGHT, but which does not allow a well-defined IMAGE to be seen through it with little or no diffusion.

See also TRANSPARENT.

transparent (chemistry) Describing a substance that allows LIGHT (or other RADIATION) to pass through it with little or no diffusion.

See also TRANSLUCENT.

transport number (physics) In ELECTROLYSIS, FRACTION of the total CURRENT carried by a particular ION in the ELECTROLYTE. Also termed: TRANSFERENCE NUMBER.

transposition (genetics) The movement of a transposer or other movable sequence of DNA from one place in the GENOME to another.

transposon (genetics) A moveable genetic ELEMENT similar to a JUMPING GENE. They are found in the GENOME of BACTERIA, and are involved in the resistance to antibiotics. Unlike JUMPING GENES, transposers leave a copy of themselves in the original position when they move to a new site. They make it possible for ANTIBIOTIC resistance to be spread very rapidly, not only within a single strain of BACTERIA, but from one GENUS to another. *See* CONJUGATION.

transtracheal aspiration (medical) The passage of needle and plastic catheter through the TRACHEA for obtaining lower respiratory tract secretions.

transudate (cytology) Similar to exudate, but with low PROTEIN content.

transversal (general terminology) Line that intersects another SET of lines.

transversion (molecular biology) A MUTATION in which a PURINE BASE (ADENINE, GUANINE) is substituted for a PYRIMIDINE one (eytosine, THYMINE), or vice versa.

See also TRANSITION.

tranylcypromine (pharmacology) An ANTIDEPRESSANT drug of the monoamine-oxidase inhibitor (MAOI) class which is administered orally.

TRAP (physiology/ biochemistry) An abbreviation of 'T'hyroid 'R'eceptor 'A'uxiliary 'P'rotein.

trauma (medical) An injury or WOUND.

travellers diarrhoea (medical) A term applied to the short attacks of DIARRHOEA which afflict many people when they first arrive in a warm country. Most cases are due to a type *of ESCHERICHIA COLI* which produces a TOXIN which affects the BOWEL. (*USA*: traveller's diarrhea).

treatment (pharmacology) *See* THERAPY.

trematodes (parasitology) FLUKES.

treponema (bacteriology) A GENUS of spirochactes, MICRO-ORGANISMS formed like a very thin coiled thread that can bend and spin on its long AXIS. *TREPONEMA pertenue* causes YAWS, *TREPONEMA pallidum* syphilis and *TREPONEMA carateum* pinta.

TRH (physiology/ biochemistry) An abbreviation of 'T'hyrotrophin-'R'eleasing 'H'ormone (USA: thyrotropin-releasing hormone).

triamcinolone acetonide (pharmacology) A synthetic corticosteroid with ANTI-INFLAMMATORY and anti-allergic properties.

triamterene (pharmacology) A mild DIURETIC drug of the POTASSIUM-sparing type, which causes the retention of POTASSIUM. It is used as a DIURETIC, to treat OEDEMA (*USA*: edema), as an ANTI-HYPERTENSIVE, and in congestive HEART FAILURE treatment.

triatomic molecule (chemistry) MOLECULE of an ELEMENT that consists of three atoms, *e.g.* OZONE, O_3.

triazine (chemistry) $C_3H_3N_3$ One of a GROUP of isomeric HETEROCYCLIC ORGANIC COMPOUNDS with three NITROGEN atoms and three CARBON atoms in the ring. TRIAZINE derivatives are used as plastics, dyes and herbicides.

tricarboxylic acid cycle (biochemistry) An alternative term for KREBS CYCLE.

trichinosis (parasitology) An INFECTION with the worm *Trichinella spiralis,* which infects pigs and is acquired by eating undercooked pork.

trichloroacetic acid (TCA) (chemistry) A colourless (*USA*: colorless), HYGROSCOPIC SOLID, used as a herbicide (SODIUM trichloroacetate) and as an INTERMEDIATE in PESTICIDE manufacture. TCA is also used in *in vitro* LABORATORY studies to stop ENZYME reactions by PRECIPITATION of proteins. It is corrosive to the SKIN and eyes, but is not otherwise hazardous.

trichloroacetaldehyde (chemistry) An alternative term for TRICHLOROETHANAL.

trichloroethanal (chemistry) CCl_3CHO Pungent colourless (*USA*: colorless) oily LIQUID ALDEHYDE, which forms a SOLID HYDRATE (TRICHLOROETHANEDIOL). Also termed: CHLORAL; TRICHLOROACETALDEHYDE.

trichloroethanediol (chemistry) $Cl_3CCH-(OH)_2$ White CRYSTALLINE ORGANIC COMPOUND, used as a SEDATIVE. Also termed: CHLORAL HYDRATE.

trichloromethane (chemistry) $CHCl_3$ Colourless (*USA*: colorless) VOLATILE LIQUID HALOFORM, used as an ANAESTHETIC

(*USA*: anesthetic) and as a SOLVENT. Also termed: CHLOROFORM.

trichomonas (parasitology) *TRICHOMONAS vaginalis* is a protozoan PARASITE which causes INFLAMMATION of the VAGINA in women and URETHRITIS in men. It is commonly passed on in sexual intercourse.

trichuris (parasitology) The WHIPWORM, a small roundworm.

tricyclic antidepressants (pharmacology) One of the three main classes of ANTIDEPRESSANT drugs that are used to relieve the symptoms of depressive illness. Chemically they are mainly dibenzazepine or dibenzcycloheptene derivatives and examples include amitriptyline hydrochloride and imipramine hydrochloride.

triglyceride (chemistry) ESTER of GLYCEROL, in which all three HYDROXYL GROUPS have been substituted by ESTER groupings from FATTY ACIDS. Many fats are TRIGLYCERIDES.

triglycerides (biochemistry) NEUTRAL fat comprises three FATTY ACIDS esterified to GLYCEROL. The FATTY ACIDS may be saturated or UNSATURATED, and the most common ones are stearic, oleic and PALMITIC ACIDS. This is the primary STORAGE form of LIPID as an ENERGY reserve. TRIGLYCERIDES are synthesised in ADIPOSE TISSUE from GLYCEROL PHOSPHATE, derived from GLUCOSE, and from FATTY ACIDS, either derived from acetyl CoA formed from GLUCOSE or absorbed from the PLASMA after they are released from LIPOPROTEINS. TRIGLYCERIDE SYNTHESIS in adipose CELLS is dependent upon INSULIN-stimulated uptake of PLASMA GLUCOSE. Whereas the amount of GLYCOGEN that can be stored as an ENERGY reserve is

limited, the amount of TRIGLYCERIDE stored appears to be essentially unlimited.

triiodomethane (chemistry) CHI_3 Yellow CRYSTALLINE SOLID HALOFORM, used as an ANTISEPTIC. Also termed: IODOFORM.

trimer (chemistry) Chemical formed by the COMBINATION of three similar (MONOMER) molecules.

trimetaphan camsylate (pharmacology) A ganglion blocker drug which is administered by injection or INTRAVENOUS infusion and lowers BLOOD PRESSURE by reducing vascular tone normally induced by the SYMPATHETIC NERVOUS SYSTEM. It is short-acting and can be used as a hypotensive for controlled BLOOD PRESSURE during surgery.

trinitrophenol (chemistry) An alternative term for PICRIC ACID.

trinomial (chemistry) POLYNOMIAL with only three terms.

triple bond (chemistry) COVALENT BOND formed by the sharing of three pairs of electrons between two atoms.

triploidy (genetics) The condition of having three copies of every CHROMOSOME, a form of POLYPLOIDY. TRIPLOIDY does not occur in nature as a permanent feature of a SPECIES, as triploid organisms have very low fertility. This is because at MEIOSIS there are three chromosomes trying to find partners for a process that only works with two, so the DIVISION is usually a failure. However, triploid organisms are just as capable of NORMAL GROWTH as any others (MITOSIS is not impeded at all, since the process consists of each CHROMOSOME dividing itself in half, irrespective of any partner). Artificially produced triploids can be commercially useful. One example of this is the banana, the trees of which are bred as triploids from stocks of a TETRAPLOID and a DIPLOID strain. The triploid hybrids grow well, but their seeds never develop properly, so that the inside of the banana is not full of inedible seeds as it is in a NORMAL banana.

trisaccharide (chemistry) CARBOHYDRATE consisting of three joined monosaccharides.

trisomy (genetics) The state of having three representatives of a given CHROMOSOME instead of the usual pair, as in TRISOMY 21 (DOWN'S SYNDROME).

tritium (chemistry) A RADIOACTIVE ISOTOPE of HYDROGEN, with MASS NUMBER 3 and ATOMIC MASS 3.016. Its HALF-LIFE is 12.5 years. TRITIUM is used extensively as a radiolabel tracer in toxicity studies.

triton (chemistry) Atomic NUCLEUS of TRITIUM, consisting of two neutrons and one PROTON.

trivalent (chemistry) Having a VALENCE of three. Also termed: tervalent.

tRNA (molecular biology) An abbreviation of 't'ransfer (or soluble) 'R'ibo'N'ucleic 'A'cid.

trop. med. (medical) An abbreviation of 'trop'ical 'med'icine.

trophozoite (microbiology) Feeding, MOTILE stage of PROTOZOA.

tropical sore (medical) A slow-healing ulcer in the SKIN caused by *Leishmania major* or *Leishmania tropica*. *See* LEISHMANIASIS.

Tryp. (biochemistry) An abbreviation of 'Tryp'tophan.

trypan blue (biochemistry) A vital dye that is used to determine the viability of isolated CELLS. Living CELLS exclude the dye, whereas nonviable CELLS do not.

trypanosomiasis (parasitology) INFESTATION with Trypanosomes, small PARASITES spread by the TSETSE FLY. *Trypanosoma brucei gambiewe* causes sleeping sickness in West Africa, and *Trypanosoma brucei rhoesiense* causes the disease in East Africa.

See also CHAGAS DISEASE.

tryptophan (biochemistry) An ESSENTIAL AMINO ACID

tryptophan (biochemistry) An ESSENTIAL AMINO ACID which is a PRECURSOR of SEROTONIN, that contains an aromatic GROUP, needed in animals for proper GROWTH and development.

tsetse fly (parasitology) *See* TRYPANOSOMIASIS.

TSF (haematology) An abbreviation of 'T'hrombopoietic 'S'timulating 'F'actor, thrombopoietin.

TSH (physiology/ biochemistry) An abbreviation of 'T'hyroid-'S'timulating 'H'ormone.

TSI (physiology/ immunology) abbreviation of 'T'hyroid-'S'timulating 'I'mmunoglobulins.

T/S ratio (physiology/ biochemistry) An abbreviation of 'T'hyroid/ 'S'erum iodide ratio.

TSS (microbiology) An abbreviation of 'T'oxic 'S'hock 'S'yndrome.

t-test (statistics) A parametric test for assessing hypotheses about population means. It is most commonly used when the null HYPOTHESIS is that two populations have the same MEAN value on some VARIABLE of interest. The form of the test used in this case depends on whether independent samples are drawn from each population, or whether samples are matched in some way (*e.g.* thereby having the same subjects each perform under two conditions). Though the test is based on assumptions of normality and homogeneity of population variances, it is relatively robust against departures from these assumptions.

TTX (biochemistry) An abbreviation of 'T'etrodo'T'o'X'in.

Tu (chemistry) The CHEMICAL SYMBOL for THULIUM.

Tuberc. (medical) An abbreviation of 'Tuberc'ulosis.

tuberculosis (medical) A disease caused by INFECTION with the MICRO-ORGANISMS *Mycobacterium TUBERCULOSIS* or *Mycobacterium bovis,* of which the first is responsible for most human infections. The MICROORGANISMS provoke the formation of tubercles, collections of MACROPHAGES, which are WHITE BLOOD CELLS and TISSUE CELLS able to engulf BACTERIA and form epithelioid CELLS; these may FUSE to form giant CELLS, which are CHARACTERISTIC of the tubercle. The MACROPHAGES are activated by T LYMPHOCYTES, by the invading organisms and by the activity of other MACROPHAGES. When the tubercle has formed, the centre (*USA*: center) breaks down, a process called caseation. The disease process destroys the tissues which it involves, which are principally those of the LUNG.

tubocurarine chloride (pharmacology) A non-depolarising skeletal muscle relaxant drug which is administered by injection to induce muscle paralysis during surgery.

tularaemia (medical/ bacteriology) A rare disease in human beings caused by the BACTERIA *Franciselia tularensis,* named after Tulare in California where the disease was first identified. It occurs principally in rodents but may affect other animals, and is spread to man by TICKS, flies and mosquitoes, or by touching infected animals.

tumour (histology) An overt NEOPLASM, either BENIGN (*e.g.* a POLYPUS) or MALIGNANT (*i.e.* cancerous). (*USA*: tumor).

See also CARCINOGENESIS; NEOPLASM.

tumour suppressor genes (genetics) The PROTEIN products of TUMOUR SUPPRESSOR GENES inhibit the PROGRESSION of CELLS in the DIVISION CYCLE. MUTATIONS in TUMOUR SUPPRESSOR GENES may bring about the formation of proteins that cannot suppress CELL DIVISION. Inactivating MUTATIONS in the GERM CELLS bring about a predisposition to certain form of CANCER, *e.g.* familial retinoblastoma, familial polyposis, etc. SOMATIC MUTATIONS in tumor suppressor genes may also play a role in TUMOUR PRO GRESSION (*USA*: tumor progression). (*USA*: tumor suppressor genes).

Turnbull stain (histology) Histological staining technique which may be used to make FERROUS IRON visible under the microscope.

Turner's syndrome (genetics) The condition in which a female has GENOTYPE XO, *i.e.* only one SEX CHROMOSOME. A TURNER'S SYNDROME girl looks fairly NORMAL, but with short stature and a wide 'webbed' neck; the ovaries are present but undeveloped so she is not fertile.

two-tailed test (statistics) A statistical test of an HYPOTHESIS whose regions of rejection are placed at both ends (or tails) of the distribution of the test statistic, *e.g.* when the alternative to the null HYPOTHESIS is that the MEAN of one population differs from that of the other, regardless of whether it is higher or, lower. *Contrast* one-tailed test.

type I error (statistics) Rejection of the null HYPOTHESIS when it is in fact true.

type II error (statistics) Acceptance of the null HYPOTHESIS when it is in fact false.

typhoid fever (medical/ bacteriology) A serious disease caused by *Salmonella typhi,* found throughout the world but commonest where sanitation and WATER supplies are less than first CLASS. The INFECTION is spread by contamination of food or WATER by the excreta of patients suffering or recovering from the disease, or of those carrying the disease but apparently in health. It is confined to human beings.

typhoid, paratyphoid A and paratyphoid B vaccine (TAB) (medical) A triple VACCINE to prevent these infections.

typhus (Gail FEVER) (medical/ microbiology) An INFECTION caused by *Rickettsia prowazekii* and spread by lice.

Tyr (biochemistry) An abbreviation of 'Tyr'osine.

tyrosine (chemistry) White CRYSTALLINE ORGANIC COMPOUND, a naturally occurring ESSENTIAL AMINO ACID that is a PRECURSOR for ADRENERGIC transmitters, *e.g.* ADRENALINE (*USA*: epinephrine) and NORADRENALINE (*USA*: norepinephrine).

U

U (1 chemistry; 2 measurement) 1 The CHEMICAL SYMBOL for URANIUM, ELEMENT 92. 2 An abbreviation of 'U'nit(s).

UCHD (medical) An abbreviation of 'U'sual 'C'hild'H'ood 'D'iseases.

UCL (physics) An abbreviation of 'U'pper 'C'ontrol 'L'imit.

UDPG (biochemistry) An abbreviation of 'U'ridine 'D'i'P'hospho'G'lucose.

UDPGA (biochemistry) An abbreviation of 'U'ridine 'D'i'P'hospho'G'lucuronic 'A'cid.

UFA (physiology/ biochemistry) An abbreviation of 'U'nesterified free 'F'atty 'A'cid.

UHF (physics) An abbreviation of 'U'ltra'H'igh 'F'requency.

UL (histology) An abbreviation of 'U'nstirred 'L'ayer.

ulf (1, 2 physics) 1 An abbreviation of 'u'ltra 'l'ow 'f'requency. 2 An abbreviation of 'u'pper 'l'imiting 'f'requency.

ulna (anatomy) Rearmost (and usually larger) of the two bones in the lower forelimb of a tetrapod VERTEBRATE (the other BONE is the RADIUS).

ultrahigh frequency (UHF) (physics) A radio FREQUENCY between 300 and 3,000 megahertz.

ultramicroscope (microscopy) Instrument for viewing sub-microscopic objects. *e.g.* particles of smoke and fog.

ultrasonic (physics) Describing a band of sound frequencies of about 2×10^9 hertz, which are just above the upper LIMIT of NORMAL human hearing. ULTRASONIC ENERGY is used in sonar, for degreasing (in conjunction with a suitable SOLVENT) and for scanning soft tissues in medical diagnosis. Also termed: supersonic.

ultraviolet radiation (UV) (physics) ELECTROMAGNETIC RADIATION with wave-Lengths in the range 4×10^{-7} to 4×10^{-9}m, the region between VISIBLE LIGHT and X-RAYS. Also termed: ultraviolet light.

ultronics (physics) Sound waves which are of a FREQUENCY above the range of audible sound, which lies between 20 and 20,000 cycles per second.

umbilical cord (anatomy) In EMBRYOLOGY, vascular structure that contains the umbilical arteries and veins, connecting the FOETUS (*USA*: fetus) to the PLACENTA.

umbilicus (anatomy) The navel.

uncertainty principle (physics) It is impossible to determine simultaneously with ACCURACY both the position and the momentum of a moving PARTICLE. The LIMIT of ACCURACY may be given by the relation $p_x x > h/2\pi$, where p_x is the uncertainty in the momentum, x the uncertainty in position and h is PLANCK'S

CONSTANT. Also termed: Heisenberg UNCERTAINTY PRINCIPLE.

undulant fever (medical/ bacteriology) *See* BRUCELLOSIS.

uniaxial crystal (crystallography) Doubly-refracting crystal in which there is only one direction of single REFRACTION. *See* DOUBLE REFRACTION.

unicellular (biology) Describing an organism that consists of only one CELL (*e.g.* PROTOZOANS, BACTERIA).

uniform distribution (statistics) A FREQUENCY DISTRIBUTION in which all classes or values have the same FREQUENCY or probability.

unilateral (medical) Pertaining to one side of the body or one hemisphere of the BRAIN.

unimodal (statistics) Of a distribution, having only one MODE, which, if the DATA are represented graphically, corresponds to there being only one peak.

unimolecular reaction (chemistry) CHEMICAL REACTION that involves only one type of MOLECULE as the REACTANT.

unit (1, 2 measurement) 1 A standard quantity in which something is measured, *e.g.* decibel, or WAVELENGTH. 2 A single UNIT. 3 An alternative term for KILOWATT-HOUR, the UNIT that measures consumption of ELECTRICITY.

unit cell (crystallography) Smallest GROUP of atoms, ions or molecules whose three dimentional repetition at regular intervals produces a CRYSTAL LATTICE.

univalent (1 cytology; 2 chemistry) 1 Single CHROMOSOME that separates during the MEIOTIC DIVISION. *See* MEIOSIS. 2 MONOVALENT.

univariate (statistics) Having only one VARIABLE.

universal indicator (chemistry) MIXTURE of chemical indicators that give a definite for various values of PH.

unkn (general terminology) An abbreviation of 'unk'now'n'.

unpub (literary terminology) An abbreviation of 'unpub'lished.

unsaturated (1, 2 chemistry) 1 Describing an ORGANIC COMPOUND with doubly or triply bonded CARBON atoms. *See also* SATURATED COMPOUND. 2 Describing a SOLUTION that can dissolve more SOLUTE before reaching SATURATION.

up. (general terminology) An abbreviation of 'up'per.

upstream (molecular biology) Further back on a DNA MOLECULE, in respect of the direction in which the sequence is being read. *See* REPLICATION.

Ur (chemistry) An abbreviation of 'Ur'anium.

uracil (molecular biology) $C_4H_4N_2O_2$ PYRIMIDINE BASE; one of the four NUCLEOTIDE bases in RNA; in DNA the corresponding BASE is THYMINE. Also termed: 2,6-dioxypyrimidine.

uraemia (biochemistry) Excess of UREA and other NITROGEN containing compounds, principally CREATININE, in the BLOOD. The condition is the result of KIDNEY FAILURE, except in cases where there is failure of the circulation from any cause, when the state is described as pre-renal URAEMIA; such cases may recover when the circulatory collapse is remedied. Also termed 'azotaemia'.

uranium U (chemistry) RADIOACTIVE grey metallic ELEMENT in GROUP IIIA of the PERIODIC TABLE (one of the ACTINIDES), obtained mainly from its ore uraninite (which contains URANIUM(IV) OXIDE, UO_2). It has three natural and several artificial isotopes with half-lives of up to 4.5 x 10^9 years. URANIUM-235 undergoes nuclear FISSION and is used in nuclear weapons and reactors; URANIUM-238 can be converted into the fissile PLUTONIUM-239 in a breeder REACTOR. At. no. 92; r.a.m. 238.029.

urates (biochemistry) Salts of URIC ACID, the result of the breakdown of purines, which are compounds which have an important role in METABOLISM. URATES are normally present in the BLOOD, but when the BLOOD LEVEL is too high crystals may form; in the joints they give rise to GOUT, and in the kidneys to stones.

urea (biochemistry) H_2NCONH_2 White CRYSTALLINE ORGANIC COMPOUND, found naturally in the URINE of mammals as the natural end-PRODUCT of the METABOLISM of proteins. It is also manufactured commercially from CARBON DIOXIDE and AMMONIA under high PRESSURE. It is used in plastics, adhesives, fertilizers and ANIMAL-feed additives. Also termed: CARBAMIDE.

urease (chemistry) ENZYME that occurs in plants (*e.g.* soya beans) and acts as a CATALYST for the HYDROLYSIS of UREA to AMMONIA and CARBON DIOXIDE.

ureter (anatomy) One of a pair of ducts that carry URINE from the kidneys to the BLADDER.

urethane (chemistry) $CO(NH_2)OC_2H_5$ Highly toxic, inflammable organic used in veterinary medicine, biochemical research and as a chemical INTERMEDIATE. Also termed: ETHYL CARBAMATE; ETHYL URETHANE.

urethra (anatomy) Tube through which URINE is discharged to the exterior from the urinary BLADDER of most mammals.

urethritis (medical) INFLAMMATION of the URETHRA, the canal through which URINE is discharged *e.g.* gonococcal URETHRITIS.

URF (physiology) An abbreviation of 'U'terine-'R'elaxing 'F'actor; relaxin.

URI (medical) An abbreviation of 'U'pper 'R'espiratory 'I'nfection.

uric acid (biochemistry) $C_5H_4N_4O_3$ White CRYSTALLINE ORGANIC ACID of the PURINE GROUP, the end-PRODUCT and the principal excretory PRODUCT of PURINE METABOLISM. Defects in URIC ACID metabolism and EXCRETION appear to be associated with a number of disease states, and it frequently occurs as a COMPONENT of renal calculi. URIC ACID deposition in the joints is the principal cause of GOUT. Also termed: 2,6,8-trihydroxypurine.

urine (biochemistry) LIQUID, produced in the kidneys and stored in the urinary BLADDER, that contains UREA and other excretory products. It is discharged to the outside via the URETHRA.

urobilinogen (biochemistry) A DERIVATIVE of BILIRUBIN formed by the GUT microflora; this COMPOUND is colourless (*USA*: colorless).

urol. (medical) An abbreviation of 'urol'ogy.

urology (medical) The branch of medicine that deals with diseases of the urinary tract in both sexes, and those of the genital organs in the male.

urticaria (nettle-rash) (immunology) Swelling and redness of the SKIN, usually with itching, caused by an allergic REACTION which results in the liberation of HISTAMINE in the SKIN.

US (physiology) An abbreviation of 'U'nconditioned 'S'timulus.

u-shaped curve (statistics) Any GRAPH of a distribution that is shaped like a U.

USPHS (governing body) An abbreviation of 'U'nited 'S'tates 'P'ublic 'H'ealth 'S'ervice.

usu. (general terminology) An abbreviation of 'usu'ally.

uterus (anatomy) Muscular ORGAN located in the lower ABDOMEN of female mammals, in which a fertilized OVUM develops into a FOETUS (*USA*: fetus) prior to birth. Also termed: womb.

UTP (biochemistry) An abbreviation of 'U'ridine 'T'ri'P'hosphate.

UV (physics) An abbreviation of 'U'ltra'V'iolet.

UVL (physics) An abbreviation of 'U'ltra'V'iolet 'L'ight.

V

V (1 chemistry; 2 biochemistry) 1 The CHEMICAL SYMBOL for ELEMENT 23, VANADIUM. 2 A symbol for valine.

vaccination (immunology) The artificial production of ACTIVE IMMUNITY by the injection of a VACCINE. The word 'VACCINATION' is derived from the Latin for 'cow', and was coined by the British physician Edward Jenner (1749-1823) to describe his idea of injecting patients with cowpox VIRUS to protect them against smallpox (a very similar VIRUS). A VACCINE now means any SUSPENSION of dead or non-virulent VIRUSES or BACTERIA used in IMMUNISATION.

vaccine (immunology) A preparation of dead organisms, ATTENUATED live organisms, live virulent organisms, or parts of MICRO-ORGANISMS which are either injected or ingested into the body, where they stimulate the production of antibodies and so confer IMMUNITY against INFECTION. Less commonly, vaccines are used in treating a disease.

vac. pmp (physics) An abbreviation of 'vac'uum 'p'u'mp'.

vacuity (anatomy) Any gap between the bones of a SKULL.

vacuole (biology) An alternative term for a VESICLE.

See also CONTRACTILE VACUOLE.

vacuum (physics) Space containing no MATTER. A good LABORATORY VACUUM still contains about 10^{14} molecules of AIR per CUBIC METRE; intergalactic space may have an almost perfect VACUUM (although it does contain some SUBATOMIC PARTICLES).

vacuum pump (equipment) An alternative term for DIFFUSION PUMP.

vagina (anatomy) The canal which leads from the external female genitalia to the CERVIX.

vaginitis (medical) INFLAMMATION of the VAGINA. The commonest causes are INFECTION with *TRICHOMONAS vaginalis* or *Candida albicans*, or ATROPHY that occurs with age as the result of lack of OESTROGEN (*USA*: estrogen).

vagus nerve (anatomy) In vertebrates, tenth CRANIAL NERVE, which forms the major NERVE of the PARASYMPATHETIC NERVOUS SYSTEM, supplying motor NERVE FIBRES (*USA*: nerve fibers) to the STOMACH, kidneys, HEART, LIVER, lungs and other organs.

Val. (biochemistry) An abbreviation of 'Val'ine.

valence band (1, 2 chemistry) 1 Highest ENERGY LEVEL in an INSULATOR or semiconductor that can be filled with electrons. 2 Region of electronic ENERGY LEVEL that binds atoms of a crystal together.

valence bond (chemistry) CHEMICAL BOND formed by the INTERACTION of VALENCE ELECTRONS between two or more atoms.

valence electron (chemistry) ELECTRON in an outer shell of an ATOM which participates in bonding to other atoms to form molecules.

valence (chemistry) POSITIVE number that characterizes the combining POWER of an ATOM of a given ELEMENT to the number of HYDROGEN atoms or their equivalent (in a CHEMICAL REACTION). For an ION, the VALENCE equals the CHARGE on the ION. Also termed: VALENCY.

valency (chemistry) *See* VALENCE.

validation (biology) The process of establishing that a theory or test is valid.

validity (biology) The extent which a test or experiment genuinely measures what it purports to measure.

valine (biochemistry) $C_5H_{11}NO_2$ One of the ESSENTIAL AMINO ACIDS required for NORMAL GROWTH in animals. Also termed: 2-AMINOISOVALERIC ACID; 2-amino-3-methylbutyric ACID.

valve (anatomy) Flap of TISSUE that controls movement of FLUID through a tube, duct or APERTURE in one direction, *e.g.* as between the chambers of the HEART or in the veins.

van der Waals forces (physics) Very weak forces acting between the NUCLEUS of one ATOM and the electrons of another ATOM (*i.e.* between dipoles and induced dipoles). The attractive forces arise from slight distortions induced in the ELECTRON clouds surrounding each NUCLEUS as two atoms are brought close together. Named after the Dutch physicist Johannes Diderik van der Waals (1837-1923).

van Gieson stain (histology) A histological staining technique that may be used to make CONNECTIVE TISSUE visible under the MICROSCOPE.

vanadium V (chemistry) Silvery-grey metallic ELEMENT in GROUP VA of the PERIODIC TABLE (a TRANSITION ELEMENT), used to make special steels. VANADIUM(V) OXIDE, V_2O_5, is used as an industrial CATALYST and in ceramics. At. no. 23; r.a.m. 50.9414.

van't Hoff's law (physics) OSMOTIC PRESSURE of a SOLUTION is equal to the PRESSURE that would be exerted by the SOLUTE if it were in the gaseous PHASE and occupying the same VOLUME as the SOLUTION at the same TEMPERATURE. It was named after the Dutch chemist Jacobus van't Hoff (1852-1911).

vapour (chemistry) A GAS when its TEMPERATURE is below the CRITICAL TEMPERATURE; a VAPOUR can thus be condensed to a LIQUID by PRESSURE alone.

vapour density (physics) DENSITY of a GAS relative to a reference GAS, such as HYDROGEN, equal to the MASS of a VOLUME of GAS divided by the MASS of an equal VOLUME of HYDROGEN at the same TEMPERATURE and PRESSURE. It is also equal to half the RELATIVE MOLECULAR MASS.

vapour pressure (physics) PRESSURE under which a LIQUID and its VAPOUR coexist at EQUILIBRIUM. Also termed: SATURATION VAPOUR PRESSURE.

var. (1 statistics; 2 general terminology) 1 An abbreviation of 'var'iable. 2 An abbreviation of 'var'ious.

variability (statistics) The spread of scores in a SAMPLE or the extent to which they differ from the MEAN.

variable (1 mathematics; 2 computing) 1 Something that is not CONSTANT. 2 Block of DATA that is stored at different locations during the operation of a PROGRAM.

variable number tandem repeats (VNTRs) (molecular biology) The repeated sequences of DNA that vary from one individual to another and are the basis for GENETIC FINGERPRINTING.

variable region (immunology) *See* V REGION.

variance (statistics) For a SET of numbers, the MEAN of the squares of the deviations of each number from the ARITHMETIC MEAN of the SET. Its SQUARE ROOT is the STANDARD DEVIATION.

variation (biology) Differences between members of the same SPECIES, which may be either continuous (having a NORMAL DISTRIBUTION about a SPECIES MEAN, *e.g.* height and WEIGHT) or discontinuous (having different specific characteristics with no INTERMEDIATE forms, *e.g.* BLOOD types).

varicella (virology) Chicken-pox.

variety (taxonomy) Any sub-DIVISION of a SPECIES, *e.g.* breed, RACE, strain, etc.

variola (virology) Any of the diseases caused by the poxviruses. VARIOLA major is an alternative term for smallpox.

vas deferens (anatomy) One of a pair of ducts that carry SPERM from the TESTES. In mammals it joins the URETHRA and passes along the PENIS. Plural: vasa deferentia. Also termed: SPERM duct.

vas. (medical) An abbreviation of 'vas'ectomy.

vasc. (histology) An abbreviation of 'vasc'ular.

vascular accident (medical) An alternative term for STROKE.

vascular system (anatomy) A system of interlinked FLUID-filled vessels, *e.g.* the BLOOD VASCULAR SYSTEM.

vasculitis (medical) INFLAMMATION of a VESSEL.

vasoconstriction (physiology) REDUCTION in DIAMETER of a BLOOD VESSEL due to contraction of the SMOOTH MUSCLEs in its walls. It may be induced by the SECRETION of ADRENALINE (*USA*: epinephrine) in RESPONSE to pain, fear, decreased BLOOD PRESSURE, low external TEMPERATURE, etc. or result from stimulation by vasoconstrictor NERVE FIBRES (*USA*: nerve fibers).

vasodilation (physiology) Increase in DIAMETER of small BLOOD VESSELs due to relaxation of the SMOOTH MUSCLEs in their walls. It is induced in RESPONSE to exercise, HIGH BLOOD PRESSURE, high external TEMPERATURE, etc. or results from stimulation by VASODILATOR NERVE FIBRES (*USA*: nerve fibers). Also termed: vasodilatation.

vasodilator (medical) An agent that causes dilatation of the BLOOD VESSELS.

vasomotor (physiology) Pertaining to the motor control of the DIAMETER of BLOOD VESSELS.

vasomotor nerve (physiology) NERVE of the AUTONOMIC NERVOUS SYSTEM that controls the VARIATION in the DIAMETER of BLOOD VESSELS, *e.g.* causing them to become constricted or dilated.

vasopressin (biochemistry) PEPTIDE HORMONE, secreted by the PITUITARY GLAND

and HYPOTHALAMUS, that stimulates WATER resorption in the KIDNEY tubules, contraction of the SMOOTH MUSCLEs in the walls of BLOOD VESSELs. It is secreted in RESPONSE to low BLOOD PRESSURE. A lack of VASOPRESSIN results in DIABETES insipidus. Also termed: ANTIDIURETIC HORMONE (ADH).

vasopressor (biochemistry/ physiology) A substance which increases BLOOD PRESSURE by narrowing the BLOOD VESSELs.

vauqueline (chemistry) An alternative term for STRYCHNINE.

vcm (physics) An abbreviation of 'v'a'c'uu'm'.

Vd (chemistry) CHEMICAL SYMBOL for VANADIUM.

vd (physics) An abbreviation of 'v'apour 'd'ensity.

VDH (medical) An abbreviation of 'v'alvular 'd'isease of 'h'eart.

VDRL (bacteriology) A BLOOD test for syphilis named after the VENEREAL DISEASE Research Laboratories.

VDT (computing) An abbreviation of 'V'isual 'D'isplay 'T'erminal.

VDU (computing) An abbreviation of 'V'isual 'D'isplay 'U'nit.

vector (1 molecular biology; 2 medicine/ parasitology; 3 mathematics) 1 A plasmid or other self-replicating DNA MOLECULE that transfers DNA between CELLs in nature or in RECOMBINANT DNA technology. In the latter case it may be called a cloning VECTOR or cloning vehicle. 2 An organism responsible for PARASITE transmission between hosts, *e.g.* the mosquito in MALARIA. Also termed:

CARRIER. 3 A quantity having both magnitude and direction, which can be used to characterise forces.

vecuronium bromide (pharmacology) A non-depolarising skeletal muscle relaxant drug which is administered by injection to induce muscle paralysis during surgery.

vein (anatomy) BLOOD VESSEL that, with the exception of the PULMONARY VEIN, carries deoxygenated BLOOD away from CELLs and tissues.

vena cava (anatomy) Collective term for the precaval (ANTERIOR VENA CAVA) and postcaval (POSTERIOR VENA CAVA) VEIN. The precaval VEIN is paired, and carries eoxygenated BLOOD away from the HEAD and forelimbs; the postcaval VEIN is single and carries deoxygenated BLOOD away from most of the body and hind limbs (or legs) to the HEART.

venereal disease (medical) *See* SEXUALLY TRANSMITTED DISEASE.

venesection (medical) The cutting of a VEIN to draw off BLOOD or, more usually, to insert a cannula for INTRAVENOUS THERAPY.

ventral (general terminology) Describing something that is on or near the surface of an organism and, in a tetrapod, directed downwards (on a human being it is directed forwards).

ventral noradrenergic bundle (histology) A noradrenergic (*USA*: norepinephrine) tract running from the brainstem to the HYPOTHALAMUS.

ventricle (1, 2 anatomy) 1 In mammals, thick-walled muscular lower chamber of the HEART. Contraction of the right

VENTRICLE pumps deoxygenated BLOOD into the PULMONARY ARTERY, and contraction of the left VENTRICLE forces oxygenated BLOOD into the AORTA. 2 In vertebrates, one of the FLUID-filled interconnected cavities within the BRAIN.

Venturi tube (physics) Cylindrical pipe with a constriction at its centre (*USA*: center). When a FLUID flows through the tube, its rate of flow increases and FLUID PRESSURE drops in the constriction. The rate can be calculated from the difference in PRESSURE between the ends of the tube and at the constriction. It was named after the Italian physicist Giovanni Battista Venturi (1746-1822).

venule (anatomy) Small VEIN located close to CAPILLARY BLOOD VESSELs, where it collects and conveys deoxygenated BLOOD from the CAPILLARY NETWORK to a VEIN.

verapamil hydrochloride (pharmacology) A calcium-channel blocker used as an orally administered ANTI-ANGINA drug in the prevention and treatment of attacks, as an ANTI-ARRHYTHMIC to correct HEART irregularities and as an ANTIHYPERTENSIVE treatment.

verdigris green (chemistry) BASIC COPPER(II) CARBONATE, $CUCO_3.CU(OH)_2$, formed by corrosion of metallic COPPER or its ALLOYs. The term is also used for the similar BASIC COPPER(II) ACETATE, used as a PIGMENT, FUNGICIDE and mordant in dyeing.

vermiform appendix (anatomy) An alternative term for the APPENDIX.

vertebra (anatomy) One of the hollow bones or pieces of CARTILAGE that form the VERTEBRAL COLUMN.

vertebral column (anatomy) Flexible column of closely arranged vertebrae that form an axial SKELETON running from the SKULL to the tail. It provides a protective channel for the SPINAL CORD. The VERTEBRAL COLUMN becomes larger and stronger towards the POSTERIOR, which is the major weightbearing region. Also termed: SPINAL COLUMN; BACKBONE.

vertebrata (taxonomy) Major subphylum of Chordata that contains all animals with a VERTEBRAL COLUMN, *i.e.* mammals, birds, fish, reptiles and amphibians. Vertebrates are characterized by a well-developed BRAIN, complex NERVOUS SYSTEMS and a flexible endoskeleton of BONE and CARTILAGE. Also termed: Craniata.

vertebrate (taxonomy) A backboned ANIMAL; a member of the subphylum VERTEBRATA.

vertical transmission (genetics) The usual type of genetic INHERITANCE, from one generation to the next. It is contrasted with HORIZONTAL TRANSMISSION.

very high frequency (VHF) (physics) A radio FREQUENCY between 30 and 300 KILOHERTZ.

vesical (medical) Pertaining to the BLADDER.

vesicle (1 biology; 2 medical) 1 A small FLUID-filled sac of VARIABLE ORIGIN, *e.g.* GOLGI APPARATUS, pinocytotic VESICLE. Also termed: VACUOLE; AIR sac; BLADDER. 2 small blister on the SKIN.

vessel (anatomy) Tubular structure that transports FLUID (*e.g.* BLOOD, LYMPH).

VGA (computing) An abbreviation of 'V'ideo 'G'raphics 'A'rray.

VHF (physics) An abbreviation of 'V'ery 'H'igh 'F'requency.

viable (biology) Capable of living.

vibration receptor (physiology) The SKIN RECEPTOR that responds to vibration, thought to be the PACINIAN CORPUSCLE.

vibrio (bacteriology) A Gram-negative GENUS of BACTERIA which includes the organism causing cholera, *VIBRIO cholerae*. Another less important VIBRIO causing DIARRHOEA (*USA*: diarrhea) and abdominal pain is *VIBRIO parahaemalyticus,* which lives in the sea in warm climates and infects fish, crabs and prawns; the illness only lasts for a day or two.

video graphics array (VGA) (computing) A type of COMPUTER graphics circuitry that drives a COMPUTER monitor with very high resolution, or the monitor itself.

vigabatrin (pharmacology) An ANTI-EPILEPTIC drug administered orally to treat epilepsy.

villus (histology) A small protrusion from the surface of a MEMBRANE. One of many finger-like structures that line the inside of the SMALL INTESTINE. Villi increase the surface AREA for ABSORPTION. Each VILLUS contains a central LACTEAL and a NETWORK of BLOOD capillaries, which absorb the SOLUBLE products of DIGESTION into the body.

Vincent's angina (trench mouth) (medical/ bacteriology) A BACTERIAL INFECTION of the mouth and gums, which ulcerate and bleed. The INFECTION is mixed, with *Borrelia vincentii* and *Fusobacterium fusiformis* predominating.

vinyl group (chemistry) Double-bonded organic GROUP $CH_2 = CH-$.

VIP (physiology/ biochemistry) An abbreviation of 'V'asoactive 'I'ntestinal 'P'olypeptide.

viroid (microbiology) A small disease-causing agent, a tight loop of RNA lacking any form of capsid (outer coat).

virulence (microbiology) The ability of a PATHOGEN (a VIRUS, BACTERIUM or other MICRO-ORGANISM) to produce a disease. It depends partly on its CAPACITY to invade the HOST CELL and multiply, and partly on its ability to produce toxins. VIRULENCE tends to be favoured by NATURAL SELECTION, as virulent strains are often the most successful at reproducing themselves; but beyond a certain point VIRULENCE is a disadvantage to a strain of pathogens, as they may kill their hosts too soon for their own good.

virus (virology) PATHOGENIC MICRO-ORGANISM with a DIAMETER between about 20 and 400 nm, visible only under an ELECTRON MICROSCOPE. It consists of an outer coat (capsid) PROTEIN and an inner CORE of DEOXYRIBONUCLEIC ACID (DNA) or RIBONUCLEUR ACID (RNA). VIRUSES infect plants, animals and BACTERIA. Outside the HOST CELLS viruses are metabolically inactive (and may be crystallizable), and only when attached to a CELL or wholly inside it does the viral DNA interfere with the metabolic activities of the CELL, suppressing its NORMAL control processes and causing it to manufacture new PROTEIN coats and NUCLEIC ACID threads identical with those of the invading VIRUS. Viruses which actively attack and proliferate in CELLS are described as virulent. Those VIRUSES that infect animals include: DNA genomes: adenoviruses, herpesviruses, poxviruses, parvoviruses. RNA genomes: reoviruses, retroviruses. The VIRUSES that attack BACTERIA are called bacteriophages.

viscera (histology) The large internal organs of the body, *e.g.* lungs, LIVER and intestines.

visceral (anatomy) Relating to the VISCERA.

viscometer (physics) Instrument for measuring VISCOSITY.

viscosity (physics) Property of a FLUID (LIQUID or gases) that makes it resist flow, resulting in different velocities of flow at different points in the FLUID. Also termed: INTERNAL FRICTION.

visible light (physics) LIGHT that can be seen by the human EYE (the VISIBLE SPECTRUM), as opposed to INFRA-RED and ULTRAVIOLET RADIATION.

visible spectrum (physics) Range of wavelengths of visible ELECTROMAGNETIC RADIATION (LIGHT), between about 780 and 380 nm.

visual defect (medical) *See* ASTIGMATISM; HYPERMETROPIA; MYOPIA.

visual purple (biochemistry) An alternative term for RHODOPSIN.

vitamins (biochemistry) A group of substances that are necessary for METABOLISM but only in MINUTE quantities. There are two major groups, WATER-SOLUBLE (*e.g.* VITAMINS C, B) and fat-SOLUBLE (*e.g.* A, D, E, K), which are present in foodstuffs and must be taken as part of a balanced diet. VITAMINS WORK as CO-ENZYMES within the ENZYME system, enabling the various essential CHEMICAL REACTIONS within CELLS to take place, *e.g.*

the production of ENERGY, the SYNTHESIS of proteins (for TISSUE-building, HORMONES, etc). Excessive doses of VITAMINS often have a deleterious effect, such toxic overdoses being known by the general term, hypervitaminosis.

vitamin A (biochemistry) *See* RETINOL.

vitamin B$_1$ (biochemistry) *See* THIAMINE.

vitamin B$_2$ (biochemistry) *See* RIBOFLAVIN.

vitamin C (biochemistry) *See* ASCORBIC ACID.

vitamin D (biochemistry) *See* CALCIFEROL.

vitamin E (biochemistry) *See* TOCOPHEROL.

vitamin H (biochemistry) *See* BIOTIN.

vitamin K (biochemistry) An essential fat-soluble vitamin that occurs naturally in two forms, vitamin k$_1$ (phytomenadione) and vitamin K$_2$. Vitamin K$_1$ is found in food such as fresh root vegetables, fruit, dairy products and meat, while vitamin K$_2$ is synthesised in the INTESTINE by bacteria and this source supplements the dietary form. Vitamin K is required for blood-clotting factors and is also important for the proper calcification of bone. The secretion of bile salts by the LIVER and fat absorption from the INTESTINE is required by both forms of vitamin K to achieve uptake into the body. Therefore when treating vitamin K deficiency due to malabsorption disorders a synthetic form, vitamin K$_3$ (menadiol sodium phosphate), which is water-soluble and effective when administered orally, is used.

vitreous humour (anatomy) Firm TRANS-PARENT GEL-like substance in the EYE, that fills the space behind the LENS, thus maintaining the shape of the eyeball.

See also AQUEOUS HUMOUR.

vitriol (chemistry) An alternative term for SULPHURIC ACID (*USA:* sulfuric acid).

VLDL (biochemistry) An abbreviation of 'V'ery 'L'ow 'D'ensity 'L'ipoPROTEIN.

VLDLP (chemistry) An abbreviation of 'V'ery-'L'ow-'D'ensity 'L'ipo'P'rotein. *See* LIPOPROTEINS.

VLN (physics) An abbreviation of 'V'ery 'L'ow 'N'itrogen.

VMA (biochemistry) An abbreviation of 'V'anillyl'M'andelic 'A'cid (3-methoxy-4-hydroxymandelic acid).

vocal cord (anatomy) One of a pair of membranous flaps in the LARYNX that are vibrated by AIR from the lungs to produce sounds.

volatile (1 chemistry; 2 computing) 1 Describing any substance that is readily changed to a VAPOUR and hence lost through EVAPORATION. VOLATILE liquids have low BOILING POINTS. 2 Describing stored information that is lost through a POWER cut.

volt (V) (measurement) SI UNIT of POTENTIAL DIFFERENCE (**pd**) or ELECTROMOTIVE FORCE (**emf**), which equals the pd between two points when one coulomb of ELECTRICITY produces one JOULE of WORK in going from one point to the other. It was named after the Italian physicist Alessandro Volta (1745-1827).

voltage (P) (physics) Value of a POTENTIAL DIFFERENCE, or the POTENTIAL DIFFERENCE itself.

voltage divider (physics) RESISTOR that can be tapped at a point along its length to give a particular FRACTION of the VOLTAGE across it. Also termed: POTENTIOMETER.

voltaic cell (physics) Any device that produces an ELECTROMOTIVE FORCE (e.m.f.) by the conversion of chemical ENERGY to electrical ENERGY, *e.g.* a BATTERY or ACCUMULATOR. Also termed: GALVANIC CELL.

voltmeter (physics) An instrument for measuring VOLTAGE or POTENTIAL DIFFERENCE.

volume (P) (physics) Amount of space occupied by a SOLID OBJECT, or the CAPACITY of a hollow VESSEL.

volumetric analysis (chemistry) Method of chemical ANALYSIS that relies on the accurate measurement of the reacting volumes of substances in SOLUTION (*e.g.* by carrying out a TITRATION).

voluntary muscle (histology) Type of MUSCLE, connected to the bones, that is under conscious control. It is responsible for most body movements. Also termed: STRIATED MUSCLE.

Von Kossa stain (histology) A histological staining technique that may be used to make CALCIUM visible under the MICROSCOPE.

VOR (physiology) An abbreviation of 'V'estibulo-'O'cular 'R'eflex.

V region (immunology) VARIABLE REGION. Part of the heavy and LIGHT chains of an IMMUNOGLOBULIN MOLECULE. It is this region that interacts with the ANTIGEN.

Vs (medical) An abbreviation of 'V'ene's'ection.

vulgar fraction (mathematics) FRACTION in which both NUMERATOR and DENOMINATOR are integers (whole numbers).

vulva (anatomy) In female mammals, the external opening of the VAGINA.

v.v. (literary terminology) An abbreviation of *'v'ICE 'v'ersa.* Latin, meaning 'reversal of ORDER'.

W

W (1 chemistry; 2 physics; 3 biochemistry) 1 The CHEMICAL SYMBOL for the ELEMENT tungsten (from its German name: 'WOLFRAM'). 2 Symbol for the UNIT WATT. 3 A symbol for tryptophan.

Wade/Fite stain (histology) A histological staining technique that may be used to make the LEPROSY bacilli visible under the MICROSCOPE.

Wagner-nelson method (chemistry) Technique to characterise the rate and extent of ABSORPTION of a substance.

Waldenstrom's macroglobulinaemia (immunology) Disease occurring mainly in elderly males, characterised by the presence of large amounts of MONO-CLONAL IMMUNOGLOBULIN M in the BLOOD, LYMPHOID TISSUE enlargement, splenomegaly, a haemorrhagic (*USA*: hemorrhagic) tendency and depression. The IMMU-NOGLOBULIN M is occassionally found to have detectable ANTIBODY activity *e.g.* rheumatoid FACTOR. The disease is probably a relatively BENIGN and slowly progressing form of myelomatosis. (USA: Waldenstrom's macroglobulinemia).

Wallerian degeneration (histology) The degeneration of myelinated and unmyelinated axons that occurs in a NERVE distal to a transaction or crush of the NERVE. MYELIN SHEATHS also degenerate in the distal NERVE stump as a consequence of the loss of their underlying AXON. Axonal degeneration due to other causes (*e.g.* neurotoxicants) is often referred to as 'Wallerian-like' or 'Wallerian-type' if the axonal degeneration is morphologically similar to WALLERIAN DEGENERATION.

warfarin (pharmacology) ORGANIC COMPOUND used (as its SODIUM DERIVATIVE) as an ANTICOAGULANT drug and as a PESTICIDE for killing rats and mice.

warm-blooded (biology) An alternative term for HOMOIOTHERMIC.

Warthin/ Starry stain (histology) A histological staining technique that may be used to make spirochaetes visible under the MICROSCOPE.

warts (microbiology/ histology) A non-maglignant, localised TUMOUR (*USA*: tumor) of the SKIN formed by overgrowth of the prickle-CELL layer, with or without hyperkeratosis, caused by INFECTION with the human papilloma VIRUS. WARTS can affect many parts of the SKIN including the fingers and feet which can be treated with a MIXTURE of salicylic and LACTIC ACIDS in collodion, or by the use of LIQUID NITROGEN. If left they often disappear in time.

washed red cells (haematology) BLOOD COMPONENT in which PLATELET and LEUCO-CYTE (USA: leukocyte) antigens have been removed.

washing soda (chemistry) An alternative term for HYDRATED SODIUM CARBONATE.

Wass. (microbiology/ immunology) An abbreviation of 'Wass'ermann REACTION.

411

Wassermann reaction (microbiology/ immunology) A BLOOD test formerly used in the diagnosis of syphilis, introduced by the German pathologist, August Paul von Wassermann (1866-1925). A complement fixation test in which cardiolipin derived from ox HEART is used as ANTIGEN because the BLOOD of individuals with syphilis regularly contains ANTIBODY which reacts with this substance. However, the Wassermann test is not entirely specific for syphilis. False results may be obtained in cases where there are increased IMMUNOGLOBULIN levels, *e.g.* due to parasitic INFECTION or in autoimmune conditions and confirmatory tests using *TREPONEMA pallidum* itself as the ANTIGEN may need to be made for a POSITIVE diagnosis. Tests such as the *TREPONEMA pallidum* haematagglutination assay (TPHA) (*USA: Treponema pallidum* hematagglutination assay) or a FLUO-RESCEIN-labelled ANTIBODY test (FTA-ABS) are now generally used.

WAT (physics) An abbreviation of 'W'eight, 'A'ltitude and 'T'emperature.

water (chemistry) H_2O Colourless (*USA*: colorless) LIQUID, one of the oxides of HYDROGEN (the other is HYDROGEN PEROXIDE, H_2O_2) and the commonest substance on the EARTH. It can be made by burning HYDROGEN or fuels containing it in AIR or OXYGEN, or by the ACTION of an ACID on an ALKALI or ALCOHOL. It is a good (polar) SOLVENT, particularly for ionic compounds, with which it may form SOLID hydrates. It can be decomposed by the ACTION of certain reactive metals (*e.g.* the ALKALI METALS) or by ELECTROLYSIS. WATER is essential for life and forms the major part of most body fluids (*e.g.* BLOOD, LYMPH). It freezes at 0°C and BOILS at 100°C (at NORMAL ATMOSPHERIC PRESIURE), and has its maximum DENSITY at 3.98°C.

See also HARDNESS OF WATER.

water of crystallization (chemistry) Definite amount of WATER retained by a COMPOUND (usually a SALT) when crystallized from SOLUTION. The CHEMICAL FORMULA of the resulting HYDRATE shows the number of molecules of WATER OF CRYSTALLIZATION associated with each MOLECULE of HYDRATE; *e.g.* $Na_2SO_4.7H_2O$. The WATER can usually be removed by heating, and the resulting COMPOUND is termed ANHYDROUS. Also termed: WATER OF HYDRATION.

water of hydration (chemistry) The WATER present in HYDRATED compounds. These compounds when crystallized from SOLUTION in WATER retain a definite amount of WATER, *e.g.* COPPER (II) SULPHATE (*USA*: copper (II) sulfate), $CuSO_4.5H_2O$.

waterbrash (medical) Regurgitation of a watery SECRETION containing ACID fluids from the STOMACH into the OESOPHAGUS (*USA*: esophagus) and mouth.

water-in-oil emulsion adjuvant (immunology) Adjuvant in which the ANTIGEN, dissolved or suspended in WATER, is enclosed in tiny droplets within a continuous PHASE of MINERAL OIL. The ANTIGEN SOLUTION constitutes the dispersed PHASE, stabilised by an emulsifying agent such as MANNITOL mono-OLEATE.

watt (W) (measurement) SI UNIT of POWER, equal to 1 JOULE per second (j s^{-1}). 745.70 watts = 1 horsepower. Wattage is the POWER of an electrical CIRCUIT determined by multiplying the VOLTAGE by the amperage. It was named after the British engineer James Watt (1736-1819).

watt-hour (measurement) Measure of electric POWER consumption. Also termed: UNIT.

wattmeter (physics) Instrument for measuring POWER consumption in an electric CIRCUIT. POWER consumption is usually expressed in WATT-HOURS, or units.

wave (physics) Regular (periodic) disturbance in a substance or in space; *e.g.* in an airborne sound WAVE, alternate regions of high and low PRESSURE travel through the AIR, although the AIR itself does not move along. In an ELECTROMAGNETIC WAVE, such as LIGHT, electric and magnetic waves at rightangles to each other and the direction of movement travel through a medium or through space.

wave function (mathematics) Equation that expresses time and space VARIATION in AMPLITUDE for a WAVE system.

wave number (physics) RECIPROCAL of the WAVELENGTH of an ELECTROMAGNETIC WAVE. Also termed: RECIPROCAL WAVELENGTH.

wavelength (λ) (physics) The distance between two successive points at which a WAVE has the same PHASE *e.g.* VISIBLE LIGHT has a WAVELENGTH of between 400 nm (violet) to 750 nm (red).

wax (chemistry) SOLID or semi-solid organic substance that is 1 an ESTER of a FATTY ACID, produced by a plant or ANIMAL (*e.g.* beeswax, tallow), or 2 a high MOLECULAR WEIGHT HYDROCARBON (*e.g.* PARAFFIN WAX, from petroleum), also called mineral WAX.

WBC (1, 2 haematology) 1 An abbreviation of 'W'hite 'B'lood 'C'ell. 2 An abbreviation of 'W'hite 'B'lood 'C'ount.

weak acid (chemistry) ACID that shows little IONIZATION or DISSOCIATION in SOLUTION; *e.g.* CARBONIC ACID, acetic (ethanoic) ACID.

weak electrolyte (chemistry) An ELECTROLYTE which is only slightly ionised in moderately concentrated solutions.

weaning index (toxicology) An expression of survival of offspring to weaning in reproductive toxicity tests. The number of offspring surviving to weaning (*i.e.* 21 days in the rat) as a PERCENTAGE of those alive at four days.

weber (Wb) (measurement) SI UNIT of MAGNETIC FLUX, named after the German physicist Wilhelm WEBER (1804-91).

weight (physics) The FORCE of gravity (9.8 m s^{-2}) acting on an OBJECT at the EARTH's surface; *i.e.* WEIGHT = MASS X ACCELERATION of free fall (ACCELERATION due to gravity). It is measured in newtons, pounds-FORCE or dynes.

weights and measures (measurement) *See* SI UNITS.

Weil-Felix reaction (immunology) An AGGLUTINATION test used in the diagnosis of rickettsial infections (TYPHUS etc.) which depends upon a CARBOHYDRATE cross-reacting ANTIGEN shared by *RICKETTSIAE* and certain strains of *Proteus*. The AGGLUTINATION pattern of patients with rickettsial disease against O-agglutinable strains of *Proteus* OX19, OX2 and OXK is diagnostic of the various rickettsial diseases. Named after the Austrian physician, Edmund Weil (1880-1922) and the Polish BACTERIOLOGIST, Arthur Felix (1887-1956).

Weil's disease (medical/ bacteriology) Severe form of INFECTION by *LEPTOSPIRA interrogans,* a SPIROCHAETE which infects rats and other animals and is passed on to man mainly by contact with rats, their URINE, or WATER contaminated by their URINE. There are a large number of types of the SPIROCHAETE, and the type commonly responsible for WEIL'S DISEASE is *LEPTOSPIRA icterohaemorrhagica;* it causes damage to the LIVER and the kidneys. Named after the German physician Adolf Weil (1848-1916). *See* LEPTOSPIRA.

Weil's myelin stain (histology) A histological staining technique that may be used to make myelin visible under the MICROSCOPE.

Weismannism (philosophy) Idea put forward by the German biologist August Weismann (1834-1914), who expressed it in terms of the theory of the continuity of the 'germ plasm', which states that INHERITANCE is affected only by the GERM CELLS (gametes), which is in disagreement with the theory of INHERITANCE of ACQUIRED CHARACTERISTICS as in LAMARCKISM.

See also DARWINISM.

wen (histology) A sebaceous cyst.

Wernicke-Korsakoff syndrome (medical/ biochemistry) A COMBINATION of WERNICKE'S DEMENTIA and the Korsakoff SYNDROME, both of which are thought to be caused by THIAMINE deficiency. Named after the German psychiatrist and neurologist, Karl Wernicke (1848-1905), and Russian psychiatrist, Sergei Sergeevich Korsakoff (1854-1900).

Wernicke's dementia (biochemistry) A BRAIN disorder caused by lack of THIAMINE and NIACIN and marked by clouding of consciousness and ATAXIA; it can be caused by ALCOHOLISM. Named after the psychiatrist and neurologist, Karl Wernicke (1848-1905).

Western blotting (biochemistry) A technique for the ANALYSIS and identification of proteins in complex mixtures. The proteins are separated by polyacrylamide GEL ELECTROPHORESIS and the separated bands then transferred by 'blotting' onto a POLYMER MEMBRANE by ELECTROPHORESIS at 90^0 to the GEL surface. The proteins bound on the POLYMER MEMBRANE can then be identified by REACTION with specific reagents such as RADIOACTIVE or FLUORESCENT labelled antibodies. The method is very specific and can be used to confirm the results of the ELISA test. It is named by analogy with SOUTHERN BLOTTING.

See also NORTHERN BLOTTING; SOUTHERN BLOTTING.

WFN (professional body) An abbreviation of 'W'orld 'F'ederation of 'N'eurology.

Wheatstone bridge (physics) Electric CIRCUIT for measuring the resistance of a RESISTOR (by comparing it with three other resistors of known values). It was named after the British physicist Charles Wheatstone (1802-75).

whewellite (biochemistry) HYDRATED CALCIUM OXALATE $CaC_2O_4.H_2O$. It occurs uncommonly in the mineral world but is abundant in human calculi.

whipworm (parasitology) A popular name for *TRICHURIS trichiura.*

white arsenic (chemistry) An alternative term for ARSENIC(III) OXIDE (arsenious OXIDE). *See* ARSENIC.

white blood cell (haematology) *See* LEUCOCYTE.

white light (physics) LIGHT that is composed of a MIXTURE of wavelengths in the visable SPECTRUM.

white matter (histology) Those parts of the CENTRAL NERVOUS SYSTEM containing mainly myelinated fibres (*USA*: myelinated fibers), which appear white; *e.g.* the myelinated fibres of the CORTEX which run below the GREY MATTER.

white vitriol (chemistry) An alternative term for ZINC SULPHATE (*USA*: zinc sulfate).

whitlow (microbiology) A purulent INFECTION of the end of the finger involving the pulp. The term is also applied to an INFECTION of the SKIN in the region of the NAIL by *HERPES simplex* VIRUSES. Also known as FELON.

WHO (governing body) An abbreviation of 'W'orld 'H'ealth 'O'rganisation.

whole blood (haematology) BLOOD which has not been broken down into its various components. It is used in transfusion THERAPY a) in NEONATAL total BLOOD exchange and b) in cases of ACUTE massive BLOOD loss. WHOLE BLOOD is usually collected in citrate-PHOSPHATE-DEXTROSE (CPD) ANTICOAGULANT preservative SOLUTION. WHOLE BLOOD is suitable for transfusion up to a 21 day STORAGE PERIOD.

whooping cough (medical/ bacteriology) *See* PERTUSSIS.

Widal test (microbiology/ immunology) A serological AGGLUTINATION REACTION of *Salmonella typhi* and similar organisms by the patient's SERUM, used to diagnose typhoid and paratyphoid fevers. The organisms used must be MOTILE, smooth and in the specific PHASE. Formalised and alcoholised suspensions are used respectively for testing for H (flageller) and O AGGLUTININS. The WIDAL TEST is not likely to be POSITIVE until after the first 10 days of the disease. Prior IMMUNISATION with TAB VACCINE may cause FALSE POSITIVE results and for this reason the test is of limited value in countries which have an active TAB IMMUNISATION programme. Named after the Algerian born French pathologist George Fernand Isadore Widal (1862-1929).

wide-spectrum (microbiology) Of antibiotics etc. effective against a wide range of MICRO-ORGANISMS. The term 'broad-SPECTRUM' is also used.

Wilcoxon rank-sum test (statistics) A distribution-free, NON-PARAMETRIC test for two independent groups. The DATA from both groups are combined and ranked with the lowest value assigned a rank of 1. The ranks assigned to each GROUP are then summed, with the test statistic T' being the sum of the ranks for the smaller GROUP. For small groups (n < 10), the critical value for T' can be obtained from special tables. If n > 10 for both groups, the distribution approximates NORMAL, and the obtained value for T' can be assessed using the NORMAL curve table.

See also NON-PARAMETRIC.

Wilcoxon signed ranks test (statistics) *See* WILCOXON RANK-SUM TEST.

wild strain (microbiology) A strain of a particular type of MICRO-ORGANISM that has not become LABORATORY adapted.

wild type (genetics) The ALLELE that is deemed to be the one that occurs in the SPECIES in its original state, as opposed to subsequent MUTATIONS, either spontaneous or induced. The wild-type ALLELE may be either DOMINANT or RECESSIVE in relation to a MUTANT ALLELE. Its symbol is +.

Wilm's tumour (haematology) *See* NEPHROBLASTOMA.

Wilson's disease (biochemistry) A rare disease in which excessive amounts of COPPER are deposited in the BRAIN and LIVER. Named after the British neurologist, Samuel Alexander Kinnier Wilson (1878-1937).

winchester (equipment) A bottle, commonly used for LIQUID chemicals, with a CAPACITY of about 2.25 LITRES. It was named after the city of Winchester, Hampshire, UK.

winter vomiting disease (medical/ virology) A disease caused by parvoviruses characterised by nausea, vomiting, DIARRHOEA (*USA*: diarrhea) and giddiness which occurs during the winter months. Outbreaks may involve whole families or may affect communities such as schools. The INCUBATION PERIOD is 1 to 2 days, and the condition seldom lasts for more than 3 days.

Wiskott-Aldrich syndrome (medical/ haematology) An IMMUNE SYSTEM sex-linked RECESSIVE disease of infants, characterised by THROMBOCYTOPENIA, with a haemorrhagic (*USA*: hemorrhagic) tendency, eczema, and immunodeficiency with recurrent infections. Delayed HYPERSENSITIVITY reactions are absent and there is a defective ANTIBODY RESPONSE to POLYSACCHARIDE antigens, with low immunoglobulin M levels. A PROTEIN normally present in PLATELET membranes

is missing. Sufferers are particularly susceptible to infections from HERPES VIRUSES and lymphoreticular malignancies, especially of the CENTRAL NERVOUS SYSTEM.

witches' milk (physiology) The milk secreted from the breasts of a newborn baby in RESPONSE to the HORMONES of its mother.

withdrawal symptoms (toxicology) The unpleasant symptoms that are caused by ceasing to take a drug of ADDICTION. The symptoms vary with the drug but may include restlessness, inability to concentrate, IRRITABILITY, insomnia, depression, nausea, and delirium.

within-group variance (statistics) The amount of VARIANCE caused by differences within a GROUP.

w/o (literature terminology) An abbreviation of 'w'ith'o'ut.

wolfram (chemistry) Old name for tungsten.

wood spirit (chemistry) An alternative term for METHANOL.

wood sugar (chemistry) An alternative term for XYLOSE.

wool fat (chemistry) An alternative term for LANOLIN.

woolsorter's disease (medical/ bacteriology) An ACUTE LUNG disease due to INFECTION with *Bacillus anthracis*, conveyed to humans by inhalation of spores from infected sheep's wool.

See also ANTHRAX.

word processor (computing) Microcomputer that is programed to help in the preparation of text, for DATA TRANSMISSION or printing.

work (W) (physics) The measurement of a FORCE multiplied by the distance moved by the point of application of the FORCE in the direction of the FORCE. It is measured in joules.

working (mathematics) Pertaining to something assumed or approximated, *e.g.* 'WORKING HYPOTHESIS'.

World Health Organisation (WHO) (governing body) The health agency of the United Nations, WHO is based in Geneva, Switzerland. SET up in 1948 it co-ordinates international health activities, and aims to improve health, particularly of developing countries, through education and information and practical assistance with MASS VACCI-NATION programmes, public health schemes and medical facilities.

worms (microbiology/ parasitology) An imprecise term applied to elongated invertebrates with no appendages. Those that infest human beings can be divided into three groups: roundworms or nematodes, tapeworms or cestodes and FLUKES or TREMATODES.

wounds (medical) Disruption of the tissues by external agents of a mechanical nature which may be classified as incised, punctured, contusm, lacerated, perforating and penetrating.

WP (computing) An abbreviation of 'W'ord 'P'rocessing.

wt (measurement) An abbreviation of 'w'eigh't'.

Wuchereria (parasitology) *See* FILARLASIS; WORMS.

X

X (statistics) The ARITHMETIC MEAN.

xanthene (chemistry) $CH_2(C_6H_4)_2O$ Yellow CRYSTALLINE ORGANIC COMPOUND, used as a FUNGICIDE and in making dyes. Also termed: tricyclicdibenzopyran.

xanthine (chemistry) $C_5H_4N_2O_2$ ORGANIC COMPOUND that occurs in potatoes, coffee beans, BLOOD and URINE, used industrially as a chemical INTERMEDIATE. Also termed: 3 7-dihydro-1H-PURINE-2,6-dione; 2,6-DIHYDROXYPURINE.

xanthone (chemistry) $CO(C_6H_4)_2O$ Plant PIGMENT that occurs in gentian and other flowers, used commercially as an INSECTICIDE and dye INTERMEDIATE. Also termed: 9H-xanthen-9-one.

xanthophyll (chemistry) $C_{40}H_{56}O_2$ Yellow to orange PIGMENT present in the NORMAL chlorophyll MIXTURE of green plants. Also termed: lutein.

x-axis (mathematics) The horizontal AXIS on a GRAPH.

X chromosome (genetics) One of the SEX CHROMOSOMES. In humans the female has two X CHROMOSOMES and the male an X and a Y. The human X CHROMOSOME is the seventh largest in the human KARYOTYPE, nearly three times the size of the Y CHROMOSOME. It carries a large number of genes, which are said to be X-linked. *See* X LINKAGE.

x coordinate (mathematics) A value on the horizontal AXIS of a GRAPH.

Xe (chemistry) The CHEMICAL SYMBOL for the ELEMENT XENON.

xenobiotic (toxicology) A general term used to describe any chemical interacting with an organism that does not occur in the NORMAL metabolic pathways of that organism.

xenodiagnosis (parasitology) Procedure involving the feeding of LABORATORY-reared triatomid bugs on patients suspected of having Chagas' disease; after several weeks the FAECES (*USA*: feces) of the bugs are checked for INTERMEDIATE stages of *Trypanosoma cruzi*.

xenograft (biology) The grafting of TISSUE to an immunosuppressed ANIMAL of a different SPECIES. A convenient method to grow human tumours (*USA*: tumors) in experimental animals for further study.

xenon Xe (chemistry) Unreactive gaseous ELEMENT in GROUP 0 of the PERIODIC TABLE (the RARE GASes) which occurs as traces in the ATMOSPHERE, from which it is extracted. It is used in electronic flash tubes and high-INTENSITY ARC lamps. At. no. 54; r.a.m. 131.30.

xeroderma pigmentosum (medical/ genetics) A disease in which the SKIN is excessively vulnerable to bright sunlight, resulting in a high INCIDENCE of SKIN cancers. The underlying cause is an inherited inability to repair the damage to DNA in SKIN CELLS, brought about by exposure to ULTRAVIOLET RADIATION. The disorder is inherited as an autosomal

RECESSIVE, and is one of the few clear-cut examples of a genetic basis for CANCER. Fibroblasts obtained from XERODERMA PIGMENTOSUM patients nave been used in the development of MUTATION assays.

xeroradiography (radiology) A method of producing radiographs by a dry process.

xipamide (pharmacology) A DIURETIC drug of the THIAZIDE-related class. Administered orally it can be used in ANTIHYPERTENSIVE treatment and in congestive HEART FAILURE treatment and associated OEDEMA (*USA*: edema).

X linkage (genetics) The situation in which a GENE is located on the X CHROMOSOME. In males, with SEX CHROMOSOMES XY, any ALLELE on the X CHROMOSOME behaves as a DOMINANT, because there is no corresponding ALLELE to mask it on the other CHROMOSOME (the Y does not behave as HOMOLOGOUS to the X). A male passes on to all his daughters any GENE that he carries on the X CHROMOSOME, but his sons will not inherit it. A female who carries the same ALLELE on one of her X CHROMOSOMES will not be affected, if the GENE is RECESSIVE as most X-linked genes are. Such a female is known as a CARRIER, and passes on the GENE to half of her offspring, sons and daughters alike: males who receive the GENE will inherit the condition, females will be carriers. It is possible for a female to inherit an X-linked GENE simultaneously from her father (he will have the trait in question) and from her CARRIER mother, but this is rare (how rare depends on the FREQUENCY of the X-linked allele in the population). Over 100 genes are known to be X-linked in humans, including COLOUR BLINDNESS (*USA*: color blindness), Duchenne muscular dystrophy and HAEMOPHILIA (*USA*: hemophilia). Occasionally an X-linked GENE is DOMINANT; its

pattern of transmission is similar, in that a father cannot pass it on to his sons.

XPS (physics) An abbreviation of 'X'-RAY 'P'hotoelectron 'S'pectroscopy.

X-ray crystallography (biochemistry) The technique used for investigating the three dimensional structure of large molecules such as proteins and NUCLEIC ACIDS. The WAVELENGTH of the X-RAYS used is similar to the inter-atomic distances in these molecules, and the position of atoms can be deduced from the patterns of DIFFRACTION seen when X-RAYS are passed through them.

X-ray diffraction (physics) Pattern of VARIABLE intensities produced by DIFFRACTION of X-RAYS when passed through a DIFFRACTION GRATING consisting of spacings of about 10^{-8}cm, in particular that formed by the LATTICE of a crystal.

X-ray fluorescence (physics) Less penetrating, secondary X-RAYS emitted by a substance when subjected to primary X-RAYS or high-ENERGY electrons. The secondary X-RAYS are CHARACTERISTIC of the bombarded substance.

X-ray spectrum (physics) Line SPECTRUM of the INTENSITY of X-RAYS emitted when a SOLID target is bombarded with electrons. It consists of sharp superimposed lines, which are CHARACTERISTIC of the target atoms, on a continuous background.

X-ray tube (radiology) VACUUM tube designed to produce X-RAYS by using an ELECTROSTATIC FIELD which accelerates and directs electrons on to a target.

X-rays (radiology) ELECTROMAGNETIC RADIATION produced in a partial VACUUM by the sudden arrest of high-ENERGY bombarding electrons as they collide with the heavy ATOM nuclei of a target METAL. The X-RAYS produced are thus CHARACTERISTIC of the target's atoms. X-RAYS have very short wavelengths (10^{-3} to 1 nm) and can penetrate solids to varying degrees; this CHARACTERISTIC has made them useful in medicine, dentistry and X-RAY CRYSTALLOGRAPHY. Also termed: rontgen (ROENTGEN) rays; X-radiation.

xylene (chemistry) $C_6H_4(CH_3)_2$ Aromatic LIQUID ORGANIC COMPOUND that exists in three isomeric forms (*ortho-, meta-* and para-XYLENE), obtained from coaltar and petroleum. They are used as solvents in polyester SYNTHESIS, in microscopy for preparation of specimens and as cleaning agents. Also termed: DIMETHYLBENZENE.

xylose (chemistry) $C_5H_{10}O_5$ Naturally occurring PENTOSE SUGAR, found in the form of xylan or as GLYCOSIDES in many plants (*e.g.* cherry and maple wood, straw, pecan shell, corn cobs and cottonseed hulls). Also termed: WOOD SUGAR.

Y

Y (1 chemistry; 2 biochemistry) 1 The CHEMICAL SYMBOL for YTTRIUM. 2 The symbol for TYROSINE.

Y1 adrenal cells (microbiology) A commonly used continuous CELL line used in TISSUE CULTURE systems.

YAC (genetics) An abbreviation of 'Y'east 'A'rtificial 'C'hromosome.

yard (measurement) UNIT of length equal to 3 feet; there are 1,760 yards in 1 mile. 1 YARD = 0.9144 m.

Yates correction (statistics) A correction for small samples in the calculation of chi-square in a 2-by-2 table, in which 0.5 is deducted from each figure exceeding expectation, and 0.5 is added to each figure that is less than the expected value. Assuming fixed marginal totals, which is rarely appropriate, the effect is to bring the distribution of the calculated chi-square nearer to the continuous distribution from which the usual chi-square tables are derived. *Compare* correction for continuity.

yaws (medical/ microbiology) A CHRONIC disease of the tropics, especially of Africa and the West Indies, caused by *TREPONEMA pertenue,* a SPIROCHAETE. The disease is also known as FRAMBOESIA, and pian.

y-axis (mathematics) The AXIS perpendicular to and in the horizontal plane through the *X-AXIS* in any type of GRAPH.

Yb (chemistry) The CHEMICAL SYMBOL for YTTERBIUM.

Y chromosome (genetics) One of the SEX CHROMOSOMEs and the third smallest in the human KARYOTYPE. In humans the male has an X and a Y, while the female has two X CHROMOSOMEs. It is the presence of the Y CHROMOSOME that causes maleness to develop. The sex-determining GENE is on the short arm of the Y CHROMOSOME, and individuals who are XY but have lost the short arm of the Y develop as female, while the longer arm of Y CHROMOSOMEs can apparently be lost with no effect on the PHENOTYPE.

y coordinate (mathematics) A value on the vertical AXIS of a GRAPH.

yeast (mycology) A member of a GROUP of widespread UNICELLULAR FUNGI of the CLASS Ascomycota. There are a very large number of naturally occurring varieties. Some yeasts are pathogens, such as Candida albicans, and cause diseases such as THRUSH in humans. *SACCHAROMYCES CEREVISIAE* is an important LABORATORY organism, and is the FOCUS of much genetic research using RECOMBINANT DNA and DNA cloning techniques.

yeast artificial chromosome (YAC) (genetics) A system used for producing segments of DNA of more than 200,000 bases. GENETIC ENGINEERING techniques have been used to construct DNA molecules that contain a YEAST CENTROMERE and several YEAST genes. Segments of DNA can be inserted into such molecules and, when introduced into YEAST CELLS, they behave like chromosomes and divide in step with the CELL. YACs have become important HOST vectors for cloning large regions of genomes.

yeast mutation tests (toxicology) *In vitro* test systems used to detect mutagenicity that have been developed with strains of the YEAST SACCHAROMYCES CEREVISIAE which are capable of detecting FORWARD MUTATIONS, reverse MUTATIONS and recombinant events such as RECIPROCAL or non-RECIPROCAL mitotic RECOMBINATION.

yellow fever (medical/ microbiology) An ACUTE and severe disease ENDEMIC in tropical America and Africa. It is caused by a flavivirus of the togavirus FAMILY transmitted between humans by the bite of the mosquito *Aedes aegypti.*

yellow spot (MACULA lutea) (anatomy) An alternative term for FOVEA.

Yersinia (microbiology) A GENUS of gram-negative ROD-shaped BACTERIA of the FAMILY Enterobacteriaceae. This GENUS contains some important human pathogens including YERSINIA PESTIS, YERSINIA ENTEROCOLICITA and YERSINIA PSEUDOTUBERCULOSIS.

Yersinia enterocolicita (microbiology) The agent recognized as a cause of enterocolitis and mesenteric LYMPH-ADENITIS. Although some strains apparently produce a HEAT-STABLE enterotoxin that closely resembles that of ESCHERICHIA COLI, *Yersinia enterocolitica* is considered an invasive PATHOGEN. Involvement of intestinal LYMPH NODES is common, and the condition is difficult to distinguish from ACUTE appendicitis. Only strains pocessing essential VIRULENCE factors are capable of causing human intestinal disease.

Yersinia pestis (microbiology) A member of the GENUS YERSINIA. The agent responsible for bubonic plague, formerly called *Pasteurella pestis.*

Yersinia pseudotuberculosis (microbiology) An organism that is very similar biochemically to YERSINA PESTIS and that causes infections that have a broad clinical picture that closely resembles that of YERSINIA ENTEROCOLITICA.

yolk (biology) Part of an OVUM that stores the nutritive materials, or the yellow central portion of the EGG of birds and reptiles.

yolk sac (microbiology) A tiny bag attached to the EMBRYO that provides early nourishment before the PLACENTA is formed. *See* YOLK SAC ISOLATION.

yolk sac isolation (microbiology) A technique used for harvesting and increasing yields of chlamydiae and certain VIRUSES. All known chlamydiae grow in the YOLK SAC of the embryonated hen EGG. However, these techniques are relatively slow and will not provide an aetiologic diagnosis quickly enough to be clinically relevant.

ytterbium Yb (chemistry) Silvery-white metallic ELEMENT in GROUP IIIA of the PERIODIC TABLE (one of the LANTHANIDES), with no commercial uses. At. no. 70; r.a.m. 173.04.

yttrium Y (chemistry) Grey metallic ELEMENT in GROUP IIIA of the PERIODIC TABLE (one of the ALKALINE EARTHS, but often classed with the LANTHANIDES). It is used in ALLOYS for superconductors and magnets, and YTTRIUM(VI) OXIDE, Y_2O_6, is employed in lasers and phosphors. At. no.39; r.a.m. 88.9059.

Yttrium-90 (radiology) An artificially produced RADIOACTIVE ISOTOPE of the ELEMENT YTTRIUM. The ISOTOPE emits BETA RAYS and is used for the TREATMENT of tumours (*USA*: tumors).

Z

z-axis (mathematics) The vertical AXIS in any 3-dimensional CO-ORDINATE system.

Z DNA (genetics) DNA in which the double HELIX is wound left-handed rather than right-handed as NORMAL. The sugars do not fit together so well in this CONFIGURATION, giving the MOLECULE a jagged appearance. Z DNA has been studied *in Drosophila* chromosomes, and it has been suggested that it has a role in GENE REGULATION.

zearalenone (toxicology/ microbiology) A MYCOTOXIN produced by the FUNGI *Fusarium* which is oestrogenic (*USA*: estrogenic) and causes hyperoestrogenic (*USA*: hyperestrogenic) effects. It is found on corn, barley, wheat, hay, oats.

Zeeman effect (physics) Splitting of SPECTRAL LINES of a substance into components of different FREQUENCY when placed in a MAGNETIC FIELD. It was named after the Dutch physicist Pieter Zeeman (1865-1943).

Zener current (physics) CURRENT produced in an INSULATOR in a strong ELECTRIC FIELD when its VALENCE BAND electrons are raised to the CONDUCTION BAND.

Zener diode (physics) Semiconductor DIODE which at a certain negative VOLTAGE produces a sharp breakdown of CURRENT and hence may be used as a VOLTAGE control device. Also termed: AVALANCHE DIODE; breakdown DIODE.

Zenker's degeneration (histology) The degeneration of STRIATED MUSCLE CELLS,

occuring, *e.g.* in prolonged fevers such as typhoid or in HEPATITIS. Also known as hyaline necrosis. Named after the German Pathologist, Friedrich Albert von Zenker (1825-89).

zeolite (chemistry) HYDRATED ALUMINO-SILICATE mineral, from which the WATER is easily removed, used for making MOLECULAR SIEVES and for ION EXCHANGE columns.

zero method (statistics) An alternative term for NULL METHOD.

zero-order correlation (statistics) A correlation performed on the raw DATA without first removing the effects of any related variables. *Compare* partial correlation.

zeta potential (physics) POTENTIAL DIFFERENCE that exists across the INTERFACE between a SOLID PARTICLE and a LIQUID in which it is immersed. Also termed: ELECTROKINETIC POTENTIAL.

Ziehl-Neelsen stain (microbiology) Micro-biological staining technique that may be used to make ALCOHOL fast bacilli, such as *Mycobacterium tuberculosis*, visible under the MICROSCOPE.

zinc Zn (chemistry) Bluish-white metallic ELEMENT in GROUP IIB of the PERIODIC TABLE (a TRANSITION ELEMENT), used to give a corrosion-resistant coating to steel (galvanizing), to make dry batteries and in various ALLOYS (*e.g.* brass, bronze). It is an essential TRACE ELEMENT which are needed for ENZYME systems in the body.

Although sufficient is normally present in the diet, deficiency results in stunted GROWTH, SKIN disease and inadequacy of the IMMUNE SYSTEM. At. no. 30; r.a.m. 65.38.

zinc chloride (chemistry) $ZnCl_2$ White HYGROSCOPIC SALT produced commercially by heating metallic ZINC in dry CHLORINE GAS. It is used to fireproof timber, in BATTERY making, vulcanizing and galvanizing, in oil refining, and as a FUNGICIDE and CATALYST.

zinc oxide (chemistry) ZnO White CRYSTALLINE SOLID (yellow when hot) which can be produced directly by heating ZINC in AIR. It is used as a white PIGMENT (Chinese white), in ceramics, cosmetics, pharmaceuticals and floor coverings, and in the manufacture of tyres. It dissolves in ALKALIS (*USA*: alkalies) to form zincates.

zinc sulphate (chemistry) $ZnSO_4.7H_2O$ Colourless (*USA*: colorless) CRYSTALLINE SALT prepared by dissolving metallic ZINC in DILUTE SULPHURIC ACID (*USA*: sulfuric acid). It is used in the manufacture of rayon, glue, fertilizers, FUNGICIDES, wood preservatives, rubber, paint and varnishes. Also termed: white copperas; WHITE VITRIOL; ZINC VITRIOL. (*USA*: zinc sulfate).

zincate (chemistry) COMPOUND formed by the REACTION of metallic ZINC or ZINC OXIDE with an ALKALI; *e.g.* Na_2ZnO_2.

zirconium Zr (chemistry) Silvery-grey metallic ELEMENT in GROUP IVA of the PERIODIC TABLE (a TRANSITION ELEMENT). It is used to clad URANIUM fuel rods in nuclear reactors. Naturally occurring CRYSTALLINE ZIRCONIUM(IV) OXIDE, ZrO_2, is the semi-precious gemstone zircon; the OXIDE is

also used as an ELECTROLYTE in fuel CELLS. At. no. 40; r.a.m. 91.22.

zinc sulphide ZnS (chemistry) Occurs naturally as blende, an important ZINC ore, and can be prepared as a white PRECIPITATE by adding ammonium SULPHIDE (*USA*: ammonium sulfide) or HYDROGEN SULPHIDE (*USA*: hydrogen sulfide) to a SOLUTION of a ZINC SALT. It is used as the pigmentary BASE for white ZINC SULPHIDE (*USA*: zinc sulfide) which contains up to 60 per cent ZINC SULPHIDE and a BALANCE of BARIUM SULPHATE (*USA*: barlum sulfate). It is also used in FUNGICIDES and phosphors. (*USA*: zinc sulfide).

ZN (microbiology) An abbreviation of 'Z'IEHL-'N'EELSEN STAIN.

Zn (chemistry) The CHEMICAL SYMBOL for ZINC.

Zollinger-Ellison syndrome (biochemistry/ histology) A severe form of STOMACH and duodenal ulceration caused by an excessive production of ACID by the STOMACH. This is stimulated by one or more slow growing, and often maglignant, tumours (*USA*: tumors) of the PANCREAS, known as gastrinomas, that secrete a powerful HORMONE acting on the STOMACH. Named after the American surgeons Robert Milton Zollinger (b. 1903) and Edwin H. Ellison (1918-1970).

zolpidem tartrate (pharmacology) A hypnotic drug administered orally for the short term treatment of insomnia. It acts in the same way as the benzodiazepine drugs.

zone (1 chemistry; 2 crystallography; 3 mathematics) 1 Orientation of SOLUTE molecules in a SERIES of tubes in a LIQUID-LIQUID extraction procedure. 2 Crystal faces that intersect along parallel edges.

3 The part of a sphere that is enclosed between two parallel planes which intersect the sphere. Also termed: fresnel.

zool. (biology) An abbreviation of 'zool'ogy.

zoology (biology) Systematic study of the ANIMAL KINGDOM.

zoomastigophorea (microbiology) A CLASS of flagellated PROTOZOA many of which cause diseases such as LEISHMANIASIS, trichomoniasis and TRYPANOSOMIASIS.

zoonosis (microbiology) Any disease of animals which may be transmitted to human beings. Examples are plague and RABIES; ANTHRAX, Q FEVER and salmonella infections; all kinds of worm infestations, and various VIRUS, rickettsial, leptospiral and FUNGUS infections; BRUCELLOSIS, ORNITHOSIS, and GLANDERS.

zopiclone (pharmacology) A hypnotic drug, which works in the same way as the benzodiazepine drugs, which can be administered orally for the short-term treatment of insomnia.

zoster (virology) See HERPES ZOSTER.

zovirax (pharmacology) See ACYCLOVIR.

ZPP (haematology) An abbreviation of 'Z'inc 'P'roto'P'orphyrin. See FREE ERYTHROCYTE PROTOPORPHYRIN.

Zr (chemistry) The CHEMICAL SYMBOL for ELEMENT 40, ZIRCONIUM.

z-score (statistics) A score expressed as the number of units of STANDARD DEVIATION above or below the MEAN, according to the FORMULA, $z = (X-M)/SD$, where X is the score, M the MEAN,

and SD the STANDARD DEVIATION. They have the following properties: (i) their sum is zero; (ii) their STANDARD DEVIATION is 1.0.

zwitterion (chemistry) An ION carrying both a POSITIVE and a negative CHARGE, e.g. present in SOLID and LIQUID amino acids such as GLYCINE, $N^+H_3CH_2COO^-$.

zygomycocosis (microbiology) A FUNGUS INFECTION in which masses of various FUNGI form in the nasal sinuses, under the SKIN of the face and in other parts of the body especially in people with immune deficiency.

zygosis (genetics) The union of two gametes.

zygote (genetics) The individual as it exists at the moment of fertilization, i.e. the DIPLOID CELL that results from the FUSION of two gametes. See HYBRID.

zygotene (genetics) One of the stages in MEIOSIS.

zymase (chemistry) ENZYME that catalyses the FERMENTATION of carbohydrates to ETHANOL (ETHYL ALCOHOL).

zymogen (biochemistry) Inactive PRECURSOR of an ENZYME. It is activated by the ACTION of a KINASE. Also termed: PROENZYME.

zymogenesis (biochemistry) The conversion of an ENZYME PRECURSOR to the active state.

zymotic (microbiology) Describing an agent that causes an INFECTIOUS DISEASE.

Appendices

Appendix 1 Reference Ranges

Blood constituents

Values are for adults and refer to plasma/ serum except as indicated*

Electrolytes and blood gases

Osmolarity	280-298 mmol/ kg
pCO_2 (arterial)	4.5-6.1 kPa
pO_2 (arterial)	11-15 kPa
pH (arterial)	7.35-7.45
Sodium	134-147 mM
Potassium	3.5-5.0 mM
Chloride	96-106 mM
Bicarbonate	21-30 mM
Phosphate	0.7-1.4 mM
Sulphate	0.25-0.38 mM
Calcium	2.1-2.7 mM
Magnesium	0.7-1.3 mM
Copper	12-30 μM
Zinc	12-24 μM
Lead	< 2.4 μM

Haemoglobin and blood cells

Haemoglobin*	13-17 g/ dl (males)
	11-15 g/ dl (females)
Erythrocytes (red cell count)*	$4.5\text{-}6.5 \times 10^{12}/\text{ l}$ (males)
	$3.9\text{-}5.6 \times 10^{12}/\text{ l}$ (females)
Packed cell volume (PCV)*	0.41-0.53 l/ l (males)
	0.35-0.48 l/ l females)
Mean corpuscular volume (MCV)	76-96 fl
Mean corpuscular haemoglobin (MCH)	26-33 pg/ cell
Mean corpuscular haemoglobin concentration (MCHC)*	31-35 g/ dl
Leukocytes (white cell count)*	$4\text{-}6 \times 10^9/\text{ l}$
Platelets*	$2\text{-}4 \times 10^{11}/\text{ l}$
Reticulocytes*	0.5-2.5% red cells
Glucose 6-phosphate dehydrogenase (erythrocyte)*	5-15 U/ g Hb
Pyruvate kinase (erythrocyte)*	13-17 U/ g Hb
Iron	10-30 μM
Total iron-binding capacity (TIBC)	40-70 μM

Nitrogenous constituents and amino acids

Ammonia	12-60 μM
Urea	2.5-7.0 mM
Creatinine	53-124 μM
Uric Acid	0.18-0.42 μM
Alanine	0.2-0.3 mM
Glutamine	0.45-0.75 mM
Citrulline	10-30 μM
Phenylalanine	0-0.12 mM

Organic constituents

Glucose (fasting)	3.5-5.5 mM
Lactate	0.6-1.8 mM
Pyruvate	0.03-0.11 mM
Citrate	0.08-0.16 mM
Bilirubin (total)	3-15 μM

Vitamins

Ascorbic acid (C)	20-100 μM
Biotin	2.5-5.5 μM
Cholecalciferol (D_3)	0.07 μM
Cobalamin (B_{12})	0.15-0.67 nM
Folic acid	15-80 nM
Niacin (nicotinic acid)	50 μM
Pantothenic acid	1.3 μM
Retinol (A)	0.3-2.1 μM
Riboflavin (B_2)	0.07-0.1 μM
Thiamine (B_1)	0.2-0.3 μM
α-Tocopherol (E)	20-45 μM

Lipids (fasting)

Triglyceride	0.6-3.2 mM
Cholesterol	3.7-6.8 mM
Fatty acids (total)	0.2-0.8 mM

Proteins

Total protein	60-84 g/ l
Albumin	35-50 g/ l
Globulins (total)	23-35 g/ l
IgG	7-15 g/ l
Lipoprotein (HDL)	3-8 g/ l
Ceruloplasmin	0.2-0.4 g/ l

Clotting factors

Fibrinogen	2-4 g/ l
Plasminogen	0.3 g/ l
Prothrombin	0.1 g/ l

Enzymes*

Acid phosphatase	4-11
Alkaline phosphatase	100-300
Aldolase	2-12
Creatine kinase (CK)	20-150
Lactate dehydrogenase (LDH)	45-90
Amylase	70-300
γ-Glutamyl transferase (GGT)[tt]	7-45
Aspartate transaminase (AST)[s]	10-40
Alanine transaminase (ALT)[ss]	5-35
Serum lipase	28-280
Cholinesterase	39-51
α-Fucosidase	4.5-14.0
α-Galactosidase	0.22-0.50
β-Galactosidase	0.4-1.1
α-Mannosidase	0.35-0.90
N-Acetyl-α-glucosaminidase	0.15-0.40
N-Acetyl-β-glucosaminidase	12-25
p-Nitrocatechol sulphatase	0.04-0.12
α-Glucosidase	0.1-0.25

*	Enzyme activities in units/ l (U/ l)
[t]	PCV also expressed as % = l/ l x 100.
[tt]	Serum γ-glutamyl transpeptidas (γ-GT)
[s]	Serum glutamate-oxaloacetate transaminase (SGOT)
[ss]	Serum glutamate-pyruvate transaminase (SGPT)

Urinary constituents

The daily (24 hour) excretion of many constituents will vary considerably from subject to subject depending on diet, age, sex, exercise, etc. Therefore, the values listed in this Appendix are only very approximate.

Volume	1-2 l/ day
pH	4.8-7.5 (mean 6.0)

Nitrogen compounds

Total nitrogen	600-1400 mmol/ day
Urea	300-640 mmol/ day
Ammonia	60-110 mmol/ day
Uric acid	2-6 mmol/ day
Creatinine	7-17 mmol/ day
Amino acids	7-21 mmol/ day
Protein	0-150 mg/ day

Electrolytes

Titratable activity (H^+)	15-50 mmol/ day
Sodium	180-440 mmol/ day
Potassium	40-80 mmol/ day
Calcium	5-12 mmol/ day
Magnesium	4-8 mmol/ day
Chloride	100-260 mmol/ day
Sulphate (as S)	18-56 mmol/ day
Phosphate (as P)	23-52 mmol/ day
Lead	0-500 nmol/ day
Copper	0-1.6 µmol/ day

Porphyrins

δ-Aminolævulinic acid	0-40 µmol/ day
Porphobilinogen	0-16 µmol/ day
Coproporphyrin	0-380 nmol/ day
Urobilinogen	0-7 µmol/ day
Uroporphyrin	0-49 nmol/ day

Others

Glucose	negative
Ketones	negative
Citrate	1.0-5.7 mmol/ day
17-ketosteroids	3-56 µmol/ day
17-hydroxysteroids	8-22 µmol/ day

Appendix 2 Metric conversions

Distance

1 inch = 2.54 centimetres
1 foot = 0.3048 metre
1 yard = 0.9144 metre
1 rod = 5.0292 metres
1 chain = 20.117 metres
1 furlong = 201.17 metres
1 mile = 1.6093 kilometre
1 nautical mile = 1.8532 kilometre

1 millimetre = 0.03937 inch
1 centimetre = 0.3937 inch
1 decimetre = 0.3281 foot
1 metre = 3.281 feet
1 metre = 1.094 yard
1 decametre = 10.94 yards
1 kilometre = 0.6214 mile
1 kilometre = 0.539 nautical mile

Surface or area

1 square inch = 6.4516 square centimetres
1 square foot = 929.03 square centimetres
1 square yard = 0.8361 square metre
1 acre = 4046.9 square metres
1 square mile = 259.0 hectares
1 square centimetre = 0.1550 square inch
1 square metre = 1550 square inches
1 acre = 119.6 square yards
1 hectare = 2.4711 acres
1 square kilometre = 0.3861 square mile

Temperature conversion

Celsius° = 5/9 (Fahrenheit° − 32°)
Fahrenheit° = 9/5 Celsius° + 32°

Capacity

1 cubic inch = 16.387 cubic centimetres
1 cubic foot = 0.0283 cubic metre
1 cubic yard = 0.7646 cubic metre
1 cubic centimetre = 0.061 cubic inch
1 cubic decimetre = 0.035 cubic foot
1 cubic metre = 1.308 cubic yard

Dry measure (Imperial)

1 pint = 0.5506 litre
1 quart = 1.136 litres
1 gallon = 4.546 litres
1 peck = 9.092 litres
1 bushel = 36.369 litres

Liquid measure (USA)

1 pint = 0.473 litre
1 quart = 0.9463 litre
1 gallon = 3.785 litres
1 peck = 8.809 litres
1bushel = 35.24 litres

Avoirdupois weight

1 ounce = 28.35 grams
1 pound = 453.59 grams
1 hundredweight = 50.802 kilograms
1 ton = 907.18 kilograms
1 gram = 0.035 ounce
1 hectogram = 3.527 ounces
1 kilogram = 2.205 pounds
1 ton = 1.102 ton (short)

Appendix 3

Organizations of Biomedical Science

Biomedical science incorporates information from a large number of disciplines and worldwide there are many hundreds of associations, societies and other organisations dedicated to various aspects. The following information contains the contact addresses of a selection of key organisations in the United Kingdom, Ireland and the United States of America relevant to biomedical science from which specialised information and assistance may be sought. These are listed under headings indicating the scientific areas in which they are particularly involved. Although it is appreciated that some of the organisations indicated may be involved in many aspects of biomedical scientific practice and research and could legitimately be included under more than one heading, only one entry per organisation has been included. It is hoped, however, that the listing provides a useful guide, as a starting point, to identifying sources of information being sought.

Anatomy	American Association of Anatomists (AAA)
	9650 Rockville Pike
	Bethesda
	Maryland
	United States of America

British Association of Clinical Anatomists (BACA)
Department of Human Anatomy and Cell Biology
New Medical School
The University of Liverpool
Ashton Street
Liverpool L69 3GE
United Kingdom

Biochemistry	American Society for Biochemistry and Molecular Biology (ASBMB)
	9650 Rockville Pike
	Bethesda
	Maryland
	United States of America
	Association of Clinical Biochemists (ACB)
	130-132 Tooley Street
	London SE1 2TU
	United Kingdom
	Biochemical Society
	59 Portland Place
	London W1B 1QW
	United Kingdom
Biology	Institute of Biology (IOB)
	20-22 Queensberry Place
	London SW7 2DZ
	United Kingdom
Biophysics	British Biophysical Society (BBS)
	Department of Chemistry
	University of York
	Heslington
	York YO1 5DD
	United Kingdom
Cancer	American Institute for Cancer Research (AICR)
	1759 R Street NW
	Washington DC 20009
	United States of America
	British Association for Cancer Research (BACR)
	Cotswold Road
	Sutton
	Surrey SM2 5NG
	United Kingdom

Cell Biology	British Society for Cell Biology (BSCB) Department of Zoology University of Cambridge Downing Street Cambridge CB2 3EJ United Kingdom
Cytology	British Society for Clinical Cytology (BSCC) Thorn EMI Central Research Laboratories Dawley Road Hayes Middlesex UB3 1HH United Kingdom
Epidemiology	PHLS Communicable Disease Surveillance Centre (CDSC) 61 Colindale Avenue London NW9 5EQ United Kingdom
General	Institute of Biomedical Sciences (IBMS) 12 Coldbath Square London EC1R 5HL United Kingdom
Genetics	The Genetical Society Department of Biology University of York Heslinton York YO1 5DD United Kingdom
Haematology	British Society of Haematology (BSH) 2 Carlton House Terrace London SW1Y 5AF United Kingdom
Histology	Anatomical Society of Great Britain and Ireland (ASGBI) Department of Anatomy National University of Ireland Cork Ireland

Immunology	American Association of Immunologists (AAI)

Immunology

American Association of Immunologists (AAI)
9650 Rockville Pike
Bethesda
Maryland
United States of America

British Society for Allergy and Clinical Immunology
(BSACI)
66 Weston Park
Thames Ditton
Surrey KT7 0HL
United Kingdom

British Society for Immunology (BSI)
Triangle House
Broomhill Road
London SW18 4HX
United Kingdom

Medicine

American Medical Association (AMA)
515 N State Street
Chicago
Illinois 60610
United States of America

British Medical Association (BMA)
BMA House
Tavistock Square
London WC1H 9JP
United Kingdom

Royal Society of Medicine (RSM)
1 Wimpole Street
London W1M 8AE
United Kingdom

Microbiology

American Society for Microbiology (ASM)
1752 N Street NW
Washington DC 20036
United States of America

Association of Medical Microbiologists (AMM)
Public Health Laboratory
Birmingham Heartlands Hospital
Bordesley Green East
Birmingham B9 5SS
United Kingdom

Society for General Microbiology (SGM)
Marlborough House
Basingstoke Road
Spencers Wood
Reading RG7 1AE
United Kingdom

Microscopy   Royal Microscopical Society (RMS)
37/38 St Clements
Oxford OX4 1AJ
United Kingdom

Mycology   British Society for Mycopathology (BSM)
MRC Immunology Laboratories
Sully Hospital
Penarth
South Glamorgan CF6 2YA
United Kingdom

Neuroscience   British Society Clinical Neurophysiology (BSCN)
Department of Neurophysiology
Middlesex Hospital
Mortimer Street
London W1N 8AA
United Kingdom

Parasitology   British Society for Parasitology (BSP)
Triangle House
Broomhill Road
London SW18 4HX
United Kingdom

Pharmacology   British Pharmacology Society (BPS)
16 Angel Gate
City Road
London EC1V 2SG
United Kingdom

Physiology	British Biophysical Society (BBS)
	Department of Chemistry
	University of York
	Heslington
	York YO1 5DD
	United Kingdom

Physiological Society
PO Box 11319
London WC1E 7JF
United Kingdom

Public Health   Centers for Disease Control and Prevention (CDC)
1600 Clifton Road
Atlanta
GA 30333
United States of America

Public Health Laboratory Services (PHLS)
61 Colindale Avenue
London NW9 5HT
United Kingdom

Royal Institute of Health and Hygiene and Society
    of Public Health
28 Portland Place
London W1B 1DE
United Kingdom

Radiology   British Institute of Radiology (BIR)
36 Portland Place
London W1B 1AT
United Kingdom

Toxicology   British Toxicology Society (BTS)
PO Box 249
Macclesfield
Cheshire SK11 6FT
United Kingdom

Virology

American Society for Virology (ASV)
Howard Hughes Medical Institute
Department of Biochemistry, Molecular Biology
    and Cell Biology
Northwestern University
2153 North Campus Drive
Evanston
IL 60208-3500
United States of America

Appendix 4

Select Bibliography and Further Reading List

Books

Academic Press Dictionary of Science and Technology, Academic Press Inc, 1992.

Anderson KN, Anderson L, Glanze WD, Mosby's Medical, Nursing, and Allied Health Dictionary, Mosby, 1994.

Blackwell's Dictionary of Nursing, Blackwell Science (UK), 1997.

Borowski EJ, Borwein JM, Dictionary of Mathematics, HarperCollins, 1999.

Brown JAC, Pears Medical Encyclopaedia, Little, Brown and Company, 2000.

Calbreath DF, Clinical Chemistry, WB Saunders Co. Ltd, 1992.

Cassell Dictionary of Science, Ward Lock, 1999.

Chambers Dictionary of Science and Technology, Chambers, 2000.

Clugston MJ (ed), The New Penguin Dictionary of Science, Penguin Books, 1998.

Coatrieux, The Biomedical Engineering Dictionary, Academic Press Inc, 2000.

Collin PH, Dictionary of Medicine, Peter Collin Publishing, 2000.

Collin S, Dictionary of Science and Technology, Peter Collin Publishing, 2000.

Compact American Library Medical Dictionary, American Heritage Dictionaries, Houghton Mifflin Co., 1999.

Concise Science Dictionary, Oxford University Press, 1996.

Daintith J, Oxford's Dictionary of Chemistry, Oxford University Press, 1996.

Dictionary of Science, Brockhampton Press, 1997.

Dictionary of the Sciences, Harcourt Publishers Ltd, 2000.

Dupayrat J, Dictionary of Biomedical Acronyms and Abbreviations, John Wiley and Sons, 1990.

Everitt B, Cambridge Dictionary of Statistics, Cambridge University Press, 1998.

Everitt BS, The Cambridge Dictionary of Statistics in the Medical Sciences, Cambridge University Press, 1995.

Farr AD, Dictionary of Medical Laboratory Sciences, Blackwell Science (UK), 1988.

Fukui S, Schmid R, Dictionary of Biotechnology, Springer-Verlag Berlin and Heidelberg GmbH & Co. KG, 1986.

Ganong WF, Review of Medical Physiology, Appleton and Lange, 1995.

Gard P, Human Pharmacology, Taylor and Francis, 2001.

Gray H, Gray's Anatomy, Parragon, 1998.

Griffin JP, Hematology and Immunology Concepts for Nursing, Appleton Century Crofts, 1986.

Hale WG, Margham JP, Saunders VA, Dictionary of Biology, HarperCollins, 1999.

Harrap's Dictionary of Science and Technology, Harrap, 1991.

Harrison P, Waites G, Cassell Dictionary of Chemistry, Ward Lock, 1999.

Heister R, Dictionary of Abbreviations in Medical Sciences, Springer-Verlag Berlin and Heidelberg GmbH & Co. KG, 1989.

Herbert WJ, Wilkinson PC, Dictionary of Immunology, Blackwell Science (UK), 1985.

Higgins SJ, Turner AJ, Wood EJ , Biochemistry for the Medical Sciences, Longman Group Ltd, 1994.

Hodgson E, Mailman RB, Chambers JE (eds), Dictionary of Toxicology, Macmillan Reference Ltd, 1998.

Hodson A, Essential Genetics, Bloomsbury, 1992.

Howell DC, Statistical Methods for Psychology, Duxbury Press, 1997.

Hull D and Johnson DI, Essential Paediatrics, Churchill Livingstone, 1994.

Lafferty P, Rowe J, The Dictionary of Science, Prentice Hall, 1994.

Lewis RJ Sr, Hawley's Condensed Chemical Dictionary, John Wiley and Sons, 1997.

McLaren DS, Meguid MM, Nutrition and its Disorders, Churchill Livingstone, 1988.

McGraw-Hill, Dictionary of Bioscience, McGraw-Hill Publishing Company 1996.

MacPherson G, Black's Medical Dictionary, A & C Black, 1999.

Martin CR, Dictionary of Endocrinology and Related Biomedical Sciences, Oxford University Press Inc, USA, 1995.

Merrell S (ed), Medicines, Bloomsbury Publishing Plc, 1995.

Millodot M, Dictionary of Optometry and Visual Science, Butterworth-Heinemann, 2000.

Muir H, Walker P, Larousse Dictionary of Science and Technology, Kingfisher Chambers Harrap, 1995.

Oxfords' Concise Medical Dictionary, Oxford University Press, 1998.

Oxford's Science Dictionary, Oxford University Press, 1999.

Pearce EC, Pearce's Medical and Nursing Dictionary and
Encyclopaedia, Mosby, 1983.

Potparic O, Gibson J, A Dictionary of Medical and Surgical Syndromes
Parthenon Publishing, 1991.

Reuter P, Birkhauser Pocket Dictionary of Biochemistry, Birkhauser
Verlag AG, 2000.

Rowland LP, Wood DS, Schon EA, *et al.*, Molecular Genetics in
Diseases of Brain, Nerve, and Muscle, Oxford University Press,
1989.

Roper N, Churchill Livingstone Pocket Medical Dictionary, Harcourt
Publishers Ltd, 1988.

Roper N, New American Pocket Medical Dictionary, Prentice Hall,
1988.

Ross JS, Wilson KJW, Foundations of Anatomy and Physiology,
Churchill Livingstone, 1984.

Smith AD, Datta SP, Smith G, *et al.*, Oxford Dictionary of
Biochemistry and Molecular Biology, Oxford University Press,
1997.

Stedman's Concise Medical and Allied Health Dictionary, Lippincott
Williams and Wilkins, 1997.

Stenesh J, Dictionary of Biochemistry and Molecular Biology, John
Wiley and Sons, 1989.

The Hutchinson Dictionary of Science, Helicon, 1998.

The Wordsworth Dictionary of Science and Technology, Wordsworth
Editions Ltd, 1995.

Uvarov EB, Isaacs A, Penguin Dictionary of Science, Penguin Books,
1993.

Vogt WP, Dictionary of Statistics and Methodology, A Non-Technical
Guide for the Social Sciences, Sage Publications Ltd, 1993.

Walker P, Chambers Science and Technology Dictionary, Kingfisher
Chambers Harrap, 1991.

Webster's New American Dictionary, Merriam-Webster Inc, 1995.

Wilson J, Hunt T, Molecular Biology of the Cell, Garland Publishing
Inc, 1994.

Youngson RM, Dictionary of Medicine, HarperCollins, 1999.

Journals and Periodicals

Advances in Applied Probability *(Quarterly)*, Applied Probability Trust.

Analyst *(Monthly)*, The Royal Society of Chemistry.

Annals of Clinical Biochemistry *(Bi-monthly)*, The Royal Society of
Medicine Press Ltd.

Aspects of Applied Biology *(3 Issues Yearly)*, Association of Applied
Biologists.

Biochemical Society Transactions *(Bi-monthly)*, Portland Press Ltd.

Biochemist *(Bi-monthly)*, The Biochemical Society.

Biomedical Materials *(Monthly)*, International Newsletters.

Biomedical News (10 *Issues Yearly)*, Quantum Publishing Ltd.

Biomedical Scientist *(Monthly)*, Institute of Biomedical Sciences.

Brain: A Journal of Neurology *(Monthly)*, Oxford University Press.

British Journal for the Philosophy of Science *(Quarterly)*, Oxford University Press.

British Journal of Biomedical Science *(Quarterly)*, The Royal Society of Medicine Press Ltd.

British Medical Journal *(Weekly)*, British Medical Association.

CLI Clinical Laboratory International *(8 Issues Yearly)*, Pan European Publishing Co.

Clinical & Experimental Immunology *(Monthly)*, Blackwell Science Ltd.

Comparative Haematology International *(Quarterly)*, Springer-Verlag London Ltd.

Current Opinion in Neurobiology *(Bi-monthly)*, Current Biology Ltd.

European Clinical Laboratory *(Bi-monthly)*, International Scientific Communications.

Experimental Physiology *(Bi-monthly)*, Cambridge University Press.

Gene Therapy *(Monthly)*, Stockton Press.

Genes & Function *(Bi-monthly)*, Blackwell Science Ltd.

Health and Hygiene *(Quarterly)*, The Royal Institute of Public Health and Hygiene.

Human and Experimental Toxicology *(Monthly)*, Stockton Press.

Infection and Immunity *(Monthly)*, American Society for Microbiology.

Immunology Today *(Monthly)*, Elsevier Science Ltd.

International Biotechnology Laboratory *(Bi-monthly)*, International Scientific Communications.

International Journal of Systematic Bacteriology *(Quarterly)*, The Society for General Microbiology.

Journal of Applied Toxicology *(Bi-monthly)*, John Wiley and Sons Ltd.

Journal of Bacteriology *(24 issues Yearly)*, American Society for Microbiology.

Journal of Comparative Pathology (8 *Issues Yearly)*, WB Saunders Co. Ltd.

Journal of Electron Microscopy *(Bi-monthly)*, Oxford University Press.

Journal of Gene Medicine *(Bi-monthly)*, John Wiley and Sons Ltd.

Journal of Medical Engineering & Technology *(Bi-monthly)*, Taylor and Francis Ltd.

Journal of Molecular Recognition *(Bi-monthly)*, John Wiley and Sons Ltd.

Journal of Neurovirology *(Bi-monthly)*, Stockton Press.

Journal of Pathology *(Monthly)*, John Wiley and Sons Ltd.

Journal of Virology *(24 issues Yearly)*, American Society for Microbiology.

Laboratory News *(Monthly)*, Quantum Publishing Ltd.

Lancet *(Weekly)*, The Lancet Ltd.

Luminescence: The Journal of Bioluminescence and Chemical Luminescence *(Bi-monthly)*, John Wiley and Sons Ltd.

Medical & Biological Engineering & Computing *(Bi-monthly)*, Peter Peregrinus Ltd.

Medical Computing *(Bi-monthly)*, Healthworks Ltd.

Medical Mycology *(Bi-monthly)*, Blackwell Science Ltd.

Microbial Pathogenesis *(Monthly)*, Academic Press Ltd.

Microscopy & Imaging News *(Quarterly)*, Quantum Publishing Ltd.

Nature: International Weekly Journal of Science *(Weekly)*, Macmillan Magazines Ltd.

Neuropathology and Applied Neurobiology *(Bi-monthly)*, Blackwell Science Ltd.

New Scientist *(Weekly)*, Reed Business Information Ltd.

NMR in Biomedicine *(8 Issues Yearly)*, John Wiley and Sons Ltd.

Optics and Laser Technology *(8 Issues Yearly)*, Elsevier Science Ltd.

Optometry Today Inc., The Scottish Optometrist *(24 Issues Yearly)*, Association of Optometrists.

Radiology Now *(3 Issues Yearly)*, Franklin Scientific Projects.

Receptor & Ion Channel Nomenclature Supplement *(Annual)*, Elsevier Trends Journals.

RNA *(Monthly)*, Cambridge University Press.

Science *(Weekly)*, American Association for the Advancement of Science.

Trends in Neurosciences *(Monthly)*, Elsevier Trends Journals.

Ultrasound in Obstetrics & Gynecology *(Monthly)*, The Parthenon Publishing Group Ltd.

Visual Neuroscience *(Bi-monthly)*, Cambridge University Press.